HEMATOLOGY, IMMUNOLOGY AND INFECTIOUS DISEASE

Neonatology Questions and Controversies

HEMATOLOGY, IMMUNOLOGY AND INFECTIOUS DISEASE
Neonatology Questions and Controversies

Series Editor

Richard A. Polin, MD
Professor of Pediatrics
College of Physicians and Surgeons
Columbia University
Vice Chairman for Clinical and Academic Affairs, Department of Pediatrics
Director, Division of Neonatology
Morgan Stanley Children's Hospital of NewYork-Presbyterian
Columbia University Medical Center
New York, New York

Other Volumes in the Neonatology Questions and Controversies Series

HEMATOLOGY, IMMUNOLOGY AND INFECTIOUS DISEASE

Neonatology Questions and Controversies

Robin K. Ohls, MD
Professor of Pediatrics
University of New Mexico
Associate Director, Pediatrics
Clinical Translational Science Center
University of New Mexico Health Sciences
Albuquerque, New Mexico

Akhil Maheshwari, MD
Associate Professor of Pediatrics and Pharmacology
Chief, Division of Neonatology
Director, Neonatology Fellowship Program
Director, Center for Neonatology and Pediatric Gastrointestinal Disease
University of Illinois at Chicago;
Medical Director,
Neonatology Intensive Care Unit and Intermediate Care Nursery
Children's Hospital of University of Illinois
Chicago, Illinois

Consulting Editor

Richard A. Polin, MD
Professor of Pediatrics
College of Physicians and Surgeons
Columbia University
Vice Chairman for Clinical and Academic Affairs, Department of Pediatrics
Director, Division of Neonatology
Morgan Stanley Children's Hospital of NewYork-Presbyterian
Columbia University Medical Center
New York, New York

SECOND EDITION

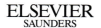

ELSEVIER
SAUNDERS

1600 John F. Kennedy Blvd.
Ste 1800
Philadelphia, PA 19103-2899

HEMATOLOGY, IMMUNOLOGY AND INFECTIOUS DISEASE:
NEONATOLOGY QUESTIONS AND CONTROVERSIES

ISBN: 978-1-4377-2662-6

Copyright © 2012, 2008 by Saunders, an imprint of Elsevier Inc.

Notices

Knowledge and best practice in this field are constantly changing. As new research and experience broaden our understanding, changes in research methods, professional practices, or medical treatment may become necessary.

Practitioners and researchers must always rely on their own experience and knowledge in evaluating and using any information, methods, compounds, or experiments described herein. In using such information or methods, they should be mindful of their own safety and the safety of others, including parties for whom they have a professional responsibility.

With respect to any drug or pharmaceutical products identified, readers are advised to check the most current information provided (i) on procedures featured or (ii) by the manufacturer of each product to be administered to verify the recommended dose or formula, the method and duration of administration, and contraindications. It is the responsibility of practitioners, relying on their own experience and knowledge of their patients, to make diagnoses, to determine dosages and the best treatment for each individual patient, and to take all appropriate safety precautions.

To the fullest extent of the law, neither the Publisher nor the authors, contributors, or editors assume any liability for any injury and/or damage to persons or property as a matter of products liability, negligence or otherwise, or from any use or operation of any methods, products, instructions, or ideas contained in the material herein.

Library of Congress Cataloging-in-Publication Data
Hematology, immunology, and infectious disease : neonatology questions and controversies / [edited by Robin K. Ohls]. — 2nd ed.
    p.   cm. — (Neonatology questions and controversies series)
    Includes bibliographical references and index.
    ISBN 978-1-4377-2662-6 (alk. paper)
    1. Neonatal hematology. 2. Newborn infants—Immunology. 3. Communicable diseases in newborn infants.   I. Ohls, Robin K.
    RJ269.5.H52 2012
    618.92′01—dc23

                                                                                          2011053382

Senior Content Strategist: Stefanie Jewell-Thomas
Content Development Specialist: Lisa Barnes
Publishing Services Manager: Anne Altepeter
Team Manager: Hemamalini Rajendrababu
Project Manager: Siva Raman Krishnamoorthy
Design Direction: Ellen Zanolle

Printed in The United States of America

Last digit is the print number: 9 8 7 6 5 4 3 2 1

Contributors

Jennifer L. Armstrong-Wells, MD
Director
Perinatal and Hemorrhagic Stroke
    Programs
Department of Pediatrics
Section of Neurology
Hemophilia and Thrombosis Center;
Assistant Professor
Pediatric Neurology
University of Colorado
Aurora, Colorado;
Assistant Adjunct Professor
Neurology
University of California, San Francisco
San Francisco, California
    Hematology and Immunology:
    Coagulation Disorders

Nader Bishara, MD
Attending Neonatologist
Pediatrix Medical Group
Huntington Memorial Hospital
Pasadena, California
    The Use of Biomarkers for Detection of
    Early- and Late-Onset Neonatal Sepsis

L. Vandy Black, MD
Instructor, Division of Pediatric
    Hematology
The Johns Hopkins University
Baltimore, Maryland
    A Practical Approach to the
    Neutropenic Neonate

Suresh B. Boppana, MD
Professor, Pediatrics and Microbiology
University of Alabama at Birmingham
Birmingham, Alabama
    CMV: Diagnosis, Treatment, and
    Considerations on Vaccine-Mediated
    Prevention

Catalin S. Buhimschi, MD
Associate Professor, Director
Perinatal Research
Interim Division Director
Maternal Fetal Medicine
Obstetrics, Gynecology, and
    Reproductive Sciences
Yale University School of Medicine;
Interim Chief of Obstetrics
Obstetrics, Gynecology, and
    Reproductive Sciences
Yale New Haven Hospital
New Haven, Connecticut
    Chorioamnionitis and Its Effects on the
    Fetus/Neonate: Emerging Issues and
    Controversies

Irina A. Buhimschi, MD, MMS
Associate Professor
Obstetrics, Gynecology, and
    Reproductive Sciences
Yale University School of Medicine
New Haven, Connecticuit
    Chorioamnionitis and Its Effects on the
    Fetus/Neonate: Emerging Issues and
    Controversies

Robert D. Christensen, MD
Director of Research
Women and Newborns
Intermountain Healthcare
Salt Lake City, Utah
    The Role of Recombinant Leukocyte
    Colony-Stimulating Factors in the
    Neonatal Intensive Care Unit

Misti Ellsworth, DO
Pediatric Infectious Disease
San Antonio, Texas
    Neonatal Fungal Infections

Björn Fischler, MD, PhD
Associate Professor
Pediatrics CLINTEC
Karolinska Institutet;
Senior Consultant
Pediatric Hepatology
Pediatrics
Karolinska University Hospital
Stockholm, Sweden
  Breast Milk and Viral Infection

Marianne Forsgren, MD, PhD
Associate Professor of Virology
Department of Clinical Microbiology
Karolinska University Hospital,
  Huddinge
Stockholm, Sweden
  Breast Milk and Viral Infection

Peta L. Grigsby, PhD
Assistant Scientist
Division of Reproductive Sciences
Oregon National Primate Research
  Center;
Assistant Research Professor
Department of Obstetrics and
  Gynecology
Oregon Health and Science University
Portland, Oregon
  *The Ureaplasma Conundrum: Should
  We Look or Ignore?*

Sandra E. Juul, MD, PhD
Professor, Pediatrics
University of Washington;
Professor, Pediatrics
Seattle Children's Hospital
Seattle, Washington
  *Nonhematopoietic Effects of
  Erythropoietin*

David B. Lewis, MD
Professor and Chief, Division of
  Immunology and Allergy
Department of Pediatrics
Stanford University School of Medicine
Stanford, California;
Attending Physician in Immunology
  and Infectious Diseases
Department of Pediatrics
Lucile Packard Children's Hospital
Palo Alto, California
  *Neonatal T Cell Immunity and Its
  Regulation by Innate Immunity and
  Dendritic Cells*

Akhil Maheshwari, MD
Associate Professor of Pediatrics
  and Pharmacology
Chief, Division of Neonatology
Director, Neonatology Fellowship
  Program
Director, Center for Neonatology
  and Pediatric Gastrointestinal Disease
University of Illinois at Chicago;
Medical Director, Neonatology
  Intensive Care Unit and Intermediate
  Care Nursery
Children's Hospital of University
  of Illinois
Chicago, Illinois
  *A Practical Approach to the
  Neutropenic Neonate*

Marilyn J. Manco-Johnson, MD
Professor, Pediatrics
Hemophilia and Thrombosis Center
University of Colorado and Children's
  Hospital
Aurora, Colorado
  *Hematology and Immunology:
  Coagulation Disorders*

Cynthia T. McEvoy, MD
Associate Professor of Pediatrics
Division of Neonatology
Oregon Health and Science University
Portland, Oregon
  *The Ureaplasma Conundrum: Should
  We Look or Ignore?*

Neelufar Mozaffarian, MD, PhD
Medical Director
Immunology Development Global
  Pharmaceutical Research
  and Development
Abbott
Abbott Park, Illinois
  *Maternally Mediated Neonatal
  Autoimmunity*

Lars Navér, MD, PhD
Senior Consultant in Pediatrics
  and Neonatology
Departments of Pediatrics
  and Neonatology
Karolinska University Hospital
Stockholm, Sweden
  Breast Milk and Viral Infection

Robin K. Ohls, MD
Professor of Pediatrics
University of New Mexico
Associate Director, Pediatrics
Clinical Translational Science Center
University of New Mexico Health
  Sciences
Albuquerque, New Mexico
  *Why, When, and How Should We
  Provide Red Cell Transfusions and
  Erythropoiesis-Stimulating Agents to
  Support Red Cell Mass in Neonates?*

**David A. Osborn, MBBS, MMed
  (Clin Epi), FRACP, PhD**
Clinical Associate Professor
Central Clinical School
University of Sydney;
Senior Neonatalogist and Director
Neonatal Intensive Care Unit
Royal Prince Alfred Newborn Care
Royal Prince Alfred Hospital
Sydney, Austrailia
  *What Evidence Supports Dietary
  Interventions to Prevent Infant Food
  Hypersensitivity and Allergy?*

**Luis Ostrosky-Zeichner, MD, FACP,
  FIDSA**
Associate Professor of Medicine
  and Epidemiology
Division of Infectious Diseases
University of Texas Medical School
  at Houston
Houston, Texas
Neonatal Fungal Infections

Shrena Patel, MD
Assistant Professor
Department of Pediatrics
Division of Neonatology
University of Utah
Salt Lake City, Utah
  *Diagnosis and Treatment of Immune-
  Mediated and Non–Immune-Mediated
  Hemolytic Disease of the Newborn*

**Sanjay Patole, MD, DCH, FRACP,
  MSc, DrPH**
Clinical Associate Professor
Department of Neonatal Paediatrics
King Edward Memorial Hospital
  for Women
Subiaco, Australia;
University of Western Australia
Perth, Australia
  *Probiotics for the Prevention of Necrotizing
  Enterocolitis in Preterm Neonates*

Simon Pirie, MBBS, MRCPCH
Consultant Neonatologist
Neonatal Unit
Gloucestershire Hospital
National Health Service Foundation
  Trust
Gloucester, England
  *Probiotics for the Prevention of
  Necrotizing Enterocolitis in Preterm
  Neonates*

Nutan Prasain, PhD
Postdoctoral Fellow
Pediatrics
Herman B. Well Center for Pediatric
  Research
Indiana University School of Medicine
Indianapolis, Indiana
  *Updated Information on Stem Cells for
  the Neonatologist*

Victoria H.J. Roberts, PhD
Staff Scientist II
Oregon National Primate Research
  Center
Oregon Health and Science University
Portland, Oregon
  *The Ureaplasma Conundrum: Should
  We Look or Ignore?*

Shannon A. Ross, MD, MSPH
Assistant Professor
Pediatrics
University of Alabama School of Medicine
Birmingham, Alabama
  *CMV: Diagnosis, Treatment, and
  Considerations on Vaccine-Mediated
  Prevention*

Matthew A. Saxonhouse, MD
Attending Neonatologist, Pediatrics
Pediatrix Medical Group;
Attending Neonatologist, Pediatrics
Jeff Gordon Children's Hospital
Concord, North Carolina
  *Current Issues in the Pathogenesis,
  Diagnosis, and Treatment of Neonatal
  Thrombocytopenia*

Robert L. Schelonka, MD
Associate Professor and Chief
Division of Neonatology
Pediatrics
Department of Oregon Health
  and Science University
Portland, Oregon
  *The Ureaplasma Conundrum: Should
  We Look or Ignore?*

Elizabeth A. Shaw, DO
Acting Assistant Professor of Pediatrics
Division of Pediatric Rheumatology
Seattle Children's Hospital
University of Washington
Seattle, Washington
   *Maternally Mediated Neonatal
   Autoimmunity*

Charles R. Sims, MD
Division of Infectious Diseases
The University of Texas Health
   Science Center at Houston
Laboratory of Mycology Research
Houston, Texas
   Neonatal Fungal Infections

**John K.H. Sinn, MBBS, FRACP,
MMed (Clin Epi)**
Assistant Professor
Neonatology and Pediatric and Child
   Health
University of Sydney;
Assistant Professor
Neonatology
Royal North Shore Hospital;
Assistant Professor
Pediatric and Child Health
The Children's Hospital at Westmead
Sydney, Australia
   *What Evidence Supports Dietary
   Interventions to Prevent Infant Food
   Hypersensitivity and Allergy?*

Martha C. Sola-Visner, MD
Assistant Professor of Pediatrics
Department of Medicine
Division of Newborn Medicine
Children's Hospital Boston;
Harvard Medical School
Boston, Massachusetts
   *Current Issues in the Pathogenesis,
   Diagnosis, and Treatment of Neonatal
   Thrombocytopenia*

Anne M. Stevens, MD, PhD
Associate Professor
Pediatrics
University of Washington
Center for Immunity
   and Immunotherapies
Seattle Children's Research Institute
Seattle, Washington
   *Maternally Mediated Neonatal
   Autoimmunity*

Philip Toltzis, MD
Professor of Pediatrics
Pediatrics
Rainbow Babies and Children's Hospital
Cleveland, Ohio
   *Control of Antibiotic-Resistant Bacteria
   in the Neonatal Intensive Care Unit*

Christopher Traudt, MD
Acting Assistant Professor of Pediatrics
University of Washington
Seattle, Washington
   *Nonhematopoietic Effects of
   Erythropoietin*

Mervin C. Yoder, Jr., MD
Richard and Pauline Klingler Professor
   of Pediatrics
Professor of Biochemistry
   and Molecular Biology
Professor of Cellular and Integrative
   Physiology
Director, Herman B. Wells Center
   for Pediatric Research
Indiana Universitiy School of Medicine
Indianapolis, Indiana
   *Updated Information on Stem Cells for
   the Neonatologist*

Series Foreword

Richard A. Polin, MD

"Medicine is a science of uncertainty and an art of probability."

—William Osler

Controversy is part of everyday practice in the neonatal intensive care unit (NICU). Good practitioners strive to incorporate the best evidence into clinical care. However, for much of what we do, the evidence is either inconclusive or nonexistent. In those circumstances, we have come to rely on experienced practitioners who have taught us the importance of clinical expertise. This series, "Neonatology Questions and Controversies," provides clinical guidance by summarizing the best evidence and tempering those recommendations with the art of experience.

To quote David Sackett, one of the founders of evidence-based medicine:

> *Good doctors use both individual clinical expertise and the best available external evidence*, and neither alone is enough. *Without clinical expertise, practice risks become tyrannized by evidence, for even excellent external evidence may be inapplicable to or inappropriate for an individual patient. Without current best evidence, practice risks become rapidly out of date to the detriment of patients.*

This series focuses on the challenges faced by care providers who work in the NICU. When should we incorporate a new technology or therapy into everyday practice, and will it have a positive impact on morbidity or mortality? For example, is the new generation of ventilators better than older technologies such as continuous positive airway pressure, or do they merely offer more choices with uncertain value? Similarly, the use of probiotics to prevent necrotizing enterocolitis is supported by sound scientific principles (and some clinical studies). However, at what point should we incorporate them into everyday practice given that the available preparations are not well characterized or proven safe? A more difficult and common question is when to use a new technology with uncertain value in a critically ill infant. As many clinicians have suggested, sometimes the best approach is to do nothing and "stand there."

The "Neonatal Questions and Controversies" series was developed to highlight the clinical problems of most concern to practitioners. The editors of each volume (Drs. Bancalari, Oh, Guignard, Baumgart, Kleinman, Seri, Ohls, Maheshwari, Neu, and Perlman) have done an extraordinary job in selecting topics of clinical importance to everyday practice. When appropriate, less controversial topics have been eliminated and replaced by others thought to be of greater clinical importance. In total, there are 56 new chapters in the series. During the preparation of the *Hemodynamics and Cardiology* volume, Dr. Charles Kleinman died. Despite an illness that would have caused many to retire, Charlie worked until near the time of his death. He came to work each day, teaching students and young practitioners and offering his wisdom and expertise to families of infants with congenital heart disease. We dedicate the second edition of the series to his memory. As with the first edition, I am indebted to the exceptional group of editors who chose the content and edited each of the volumes. I also wish to thank Lisa Barnes (content development specialist at Elsevier) and Judith Fletcher (global content development director), who provided incredible assistance in bringing this project to fruition.

Preface

Just like every other organ in the body, the hematological and immune systems in the newborn are in a state of maturational flux. Exposed to a continuous barrage of environmental antigens at birth, the neonatal immune system has to protect the host from potentially harmful pathogens while developing tolerance to commensal microbes and dietary macromolecules. Although many components of the innate immune system are reasonably mature at full-term birth, the neonate remains highly susceptible to specific pathogens because of developmental constraints in the adaptive branch of immunity. Not surprisingly, despite major strides in neonatal care, neonatal sepsis remains the leading cause of death at any point of time in human life.

In the second edition of this volume of the series "Neonatology Questions and Controversies," our original goals remain unchanged: we seek to update physicians, nurse practitioners, nurses, residents, and students on (1) developmental physiology of the immune response in the human fetus and neonate that are not typically high-lighted, (2) cellular or cytokine replacement therapies for treatment of hematological deficiencies or infectious disease, and (3) controversies in immune modulation that may play a role in preventing allergic disorders in the developing infant. Each chapter provides an overview of how the neonate must utilize cells of the hemato-logical and immune systems to thwart the onslaught of microbial challenges and a roadmap for the clinician to quickly diagnose and intervene to augment neonatal hematological or immunological defenses. We further provide information about how distortions in the immune response can result in allergy or autoimmunity in the neonate. In this extensively revised edition, we have also added several new chapters on infectious diseases specific to the perinatal/neonatal period.

We wish to thank Judith Fletcher, global content development director at Else-vier; Lisa Barnes, content development specialist at Elsevier; and Dr. Richard Polin, chairman of the Department of Pediatrics at Morgan Stanley Children's Hospital of New York Presbyterian, for their encouragement to write this volume. We, of course, are indebted and grateful to the authors of each chapter whose contributions from around the world will be fully appreciated by the readers and to our families (Daniel, Erin, and Fiona and Ritu, Jayant, and Vikram) for their enduring support. Finally, we would like to acknowledge Dr. Robert Christensen for his ongoing inspiration, enthusiasm, and generosity and for being the best mentor and role model we could ever ask for.

Robin K. Ohls, MD
Akhil Maheshwari, MD

Contents

CHAPTER 1

Updated Information on Stem Cells for the Neonatologist

Nutan Prasain, PhD, and Mervin C. Yoder, Jr., MD

Introduction

As a normal process of human growth and development, many organs and tissues display a need for continued replacement of mature cells that are lost with aging or injury. For example, billions of red blood cells, white blood cells, and platelets are produced per kilogram of body weight daily. The principal site of blood cell production, the bone marrow, harbors the critically important stem cells that serve as the regenerating source for all manufactured blood cells. These hematopoietic stem cells share several common features with all other kinds of stem cells.[1] Stem cells display the ability to self-renew (to divide and give rise to other stem cells) and to produce offspring that mature along distinct differentiation pathways to form cells with specialized functions.[1] Stem cells have classically been divided into two groups: *embryonic stem cells (ESCs)* and *nonembryonic stem cells,* also called *somatic* or *adult stem cells.*[1] The purpose of this review is to introduce and provide up-to-date information on stem cell facts that should be familiar to all clinicians caring for sick neonates regarding selected aspects of ESC and adult stem cell research. We will also review several new methods for inducing pluripotent stem cells from differentiated somatic cells and methods for direct reprogramming of one cell type to another. These latest approaches offer entirely novel, patient-specific, non–ethically charged approaches to tissue repair and regeneration in human subjects.

The fertilized oocyte (zygote) is the "mother" of all stem cells. All the potential for forming all cells and tissues of the body, including the placenta and extraembryonic membranes, is derived from this cell (reviewed in Reference 1). Furthermore, the zygote possesses unique information leading to the establishment of the overall body plan and organogenesis. Thus, the zygote is a totipotent cell. The first few cleavage stage divisions also produce blastomere cells retaining totipotent potential. However, by the blastocyst stage, many of these cells have adopted specific developmental pathways. One portion of the blastocyst, the *epiblast,* contains cells (inner cell mass cells) that will go on to form the embryo proper. Trophectoderm cells make up the cells at the opposite pole of the blastocyst; these cells will differentiate to form the placenta. Cells within the inner cell mass of the blastocyst are pluripotent, that is, each cell possesses the potential to give rise to types of cells that develop from the three embryonic germ layers (mesoderm, endoderm, and ectoderm). ESCs do not technically exist in the developing blastocyst, but are derived upon ex vivo culture of inner cell mass cells from the epiblast using specific methods and reagents as discussed later.

Isolation of Murine Embryonic Stem Cells

Mouse ESCs were isolated more than 20 years ago in an extension of basic studies that had been conducted on how embryonic teratocarcinoma cells could be maintained in tissue culture.[2,3] Inner cell mass cells were recovered from murine blastocysts and plated over an adherent layer of mouse embryonic fibroblasts in the presence of culture medium containing fetal calf serum and, in some instances, conditioned medium from murine teratocarcinoma cells. Over a period of several weeks, colonies of rapidly growing cells emerged. These colonies of tightly adherent but proliferating cells could be recovered from culture dishes and disaggregated with enzymes to form a single cell suspension, and the cells replated on fresh embryonic fibroblasts. Within days, the individually plated cells had formed new colonies that could in like manner be isolated and recultured with no apparent restriction in terms of proliferative potential. Cells making up the colonies were eventually defined as ESCs.

Murine (m) ESCs display several unique properties. The cells are small and have a high nuclear to cytoplasmic ratio and prominent nucleoli. When plated in the presence of murine embryonic fibroblasts, with great care taken to keep the cells from clumping at each passage (clumping of cells promotes mESC differentiation), mESCs proliferate indefinitely as pluripotent cells.[4] In fact, one can manipulate the genome of the mESC using homologous recombination to insert or remove specific genetic sequences and maintain mESC pluripotency.[5] Injection of normal mESCs into recipient murine blastocysts permits ESC-derived contribution to essentially all tissues of the embryo, including germ cells. By injecting mutant mESCs into donor blastocysts, one is able to generate genetically altered strains of mice (commonly referred to as *knockout mice*).[6]

Although the molecular regulation of mESC self-renewal divisions remains unclear, the growth factor leukemia inhibitory factor (LIF) has been determined to be sufficient to maintain mESCs in a self-renewing state in vitro, even in the absence of mouse fibroblast feeder cells. More recently, addition of the growth factor bone morphogenetic protein-4 (BMP-4) to mESC cultures (with LIF) permits maintenance of the pluripotent state in serum-free conditions.[7,8] Several transcription factors, including Oct-4 and Nanog, are required to maintain mESC self-renewal divisions.[9,10] Increasing mitogen-activated protein (MAP) kinase activity and decreasing signal transducer and activator of transcription 2 (STAT2) activity result in loss of mESC self-renewal divisions and differentiation of the mESC into multiple cell lineages.[8] Isolation and determination of the transcriptional and epigenetic molecular mechanisms controlling mESC self-renewal continues to be an active area of ongoing research.[11-14]

The strict culture conditions required for in vitro differentiation of mESCs into a wide variety of specific somatic cell types, such as neurons, hematopoietic cells, pancreatic cells, hepatocytes, muscle cells, cardiomyocytes, and endothelial cells, have been well described.[15-18] In most differentiation protocols, mESCs first are deprived of LIF; this is followed by the addition of other growth factors, vitamins, morphogens, extracellular matrix molecules, or drugs to stimulate ESCs to differentiate along specific pathways. It is also usual for the ESC differentiation protocol to give rise to a predominant but not a pure population of differentiated cells. Obtaining highly purified differentiated cell populations generally requires some form of cell selection to enhance the survival of a selected population, or to preferentially eliminate a nondesired population.[19] The ability to isolate enriched populations of differentiated cells has encouraged many investigators to postulate that ESCs may be a desirable source of cells for replacement of aged, injured, or diseased tissues in human subjects if pluripotent human (h) ESCs were readily available.[20,21]

Isolation of Human Embryonic Stem Cells

The growth conditions that have permitted isolation and characterization of hESCs have become available only in the last decade.[22] Left-over cleavage-stage human embryos originally produced by in vitro fertilization for clinical purposes are a prominent source for hESC derivation. Embryos are grown to the blastocyst stage, the inner cell mass cells isolated, and the isolated cells plated on irradiated mouse embryonic fibroblast feeder layers in vitro. After growing in culture for several cell divisions, colonies of hESCs emerge, similar to mESCs. These hESCs are very small cells with minimal cytoplasm and prominent nucleoli; similar to mouse cells, they grow very rapidly without evidence of developing senescence and possess high telomerase activity. Unlike mESCs, LIF is not sufficient to maintain hESCs in a self-renewing state in the absence of mouse fibroblast feeder cells. However, human ESCs can be grown on extracellular matrix–coated plates in the presence of murine embryonic fibroblast conditioned medium without the presence of mouse feeder cells. Recent data reveal that the use of specific recombinant molecules and peptides as a tissue culture plate coating is sufficient to maintain and/or modulate hESC into states of high self-renewal and limited differentiation.[23-26] Relatively high doses of fibroblast growth factor-2 (FGF-2) help maintain hESCs in an undifferentiated state even in the absence of feeder cells.[27,28]

The pluripotent nature of hESCs has been demonstrated by injecting the cells into an immunodeficient mouse.[22] A tumor (specifically called a *teratoma*) emerges from the site of the injected cells and histologically contains numerous cell types, including gastric and intestinal epithelium, renal tubular cells, and neurons—descendants of the endoderm, mesoderm, and ectoderm germ cell layers, respectively. At present, teratoma formation in immunodeficient mice continues to serve as the only method to document hESC pluripotency.[29] Expression of Oct-4 and alkaline phosphatase, as biomarkers of ESC pluripotency, helps to support but is inadequate alone as evidence of hESC pluripotency.[28] Recent evidence indicates that the pluripotent state is best distinguished by colonies of cells with a distinct methylation pattern of the Oct-4 and Nanog promoters, expression of TRA-1-60, and differentiation into teratomas in vivo in immunodeficient mice.[30]

Derivation of Mouse-Induced Pluripotent Stem Cells (miPSCs) by Defined Factors

Although pluripotent stem cells can be derived from a developing blastocyst to generate ESCs, direct nuclear reprogramming of differentiated adult somatic cells to a pluripotent state has more recently been achieved by ectopic expression of a defined set of transcription factors. Takahashi and Yamanaka reported breakthrough studies in 2006 demonstrating that the retroviral transduction of mouse fibroblast cells with four transcription factors—Oct4, Sox2, Klf4, and c-Myc—induced a stable fate change, converting differentiated cells into pluripotent stem cells.[31] These four transcription factors were identified as sufficient factors for direct reprogramming when systematic screening of 24 ESC genes believed to be essential for the maintenance of ESC pluripotency and self-renewal was conducted. Reprogrammed cells were selected by expression of a fusion cassette of β-galactosidase and neomycin resistance genes driven by the promoter of the ESC-specific, but nonessential, pluripotency gene *Fbx15*. Although *Fbx15*-expressing induced pluripotent stem calls (iPSCs) shared phenotypic characteristics of mESCs and formed teratoma tumors in nude mice upon implantation (with histologic evidence of cells differentiating into all three germ layers), these cells were significantly different in genetic and epigenetic signatures from naïve mESCs and failed to produce germline transmissible chimeric mice.[31] However, when promoter sequences from ESC-specific and essential pluripotency genes (Oct4 or Nanog) were used as selection markers, iPSCs closely resembling ESCs capable of germline transmissible chimera formation were generated.[32-34]

Although the exact molecular mechanism that led to reprogramming of these somatic cells to pluripotent stem cells is unknown, ectopic expression of these factors eventually resulted in reactivation of endogenous pluripotency genes to mediate the activation of autoregulatory loops that maintain the pluripotent state. Transgene expression of these factors was determined to be required only transiently to reactivate the endogenous pluripotent genes; once the pluripotent state was established, the exogenous transgenes were epigenetically silenced.[33,34] Completely reprogrammed mouse iPSCs share all defining features with naïve mESCs, including expression of pluripotency markers, global patterns of gene expression, DNA methylation of the promoter regions of Oct4 and Nanog, reactivation of both X chromosomes, global patterns of histone methylation (H3 lysine 4 and lysine 27 trimethylation), ability to produce germline transmissible chimeric mice,[32-35] and development of transgenic mice following tetraploid complementation in which the whole embryo is iPSC derived.[36-38]

Although original methods of reprogramming factor delivery using retroviral or lentiviral vectors provided proof-of-principle for induced pluripotency, low reprogramming efficiencies, safety concerns associated with the use of randomly integrating viral vectors, and the known oncogenic potential of *c-Myc* and *Klf4* genes have been limiting factors in the clinical applicability of the translation of iPSCs for human cell therapy. Although the most recent studies have reported the ability to reprogram fibroblasts with greater than 2% reprogramming efficiency,[39] two orders of magnitude higher than those typically reported for virus-based reprogramming efficiency, a significant increase in reprogramming efficiency is needed for effective clinical utility. Nonintegrative reprogramming factor delivery approaches (to avoid risks of vector insertional mutagenesis), such as use of adenoviral vectors,[40] repeated transfection with reprogramming of plasmid vectors,[41] excision of reprogramming factors with Cre-loxP[42,43] or piggyBAC transposition approaches,[44,45] recombinant protein transduction of reprogramming factors,[46] transient expression of reprogramming factors with nonviral minicircle DNA vectors,[47] and, most recently, use of synthetic modified mRNA encoding the reprogramming factors,[39] have made it possible to generate iPSCs through transient expression of reprogramming factors. Further, attempts have been made to remove one or more reprogramming transcription factors, specifically avoiding the known oncogenes *c-Myc* and *Klf4,* by substitution with small molecules, such as valproic acid, which modulate the epigenetic status of the cells undergoing reprogramming.[48,49] In addition, small molecule inhibitors of transforming growth factor (TGF)-β_1, extracellular signal–related kinase (ERK), and glycogen synthase kinase 3 (GSK3) signaling pathways have been shown to facilitate efficient reprogramming of somatic cells into iPSCs.[50,51]

Derivation of Human-Induced Pluripotent Stem Cells (hiPSCs) by Defined Factors

One of the ultimate goals of regenerative medicine is to have a renewable source of patient- and disease-specific cells to replace or repair diseased or impaired cells in tissues and organs. Although pluripotent hESCs have the potential to give rise to cells from all three embryonic germ layers, they have yet to overcome numerous ethical and scientific barriers. The fact that derivation of hESCs requires the death of an embryo is an ethical dilemma that does not appear to be resolvable. Among the scientific barriers, effective therapies have not yet been developed to overcome host adaptive immune responses because hESC-derived cells are allogeneic in origin. In light of these limitations, Shinya Yamanaka's announcement of directed reprogramming of mouse[31] and human[52] fibroblast cells to pluripotent stem cells by a set of defined transcription factors paved the way for overcoming these two major obstacles surrounding the promise of hESCs. The promise of iPSC derivation has profound implications for basic research and clinical therapeutics in that this approach provides patient- and disease-specific cells for the study of disease pathogenesis and the therapeutic efficacy of pharmacologic agents against the disease; it also provides an autologous source of patient cells for cell-based therapeutics (Fig. 1-1).

Although hiPSCs closely resemble hESCs in their morphology, gene expression, epigenetic states, pluripotency, and ability to form teratomas in immune-deficient mice,[52,53] more studies are needed to access the functional similarity

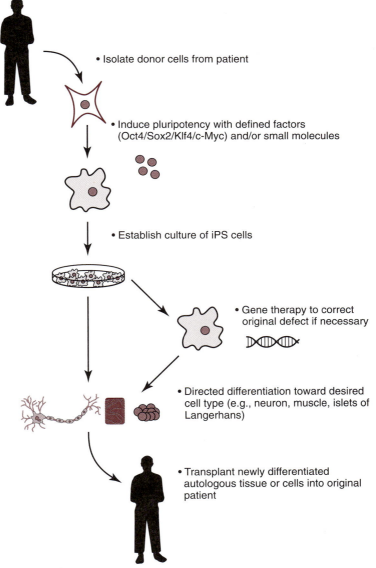

• Isolate donor cells from patient

• Induce pluripotency with defined factors (Oct4/Sox2/Klf4/c-Myc) and/or small molecules

• Establish culture of iPS cells

• Gene therapy to correct original defect if necessary

• Directed differentiation toward desired cell type (e.g., neuron, muscle, islets of Langerhans)

• Transplant newly differentiated autologous tissue or cells into original patient

Figure 1-1 Diagram depicting generation of induced pluripotent stem cells (iPSCs) from patient somatic cells, correction of original genetic defects if necessary, and directed differentiation of patient iPSCs to generate autologous cells of therapeutic importance. (Diagram adapted from Robbins RD, Prasain N, Maier BF, et al. Inducible pluripotent stem cells: Not quite ready for prime time? *Curr Opin Organ Transplant.* 2010;15:61-67.)

between hiPSCs and hESCs. However, significant strides have been made in iPSC research in the last few years since the original description of iPSC induction by Yamanaka from mouse cells in 2006[31] and from human cells[52] by Yamanaka and, independently, by Thomson in 2007.[53] Although the Yamanaka group used Oct4, Sox2, Klf4, and c-Myc as reprogramming factors, the Thomson group used Oct4, Sox2, Nanog, and Lin28 to reprogram human fibroblasts to iPSCs. Subsequently, a number of human diseases and patient-specific iPSCs were established,[54-58] and some of these cells were subjected to directed differentiation to generate healthy functional autologous cells of therapeutic importance. Moreover, other studies have successfully described the differentiation of iPSCs into a diversity of cell types of therapeutic importance, including endothelial cells,[59,60] cardiomyocytes,[61,62] neuronal cells,[63,64] retinal cells,[65-67] and hematopoietic cells.[23,57,59]

Human iPSCs have been generated from patients with a variety of genetic diseases, including Parkinson disease, Huntington disease, juvenile-onset type 1 diabetes mellitus, and Down syndrome.[56] Although intense focus has been placed on improving ease, safety, and efficiency for generation of disease- and patient-specific iPSCs, equally impressive progress has been made in the directed differentiation of iPSCs to cell types of therapeutic importance. Particularly promising examples include derivation of glucose-responsive pancreatic islet–like cell clusters from human skin fibroblast-derived iPSCs,[58] paving the way for generation of autologous pancreatic islet–like cells for possible cell-based therapy to treat diabetic individuals. Also, disease-free motor neurons have been derived from iPSCs generated from skin cells obtained from elderly patients with amyotrophic lateral sclerosis,[54] suggesting that cellular aging and long-term environmental exposure do not hinder the iPSC induction and directed differentiation processes. Equally important, motor neurons with a preserved patient-specific disease phenotype have been derived from iPSCs generated from primary fibroblasts obtained from a patient with spinal muscular atrophy.[55] When these motor neurons were treated in vitro with valproic acid and tobramycin, they exhibited upregulation in survival motor neuron protein synthesis, and they displayed selective deficits when compared with normal motor neurons, suggesting that patient-specific iPSC-derived cells can be used to study patient-specific disease processes in vitro, before specific drug therapies are initiated. In fact, use of iPSCs from patients with specific diseases may permit large-scale small-molecule screening efforts to discover completely novel patient therapies. Thus, the discovery of nuclear reprogramming of differentiated somatic cells into pluripotent stem cells is potentially one of the most paradigm-changing discoveries in biomedical research in several decades.

Alternative Approaches to Reprogramming Somatic Cells to a Pluripotent State

In addition to the use of transcription factors to induce nuclear reprogramming to a pluripotent stem cell state, at least two other general approaches—nuclear transfer and cell fusion—have been utilized to accomplish the same feat.[68] Nuclear transfer is accomplished by removing the nucleus from an oocyte, isolating a somatic cell nucleus, transferring the donor somatic cell nucleus into the oocyte, and electrically fusing the donor nucleus with the enucleated oocyte. The created zygote may be grown to the blastocyst stage, where the embryo is disaggregated and cells from the inner cell mass are harvested for creation of ESC in vitro, or the blastocyst is implanted into a recipient female. Such a procedure is technically challenging but possible; a variety of domestic animals and laboratory rodents have been successfully cloned in this fashion.[69]

Some of the challenges that need to be overcome when nuclear transfer technology is used to create viable cloned animals include the great inefficiency of the process (hundreds to thousands of oocytes are often injected, with only a few viable animals surviving beyond birth as an outcome). Much of this inefficiency may be the result of poor epigenetic reprogramming of the donor somatic nucleus in the oocyte.[70] In adult somatic tissues, epigenetic modifications of DNA and chromatin are stably maintained and are characteristic of each specialized tissue or organ. During nuclear transfer, epigenetic reprogramming of the somatic nucleus must occur, similar to the epigenetic reprogramming that normally occurs during oocyte activation following fertilization.[71] Epigenetic reprogramming deficiencies during animal cloning may lead to a host of problems, including epigenetic mutations and altered epigenetic inheritance patterns, causing altered gene expression and resulting in embryonic lethality or maldeveloped fetuses with poor postnatal survival. Although great strides have been made in identifying the molecules involved in chromatin remodeling and in epigenetic programming, considerable work remains to identify strategies to facilitate this process. It is interesting that hESCs have been used to reprogram human somatic cells and may offer an alternative to the use of oocytes.[72]

A more simplified approach in generating reprogrammed somatic cells is to fuse two or more cell types into a single cellular entity. The process of cell fusion may generate hybrid cells in which the donor nuclei fuse and cell division is retained, or heterokaryons that lose the ability to divide contain multiple nuclei per cell. Studies performed four decades ago revealed that the fusing of two distinctly different cell types resulted in changes in gene expression, suggesting that not only *cis*-acting DNA elements but also *trans*-acting factors are capable of modulating the cellular proteome.[73] Fusion of female embryonic germ cells with adult thymocytes yielded fused tetraploid cells that displayed pluripotent properties and heralded more recent studies, in which male thymocytes fused with female ESCs resulted in reactivation of certain genes in the thymocytes that are required for ESC self-renewal but are silenced in mature thymocytes.[74] These and other studies have revealed that factors regulating pluripotency in general can override factors regulating cellular differentiation and exemplify the potential for cell fusion studies to illuminate the mechanisms that underpin successful nuclear reprogramming.

Somatic Stem Cells

Adult (also called *somatic, postnatal,* or *nonembryonic*) stem cells are multipotent cells that reside in specialized tissues and organs and retain the ability to self-renew and to develop into progeny that yield all the differentiated cells that make up the tissue or organ of residence. For example, intestinal stem cells replenish the intestinal villous epithelium several times a week, skin stem cells give rise to cells that replace the epidermis in 3-week cycles, and hematopoietic stem cells replace billions of differentiated blood cells every hour for the life of the subject. Other sources of self-renewing adult stem cells include the cornea, bone marrow, retina, brain, skeletal muscle, dental pulp, pancreas, and liver (reviewed in Reference 1). Adult stem cells differ from their ESC and iPSC counterparts in several ways, including existence in a quiescent state in specified microenvironmental niches that protect the cells from noxious agents and facilitate such stem cell functions as orderly self-renewal, on-demand differentiation, occasional migration (for some stem cell types), and apoptosis (to regulate stem cell number). Although ESCs and iPSCs predominantly execute self-renewal divisions with maintenance of pluripotency, adult stem cells are required to maintain their stem cell pool size through self-renewal, while giving rise to daughter cells that differentiate into the particular lineage of cells needed for homeostasis at that moment—a feat requiring adult stem cells to execute asymmetric stem cell divisions. ESCs and iPSCs are easily expanded into millions of cells, but adult stem cells are limited in number in vivo, are difficult to extricate from their niches for in vitro study or for collection, and often are extremely sensitive to loss of proliferative potential and are skewed toward differentiation rather than maintaining self-renewal during in vitro propagation. Thus, obtaining sufficient numbers of adult stem cells for transplantation can be challenging. Strategies for improving adult stem cell mobilization, isolation, and expansion in vitro are all intense areas of investigation.[23,75,76] Nonetheless, adult stem cells are the primary sources of hematopoietic stem cells (adult bone marrow, mobilized peripheral blood, or umbilical cord blood) for human transplantation for genetic, acquired, or malignant disease.

Stem Cell Plasticity

Various studies have reported that adult stem cells isolated from one organ (in fact, specified to produce differentiated progeny for the cells making up that organ) possess the ability to differentiate into cells normally found in completely different organs following transplantation.[77] For example, bone marrow cells have been demonstrated to contribute to muscle, lung, gastric, intestinal, lung, and liver cells following adoptive transfer,[78-81] and neuronal stem cells can contribute to blood, muscle, and neuronal tissues.[82,83] More recent studies suggest that stem cell plasticity is an extremely rare event, and that in most human or animal subjects, the apparent donor stem cell differentiation event was in fact a monocyte-macrophage fusion event with epithelial cells of recipient tissues.[84-87] At present, enthusiasm for therapeutic multitissue repair in ill patients, from infusion of a single population of multipotent stem cells that would differentiate into the appropriate lineage required for organ repair, has waned considerably.[82,88] However, there is intense interest in understanding and utilizing novel recently developed tools to reprogram somatic cells into pluripotent cells (see earlier) or to directly reprogram one cellular lineage into another.

Direct Reprogramming of Somatic Cells from One Lineage to Another

One of the long-held tenets of developmental biology is that as an organism progresses through development to reach a final mature organized state, cells originating from embryonic precursors become irreversibly differentiated within the tissues and organs. However, in some rare examples, one cell type may be changed into another cell type; these events have been called *cellular reprogramming*. This biologic phenomenon occurs most prominently in amphibian organisms (e.g., axolotls, newts, lampreys, frogs) during limb regeneration, where fully differentiated cells dedifferentiate into progenitor cells with reactivation of embryonic patterns of gene expression. As noted previously, it has become evident through nuclear transfer, cell fusion, and transcription factor–induced reprogramming studies that differentiated somatic cells can become pluripotent cells with requisite changes in gene expression. Thus, cellular differentiation is not a fixed unalterable state, as was once thought.

Several years ago, Zhou and associates[89] rationalized that re-expression of certain embryonic genes may be a sufficient stimulus to reprogram somatic cells into different but related lineages. As a target tissue, this group chose to examine pancreatic β-cell regeneration, because it is known that exocrine cells present in the adult organ are derived from pancreatic endoderm, similarly to β-cells, and that exocrine cells could become endocrine cells upon in vitro culture. Upon screening for transcription factors specific for cells within the embryonic pancreas, several dozen were identified that were enriched in β-cells or in their endocrine progenitor precursors. Further examination revealed that nine of these transcription factors were important for normal β-cell development because mutation of these factors altered the normal developmental process. Adenoviral vectors were developed that would express each of the nine transcription factors and a reporter gene upon cellular infection. All nine of the recombinant viruses were pooled and injected into the pancreata of adult immunodeficient mice. One month later, extra-islet insulin expression was identified among some of the infected cells of the pancreas in host animals. Upon sequential elimination of one experimental construct at a time, it became evident that three transcription factors—*Ngn3, Pdx1,* and *Mafa*—were essential for the reprogramming event. Evidence was presented that the new insulin-producing cells were derived from exocrine cells, and that the induced β-cells were similar to endogenous β-cells in size, shape, and ultrastructural morphology. Induced β-cells expressed vascular endothelial growth factor and remodeled the existing vasculature within the organ in patterns similar to those of endogenous β-cells. Finally, injection of the three transcription factors via an adenoviral vector into the pancreas in diabetic mice improved fasting blood glucose levels, demonstrating that induced β-cells could produce and secrete insulin in vivo. Thus, β-cells may be regenerated directly from reprogrammed exocrine cells within the pancreas in vivo through introduction and expression of certain transcription factors. This work further postulated that reliance on knowledge of normal developmental pathways to reprogram adult somatic cells to stem/progenitor cells or another mature cell type may be a general strategy for adult cell reprogramming.

As predicted, the direct conversion of mouse fibroblast cells into functional neurons, cardiomyocytes, and multilineage blood cell progenitors has been reported. Vierbuchen and colleagues[90] reasoned that expression of multiple neural-lineage specific transcription factors may be sufficient to reprogram murine embryonic and postnatal fibroblasts into functional neurons in vitro. This group chose a strategy of using TauEGFP knock-in transgenic mice, which express enhanced green fluorescence protein (EGFP) in neurons, as a source of embryonic fibroblasts to permit reporting of new-onset EGFP expression in fibroblasts infected with a pool of 19 genes (chosen as neural specific or important in neural development) as an indicator of induced neuronal (iN) cells. A combination of three transcription factors—*Ascl1, Brn2,* and *Myt1l*—was determined to be required to rapidly and efficiently convert mouse embryonic fibroblasts into iN cells. These iN cells expressed multiple neuron-specific proteins, generated action potentials, and formed functional synapses in vitro. These studies suggest that iN cells can be generated in a timely and efficient manner for additional studies of neuronal cell identity and plasticity, neurologic disease modeling, and drug discovery, and as a potential source of cells for regenerative cell therapy.

Direct reprogramming of murine postnatal cardiac or dermal fibroblasts into functional cardiomyocytes has been reported by Ieda and coworkers.[91] Investigators developed an assay system in which induction of cardiomyocytes in vitro could be identified by new-onset expression of EGFP in fibroblasts isolated from neonatal transgenic mice in which only mature cardiomyocytes normally express the transgene. A total of 14 transcription or epigenetic remodeling factors were selected for testing as reprogramming factors in this assay system. All factors were cloned into retroviral vectors, and the retroviruses generated were used to infect the postnatal fibroblasts. A combination of three transcription factors—*Gata4, Mef2c,* and *Tbx5*—was sufficient to induce cardiac gene expression in the fibroblasts. Evidence was presented that induced cardiomyocyte-like (iCM) cells directly originated from the fibroblasts, and not through an intermediary cardiac progenitor cell state. Comparison of global gene expression patterns in the iCM, neonatal cardiomyocytes, and cardiac fibroblast cells yielded support for the contention that iCMs were similar, but not identical, to neonatal cardiomyocytes, and that the reprogramming process was generally reflected in the sweeping changes in gene expression displayed by these three different cell populations. Finally, iCMs displayed spontaneous contractile activity at 2 to 4 and at 4 to 5 weeks in culture, and intracellular electrical recordings of the iCM revealed action potentials resembling those detected in adult mouse ventricular cardiomyocytes. Proof that reprogramming events could be enacted in vivo was provided by harvesting adult cardiac fibroblasts, infecting the cells with retroviruses encoding the reprogramming transcription factors and a reporter gene (or the reporter gene control), and injecting into the heart. Some of the infected and engrafted myocardial fibroblast cells expressed the cardiomyocyte-specific reporter gene in vivo, indicating that transcription factors can reprogram the fibroblast within 2 weeks in vivo. Further studies on the ability of transcription factors to directly reprogram fibroblasts into iCMs in vivo are certainly warranted; future studies will need to test the in vivo physiologic functionality of iCM cells.

Szabo and associates[92] observed that a portion of human fibroblast cells undergoing the process of transcription factor–induced reprogramming toward pluripotency fail to fully reach the pluripotent state, but instead form colonies in which some of the progeny display morphologic characteristics similar to those of hematopoietic cells, expressing the human pan-hematopoietic marker CD45 and lacking expression of the pluripotency marker Tra-1-60. Upon comparing the role of Oct4 with those of Nanog and Sox2 in terms of ability to reprogram human fibroblast cells, these investigators determined that only Oct4 was capable of giving rise to hematopoietic-like CD45+ cells, and that once formed, CD45+ cells become responsive to hematopoietic growth factors with a fourfold to sixfold increase in hematopoietic colony formation in vitro. Evidence was presented that formation of hematopoietic colonies was not dependent on reprogramming to the pluripotent state and then differentiation to the hematopoietic lineage, but was a direct effect of Oct4 on fibroblast cells to become hematopoietic-like cells. Induced CD45+ cells displayed colony-forming activity (clonal colony growth in semi-solid medium) for myeloid, erythroid, and megakaryocytic lineages and for cells engrafted in the marrow of immunodeficient mice upon transplantation. As compared with engrafted adult bone marrow or cord blood progenitor cells, engrafted induced CD45+ cells revealed a skewing toward myeloid lineages in vivo. Induced CD45+ cells did not differentiate into lymphoid lineages in vitro or in vivo. This finding suggests that reprogramming of fibroblast cells did not lead to the generation of hematopoietic stem cells. Nonetheless, these results provide a fundamental starting point from which to explore those modifications to the reprogramming process that may eventually lead to autologous blood cell replacement therapies for patients with hematopoietic dysregulation or outright bone marrow hematopoietic failure.

Summary

Until 2006, stem cells were classified as those cells derived in vitro from preimplantation mammalian blastocysts (ESCs) or cells derived from somatic tissues and organs (adult stem cells).[1] Since 2006, it has become clear that iPSCs may be derived from differentiated somatic cells.[93] Although iPSCs and ESCs have displayed certain properties that generate enthusiasm for these stem cells as a source of differentiated cells for future applications of cell-based therapies for human diseases, iPSCs have recently emerged with greater appeal as a potential autologous approach to tissue repair and regeneration in human subjects.[93] Adult stem cell populations are also being investigated as potential sources for clinical cell-based therapies. Although ESC and iPSC approaches may offer many theoretical advantages over current adult stem cell approaches, the use of adult stem cells to treat patients with certain ailments is a current treatment of choice. No current or prior approved indications are known for the use of an hESC- or hiPSC-derived cell type for a human clinical disorder. Investigators working on adult stem cells, hESCs, and hiPSCs will continue to focus on improvements in cell isolation, in vitro stem cell expansion, regulating stem cell commitment to specific cell lineages, facilitating in vitro cellular differentiation, tissue engineering using synthetic matrices and stem cell progeny, optimizing transplantation protocols, and in vivo stem cell or stem cell–derived tissue testing for safety and efficacy in appropriate animal models of human disease. The recently acquired ability to directly reprogram one cell lineage into another cell lineage perhaps provides the most exciting possibilities for developing small molecules that someday may become drugs for administration to patients to repair or regenerate a dysfunctional or deficient cellular population. One may speculate that these approaches may permit arrest of human disease progression and may serve as methods of disease prevention as we learn how to tailor patient-specific disease risk detection with cellular reprogramming for tissue and organ regeneration.

This is an optimistic view of the potential benefit that mankind may derive from this basic research; however, we believe it is important to caution against unsubstantiated claims that such benefits can now be derived from these cells. The hope for medical benefit from a stem cell therapy is a powerful drug for many patients and their families suffering from currently incurable diseases, but as indicated previously, no indications are currently approved for the use of hESC- or hiPSC-derived cell therapy for any patient disorder. Likewise, indications for the use of adult stem cells as cell therapy are quite specific and, in general, are largely restricted to hematopoietic stem cell transplantation for human blood disorders. Several recent publications have addressed the issues that surround the phenomenon of "stem cell tourism" and provide some helpful considerations for subjects or families of subjects contemplating travel to seek medical benefits from "stem cell treatments" that may not be available in their own country.[94-96]

References

1. National Institutes of Health, Stem Cells. Scientific Progress and Future Research Directions. 2001, www.nih.gov.news/stemcell.scireport.htm. Accessed on 7/18/2011.
2. Evans M, Kaufman M. Establishment in culture of pluripotential cells from mouse embryos. *Nature*. 1981;292:145-147.
3. Martin G. Isolation of a pluripotent cell line from early mouse embryos cultured in medium conditioned by teratocarcinoma stem cells. *Proc Natl Acad Sci*. 1981;78:7634-7638.
4. Roach ML, McNeish JD. Methods for the isolation and maintenance of murine embryonic stem cells. *Methods Mol Biol*. 2002;185:1-16.
5. Capecchi M. The new mouse genetics: Altering the genome by gene targeting. *Trends in Genetics*. 1989;5:70-76.
6. Robertson EJ. Using embryonic stem cells to introduce mutations into the mouse germ line. *Biol Reprod*. 1991;44(2):238-245.
7. Bouhon IA, Kato H, Chandran S, et al. Neural differentiation of mouse embryonic stem cells in chemically defined medium. *Brain Res Bull*. 2005;68(1-2):62-75.
8. Keller G. Embryonic stem cell differentiation: Emergence of a new era in biology and medicine. *Genes Dev*. 2005;19(10):1129-1155.
9. Buehr M, Nichols J, Stenhouse F, et al. Rapid loss of Oct-4 and pluripotency in cultured rodent blastocysts and derivative cell lines. *Biol Reprod*. 2003;68(1):222-229.
10. Mitsui K, Tokuzawa Y, Itoh H, et al. The homeoprotein Nanog is required for maintenance of pluripotency in mouse epiblast and ES cells. *Cell*. 2003;113(5):631-642.
11. Heng JC, Orlov YL, Ng HH. Transcription factors for the modulation of pluripotency and reprogramming. *Cold Spring Harb Symp Quant Biol*. 2010;75:237-244.
12. Rao S, Zhen S, Roumiantsev S, et al. Differential roles of Sall4 isoforms in embryonic stem cell pluripotency. *Mol Cell Biol*. 2010;30(22):5364-5380.
13. Ruiz S, Panopoulos AD, Herrerías A, et al. A high proliferation rate is required for cell reprogramming and maintenance of human embryonic stem cell identity. *Curr Biol*. 2011;21:45-52.
14. Chan YS, Yang L, Ng HH. Transcriptional regulatory networks in embryonic stem cells. *Prog Drug Res*. 2011;67:239-252.
15. Bautch VL. Embryonic stem cell differentiation and the vascular lineage. *Methods Mol Biol*. 2002; 185:117-125.
16. Fraser ST, Ogawa M, Nishikawa S. Embryonic stem cell differentiation as a model to study hematopoietic and endothelial cell development. *Methods Mol Biol*. 2002;185:71-81.
17. Li M. Lineage selection for generation and amplification of neural precursor cells. *Methods Mol Biol*. 2002;185:205-215.
18. Wobus AM, Boheler KR, Czyz J, et al. Embryonic stem cells as a model to study cardiac, skeletal muscle, and vascular smooth muscle cell differentiation. *Methods Mol Biol*. 2002;185:127-156.
19. Pasumarthi KB, Field LJ. Cardiomyocyte enrichment in differentiating ES cell cultures: Strategies and applications. *Methods Mol Biol*. 2002;185:157-168.
20. Kassem M. Stem cells: Potential therapy for age-related diseases. *Ann N Y Acad Sci*. 2006;1067: 436-442.
21. Srivastava D, Ivey KN. Potential of stem-cell-based therapies for heart disease. *Nature*. 2006; 441(7097):1097-1099.
22. Thomson JA, Itskovitz-Eldor J, Shapiro SS, et al. Embryonic stem cell lines derived from human blastocysts. *Science*. 1998;282(5391):1145-1147.
23. Abraham S, Riggs MJ, Nelson K, et al. Characterization of human fibroblast-derived extracellular matrix components for human pluripotent stem cell propagation. *Acta Biomater*. 2010;6(12): 4622-4633.
24. Kolhar P, Kotamraju VR, Hikita ST, et al. Synthetic surfaces for human embryonic stem cell culture. *J Biotechnol*. 2010;146(3):143-146.
25. Rodin S, Domogatskaya A, Ström S, et al. Long-term self-renewal of human pluripotent stem cells on human recombinant laminin-511. *Nat Biotechnol*. 2010;28(6):611-615.
26. Xu Y, Zhua X, Hahm HS, et al. Revealing a core signaling regulatory mechanism for pluripotent stem cell survival and self-renewal by small molecules. *Proc Natl Acad Sci U S A*. 2010;107(18): 8129-8134.
27. Levenstein ME, Ludwig TE, Xu R, et al. Basic fibroblast growth factor support of human embryonic stem cell self-renewal. *Stem Cells*. 2006;24(3):568-574.
28. Ludwig TE, Bergendahl V, Levenstein ME, et al. Feeder-independent culture of human embryonic stem cells. *Nat Methods*. 2006;3(8):637-646.
29. Lensch MW, Schlaeger TM, Zon LI, et al. Teratoma formation assays with human embryonic stem cells: A rationale for one type of human-animal chimera. *Cell Stem Cell*. 2007;1(3):253-258.
30. Chan EM, Ratanasirintrawoot S, Park I, et al. Live cell imaging distinguishes bona fide human iPS cells from partially reprogrammed cells. *Nat Biotechnol*. 2009;27(11):1033-1037.
31. Takahashi K, Yamanaka S. Induction of pluripotent stem cells from mouse embryonic and adult fibroblast cultures by defined factors. *Cell*. 2006;126(4):663-676.
32. Meissner A, Wernig M, Jaenisch R. Direct reprogramming of genetically unmodified fibroblasts into pluripotent stem cells. *Nat Biotechnol*. 2007;25(10):1177-1181.

1

33. Okita K, Ichisaka T, Yamanaka S. Generation of germline-competent induced pluripotent stem cells. *Nature*. 2007;448(7151):313-317.
34. Wernig M, Meissner A, Foreman R, et al. In vitro reprogramming of fibroblasts into a pluripotent ES-cell-like state. *Nature*. 2007;448(7151):318-324.
35. Maherali N, Sridharan R, Xie W, et al. Directly reprogrammed fibroblasts show global epigenetic remodeling and widespread tissue contribution. *Cell Stem Cell*. 2007;1(1):55-70.
36. Boland MJ, Hazen JL, Nazor KL, et al. Adult mice generated from induced pluripotent stem cells. *Nature*. 2009;461(7260):91-94.
37. Kang L, Wang J, Zhang Y, et al. iPS cells can support full-term development of tetraploid blastocyst-complemented embryos. *Cell Stem Cell*. 2009;5(2):135-138.
38. Zhao XY, Li W, Lv Z, et al. iPS cells produce viable mice through tetraploid complementation. *Nature*. 2009;461(7260):86-90.
39. Warren L, Manos PD, Ahfeldt T, et al. Highly efficient reprogramming to pluripotency and directed differentiation of human cells with synthetic modified mRNA. *Cell Stem Cell*. 2010;7(5):618-630.
40. Stadtfeld M, Nagaya M, Utikal J, et al. Induced pluripotent stem cells generated without viral integration. *Science*. 2008;322(5903):945-949.
41. Okita K, Nakagawa M, Hyenjong H, et al. Generation of mouse induced pluripotent stem cells without viral vectors. *Science*. 2008;322(5903):949-953.
42. Kaji K, Norrby K, Paca A, et al. Virus-free induction of pluripotency and subsequent excision of reprogramming factors. *Nature*. 2009;458(7239):771-775.
43. Soldner F, Hockemeyer D, Beard C, et al. Parkinson's disease patient-derived induced pluripotent stem cells free of viral reprogramming factors. *Cell*. 2009;136(5):964-977.
44. Woltjen K, Michaell P, Mohseni P, et al. piggyBac transposition reprograms fibroblasts to induced pluripotent stem cells. *Nature*. 2009;458(7239):766-770.
45. Yusa K, Rad R, Takeda J, et al. Generation of transgene-free induced pluripotent mouse stem cells by the piggyBac transposon. *Nat Methods*. 2009;6(5):363-369.
46. Kim D, Kim C, Moon J, et al. Generation of human induced pluripotent stem cells by direct delivery of reprogramming proteins. *Cell Stem Cell*. 2009;4(6):472-476.
47. Jia F, Wilson KD, Sun N, et al. A nonviral minicircle vector for deriving human iPS cells. *Nat Methods*. 2010;7(3):197-199.
48. Huangfu D, Maehr R, Guo W, et al. Induction of pluripotent stem cells by defined factors is greatly improved by small-molecule compounds. *Nat Biotechnol*. 2008;26(7):795-797.
49. Huangfu D, Maehr R, Guo W, et al. Induction of pluripotent stem cells from primary human fibroblasts with only Oct4 and Sox2. *Nat Biotechnol*. 2008;26(11):1269-1275.
50. Lin T, Ambasudhan R, Yuan X, et al. A chemical platform for improved induction of human iPSCs. *Nat Methods*. 2009;6(11):805-808.
51. Silva J, Barrandon O, Nichols J, et al. Promotion of reprogramming to ground state pluripotency by signal inhibition. *PLoS Biol*. 2008;6(10):e253.
52. Takahashi K, Tanabe K, Ohnuki M, et al. Induction of pluripotent stem cells from adult human fibroblasts by defined factors. *Cell*. 2007;131(5):861-872.
53. Yu J, Vodyanik MA, Smuga-Otto K, et al. Induced pluripotent stem cell lines derived from human somatic cells. *Science*. 2007;318(5858):1917-1920.
54. Dimos JT, Rodolfa KT, Niakan KK, et al. Induced pluripotent stem cells generated from patients with ALS can be differentiated into motor neurons. *Science*. 2008;321(5893):1218-1221.
55. Ebert AD, Yu J, Rose FF, et al. Induced pluripotent stem cells from a spinal muscular atrophy patient. *Nature*. 2009;457(7227):277-280.
56. Park IH, Arora N, Huo H, et al. Disease-specific induced pluripotent stem cells. *Cell*. 2008;134(5):877-886.
57. Raya A, Rodríguez-Pizà I, Guenechea G, et al. Disease-corrected haematopoietic progenitors from Fanconi anaemia induced pluripotent stem cells. *Nature*. 2009;460(7251):53-59.
58. Tateishi K, He J, Taranova O, et al. Generation of insulin-secreting islet-like clusters from human skin fibroblasts. *J Biol Chem*. 2008;283(46):31601-31607.
59. Choi KD, Yu J, Smuga-Otto K, et al. Hematopoietic and endothelial differentiation of human induced pluripotent stem cells. *Stem Cells*. 2009;27(3):559-567.
60. Taura D, Sone M, Homma K, et al. Induction and isolation of vascular cells from human induced pluripotent stem cells–brief report. *Arterioscler Thromb Vasc Biol*. 2009;29(7):1100-1103.
61. Tanaka T, Tohyama S, Murata M, et al. In vitro pharmacologic testing using human induced pluripotent stem cell-derived cardiomyocytes. *Biochem Biophys Res Commun*. 2009;385(4):497-502.
62. Zhang J, Wilson GF, Soerens AG, et al. Functional cardiomyocytes derived from human induced pluripotent stem cells. *Circ Res*. 2009;104(4):e30-41.
63. Karumbayaram S, Novitch BG, Patterson M, et al. Directed differentiation of human-induced pluripotent stem cells generates active motor neurons. *Stem Cells*. 2009;27(4):806-811.
64. Wernig M, Zhao JP, Pruszak J, et al. Neurons derived from reprogrammed fibroblasts functionally integrate into the fetal brain and improve symptoms of rats with Parkinson's disease. *Proc Natl Acad Sci U S A*. 2008;105(15):5856-5861.
65. Buchholz DE, Hikita ST, Rowland TJ, et al. Derivation of functional retinal pigmented epithelium from induced pluripotent stem cells. *Stem Cells*. 2009;27(10):2427-2434.
66. Hirami Y, Osakada F, Takahashi K, et al. Generation of retinal cells from mouse and human induced pluripotent stem cells. *Neurosci Lett*. 2009;458(3):126-131.
67. Osakada F, Jin Z, Hirami Y, et al. In vitro differentiation of retinal cells from human pluripotent stem cells by small-molecule induction. *J Cell Sci*. 2009;122(Pt 17):3169-3179.

68. Yamanaka S, Blau HM. Nuclear reprogramming to a pluripotent state by three approaches. *Nature*. 2010;465(7299):704-712.
69. Hochedlinger K, Jaenisch R. Nuclear reprogramming and pluripotency. *Nature*. 2006;441(7097): 1061-1067.
70. Jouneau A, Renard JP. Reprogramming in nuclear transfer. *Curr Opin Genet Dev*. 2003;13(5): 486-491.
71. Armstrong L, Lako M, Dean W, et al. Epigenetic modification is central to genome reprogramming in somatic cell nuclear transfer. *Stem Cells*. 2006;24(4):805-814.
72. Cowan CA, Atienza J, Melton DA, et al. Nuclear reprogramming of somatic cells after fusion with human embryonic stem cells. *Science*. 2005;309(5739):1369-1373.
73. Davidson RL, Ephrussi B, Yamamoto K. Regulation of pigment synthesis in mammalian cells, as studied by somatic hybridization. *Proc Natl Acad Sci U S A*. 1966;56(5):1437-1440.
74. Tada M, Takahama Y, Abe K, et al. Nuclear reprogramming of somatic cells by in vitro hybridization with ES cells. *Curr Biol*. 2001;11(19):1553-1558.
75. Damon LE. Mobilization of hematopoietic stem cells into the peripheral blood. *Expert Rev Hematol*. 2009;2(6):717-733.
76. Greenbaum AM, Link DC. Mechanisms of G-CSF-mediated hematopoietic stem and progenitor mobilization. *Leukemia*. 2011;25:211-217.
77. Gruh I, Martin U. Transdifferentiation of stem cells: A critical view. *Adv Biochem Eng Biotechnol*. 2009;114:73-106.
78. Grove JE, Bruscia E, Krause DS. Plasticity of bone marrow-derived stem cells. *Stem Cells*. 2004; 22(4):487-500.
79. Kassmer SH, Krause DS. Detection of bone marrow-derived lung epithelial cells. *Exp Hematol*. 2010;38(7):564-573.
80. Pelacho B, Aranguren XL, Mazo M, et al. Plasticity and cardiovascular applications of multipotent adult progenitor cells. *Nat Clin Pract Cardiovasc Med*. 2007;4(Suppl 1):S15-S20.
81. Ross JJ, Verfaillie CM. Evaluation of neural plasticity in adult stem cells. *Philos Trans R Soc Lond B Biol Sci*. 2008;363(1489):199-205.
82. Anderson DJ, Gage FH, Weissman IL. Can stem cells cross lineage boundaries? *Nat Med*. 2001; 7(4):393-395.
83. Bjornson CR, Rietze RL, Reynolds BA, et al. Turning brain into blood: A hematopoietic fate adopted by adult neural stem cells in vivo. *Science*. 1999;283(5401):534-537.
84. Wang X, Lub Y, Zhang H, et al. Distinct efficacy of pre-differentiated versus intact fetal mesencephalon-derived human neural progenitor cells in alleviating rat model of Parkinson's disease. *Int J Dev Neurosci*. 2004;22(4):175-183.
85. Vassilopoulos G, Wang PR, Russell DW. Transplanted bone marrow regenerates liver by cell fusion. *Nature*. 2003;422(6934):901-904.
86. Rizvi AZ, Swain JR, Davies PS, et al. Bone marrow-derived cells fuse with normal and transformed intestinal stem cells. *Proc Natl Acad Sci U S A*. 2006;103(16):6321-6325.
87. Willenbring H, Bailey AS, Foster M, et al. Myelomonocytic cells are sufficient for therapeutic cell fusion in liver. *Nat Med*. 2004;10(7):744-748.
88. Wagers AJ, Sherwood RI, Christensen JL, et al. Little evidence for developmental plasticity of adult hematopoietic stem cells. *Science*. 2002;297(5590):2256-2259.
89. Zhou Q, Brown J, Kanarek A, et al. In vivo reprogramming of adult pancreatic exocrine cells to beta-cells. *Nature*. 2008;455(7213):627-632.
90. Vierbuchen T, Ostermeier A, Pang ZP, et al. Direct conversion of fibroblasts to functional neurons by defined factors. *Nature*. 2010;463(7284):1035-1041.
91. Ieda M, Fu J, Delgado-Olguin P, et al. Direct reprogramming of fibroblasts into functional cardio-myocytes by defined factors. *Cell*. 2010;142(3):375-386.
92. Szabo E, Rampalli S, Risueño RM, et al. Direct conversion of human fibroblasts to multilineage blood progenitors. *Nature*. 2010;468(7323):521-526.
93. Hwang WS, Ryu YJ, Park JH, et al. Evidence of a pluripotent human embryonic stem cell line derived from a cloned blastocyst. *Science*. 2004;303(5664):1669-1674.
94. Alleman BW, Luger T, Reisinger HS, et al. Medical tourism services available to residents of the United States. *J Gen Intern Med*. 2011;27:492-497.
95. Hyun I. Allowing innovative stem cell-based therapies outside of clinical trials: Ethical and policy challenges. *J Law Med Ethics*. 2010;38(2):277-285.
96. Lindvall O, Hyun I. Medical innovation versus stem cell tourism. *Science*. 2009;324(5935): 1664-1665.

CHAPTER 2

Current Issues in the Pathogenesis, Diagnosis, and Treatment of Neonatal Thrombocytopenia

Matthew A. Saxonhouse, MD, and Martha C. Sola-Visner, MD

- ● **Platelet Production in Neonates**
- ● **Neonatal Platelet Function**
- ● **Approach to the Neonate With Thrombocytopenia**
- ● **Treatment/Management of Neonatal Thrombocytopenia**

Evaluation and management of thrombocytopenic neonates present frequent challenges for neonatologists, because 22% to 35% of infants admitted to the neonatal intensive care unit (NICU) are affected by thrombocytopenia at some point during their hospital stay.[1] In 2.5% to 5% of all NICU admissions, thrombocytopenia is severe, which is defined as a platelet count lower than 50×10^9.[2,3] These patients are usually treated with platelet transfusions in an attempt to diminish the occurrence, or severity, of hemorrhage. However, considerable debate continues on what constitutes an "at risk" platelet count, particularly because a number of other variables (e.g., gestational age, mechanism of thrombocytopenia, platelet function) may significantly influence bleeding risk. In the absence of randomized trials to address this question, we have only limited data available to guide treatment decisions in this population. In this chapter, we will review current concepts on normal and abnormal neonatal thrombopoiesis and current methods of evaluating platelet production and function. We then will provide a step-wise approach to evaluation of the thrombocytopenic neonate, and finally will review current controversies regarding neonatal platelet transfusions and the potential use of thrombopoietic growth factors.

Platelet Production in Neonates

Platelet production can be schematically represented as consisting of four main steps (Fig. 2-1). The first is a thrombopoietic stimulus that drives the production of megakaryocytes and, ultimately, platelets. Although various cytokines (e.g., interleukin [IL]-3, IL-6, IL-11, granulocyte-macrophage colony-stimulating factor [GM-CSF]) contribute to this process, thrombopoietin (Tpo) is now widely recognized as the most potent known stimulator of platelet production.[4] Tpo promotes the next two steps in thrombopoiesis: the proliferation of megakaryocyte progenitors (the cells that multiply and give rise to megakaryocytes), and the maturation of the megakaryocytes, which is characterized by a progressive increase in nuclear ploidy and cytoplasmic maturity that leads to the generation of large polyploid (8 N to 64 N) megakaryocytes.[4,5] Through a poorly understood process, these mature megakaryocytes then generate and release new platelets into the circulation.

Although the general steps in platelet production are similar in neonates and adults, important developmental differences need to be considered when neonates with platelet disorders are evaluated. Whereas plasma Tpo concentrations are higher in normal neonates than in healthy adults, neonates with thrombocytopenia generally have lower Tpo concentrations than adults with a similar degree and mechanism of thrombocytopenia.[6-8] Megakaryocyte progenitors from neonates have a higher

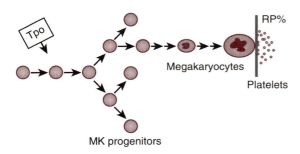

Figure 2-1 Schematic representation of neonatal megakaryocytopoiesis. Tpo acts by promoting the proliferation of megakaryocyte progenitors and the maturation of megakaryocytes. Through a poorly understood process, mature megakaryocytes release new platelets into the circulation. These new platelets represent the reticulated platelet percentage. *MK,* megakaryocyte; *RP%,* reticulated platelet percentage; *Tpo,* thrombopoietin. (Adapted from Sola MC. Fetal megakaryocytopoiesis. In: Christensen RD [ed]. *Hematologic Problems of the Neonate.* Philadelphia: WB Saunders; 2000:43–59, with permission.)

proliferative potential than those from adults and give rise to significantly larger megakaryocyte colonies when cultured in vitro.[6,9,10] Neonatal megakaryocyte progenitors are also more sensitive to Tpo than adult progenitors both in vitro and in vivo, and are present in the bone marrow and in peripheral blood (unlike adult progenitors, which reside almost exclusively in the bone marrow).[4,10,11] Finally, neonatal megakaryocytes are smaller and of lower ploidy than adult megakaryocytes.[12-17] Despite their low ploidy and small size, however, neonatal megakaryocytes have a high degree of cytoplasmic maturity and can generate platelets at very low ploidy levels. Indeed, we have recently shown that 2 N and 4 N neonatal megakaryocytes are *cytoplasmically more mature* than adult megakaryocytes of similarly low ploidy levels, challenging the paradigm that neonatal megakaryocytes are immature. At the molecular level, the rapid cytoplasmic maturation of neonatal megakaryocytes is associated with high levels of the transcription factor GATA-1 (globin transcription factor) and upregulated Tpo signaling through the mammalian target of rapamycin (mTOR) pathway.[18] Because smaller megakaryocytes produce fewer platelets than are produced by larger megakaryocytes,[19] it has been postulated that neonates maintain normal platelet counts on the basis of the increased proliferative rates of their progenitors.

An important but unanswered question involves how these developmental differences impact the ability of neonates to respond to thrombocytopenia, particularly secondary to increased platelet consumption. Specifically, it was unknown whether neonates could increase the number and/or size of their megakaryocytes, as adult patients with platelet consumptive disorders do. Finding the answer to this question has been challenging, mostly because of the limited availability of bone marrow specimens from living neonates, the rarity of megakaryocytes in the fetal marrow, the fragility of these cells, and the inability to accurately differentiate small megakaryocytes from cells of other lineages. A study using immunohistochemistry and image analysis tools to evaluate megakaryocytes in neonatal bone marrow biopsies suggested that thrombocytopenic neonates do not increase the size of their megakaryocytes.[17] In fact, most thrombocytopenic neonates evaluated in this study had a lower megakaryocyte mass than their nonthrombocytopenic counterparts. These findings were confirmed in a subsequent study using a mouse model of neonatal immune thrombocytopenia, in which thrombocytopenia of similar severity was generated in fetal and adult mice.[20] Taken together, these studies suggest that the small size of neonatal megakaryocytes represents a developmental limitation in the ability of neonates to upregulate platelet production in response to increased demand, which might contribute to the predisposition of neonates to develop severe and prolonged thrombocytopenia.

Because bone marrow studies in neonates remain technically difficult (particularly in those born prematurely), significant efforts have been aimed at developing blood tests to evaluate platelet production that would be suitable for neonates. Among these tests, Tpo concentrations,[6-8,21] circulating megakaryocyte progenitors,[6,22,23] and reticulated platelet percentages (RP%)[24-27] have been used. As shown in Figure 2-1, circulating Tpo concentrations are a measure of the thrombopoietic stimulus. Because serum Tpo levels are a reflection of both the level of Tpo production and the availability of Tpo receptor (on progenitor cells, mega-karyocytes, and platelets), elevated Tpo levels in the presence of thrombocytopenia usually indicate an inflammatory condition leading to upregulated gene expression (e.g., during infection)[28] or a hyporegenerative thrombocytopenia characterized by decreased megakaryocyte mass (such as congenital amegakaryocytic thrombo-cytopenia). Several investigators have published Tpo concentrations in healthy neonates of different gestational and postconceptional ages, and in neonates with thrombocytopenia of different causes.[6-8,29-33] Although Tpo measurements are not yet routinely available in the clinical setting, serum Tpo concentrations can provide useful information in the diagnostic evaluation of a neonate with severe thrombocytopenia.

As previously stated, megakaryocyte progenitors (the precursors for mega-karyocytes) are present both in the blood and in the bone marrow of neonates. Several investigators have attempted to measure the concentration of circulating progenitors as an indirect marker of marrow megakaryocytopoiesis, although the correlation between blood and marrow progenitors has not been clearly estab-lished.[6,22,23] The concentration of circulating megakaryocyte progenitors decreases in normal neonates with increasing postconceptional age, possibly owing to the migration of megakaryocyte progenitors from the liver to the bone marrow.[23] When applied to thrombocytopenic neonates, Murray and associates showed that preterm neonates with early-onset thrombocytopenia (secondary to placental insufficiency in most cases) had decreased concentrations of circulating megakaryocyte progeni-tors compared with their nonthrombocytopenic counterparts.[22] The number of progenitors increased during the period of platelet recovery, indicating that the thrombocytopenia observed in these neonates occurred after platelet production was decreased. It is unlikely, however, that this relatively labor-intensive test (which requires culturing of megakaryocyte progenitors for 10 days) will ever be applicable in the clinical setting.

A test that recently became available to clinicians for the evaluation of neonatal thrombocytopenia is the immature platelet fraction (IPF), which is the clinical equivalent of the reticulated platelet percentage (RP%). Reticulated platelets, or "immature platelets," are newly released platelets (<24 hours old) that contain residual RNA, which permits their detection and quantification in blood.[34-37] Unlike the RP test, which requires flow cytometry, IPF can be measured as part of the complete cell count with a standard hematologic cell counter (Sysmex 2100 XE Hematology Analyzer, Kobe, Japan), which is now available in the clinical hematol-ogy laboratories at several medical centers. In adults and children, the RP% and the IPF have been evaluated as a way of classifying thrombocytopenia kinetically, similar to the way the reticulocyte count is used to evaluate anemia, so that a low IPF would signify diminished platelet production, and an elevated IPF would signify increased platelet production. Two recent studies have shown the usefulness of the IPF in evaluating mechanisms of thrombocytopenia and in predicting platelet recovery in neonates.[38,39]

Although none of these tests has been adequately validated through concomi-tant bone marrow or platelet kinetics studies in neonates, studies in adults and children indicate that the application of several tests in combination can help dif-ferentiate between disorders of increased platelet destruction and those of decreased production, and sometimes even provide important diagnostic clues.[40-44] In neo-nates, use of these tests in combination has allowed the recognition of very specific patterns of abnormal thrombopoiesis, such as ineffective platelet production in congenital human immunodeficiency virus (HIV) infection[45] and unresponsiveness to thrombopoietin in congenital amegakaryocytic thrombocytopenia.[46]

From the clinical perspective, the IPF, if available, is likely to offer useful infor-mation to guide diagnostic evaluation in neonates with severe thrombocytopenia of unclear origin. However, bone marrow studies still provide information that cannot be obtained through any indirect measure of platelet production (e.g., marrow cel-lularity, megakaryocyte morphology, evidence of hemophagocytosis) and should be performed in selected patients.[47]

2

Neonatal Platelet Function

Although platelet transfusions are routinely provided to neonates with the goal of decreasing their risk of catastrophic hemorrhage, it is known that not only platelet count but also gestational and postconceptional age, the disease process, and platelet function at that time significantly influence an infant's risk of bleeding. Emphasizing this point, a recent study demonstrated that nearly 90% of clinically significant hemorrhages among neonates with severe thrombocytopenia occurred in infants with a gestational age less than 28 weeks and during the first 2 weeks of life.[2] Therefore, assessment of platelet function and primary hemostasis is likely to offer greater insight into an infant's bleeding risk than the platelet count alone. A limitation of this approach, however, has been the lack of a simple, rapid, and reproducible technique for the measurement of neonatal platelet function.

To evaluate the contribution of platelet function to hemostasis, two different approaches have been used. The first focuses on specific platelet functions such as adhesion, activation, or aggregation; the second involves the measurement of primary hemostasis in whole blood samples. Primary hemostasis represents the summation of the effects of platelet number and function with many other circulating factors and is a more global and physiologic measure. To measure specific platelet function, many researchers have used aggregometry to assess platelet aggregation and flow cytometry to assess platelet activation. Initial platelet aggregation studies, performed using platelet-rich plasma, demonstrated that platelets from neonatal cord blood (preterm greater than term)[48] were less responsive than adult platelets to agonists such as adenosine diphosphate (ADP), epinephrine, collagen, thrombin, and thromboxane analogues (e.g., U46619).[49-54] This hyporesponsiveness of neonatal platelets to epinephrine is probably due to the presence of fewer α_2-adrenergic receptors, which are binding sites for epinephrine, on neonatal platelets.[55] The reduced response to collagen likely reflects impairment of calcium mobilization,[51,56] whereas the decreased response to thromboxane may result from differences in signaling downstream from the receptor.[48] In contrast to these findings, ristocetin-induced agglutination of neonatal platelets was enhanced compared with that in adults, likely reflecting the higher levels and activity of circulating von Willebrand factor (vWF) in neonates.[57-61] The main limitation of platelet-rich plasma aggregometry was that large volumes of blood were needed, thus limiting its application in neonatology to cord blood samples. New platelet aggregometers, however, can accommodate whole blood samples and require smaller volumes, thus opening the door to whole blood aggregometry studies in preterm neonates.[62,63]

Activated platelets undergo a series of changes in the presence or conformation of several surface proteins, which are known as *activation markers*. Using specific monoclonal antibodies and flow cytometry to detect platelet activation markers, studies of cord blood and postnatal (term and preterm) samples demonstrated decreased platelet activation in response to platelet agonists such as thrombin, ADP, and epinephrine (concordant with aggregometry studies).[51,64-67] This platelet hyporesponsiveness appears to resolve by the 10th day after birth.[68] Flow cytometry is an attractive technique for these tests because it requires very small volumes of blood (5 to 100 μL), and it allows the evaluation of both the basal status of platelet activation and the reactivity of platelets in response to various agonists. However, data on applying this technique to neonates with thrombocytopenia, sepsis, liver failure, disseminated intravascular coagulation (DIC), and other disorders are limited.[68]

The second approach to evaluating platelet function involved methods to determine whole blood primary hemostasis, a more global and physiologic measure of platelet function in the context of whole blood. Historically, bleeding time has been considered the gold standard test of primary hemostasis in vivo. Bleeding time studies performed on healthy term neonates demonstrated shorter times than those performed on adults, suggesting enhanced primary hemostasis.[69] This finding contrasts with the platelet hyporesponsiveness observed in aggregometry and flow cytometry studies. It has been suggested that the shorter bleeding times were a result of higher hematocrits,[70] higher mean corpuscular volumes,[71] higher vWF concentrations[57,72] and a predominance of longer vWF polymers in neonates.[59,61] When bleeding times were measured in preterm neonates, they were found to be overall longer than those in healthy term neonates.[73] A recent study serially evaluated bleeding times in 240 neonates of different gestational ages and observed that preterm neonates (<33 weeks' gestation) on the first day of life had longer bleeding times than term neonates, but these differences disappeared by day 10 of life.[74]

A single study attempted to determine the relationship between bleeding times and platelet counts in thrombocytopenic neonates. This study revealed prolonged bleeding times in patients with platelet counts below 100×10^9/L but no correlation between degree of thrombocytopenia and prolongation in bleeding time.[75] However, because bleeding times are highly operator dependent and existing evidence suggests that bleeding times do not correlate well with clinically evident bleeding or the likelihood of bleeding, it was unclear whether this finding was a reflection of the limitations of the test, or whether a true lack of correlation occurred.

The cone and platelet analyzer tests whole blood platelet adhesion and aggregation on an extracellular matrix–coated plate under physiologic arterial flow conditions.[76] When a modified technique was applied to healthy full-term neonatal platelets, they demonstrated more extensive adhesion properties than adult platelets, with similar aggregate formation.[60] Healthy preterm platelets had decreased platelet adhesion compared with those of term infants, but it was still greater than that seen in adults.[77,78] Adherence in preterm infants correlated with gestational age in the first 48 hours of life and did not increase with increasing postconceptional age even up to 10 weeks of life.[78] It is interesting to note that when the cone and platelet analyzer was used, septic preterm infants displayed lower adherence than healthy preterm infants, suggesting a mechanism for bleeding tendencies in this population.[77] Similarly, term neonates born to mothers with pregnancy-induced hypertension and gestational diabetes displayed poorer platelet function compared with healthy term neonates.[79] Unfortunately, the cone and platelet analyzer is not available for clinical use in most institutions, thus limiting its use to research purposes.

More recently, a highly reproducible, automated measure of primary hemostasis was developed and commercialized as a substitute for bleeding time. The platelet function analyzer (PFA-100) measures primary hemostasis by simulating in vivo quantitative measurement of platelet adhesion, activation, and aggregation. Specifically, anticoagulated blood is aspirated under high shear rates through an aperture cut into a membrane coated with collagen and either ADP or epinephrine, which mimics exposed subendothelium. Platelets are activated upon exposure to shear stress and physiologic agonists (collagen + ADP or epinephrine), adhere to the membrane, and aggregate until a stable platelet plug occludes blood flow through the aperture.[80] The time to reach occlusion is recorded by the instrument as closure time. Two closure times are measured with each instrument run: one is obtained with collagen and epinephrine, and the other with collagen and ADP.[81,82]

The PFA-100 test offers the advantages of being rapid, accurate, and reproducible, while only requiring 1.8 mL of citrated blood. Four studies applied this method to neonates and demonstrated shorter closure times in term neonates compared with adults, in concordance with previous bleeding time studies.[80,83-85] However, these studies were performed on term cord blood samples, which makes interpretation of this diagnostic test in neonates of different gestational and postconceptional ages very difficult (in the absence of reference values). To address this issue, our group recently evaluated serial closure times in blood samples obtained from a group of nonthrombocytopenic neonates of different gestational ages. We observed that both ADP and epinephrine closure times were significantly longer in neonatal samples than in cord blood samples, and that an inverse correlation was evident between ADP closure times and gestational age in samples obtained on the first 2 days of life.[86] Several recent studies have also examined the effects of common neonatal medications on neonatal closure and bleeding times. In these studies, ampicillin tended to prolong bleeding times after three or four doses, but it did not significantly affect neonatal closure times.[87] Ibuprofen, in contrast, was found to slightly prolong closure times, but it did not affect neonatal bleeding times.[88] The clinical significance of these findings remains to be determined.

Approach to the Neonate With Thrombocytopenia

The fetal platelet count reaches a level of 150×10^9/L by the end of the first trimester of pregnancy.[89] Thus, traditionally, any neonate with a platelet count lower than 150×10^9/L, regardless of gestational age (23 to 42 weeks), is defined as having thrombocytopenia. This definition was challenged by a recent large population study involving 47,291 neonates treated in a multihospital system. In this study, reference ranges for platelet counts at different gestational and postconceptional ages were determined by excluding the top and lower 5th percentiles of all platelet counts.[90] Through this approach, the lowest limit (5th percentile) of platelet counts for infants at less than 32 weeks' gestation was found to be 104×10^9/L, compared with 123×10^9/L for neonates older than 32 weeks. Although this is the largest study of platelet counts in neonates published to date, the investigators did not exclude critically ill neonates from the study; therefore, these values may be appropriate as epidemiologic "reference ranges" for neonates admitted to the NICU rather than as "normal values" for this population. An additional finding from this study was that the mean platelet counts of the most immature infants (born at 22 to 25 weeks) always remained below the mean levels measured in more mature infants. The mechanisms underlying these observations are unknown, but they are likely related to developmental differences in megakaryocytopoiesis. Nevertheless, because platelet counts in the 100 to 150×10^9/L range can be found in healthy neonates more frequently than in healthy adults, careful follow-up and expectant management in otherwise healthy-appearing neonates with transient thrombocytopenia in this range are considered acceptable, although lack of resolution or worsening should prompt further evaluation.

For practicing neonatologists, the first step in the evaluation of a thrombocytopenic neonate is to try to identify patterns that have been associated with specific illnesses. Table 2-1 lists the diagnoses most commonly reported in the literature as potential causes of neonatal thrombocytopenia, as well as their presentations. If the pattern of thrombocytopenia fits any of the listed categories, then confirmatory testing is indicated. Some overlap in these processes is obvious, as with sepsis and necrotizing enterocolitis (NEC), or birth asphyxia and DIC.

Figures 2-2 and 2-3 provide algorithms for the evaluation of a neonate with severe (platelet count $<50 \times 10^9$/L) or mild (100 to 150×10^9/L) to moderate (50 to 100×10^9/L) thrombocytopenia, respectively. In addition to severity, this approach uses time of presentation to classify the different causes of thrombocytopenia as early (onset at <72 hours of life) versus late (onset at >72 hours of life) thrombocytopenia. When severe, early thrombocytopenia occurs (see Fig. 2-2) in a term or preterm neonate, infection (usually bacterial) should be suspected and evaluated. If the neonate is well appearing and infection has been ruled out, then a careful family history and physical examination can provide critical clues to the diagnosis. For example, a prior sibling with a history of neonatal alloimmune thrombocytopenia (NAIT) strongly supports this diagnosis, prompting immediate evaluation and treatment (see next section). A family history of any form of congenital thrombocytopenia warrants further investigation in this direction (Table 2-2). The presence of physical findings of trisomy 13 (i.e., cutis aplasia, cleft lip and palate), 18 (i.e., clinodactyly, intrauterine growth retardation [IUGR], rocker-bottom feet), or 21 (i.e., macroglossia, single palmar crease, atrioventricular [AV] canal, hypotonia), or Turner syndrome (edema, growth retardation, congenital heart defects), dictates chromosomal evaluation. Decreased ability to pronate/supinate the forearm in an otherwise normal-appearing neonate could suggest congenital amegakaryocytic thrombocytopenia with proximal radioulnar synostosis.[91] The presence of hepatosplenomegaly suggests the possibility of viral infection; an abdominal mass should prompt an abdominal ultrasound to evaluate for renal vein thrombosis.

Table 2-1 SPECIFIC ILLNESSES AND PATTERNS ASSOCIATED WITH NEONATAL THROMBOCYTOPENIA

Categories	Subtypes	Differential Diagnoses (Where Applicable)	Severity	Onset
Immune	Alloimmune	Neonatal alloimmune thrombocytopenia	Severe	Early
	Autoimmune	Maternal ITP, lupus, other collagen vascular disorder	Severe to moderate	Early
Infectious	Bacterial	GBS, *Escherichia coli, Klebsiella, Serratia, Enterobacter, Haemophilus* flu, *Staphylococcus aureus, Staphylococcus epidermidis, Enterococcus*	Variable	Variable
	Viral	CMV, HSV, HIV, parvovirus, coxsackie, EBV	Variable	Usually early
	Fungal	Candida, other	Severe	Usually late
	Parasite	Toxoplasmosis	Variable	Early
Placental insufficiency		Preeclampsia, eclampsia, chronic hypertension	Mild to moderate	Early
Medication-induced*	Antibiotic		Variable	Late
	Heparin		Variable	Late
	Anticonvulsants		Variable	Late
	NSAIDs		Variable	Late
	Histamine H$_2$-receptor antagonists		Variable	Late
DIC		Asphyxia	Severe	Early
		Sepsis	Severe	Variable
		Congenital TTP (rare)	Severe	Variable
Genetic disorders†	Chromosomal	Trisomy 13, trisomy 18, trisomy 21, Turner syndrome, Jacobsen syndrome	Variable	Early
	Familial	Macrothrombocytopenias, Wiskott-Aldrich syndrome, X-linked thrombocytopenias, amegakaryocytic thrombocytopenia, TAR, Fanconi anemia,‡ Noonan syndrome	Variable	Early‡
	Metabolic	Proprionic acidemia, methylmalonic acidemia, hyperthyroidism, infant of diabetic mother	Mild-moderate	Variable
Miscellaneous	Thrombosis	RVT, line-associated thrombosis, sagittal sinus thrombosis	Moderate	Variable
	Tumor	Kasabach-Merritt, hepatic hemangioendothelioma	Moderate	Variable
	NEC		Severe-moderate	Usually late
	Polycythemia		Mild-moderate	Early
	ECMO		Variable	Variable

Adapted from Sola MC. Evaluation and treatment of severe and prolonged thrombocytopenia in neonates. In: Christensen RD (ed). *Hematopoietic Growth Factors in Neonatal Medicine.* Philadelphia: WB Saunders; 2004:1–14, with permission.

CMV, Cytomegalovirus; *DIC,* disseminated intravascular coagulation; *EBV,* Epstein-Barr virus; *ECMO,* extracorporeal membrane oxygenation; *GBS,* Guillain-Barré syndrome; *HIV,* human immunodeficiency virus; *HSV,* herpes simplex virus I and II; *ITP,* immune thrombocytopenic purpura; *NEC,* necrotizing enterocolitis; *NSAIDs,* nonsteroidal anti-inflammatory medications; *RVT,* renal vein thrombosis; *TAR,* thrombocytopenia absent-radii syndrome; *TTP,* thrombotic thrombocytopenic purpura.

*Refer to Table 2-3 for further description.

†Refer to Table 2-2 for further description.

‡Most familial thrombocytopenias are present at birth except for Fanconi anemia, which usually does not appear until childhood.

2

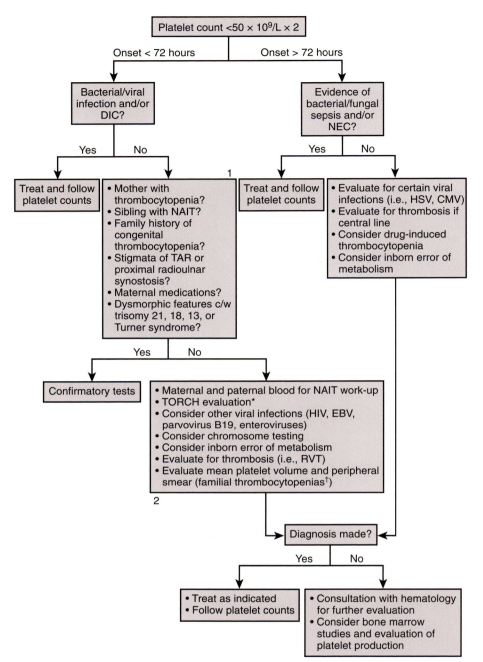

Figure 2-2 Evaluation of the neonate with severe thrombocytopenia ($<50 \times 10^9$/L) of early (<72 hours of life) versus late (>72 hours of life) onset. *DIC*, Disseminated intravascular coagulation; *EBV*, Epstein-Barr virus; *ITP*, immune thrombocytopenic purpura; *NAIT*, neonatal alloimmune thrombocytopenia; *NEC*, necrotizing enterocolitis; *RVT*, renal vein thrombosis; *TAR*, thrombocytopenia absent-radii syndrome. *TORCH evaluation consisting of diagnostic work-up for toxoplasmosis, rubella, cytomegalovirus (CMV), herpes simplex virus (HSV), and syphilis. **Refer to Table 2-2 for a listing of disorders.

In the absence of any obvious diagnostic clues, the most likely cause of thrombocytopenia in an otherwise well-appearing infant is immune (allo- or auto-) thrombocytopenia caused by the passage of antiplatelet antibodies from the mother to the fetus. If the antiplatelet antibody work-up is negative, then a more detailed evaluation is indicated. This should consist of TORCH (toxoplasmosis, rubella,

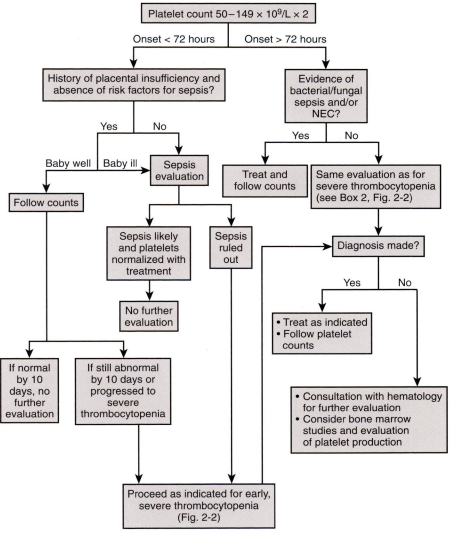

Figure 2-3 Evaluation of the neonate with mild to moderate thrombocytopenia (50 to 149 × 10⁹/L) of early (<72 hours of life) versus late (>72 hours of life) onset. *NEC*, Necrotizing enterocolitis.

cytomegalovirus [CMV], herpes simplex virus [HSV], and syphilis) evaluation, including HIV testing.[45] Rarer diagnoses such as thrombosis (renal vein thrombosis, sagittal sinus thrombosis), Kasabach-Merritt syndrome, and inborn errors of metabolism (mainly propionic acidemia and methylmalonic acidemia) should be considered if clinically indicated. Thrombocytopenia in these disorders may range from severe to mild, depending on the particular presentation. It is important to recognize that some chromosomal disorders have very subtle phenotypic features, such as can be the case in the 11q terminal deletion disorder (also referred to as *Paris-Trousseau thrombocytopenia* or *Jacobsen syndrome*),[92] which has a wide range of phenotypes (including any combination of growth retardation, genitourinary anomalies, limb anomalies, mild facial anomalies, abnormal brain imaging, heart defects, and ophthalmologic problems).[92,93] Therefore, a growth-restricted neonate with no obvious reason for growth restriction or an infant with subtle dysmorphic features and thrombocytopenia warrants chromosomal analysis. Severe and persistent isolated thrombocytopenia in an otherwise normal neonate can also represent congenital amegakaryocytic thrombocytopenia. If the thrombocytopenia is part of a

Table 2-2 FAMILIAL THROMBOCYTOPENIAS, INCLUDING PLATELET SIZE, MODE OF INHERITANCE, AND ASSOCIATED PHYSICAL FINDINGS

Syndrome	Platelet Size	Mode of Inheritance	Associated Clinical Findings
Wiskott-Aldrich syndrome	Small	X-linked	Immunodeficiency, eczema
X-linked thrombocytopenia	Small	X-linked	None
Congenital amegakaryocytic thrombocytopenia	Normal	AR	None
Congenital amegakaryocytic thrombocytopenia and radioulnar synostosis	Normal	AR	Restricted forearm pronation, proximal radioulnar synostosis in forearm X-ray
Fanconi anemia	Normal	AR	Hypopigmented and hyperpigmented skin lesions, urinary tract abnormalities, microcephaly, upper extremity radial-side abnormalities involving the thumb, pancytopenia (rarely present in the neonatal period)
Chromosome 10/THC2*	Normal	AD	None
Thrombocytopenia and absent radii	Normal	AR	Shortened/absent radii bilaterally, normal thumbs, ulnar and hand abnormalities, abnormalities of the humerus, cardiac defects (TOF, ASD, VSD), eosinophilia, leukemoid reaction
May-Hegglin anomaly	Large/giant	AD	Neutrophilic inclusions
Fechtner syndrome	Large/giant	AD	Sensorineural hearing loss, cataracts, nephritis, neutrophilic inclusions
Epstein syndrome	Large/giant	AD	Sensorineural hearing loss, nephritis
Sebastian syndrome	Large/giant	AD	Neutrophilic inclusions
Mediterranean thrombocytopenia	Large/giant	AD	None
Bernard-Soulier syndrome	Large/giant	AR	None
GATA-1 mutation	Large/giant or normal	X-linked	Anemia, genitourinary abnormalities (cryptorchidism)
Gray platelet syndrome	Large/giant	AD	None
11q terminal deletion disorder (Jacobsen syndrome)	Large/giant	AD	Congenital heart defects, genitourinary abnormalities, growth retardation, mild facial anomalies, limb anomalies, abnormal brain imaging

Adapted from Drachman JG. Inherited thrombocytopenia: When a low platelet count does not mean ITP. *Blood.* 2004;13:390–398, with permission.

AD, Autosomal dominant; *AR,* autosomal recessive; *ASD,* atrial septal defect; *TOF,* tetralogy of Fallot; *VSD,* ventricular septal defect.

*Mild to moderate thrombocytopenia associated with genetic linkage to the short arm of chromosome 10, 10p11-12.

pancytopenia, osteopetrosis and other bone marrow failure syndromes should be considered.

When a neonate presents with severe thrombocytopenia after 72 hours of life (see Fig. 2-2), prompt evaluation and treatment for bacterial/fungal sepsis and/or NEC must be initiated. If all cultures are negative and there is no clinical evidence of NEC, but the platelet count is still severely low, then the evaluation must be expanded. Appropriate testing should include evaluations for (1) DIC and liver

Table 2-3   MEDICATIONS FREQUENTLY USED IN NEONATES THAT MAY CAUSE THROMBOCYTOPENIA*

Medication Class	Examples
Antibiotics	Penicillin and derivatives Ciprofloxacin Cephalosporin Metronidazole Vancomycin Rifampin
Nonsteroidals	Indomethacin
Anticoagulants	Heparin
Histamine H_2-receptor antagonists	Famotidine, cimetidine
Anticonvulsants	Phenobarbital, phenytoin

*Most of the medications listed have been reported to cause neonatal thrombocytopenia in isolated case reports.[99-106]

dysfunction; (2) certain viral infections (i.e., HSV, CMV, Epstein-Barr virus [EBV]); (3) thrombosis, especially with a history of a central line; (4) drug-induced thrombocytopenia (Table 2-3)[94-101]; (5) inborn errors of metabolism; and (6) Fanconi anemia (rare).[102,103]

The presentation of mild to moderate thrombocytopenia (see Fig. 2-3) within the first 72 hours of life in a well-appearing preterm infant without risk factors for infection and with a maternal history of preeclampsia or chronic hypertension is most likely related to placental insufficiency.[7,22] If the platelet count normalizes within 10 days, no further evaluation is necessary. However, if thrombocytopenia becomes severe or the platelet count does not return to normal, further evaluation (especially for infection or immune thrombocytopenia) is required. Mild to moderate thrombocytopenia within the first 72 hours of life in an ill-appearing term or preterm neonate warrants an immediate evaluation for sepsis. If sepsis is ruled out, the evaluation should be very similar to the one described for early, severe thrombocytopenia in a nonseptic neonate (see Fig. 2-2). If thrombocytopenia is persistent, the differential diagnosis should be expanded to include familial thrombocytopenias, which frequently (but not always) are in the mild to moderate range. Many familial thrombocytopenias can be identified on the basis of platelet size, mode of inheritance, and associated clinical findings (see Table 2-2). Platelet size can be evaluated by using the mean platelet volume (MPV; normal, 7 to 11 fL),[93] which frequently is reported on routine complete blood counts, or by reviewing the blood smear and looking for large or small platelets. For example, the May-Hegglin anomaly, Fechtner syndrome, and Epstein syndrome present with large platelets (MPV >11 fL),[93] as well as with other associated clinical findings that may be identified during the neonatal period.[93] In contrast, Wiskott-Aldrich syndrome and X-linked thrombocytopenia present with abnormally small platelets (MPV <7 fL).[93] Certain physical findings on examination may provide key diagnostic clues as to the underlying diagnosis (see Table 2-2). The inability to supinate/pronate the forearm may be a sign of congenital amegakaryocytic thrombocytopenia with proximal radioulnar synostosis, which can be easily confirmed by forearm X-rays.[91]

If the presentation of thrombocytopenia occurs at greater than 72 hours of life, the most likely diagnosis is bacterial or fungal sepsis with or without NEC. Late-onset thrombocytopenia associated with sepsis has been reported to occur in 6% of all admissions to the NICU in some institutions.[104] However, if these are ruled out, then an approach similar to that outlined for late-onset severe thrombocytopenia should be followed (see Fig. 2-2).

In neonates with thrombocytopenia of unclear origin, identifying the responsible mechanisms (increased destruction, decreased production, sequestration, or a combination) may aid in narrowing the differential diagnosis. Neonatal alloimmune and autoimmune thrombocytopenias are examples of increased destruction, whereas infants born to mothers with placental insufficiency, or who have inherited bone marrow failure syndromes, are examples of decreased platelet production. The exact mechanism remains unknown for a large percentage of neonates with thrombocytopenia. In adults, bone marrow studies and radiolabeled platelet survival studies provide a thorough mechanistic evaluation. Unfortunately, these studies are cumbersome and technically difficult in neonates. For this reason, use of the tests described in the first section may prove to be of particular value in the evaluation of neonates with thrombocytopenia of unknown origin.

Treatment/Management of Neonatal Thrombocytopenia

Despite the frequency of thrombocytopenia in the NICU, and the severity of its potential consequences, only one prospective, randomized trial has evaluated different thresholds for platelet transfusions in neonates. In this study, performed by Andrew and associates in 1993,[105] thrombocytopenic premature infants were randomly assigned to maintain a platelet count greater than 150×10^9/L at all times, or to receive platelet transfusions only for clinical indications or for a platelet count lower than 50×10^9/L. Overall, these investigators found no differences in the frequency or severity of intracranial hemorrhages between the two groups, suggesting that nonbleeding premature infants with platelet counts greater than 50×10^9/L did not benefit from prophylactic platelet transfusions. Because this study included neonates with a platelet count greater than 50×10^9/L, it remained unclear whether lower platelet counts could be safely tolerated in otherwise stable neonates. To answer this question, Murray and colleagues[104] performed a retrospective review on their use of platelet transfusions among neonates with platelet counts lower than 50×10^9/L ($n = 53$ of 901 admissions over a 3-year period). They reported that 51% of these neonates (27/53) received at least one platelet transfusion (all infants with a platelet count lower than 30×10^9/L, and those with platelet counts between 30 and 50×10^9/L who had a previous hemorrhage or were clinically unstable). No major hemorrhages were observed in this group of severely thrombocytopenic neonates, indicating that a prophylactic platelet transfusion trigger threshold of less than 30×10^9/L probably represents safe practice for clinically stable intensive care unit (ICU) patients.[104] As the authors themselves recognized, however, this was a relatively small retrospective study that should be interpreted with caution.

In the absence of high-quality evidence to guide our transfusion decisions, numerous experts and consensus groups have published guidelines for the administration of platelet transfusions to neonates. The most recent guidelines are summarized in Table 2-4, although it is important to recognize that these represent only educated opinions based on limited existing evidence. This lack of evidence is clearly reflected in the variability of neonatal platelet transfusion practices worldwide, as exposed by recent papers describing platelet transfusion usage in different NICUs.[104-108] Three recent reports have retrospectively documented platelet transfusion practice in NICUs from the United States, the United Kingdom, and Mexico.[104,106,107] In summary, these reports highlighted that approximately 2% to 9% of neonates admitted to the NICU receive at least one platelet transfusion, that most platelet transfusions are given to nonbleeding patients with platelet counts lower than 50×10^9/L, and that more than 50% of neonates who receive a transfusion will receive more than one. A recent survey of neonatal platelet transfusion practices among neonatologists in the United States further confirmed the extraordinary variability in neonatal platelet transfusion thresholds used by clinicians in this country.[109]

Although the threshold for platelet transfusions remains controversial, there is better agreement on the desired characteristics of transfused platelets. Experts agree that neonates should receive 10 to 15 mL/kg of a CMV-safe standard platelet suspension, derived from a random donor platelet unit (whole blood–derived) or from a plateletpheresis unit. Regardless of the source, a dose of 10 to 15 mL/kg should

Table 2-4 SUMMARY OF RECENT GUIDELINES FOR PLATELET TRANSFUSIONS IN TERM AND PRETERM NEONATES (PLATELET COUNTS × 10^9/L)

Author	Nonbleeding Sick Preterm	Nonbleeding Stable Preterm	Nonbleeding Term	Before Invasive Procedure	Active Bleeding
Blanchette et al, 1991	<100	<50	<20	<50 if failure of production <100 if DIC	<50 if failure of production <100 if DIC
Blanchette et al, 1995	<50	<30	<20 if stable <30 if sick	<50 for minor procedure <100 for major surgery	<50 in all cases <100 if DIC Any platelet count if functional disorder
Roberts et al, 1999	<50 if DIC <100 if falling rapidly	<50	<30	<100	<100 if major organ bleeding <50 if minor bleeding
Calhoun et al, 2000	<50	<25	Same as preterm	<50	Not addressed
Strauss, 2000	<100	<20	<20	<50	<100
Murray et al, 2002	<50	<30	<30	<50	<100
Roseff et al, 2002	<100	<50	<30	<50 if failure of production <100 if DIC	<50 if stable <100 if sick
Gibson et al, 2004*	<30	<20	Same as preterm	Not addressed	<50
Strauss, 2008	Maintain >50 to >100 if unstable	<20	Not addressed	<50	<50
Roberts and Murray, 2008	<50	<30	Not addressed	Not addressed	<100

Reproduced from Poterjoy B, Josephson C: Platelets, frozen plasma, and cryoprecipitate: What is the clinical evidence for their use in the neonatal intensive care unit? *Semin Perinatol.* 2009;33:1.
  DIC, Disseminated intravascular coagulation.
  *Guidelines from the British Committee for Standards in Haematology Transfusion Task Force.

provide enough platelets to increase the blood platelet count to greater than 100 × 10^9/L. Volume reduction is not routinely recommended. The use of more than one random donor platelet unit in a transfusion is discouraged because this increases the number of donor exposures without conferring benefit.

Because of concerns of CMV infection, most institutions transfuse infants with blood products obtained from donors without detectable antibodies to CMV.[110] However, the incidence of CMV infection following transfusion with CMV-negative platelets is still 1% to 4% owing to an intrinsic false-negative rate of the test for antibody to CMV, a low antibody titer, or transient viremia quenching the circulating antibody.[111-113] A major limitation of the use of CMV-negative blood is that less than 50% of the blood donor population is CMV antibody negative. An alternative to CMV-negative blood is leukocyte reduction, although whether this offers comparable safety is controversial.[114-118]

Another concern involves transfusion-associated graft-versus-host disease (TA-GVHD), which is caused by contaminating T lymphocytes in platelet concentrates. TA-GVHD presents between 8 and 10 days after a transfusion and is characterized by rash, diarrhea, elevated hepatic transaminases, hyperbilirubinemia, and pancytopenia. TA-GVHD is also characterized by an extremely high mortality rate (>90%).

Exposure of platelets to 2500 cGy of gamma irradiation before transfusion effectively prevents GVHD; irradiated cellular products are definitely indicated in cases of suspected or confirmed underlying immunodeficiency (e.g., DiGeorge syndrome, Wiskott-Aldrich syndrome), intrauterine or exchange transfusions, or blood transfusions from a first- or second-degree relative or a human leukocyte antigen (HLA)-matched donor.[119] However, because an underlying primary immunodeficiency disorder may not be apparent in the neonatal period, many institutions choose to irradiate all cellular blood products administered to neonates.

When a full-term, well-appearing neonate presents at birth with severe thrombocytopenia, a diagnosis of NAIT must be considered. NAIT is caused by fetomaternal mismatch for human platelet alloantigens; the pathogenesis resembles that of erythroblastosis fetalis. Platelets exhibit a large number of antigens on their membranes, including ABO, HLA antigens, and platelet-specific antigens, referred to as *human platelet antigens (HPAs)*. If incompatibility between parental platelet antigens exists, the mother can become sensitized to an antigen expressed on the fetal platelets. These maternal antibodies then may cross the placenta, bind to fetal platelets, and induce platelet removal by the reticuloendothelial system, resulting in severe thrombocytopenia as early as 24 weeks' gestation.[120] Intracranial hemorrhage has been reported in 10% to 15% of cases of NAIT[121]; it is therefore important to provide effective therapy as soon as possible. A recent large study evaluating HPA-specific antibodies showed that in approximately 31% of cases in which NAIT was suspected, a specific antiplatelet antibody was identified.[122] In these cases, maternal HPA-1 (previously known as PLA-1) alloimmunization accounted for most cases (79%),[122] but many other specific platelet alloantigens have been implicated in the pathogenesis of NAIT and should be considered, particularly when maternal serum is shown to react with paternal platelets.[122-127]

The treatment of neonates with NAIT depends on whether the diagnosis is suspected or known prenatally. If the diagnosis is clinically suspected (i.e., first affected pregnancy), **random donor platelet transfusions are now considered the first line of therapy,** based on recent data demonstrating that a large proportion of infants with NAIT respond to random donor platelet transfusions.[128] If the patient is clinically stable and does not have evidence of an intracranial hemorrhage, platelets are usually given when the platelet count is lower than 30×10^9/L, although this is arbitrary. If the patient shows evidence of an intracranial hemorrhage, the goal is to maintain a platelet count greater than 100×10^9/L, although this can be challenging in neonates with NAIT. In addition to platelets, if the diagnosis of NAIT is confirmed or is strongly suspected, intravenous immune globulin (IVIG) (1 g/kg/day for up to 2 consecutive days) may be infused to increase the patient's own platelets and potentially to protect the transfused platelets.[129] Because in NAIT, the platelet count usually falls after birth, IVIG can also be infused when the platelet count is between 30 and 50×10^9/L to try to prevent a further drop.

The blood bank should be alerted immediately about any infant with suspected NAIT. Some of these infants will fail to respond to random donor platelets and IVIG,[128] and arrangements should be made to secure as soon as possible a source of antigen-negative platelets (either from HPA-1b1b and 5a5a donors, which should be compatible in >90% of cases, or from the mother) for the "nonresponders." If maternal platelets are used, these should be concentrated to minimize the amount of maternal plasma, which contains antiplatelet antibodies. Maternal plasma can also be eliminated by washing the platelets, although this procedure has been shown to cause significant damage to the platelets.[130] In some European countries, HPA-1b1b and 5a5a platelets are maintained in the blood bank inventory and are immediately available for use. In those cases, they are preferable to random donor platelets and/or IVIG and should be the first line of therapy. Methylprednisolone (1 mg/kg twice a day for 3 to 5 days) has been used in individual case reports and small series, but should be considered only if the infant does not respond to random platelets and IVIG, and if antigen-matched platelets are not readily available. Some experts recommend intravenous methylprednisolone at a low dose (1 mg every 8 hours) on the days that IVIG is given.[130]

When a neonate is born to a mother who had a previous pregnancy affected by confirmed NAIT, genotypically matched platelets (e.g., HPA-1b1b platelets in case of a mother with known anti–HPA-1a antibodies) should be available in the blood bank at the time of delivery and should be the first line of therapy if the infant is thrombocytopenic. In addition, mothers who delivered an infant with NAIT should be followed in high-risk obstetrics clinics during all future pregnancies and should receive prenatal treatment to reduce the incidence and severity of fetal/neonatal thrombocytopenia in subsequent pregnancies. The intensity of prenatal treatment will be based on the severity of thrombocytopenia and on the presence or absence of intracranial hemorrhage (ICH) in the previously affected fetus. This is particularly important in assessing the risk of ICH in the current pregnancy and in minimizing this risk. Current recommendations involve maternal treatment with IVIG (1 to 2 g/kg/wk) with or without steroids, starting at 12 or at 20 to 26 weeks' gestation, depending on whether the previously affected fetus suffered an ICH, and if so, at what time during pregnancy.[130]

Because of the risks associated with blood products, the potential use of thrombopoietic growth factors has been explored as an appealing therapeutic alternative for thrombocytopenia. IL-3, IL-6, IL-11, stem cell factor (SCF), and thrombopoietin (Tpo) all support megakaryocyte development in vitro and have been touted for their preclinical thrombopoietic activity, but have led to limited platelet recovery or excessive toxicity in the adult patient care setting.[131] No trials have so far been conducted in neonates.

Recombinant IL-11 was the first thrombopoietic growth factor to be approved by the Food and Drug Administration (FDA) for the prevention of severe thrombocytopenia after myelosuppressive chemotherapy for nonmyeloid malignancies,[132] although significant side effects such as fluid retention and atrial arrhythmias may limit its use.[133,134] Reports of experimental benefits for NEC[135,136] and sepsis[137] in animal models have made the thought of using this cytokine in neonates somewhat appealing. However, safety and efficacy in neonates have never been investigated, and its use should be restricted to well-controlled clinical trials.

The cloning of Tpo (the most potent known stimulator of platelet production) led to a flurry of studies that quickly progressed from bench research to clinical trials. Unfortunately, a few of the subjects treated with a truncated form of recombinant Tpo (PEG-rHMGDG) developed neutralizing antibodies against endogenous Tpo, resulting in severe thrombocytopenia and aplastic anemia.[138] This led pharmaceutical companies to discontinue all clinical trials involving Tpo. As an alternative, much interest was devoted to the development of Tpo-mimetic molecules. Most of these are small molecules that have no molecular homology to Tpo but bind to the Tpo receptor and have biologically comparable effects. In 2008, the FDA approved the use of two novel Tpo receptor agonists—romiplostim (AMG-531, Nplate) and eltrombopag (SB497115, Promacta)—for the treatment of adults with chronic immune thrombocytopenic purpura (ITP) not responsive to standard treatment. Although initially restricted to second-line treatment of ITP in adult patients, it is anticipated that both agents will become part of the treatment for other thrombocytopenic disorders and/or other patient populations. In neonates, these agents offer the opportunity to decrease platelet transfusions and potentially improve the outcomes of neonates with severe and prolonged thrombocytopenia. Neonates may be suitable candidates for treatment with Tpo-mimetics for two reasons: (1) neonates have developmental limitations in their ability to increase platelet production, and perhaps Tpo concentrations, in response to increased platelet demand; and (2) neonatal megakaryocyte progenitors are more sensitive to Tpo than adult progenitors, suggesting that doses lower than those used in adults might be sufficient to achieve the desired response.

The use of Tpo-mimetic agents in neonatal care in the future will require careful consideration of several developmental issues. First, we need to identify the subgroup of thrombocytopenic neonates who are most likely to benefit from such therapy. We know that after administration of Tpo-mimetics, platelet counts start to rise about 4 to 6 days after the initiation of therapy, peak at around 10 to 14 days, and return to baseline by 21 to 28 days. Therefore, infants who are likely to continue to require platelet transfusions for a period longer than 10 to 14 days would be appropriate candidates for treatment. Given that approximately 80% of cases of severe thrombocytopenia in the NICU resolve within 14 days,[104] this would constitute only a minority of thrombocytopenic neonates. Unfortunately, no good clinical markers currently allow us to predict the duration of thrombocytopenia in affected infants, with the exception of the association between liver disease and prolonged neonatal thrombocytopenia as described in two studies.[106,107] Because liver is the main site of Tpo production, infants with severe liver disease and thrombocytopenia might be attractive candidates. However, caution is needed in this subgroup of patients because portal vein thrombosis has been reported in adults with thrombocytopenia due to HCV-related cirrhosis treated with romiplostim.[139] Along these lines, neonates who receive the largest numbers of platelet transfusions ("very high users," >20 platelet transfusions) most frequently have thrombocytopenia due to extracorporeal membrane oxygenation (ECMO), sepsis, or NEC[140]—all conditions associated with high levels of platelet activation. In vitro studies have shown that Tpo and romiplostim, but not eltrombopag,[141] increase the degree of platelet reactivity to agonists. Thus, the theoretical potential of Tpo-mimetic agents to increase the risk of thrombosis needs to be carefully evaluated, particularly during the acute phase of clinical conditions already characterized by high levels of platelet activation.

A major consideration in the use of hematopoietic cytokines (and mimetics) in neonates is their effects on cells and tissues outside the hematopoietic system. Erythropoietin, for example, has pro-angiogenic properties on vascular cells that might explain the higher incidence of retinopathy of prematurity found in infants treated with erythropoietin during the first week of life.[142] The nonhematopoietic effects of Tpo are not yet well defined, particularly in a developing organism. Tpo and its receptor are expressed in the brain,[143] and available data indicate that Tpo might have pro-apoptotic and differentiation-blocking effects on neuronal cells.[144,145] Newer TPO mimetics, particularly eltrombopag, have a significantly lower molecular weight than endogenous Tpo, which might make these agents more likely to cross the blood–brain barrier. Thus, careful evaluation of the hematopoietic and potential nonhematopoietic effects of Tpo on the developing organism is warranted before these novel compounds are introduced into the NICU.

The use of recombinant Factor VIIa (rFVIIa), which is approved for use in severe, life-threatening bleeding episodes in patients with hemophilia A and B,[146,147] has been debated in conditions associated with thrombocytopenia. High-dose rFVIIa can shorten bleeding time in adult patients with thrombocytopenia, and recent studies have explored the use of rFVIIa in the treatment and prevention of bleeding in patients with inherited and acquired platelet function disorders.[148-150] Whether rFVIIa can improve platelet function in thrombocytopenic neonates remains to be determined. Several published case reports used rFVIIa in bleeding preterm neonates as a desperate measure, in most cases with some success.[151-154] However, until the results of further well-designed randomized clinical trials on the physiology of rFVIIa and its effects on neonates become available, its use should be reserved for select circumstances.

In conclusion, although most cases of neonatal thrombocytopenia are mild to moderate and do not warrant aggressive treatment, this condition constitutes a significant problem in the NICU and may be the presenting sign of a serious diagnosis. Recent studies indicate that neonates may have a relative inability to increase platelet production when faced with thrombocytopenia. Novel indirect tests of thrombopoiesis, such as the IPF, are currently available, and it is likely that their increasing use in neonates will lead to a better understanding of the pathophysiology of the different varieties of thrombocytopenia. In addition, application of the PFA-100 to neonates may eventually provide a better screening mechanism for evaluating platelet function, thus allowing neonatologists to determine an infant's risk of bleeding when faced with a low platelet count. Platelet transfusions remain the only current treatment for thrombocytopenia, but no solid evidence is available to guide our decisions regarding when to administer transfusions. Well-designed randomized controlled trials are required to determine what constitutes a safe platelet count and to better balance the risks of significant hemorrhage versus additional donor exposure in individual situations.

References

1. Sola-Visner M, Saxonhouse MA, Brown RE. Neonatal thrombocytopenia: What we do and don't know. *Early Hum Dev.* 2008;84:499-506.
2. Stanworth SJ, Clarke P, Watts T, et al. Prospective, observational study of outcomes in neonates with severe thrombocytopenia. *Pediatrics.* 2009;124:e826-834.
3. Baer VL, Lambert DK, Henry E, et al. Severe thrombocytopenia in the NICU. *Pediatrics.* 2009;124:e1095-e1100.
4. Kaushansky K, Broudy VC, Lin N, et al. Thrombopoietin, the mpl ligand, is essential for full megakaryocyte development. *Proc Natl Acad Sci U S A.* 1995;92:3234-3238.
5. Kaushansky K. Thrombopoietin: The primary regulator of platelet production. *Blood.* 1995;86:419-431.
6. Murray NA, Watts TL, Roberts IA. Endogenous thrombopoietin levels and effect of recombinant human thrombopoietin on megakaryocyte precursors in term and preterm babies. *Pediatr Res.* 1998;43:148-151.
7. Sola MC, Calhoun DA, Hutson AD, et al. Plasma thrombopoietin concentrations in thrombocytopenic and non-thrombocytopenic patients in a neonatal intensive care unit. *Br J Haematol.* 1999;104:90-92.
8. Sola MC, Juul SE, Meng YG, et al. Thrombopoietin (tpo) in the fetus and neonate: Tpo concentrations in preterm and term neonates, and organ distribution of tpo and its receptor (c-mpl) during human fetal development. *Early Hum Dev.* 1999;53:239-250.
9. Nishihira H, Toyoda Y, Miyazaki H, et al. Growth of macroscopic human megakaryocyte colonies from cord blood in culture with recombinant human thrombopoietin (c-mpl ligand) and the effects of gestational age on frequency of colonies. *Br J Haematol.* 1996;92:23-28.
10. Sola MC, Du Y, Hutson AD, et al. Dose-response relationship of megakaryocyte progenitors from the bone marrow of thrombocytopenic and non-thrombocytopenic neonates to recombinant thrombopoietin. *Br J Haematol.* 2000;110:449-453.
11. Sola MC, Christensen RD, Hutson AD, et al. Pharmacokinetics, pharmacodynamics, and safety of administering pegylated recombinant megakaryocyte growth and development factor to newborn rhesus monkeys. *Pediatr Res.* 2000;47:208-214.
12. de Alarcon PA, Graeve JL. Analysis of megakaryocyte ploidy in fetal bone marrow biopsies using a new adaptation of the feulgen technique to measure DNA content and estimate megakaryocyte ploidy from biopsy specimens. *Pediatr Res.* 1996;39:166-170.
13. Hegyi E, Nakazawa M, Debili N, et al. Developmental changes in human megakaryocyte ploidy. *Exp Hematol.* 1991;19:87-94.
14. Levine RF, Olson TA, Shoff PK, et al. Mature micromegakaryocytes: An unusual developmental pattern in term infants. *Br J Haematol.* 1996;94:391-399.
15. Ma DC, Sun YH, Chang KZ, et al. Developmental change of megakaryocyte maturation and DNA ploidy in human fetus. *Eur J Haematol.* 1996;57:121-127.
16. Olson TA, Levine RF, Mazur EM, et al. Megakaryocytes and megakaryocyte progenitors in human cord blood. *Am J Pediatr Hematol Oncol.* 1992;14:241-247.
17. Sola-Visner MC, Christensen RD, Hutson AD, et al. Megakaryocyte size and concentration in the bone marrow of thrombocytopenic and nonthrombocytopenic neonates. *Pediatr Res.* 2007;61:479-484.
18. Liu ZJ, Italiano J, Jr, Ferrer-Marin F, et al. Developmental differences in megakaryocytopoiesis are associated with up-regulated tpo signaling through mtor and elevated gata-1 levels in neonatal megakaryocytes. *Blood* 2011;117:4106-4117.
19. Mattia G, Vulcano F, Milazzo L, et al. Different ploidy levels of megakaryocytes generated from peripheral or cord blood cd34+ cells are correlated with different levels of platelet release. *Blood.* 2002;99:888-897.
20. Hu Z, Slayton WB, Rimsza LM, et al. Differences between newborn and adult mice in their response to immune thrombocytopenia. *Neonatology.* 2010;98:100-108.
21. Emmons RV, Reid DM, Cohen RL, et al. Human thrombopoietin levels are high when thrombocytopenia is due to megakaryocyte deficiency and low when due to increased platelet destruction. *Blood.* 1996;87:4068-4071.
22. Murray NA, Roberts IA. Circulating megakaryocytes and their progenitors in early thrombocytopenia in preterm neonates. *Pediatr Res.* 1996;40:112-119.
23. Saxonhouse MA, Christensen RD, Walker DM, et al. The concentration of circulating megakaryocyte progenitors in preterm neonates is a function of post-conceptional age. *Early Hum Dev.* 2004;78:119-124.
24. Joseph MA, Adams D, Maragos J, et al. Flow cytometry of neonatal platelet RNA. *J Pediatr Hematol Oncol.* 1996;18:277-281.
25. Kienast J, Schmitz G. Flow cytometric analysis of thiazole orange uptake by platelets: A diagnostic aid in the evaluation of thrombocytopenic disorders. *Blood.* 1990;75:116-121.
26. Peterec SM, Brennan SA, Rinder HM, et al. Reticulated platelet values in normal and thrombocytopenic neonates. *J Pediatr.* 1996;129:269-274.

27. Saxonhouse MA, Sola MC, Pastos KM, et al. Reticulated platelet percentages in term and preterm neonates. *J Pediatr Hematol Oncol*. 2004;26:797-802.
28. Kaser A, Brandacher G, Steurer W, et al. Interleukin-6 stimulates thrombopoiesis through thrombopoietin: Role in inflammatory thrombocytosis. *Blood*. 2001;98:2720-2725.
29. Dame C. Thrombopoietin in thrombocytopenias of childhood. *Semin Thromb Hemost*. 2001;27:215-228.
30. Dame C. Developmental biology of thrombopoietin in the human fetus and neonate. *Acta Paediatr Suppl*. 2002;91:54-65.
31. Dame C, Cremer M, Ballmaier M, et al. Concentrations of thrombopoietin and interleukin-11 in the umbilical cord blood of patients with fetal alloimmune thrombocytopenia. *Am J Perinatol*. 2001;18:335-344.
32. Dame C, Sutor AH. Primary and secondary thrombocytosis in childhood. *Br J Haematol*. 2005;129:165-177.
33. Sola MC, Dame C, Christensen RD. Toward a rational use of recombinant thrombopoietin in the neonatal intensive care unit. *J Pediatr Hematol Oncol*. 2001;23:179-184.
34. Ault KA, Rinder HM, Mitchell J, et al. The significance of platelets with increased RNA content (reticulated platelets). A measure of the rate of thrombopoiesis. *Am J Clin Pathol*. 1992;98:637-646.
35. Bonan JL, Rinder HM, Smith BR. Determination of the percentage of thiazole orange (to)-positive, "reticulated" platelets using autologous erythrocyte to fluorescence as an internal standard. *Cytometry*. 1993;14:690-694.
36. Matic GB, Chapman ES, Zaiss M, et al. Whole blood analysis of reticulated platelets: Improvements of detection and assay stability. *Cytometry*. 1998;34:229-234.
37. Richards EM, Baglin TP. Quantitation of reticulated platelets: Methodology and clinical application. *Br J Haematol*. 1995;91:445-451.
38. Cremer M, Paetzold J, Schmalisch G, et al. Immature platelet fraction as novel laboratory parameter predicting the course of neonatal thrombocytopenia. *Brit J Haematol*. 2009;144:619-621.
39. Cremer M, Weimann A, Schmalisch G, et al. Immature platelet values indicate impaired megakaryopoietic activity in neonatal early-onset thrombocytopenia. *Thromb Haemost*. 2010;103:1016-1021.
40. Fabris F, Cordiano I, Steffan A, et al. Indirect study of thrombopoiesis (tpo, reticulated platelets, glycocalicin) in patients with hereditary macrothrombocytopenia. *Eur J Haematol*. 2000;64:151-156.
41. Robinson M, Machin S, Mackie I, et al. Comparison of glycocalicin, thrombopoietin and reticulated platelet measurement as markers of platelet turnover in HIV+ samples. *Platelets*. 2001;12:108-113.
42. van den Oudenrijn S, Bruin M, Folman CC, et al. Three parameters, plasma thrombopoietin levels, plasma glycocalicin levels and megakaryocyte culture, distinguish between different causes of congenital thrombocytopenia. *Br J Haematol*. 2002;117:390-398.
43. Koike Y, Yoneyama A, Shirai J, et al. Evaluation of thrombopoiesis in thrombocytopenic disorders by simultaneous measurement of reticulated platelets of whole blood and serum thrombopoietin concentrations. *Thromb Haemost*. 1998;79:1106-1110.
44. Kurata Y, Hayashi S, Kiyoi T, et al. Diagnostic value of tests for reticulated platelets, plasma glycocalicin, and thrombopoietin levels for discriminating between hyperdestructive and hypoplastic thrombocytopenia. *Am J Clin Pathol*. 2001;115:656-664.
45. Tighe P, Rimsza LM, Christensen RD, et al. Severe thrombocytopenia in a neonate with congenital HIV infection. *J Pediatr*. 2005;146:408-413.
46. Sola MC, Rimsza LM. Mechanisms underlying thrombocytopenia in the neonatal intensive care unit. *Acta Paediatr Suppl*. 2002;91:66-73.
47. Sola MC, Rimsza LM, Christensen RD. A bone marrow biopsy technique suitable for use in neonates. *Br J Haematol*. 1999;107:458-460.
48. Israels SJ, Odaibo FS, Robertson C, et al. Deficient thromboxane synthesis and response in platelets from premature infants. *Pediatr Res*. 1997;41:218-223.
49. Corby DG, O'Barr TP. Neonatal platelet function: A membrane-related phenomenon? *Haemostasis*. 1981;10:177-185.
50. Corby DG, Schulman I. The effects of antenatal drug administration on aggregation of platelets of newborn infants. *J Pediatr*. 1971;79:307-313.
51. Israels SJ, Daniels M, McMillan EM. Deficient collagen-induced activation in the newborn platelet. *Pediatr Res*. 1990;27:337-343.
52. Louden KA, Broughton Pipkin F, Heptinstall S, et al. Neonatal platelet reactivity and serum thromboxane b2 production in whole blood: The effect of maternal low dose aspirin. *Br J Obstet Gynaecol*. 1994;101:203-208.
53. Mull MM, Hathaway WE. Altered platelet function in newborns. *Pediatr Res*. 1970;4:229-237.
54. Ts'ao CH, Green D, Schultz K. Function and ultrastructure of platelets of neonates: Enhanced ristocetin aggregation of neonatal platelets. *Br J Haematol*. 1976;32:225-233.
55. Corby DG, O'Barr TP. Decreased alpha-adrenergic receptors in newborn platelets: Cause of abnormal response to epinephrine. *Dev Pharmacol Ther*. 1981;2:215-225.
56. Gelman B, Setty BN, Chen D, et al. Impaired mobilization of intracellular calcium in neonatal platelets. *Pediatr Res*. 1996;39:692-696.

57. Andrew M, Paes B, Milner R, et al. Development of the human coagulation system in the healthy premature infant. *Blood*. 1988;72:1651-1657.

58. Andrew M, Paes B, Milner R, et al. Development of the human coagulation system in the full-term infant. *Blood*. 1987;70:165-172.

59. Katz JA, Moake JL, McPherson PD, et al. Relationship between human development and disappearance of unusually large von Willebrand factor multimers from plasma. *Blood*. 1989;73:1851-1858.

60. Shenkman B, Linder N, Savion N, et al. Increased neonatal platelet deposition on subendothelium under flow conditions: The role of plasma von Willebrand factor. *Pediatr Res*. 1999;45:270-275.

61. Weinstein MJ, Blanchard R, Moake JL, et al. Fetal and neonatal von Willebrand factor (vWF) is unusually large and similar to the vwf in patients with thrombotic thrombocytopenic purpura. *Br J Haematol*. 1989;72:68-72.

62. Watala C, Golanski J, Rozalski M, et al. Is platelet aggregation a more important contributor than platelet adhesion to the overall platelet-related primary haemostasis measured by pfa-100? *Thromb Res*. 2003;109:299-306.

63. Ferrer-Marin F, Chavda C, Lampa M, et al. Effects of in-vitro adult platelet transfusions on neonatal hemostasis. *J Thromb Haemost*. 2011;9:1020-1028.

64. Pietrucha T, Wojciechowski T, Greger J, et al. Differentiated reactivity of whole blood neonatal platelets to various agonists. *Platelets*. 2001;12:99-107.

65. Rajasekhar D, Barnard MR, Bednarek FJ, et al. Platelet hyporeactivity in very low birth weight neonates. *Thromb Haemost*. 1997;77:1002-1007.

66. Rajasekhar D, Kestin AS, Bednarek FJ, et al. Neonatal platelets are less reactive than adult platelets to physiological agonists in whole blood. *Thromb Haemost*. 1994;72:957-963.

67. Sitaru AG, Holzhauer S, Speer CP, et al. Neonatal platelets from cord blood and peripheral blood. *Platelets*. 2005;16:203-210.

68. Gatti L, Guarneri D, Caccamo ML, et al. Platelet activation in newborns detected by flow-cytometry. *Biol Neonate*. 1996;70:322-327.

69. Andrew M, Paes B, Bowker J, et al. Evaluation of an automated bleeding time device in the newborn. *Am J Hematol*. 1990;35:275-277.

70. Fernandez F, Goudable C, Sie P, et al. Low haematocrit and prolonged bleeding time in uraemic patients: Effect of red cell transfusions. *Br J Haematol*. 1985;59:139-148.

71. Aarts PA, Bolhuis PA, Sakariassen KS, et al. Red blood cell size is important for adherence of blood platelets to artery subendothelium. *Blood*. 1983;62:214-217.

72. Andrew M, Paes B, Johnston M. Development of the hemostatic system in the neonate and young infant. *Am J Pediatr Hematol Oncol*. 1990;12:95-104.

73. Sola MC, del Vecchio A, Edwards TJ, et al. The relationship between hematocrit and bleeding time in very low birth weight infants during the first week of life. *J Perinatol*. 2001;21:368-371.

74. Del Vecchio A, Latini G, Henry E, et al. Template bleeding times of 240 neonates born at 24 to 41 weeks gestation. *J Perinatol*. 2008;28:427-431.

75. Andrew M, Castle V, Saigal S, et al. Clinical impact of neonatal thrombocytopenia. *J Pediatr*. 1987;110:457-464.

76. Varon D, Dardik R, Shenkman B, et al. A new method for quantitative analysis of whole blood platelet interaction with extracellular matrix under flow conditions. *Thromb Res*. 1997;85:283-294.

77. Finkelstein Y, Shenkman B, Sirota L, et al. Whole blood platelet deposition on extracellular matrix under flow conditions in preterm neonatal sepsis. *Eur J Pediatr*. 2002;161:270-274.

78. Linder N, Shenkman B, Levin E, et al. Deposition of whole blood platelets on extracellular matrix under flow conditions in preterm infants. *Arch Dis Child Fetal Neonatal Ed*. 2002;86:F127-F130.

79. Strauss T, Maayan-Metzger A, Simchen MJ, et al. Impaired platelet function in neonates born to mothers with diabetes or hypertension during pregnancy. *Klin Padiatr*. 2010;222:154-157.

80. Roschitz B, Sudi K, Kostenberger M, et al. Shorter PFA-100 closure times in neonates than in adults: Role of red cells, white cells, platelets and von Willebrand factor. *Acta Paediatr*. 2001;90:664-670.

81. Mammen EF, Alshameeri RS, Comp PC. Preliminary data from a field trial of the PFA-100 system. *Semin Thromb Hemost*. 1995;21(Suppl 2):113-121.

82. Kundu SK, Heilmann EJ, Sio R, et al. Description of an in vitro platelet function analyzer—PFA-100. *Semin Thromb Hemost*. 1995;21(Suppl 2):106-112.

83. Carcao MD, Blanchette VS, Dean JA, et al. The platelet function analyzer (PFA-100): A novel in-vitro system for evaluation of primary haemostasis in children. *Br J Haematol*. 1998;101:70-73.

84. Boudewijns M, Raes M, Peeters V, et al. Evaluation of platelet function on cord blood in 80 healthy term neonates using the platelet function analyser (PFA-100); shorter in vitro bleeding times in neonates than adults. *Eur J Pediatr*. 2003;162:212-213.

85. Israels SJ, Cheang T, McMillan-Ward EM, et al. Evaluation of primary hemostasis in neonates with a new in vitro platelet function analyzer. *J Pediatr*. 2001;138:116-119.

86. Saxonhouse MA, Garner R, Mammel L, et al. Closure times measured by the platelet function analyzer pfa-100 are longer in neonatal blood compared to cord blood samples. *Neonatology*. 2010;97:242-249.

87. Sheffield MJ, Lambert DK, Henry E, et al. Effect of ampicillin on the bleeding time of neonatal intensive care unit patients. *J Perinatol*. 2011;30:527-530.

88. Sheffield MJ, Schmutz N, Lambert DK, et al. Ibuprofen lysine administration to neonates with a patent ductus arteriosus: Effect on platelet plug formation assessed by in vivo and in vitro measurements. *J Perinatol*. 2009;29:39-43.

89. Pahal GS, Jauniaux E, Kinnon C, et al. Normal development of human fetal hematopoiesis between eight and seventeen weeks' gestation. *Am J Obstet Gynecol*. 2000;183:1029-1034.

90. Wiedmeier SE, Henry E, Sola-Visner MC, et al. Platelet reference ranges for neonates, defined using data from over 47,000 patients in a multihospital healthcare system. *J Perinatol*. 2009;29: 130-136.

91. Sola MC, Slayton WB, Rimsza LM, et al. A neonate with severe thrombocytopenia and radio-ulnar synostosis. *J Perinatol*. 2004;24:528-530.

92. Grossfeld PD, Mattina T, Lai Z, et al. The 11q terminal deletion disorder: A prospective study of 110 cases. *American journal of medical genetics*. 2004;129A:51-61.

93. Drachman JG. Inherited thrombocytopenia: When a low platelet count does not mean ITP. *Blood*. 2004;103:390-398.

94. Aranda JV, Portuguez-Malavasi A, Collinge JM, et al. Epidemiology of adverse drug reactions in the newborn. *Dev Pharmacol Ther*. 1982;5:173-184.

95. Aster RH. Drug-induced immune cytopenias. *Toxicology*. 2005;209:149-153.

96. Dlott JS, Danielson CF, Blue-Hnidy DE, et al. Drug-induced thrombotic thrombocytopenic purpura/hemolytic uremic syndrome: A concise review. *Ther Apher Dial*. 2004;8:102-111.

97. Kumar P, Hoppensteadt DA, Prechel MM, et al. Prevalence of heparin-dependent platelet-activating antibodies in preterm newborns after exposure to unfractionated heparin. *Clin Appl Thromb Hemost*. 2004;10:335-339.

98. Nguyen TN, Gal P, Ransom JL, et al. Lepirudin use in a neonate with heparin-induced thrombocytopenia. *Ann Pharmacother*. 2003;37:229-233.

99. Pedersen-Bjergaard U, Andersen M, Hansen PB. Drug-specific characteristics of thrombocytopenia caused by non-cytotoxic drugs. *Eur J Clin Pharmacol*. 1998;54:701-706.

100. Schmugge M, Risch L, Huber AR, et al. Heparin-induced thrombocytopenia-associated thrombosis in pediatric intensive care patients. *Pediatrics*. 2002;109:E10.

101. Spadone D, Clark F, James E, et al. Heparin-induced thrombocytopenia in the newborn. *J Vasc Surg*. 1992;15:306-311; discussion 11-2.

102. Butturini A, Gale RP, Verlander PC, et al. Hematologic abnormalities in Fanconi anemia: An international Fanconi anemia registry study. *Blood*. 1994;84:1650-1655.

103. Landmann E, Bluetters-Sawatzki R, Schindler D, et al. Fanconi anemia in a neonate with pancytopenia. *J Pediatr*. 2004;145:125-127.

104. Murray NA, Howarth LJ, McCloy MP, et al. Platelet transfusion in the management of severe thrombocytopenia in neonatal intensive care unit patients. *Transfus Med*. 2002;12:35-41.

105. Andrew M, Vegh P, Caco C, et al. A randomized, controlled trial of platelet transfusions in thrombocytopenic premature infants. *J Pediatr*. 1993;123:285-291.

106. Del Vecchio A, Sola MC, Theriaque DW, et al. Platelet transfusions in the neonatal intensive care unit: Factors predicting which patients will require multiple transfusions. *Transfusion*. 2001;41: 803-808.

107. Garcia MG, Duenas E, Sola MC, et al. Epidemiologic and outcome studies of patients who received platelet transfusions in the neonatal intensive care unit. *J Perinatol*. 2001;21:415-420.

108. Gibson BE, Todd A, Roberts I, et al. Transfusion guidelines for neonates and older children. *Br J Haematol*. 2004;124:433-453.

109. Josephson CD, Su LL, Christensen RD, et al. Platelet transfusion practices among neonatologists in the United States and Canada: Results of a survey. *Pediatrics*. 2009;123:278-285.

110. Strauss RG, Levy GJ, Sotelo-Avila C, et al. National survey of neonatal transfusion practices: Ii. Blood component therapy. *Pediatrics*. 1993;91:530-536.

111. Lang DJ EP, Rodgers BM, Boggess HP, et al. Reduction of postperfusion cytomegalovirus-infections following the use of leukocyte-depleted blood. *Transfusion*. 1977;17:391-395.

112. Miller WJ, McCullough J, Balfour HH Jr, et al. Prevention of cytomegalovirus infection following bone marrow transplantation: A randomized trial of blood product screening. *Bone Marrow Transplant*. 1991;7:227-234.

113. Strauss RG. Blood banking and transfusion issues in perinatal medicine. In: Christensen R, ed. *Hematologic problems of the neonate*. Philadelphia: W.B. Saunders; 2000:405-425.

114. Blajchman MA, Goldman M, Freedman JJ, et al. Proceedings of a consensus conference: Prevention of post-transfusion cmv in the era of universal leukoreduction. *Transfus Med Rev*. 2001;15: 1-20.

115. Eisenfeld L, Silver H, McLaughlin J, et al. Prevention of transfusion-associated cytomegalovirus infection in neonatal patients by the removal of white cells from blood. *Transfusion*. 1992;32: 205-209.

116. Gilbert GL, Hayes K, Hudson IL, et al. Prevention of transfusion-acquired cytomegalovirus infection in infants by blood filtration to remove leucocytes. Neonatal cytomegalovirus infection study group. *Lancet*. 1989;1:1228-1231.

117. Strauss RG. Selection of white cell-reduced blood components for transfusions during early infancy. *Transfusion*. 1993;33:352-357.

118. Zwicky C, Tissot JD, Mazouni ZT, et al. [Prevention of post-transfusion cytomegalovirus infection: Recommendations for clinical practice]. *Schweiz Med Wochenschr*. 1999;129:1061-1066.

119. Strauss RG. Data-driven blood banking practices for neonatal RBC transfusions. *Transfusion*. 2000;40:1528-1540.

2

120. Bussel JB. Fetal neonatal thrombocytopenia. *Thromb Haemost*. 1995;74:426-428.
121. Blanchette VS. Neonatal alloimmune thrombocytopenia: A clinical perspective. *Curr Stud Hematol Blood Transfus*. 1988:112-126.
122. Davoren A, Curtis BR, Aster RH, et al. Human platelet antigen-specific alloantibodies implicated in 1162 cases of neonatal alloimmune thrombocytopenia. *Transfusion*. 2004;44:1220-1225.
123. Ertel K, Al-Tawil M, Santoso S, et al. Relevance of the hpa-15 (gov) polymorphism on cd109 in alloimmune thrombocytopenic syndromes. *Transfusion*. 2005;45:366-373.
124. Kaplan C. Immune thrombocytopenia in the foetus and the newborn: Diagnosis and therapy. *Transfus Clin Biol*. 2001;8:311-314.
125. Kroll H, Yates J, Santoso S. Immunization against a low-frequency human platelet alloantigen in fetal alloimmune thrombocytopenia is not a single event: Characterization by the combined use of reference DNA and novel allele-specific cell lines expressing recombinant antigens. *Transfusion*. 2005;45:353-358.
126. Mandelbaum M, Koren D, Eichelberger B, et al. Frequencies of maternal platelet alloantibodies and autoantibodies in suspected fetal/neonatal alloimmune thrombocytopenia, with emphasis on human platelet antigen-15 alloimmunization. *Vox Sang*. 2005;89:39-43.
127. Peterson JA, Balthazor SM, Curtis BR, et al. Maternal alloimmunization against the rare platelet-specific antigen hpa-9b (max a) is an important cause of neonatal alloimmune thrombocytopenia. *Transfusion*. 2005;45:1487-1495.
128. Kiefel V, Bassler D, Kroll H, et al. Antigen-positive platelet transfusion in neonatal alloimmune thrombocytopenia (NAIT). *Blood*. 2006;107:3761-3763.
129. Mueller-Eckhardt C, Kiefel V, Grubert A. High-dose IgG treatment for neonatal alloimmune thrombocytopenia. *Blood*. 1989;59:145-146.
130. Bussel JB, Sola-Visner M. Current approaches to the evaluation and management of the fetus and neonate with immune thrombocytopenia. *Semin Perinatol*. 2009;33:35-42.
131. Kurzrock R. Thrombopoietic factors in chronic bone marrow failure states: The platelet problem revisited. *Clin Cancer Res*. 2005;11:1361-1367.
132. Isaacs C, Robert NJ, Bailey FA, et al. Randomized placebo-controlled study of recombinant human interleukin-11 to prevent chemotherapy-induced thrombocytopenia in patients with breast cancer receiving dose-intensive cyclophosphamide and doxorubicin. *J Clin Oncol*. 1997;15:3368-3377.
133. Bussel JB, Mukherjee R, Stone AJ. A pilot study of rhuil-11 treatment of refractory itp. *Am J Hematol*. 2001;66:172-177.
134. Smith JW 2nd. Tolerability and side-effect profile of rhil-11. *Oncology (Huntingt)*. 2000;14:41-47.
135. Dickinson EC, Tuncer R, Nadler EP, et al. Recombinant human interleukin-11 prevents mucosal atrophy and bowel shortening in the defunctionalized intestine. *J Pediatr Surg*. 2000;35:1079-1083.
136. Nadler EP, Stanford A, Zhang XR, et al. Intestinal cytokine gene expression in infants with acute necrotizing enterocolitis: Interleukin-11 mRNA expression inversely correlates with extent of disease. *J Pediatr Surg*. 2001;36:1122-1129.
137. Chang M, Williams A, Ishizawa L, et al. Endogenous interleukin-11 (il-11) expression is increased and prophylactic use of exogenous il-11 enhances platelet recovery and improves survival during thrombocytopenia associated with experimental group b streptococcal sepsis in neonatal rats. *Blood Cells Mol Dis*. 1996;22:57-67.
138. Li Z, Godinho FJ, Klusmann JH, et al. Developmental stage-selective effect of somatically mutated leukemogenic transcription factor gata1. *Nat Genet*. 2005;37:613-619.
139. Dultz G, Kronenberger B, Azizi A, et al. Portal vein thrombosis as complication of romiplostim treatment in a cirrhotic patient with hepatitis c-associated immune thrombocytopenic purpura. *J Hepatol*. 2011;55:229-232.
140. Dohner ML, Wiedmeier SE, Stoddard RA, et al. Very high users of platelet transfusions in the neonatal intensive care unit. *Transfusion*. 2009;49:869-872.
141. Erhardt JA, Erickson-Miller CL, Aivado M, et al. Comparative analyses of the small molecule thrombopoietin receptor agonist eltrombopag and thrombopoietin on in vitro platelet function. *Exp Hematol*. 2009;37:1030-1037.
142. Aher SM, Ohlsson A. Early versus late erythropoietin for preventing red blood cell transfusion in preterm and/or low birth weight infants. *Cochrane database of systematic reviews (Online)*. 2006;3:CD004865.
143. Dame C, Wolber EM, Freitag P, et al. Thrombopoietin gene expression in the developing human central nervous system. *Brain Res Dev Brain Res*. 2003;143:217-223.
144. Ehrenreich H, Hasselblatt M, Knerlich F, et al. A hematopoietic growth factor, thrombopoietin, has a proapoptotic role in the brain. *Proc Natl Acad Sci U S A*. 2005;102:862-867.
145. Samoylenko A, Byts N, Rajalingam K, et al. Thrombopoietin inhibits nerve growth factor-induced neuronal differentiation and ERK signalling. *Cellular Signalling*. 2008;20:154-162.
146. Lusher JM. Early treatment with recombinant factor VIIa results in greater efficacy with less product. *Eur Haematol*. 1998;63:7-10.
147. Lusher JM, Roberts HR, Davignon G, et al. A randomized, double-blind comparison of two dosage levels of recombinant factor VIIa in the treatment of joint, muscle and mucocutaneous haemorrhages in persons with haemophilia a and b, with and without inhibitors. RFVIIa study group. *Haemophilia*. 1998;4:790-798.
148. Almeida AM, Khair K, Hann I, et al. The use of recombinant factor VIIa in children with inherited platelet function disorders. *Br J Haematol*. 2003;121:477-481.

149. Kristensen J, Killander A, Hippe E, et al. Clinical experience with recombinant factor VIIa in patients with thrombocytopenia. *Haemostasis.* 1996;26(Suppl 1):159-164.
150. Laurian Y. Treatment of bleeding in patients with platelet disorders: Is there a place for recombinant factor VIIa? *Pathophysiol Haemostas Thromb.* 2002;32(Suppl 1):37-40.
151. Chuansumrit A, Nuntnarumit P, Okascharoen C, et al. The use of recombinant activated factor VII to control bleeding in a preterm infant undergoing exploratory laparotomy. *Pediatrics.* 2002;110:169-171.
152. Chuansumrit A, Visanuyothin N, Puapunwattana S, et al. Outcome of intracranial hemorrhage in infants with congenital factor VII deficiency. *J Med Assoc Thai.* 2002;85(Suppl 4):S1059-S1064.
153. Olomu N, Kulkarni R, Manco-Johnson M. Treatment of severe pulmonary hemorrhage with activated recombinant factor VII (rFVIIa) in very low birth weight infants. *J Perinatol.* 2002;22:672-674.
154. Wong WY, Huang WC, Miller R, et al. Clinical efficacy and recovery levels of recombinant FVIIa (Novoseven) in the treatment of intracranial haemorrhage in severe neonatal FVII deficiency. *Haemophilia.* 2000;6:50-54.

2

CHAPTER 3

The Role of Recombinant Leukocyte Colony-Stimulating Factors in the Neonatal Intensive Care Unit

Robert D. Christensen, MD

- Neutrophils and Host Defense
- Neutropenia in a Neonate
- Severe Chronic Neutropenia (SCN) in the Neonate
- Neonatal Neutropenia Not Categorized as Severe Chronic Neutropenia
- Other Proposed Uses for rG-CSF in the NICU
- A Consistent Approach to the Use of rG-CSF in the NICU

Neutrophils and Host Defense

Neutrophils are pivotal to antibacterial host defense.[1] People who lack neutrophils, whether by a congenital or an acquired defect, will experience a natural history that includes repeated local and systemic infections and early death.[1-3] Severe chronic neutropenia (SCN) consists of a cluster of diagnoses that bear the common feature of very low circulating neutrophil concentrations from birth.[3,4] The advent of recombinant granulocyte colony-stimulating factor (rG-CSF) dramatically improved the lives of patients with SCN, in most cases elevating their circulating neutrophil concentrations, reducing infectious illnesses, and extending their life expectancy.[5]

Rarely, patients with SCN are diagnosed as neonates, or even as patients in neonatal intensive care units.[6,7] However, most patients with SCN are not diagnosed until several months of age, after infectious episodes have prompted an investigation into immunologic deficiencies. When SCN is diagnosed in a neonate, that patient should receive the benefit of rG-CSF treatment.[1-5] Whether neonates who have other varieties of neutropenia, distinct from SCN, benefit from rG-CSF treatment is less clear. This chapter will review biologic plausibility and clinical trials aimed at testing rG-CSF treatment for neonates with neutropenia of the SCN category and for those with neutropenia of non-SCN categories. The chapter is divided into the diagnosis of neutropenia in neonates, the use of rG-CSF in neonates with SCN, and the proposed uses of rG-CSF in neonates with varieties of neutropenia distinct from SCN.

Neutropenia in a Neonate

Neutropenia can be defined statistically as a blood neutrophil concentration below the 5th percentile of the reference range population. For neonates, this definition is complicated because the reference range varies according to several situations, including gestational age, postnatal age, gender, type of delivery (vaginal delivery vs. cesarean section), and altitude (meters above sea level).[8] Figure 3-1 shows the 5th and 95th percentile limits for blood neutrophil counts during the first 72 hours after birth of term and late preterm neonates among neonates in the Intermountain Healthcare hospitals in the Western United States.[8] Reference ranges for blood

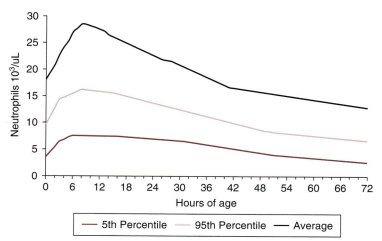

Figure 3-1 Reference range for blood neutrophil concentrations during the first 72 hours after birth of term and late-preterm neonates. A total of 12,149 values were used in this analysis. The 5th percentile, mean, and 95th percentile values are shown. (From Schmutz N, Henry E, Jopling J, et al. Expected ranges for blood neutrophil concentrations of neonates: The Manroe and Mouzinho charts revisited. *J Perinatol.* 2008;28:275–281.)

neutrophil counts at altitudes of 4000 to 5000 feet above sea level have a wider range of values than do those at sea level. This is illustrated in Figure 3-2, which shows the reference range at sea level and the range at high altitude superimposed. Dots on the graph show counts of neonates at Intermountain Healthcare hospitals who would have been judged to have an elevated neutrophil count if the sea level range was used, but who are seen to have a normal count when the appropriate reference range is used.[9] The largest altitude-dependent discrepancy is noted in the 95th percentile value. The definition of neutropenia is very similar in the sea level[10,11] and high-altitude[8,9] reference ranges (see Fig. 3-2).

A much simpler approach to defining neutropenia in a neonate is to use a neutrophil concentration less than 1000/µL, and to define *severe* neutropenia by a count less than 500/µL.[4,5] Although this approach lacks the accuracy of data-derived reference range approaches, it offers the advantages that it is easy to remember, and

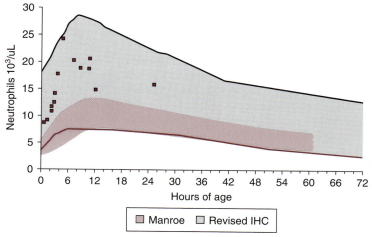

Figure 3-2 Reference range for blood neutrophil concentrations, with superimposition of the Manroe (Dallas, Tex) and Schmutz (Intermountain Healthcare) curves. The dots represent neonates in Utah who would have been regarded as having an elevated neutrophil count using the sea level (Dallas) curve, but who fell within the high-altitude (Intermountain) Schmutz curve. (From Lambert RM, Baer VL, Wiedmeier SE, et al. Isolated elevated blood neutrophil concentration at altitude does not require NICU admission if appropriate reference ranges are used. *J Perinatol.* 2009;29:822–825.)

it is in keeping with the standard definitions for neutropenia used in pediatric and adult medicine.[12] Furthermore, it is not clear whether blood neutrophil counts labeled as low by the reference range approach actually convey a host-defense deficiency, unless they are less than $1000/\mu L$.

Severe Chronic Neutropenia (SCN) in the Neonate

Kostmann Syndrome (Including Autosomal Recessive Severe Congenital Neutropenia [MIM #610738] and Autosomal Dominant Severe Congenital Neutropenia [MIM #202700])

Table 3-1 lists varieties of neutropenia that generally are considered as part of the SCN syndrome. The prototype for SCN is Kostmann syndrome, initially described in 1956 in a kindred in northern Sweden.[13-16] Patients with this variety of SCN generally have circulating neutrophil concentrations less than $200/\mu L$ and a marrow aspirate or biopsy with a "maturation arrest," where few neutrophilic cells are seen beyond the promyelocyte stage. The original family had what appeared to be an autosomal recessive disorder, but most kindreds subsequently reported seem to have an autosomal dominant inheritance. The condition is the result of mutations in the *ELA2* (neutrophil elastase) gene.[2,3,5] rG-CSF treatment is almost always effective in increasing blood neutrophil concentrations and reducing febrile illnesses; however, it does not usually correct the gingivitis that is a prominent feature of this condition in some families. This is probably because rG-CSF does not increase the natural antimicrobial peptide (LL-37) deficiency in these patients.[17,18]

Shwachman-Diamond Syndrome (MIM #260400)

This variety of severe chronic neutropenia generally is diagnosed after manifestations of exocrine pancreatic insufficiency, with diarrhea and failure to thrive. It is generally inherited as an autosomal recessive marrow failure and cancer predisposition syndrome. Patients with this condition are compound heterozygotes or homozygotes for mutations in the Shwachman-Bodian-Diamond syndrome gene at 7q11, but the molecular function of the affected protein product remains unclear.[19] Some children with this syndrome respond favorably to rG-CSF; others progress to bone marrow failure and require bone marrow transplantation.[19,20]

Barth Syndrome (MIM #302060)

These patients are usually males with dilated cardiomyopathy, organic aciduria, growth failure, muscle weakness, and neutropenia.[21] The underlying genetic abnormality involves mutations in the tafazzin gene *(TAZ)* at Xq28. G-CSF can be helpful in patients as an adjunct to treatment of infection, or as a preventive measure if the neutropenia is severe.[22,23]

Cartilage-Hair Hypoplasia (MIM #250250)

This is a form of short-limbed dwarfism mapping to 9p21-p12. The condition is associated with neutropenia and frequent infections. Patients have short pudgy hands, redundant skin, and hyperextensible joints in the hands and feet and flexor

Table 3-1 VARIETIES OF NEUTROPENIA AMONG NEONATES WHO GENERALLY ARE CONSIDERED TO HAVE SEVERE CHRONIC NEUTROPENIA

Kostmann syndrome, autosomal recessive type
Severe congenital neutropenia, autosomal dominant type
Shwachman-Diamond syndrome
Barth syndrome
Cartilage-hair hypoplasia
Cyclic neutropenia
Glycogen storage disease type 1b
Severe neonatal immune-mediated neutropenias

contractions at the elbow. Neutropenia occurs in some of these patients, who have been reported to benefit from rG-CSF administration.[24]

Cyclic Hematopoiesis (MIM #162800)

This condition is caused by mutation in the *ELA2* (neutrophil elastase) gene, mapping to 19p13.3. The disorder is characterized by regular 21-day cyclic fluctuations in the blood concentrations of neutrophils, monocytes, eosinophils, lymphocytes, platelets, and reticulocytes. Neutropenia can be severe, leading to serious infection.[2,3,5] Because it generally takes several cycles before the diagnosis is considered, most cases are not discovered during the neonatal period. rG-CSF administration is useful in preventing very low nadir neutrophil counts and in preventing infectious complications.[2,3,5]

Glycogen Storage Disease Type 1b (MIM #232220)

Von Gierke disease is an autosomal recessive disorder caused by a deficiency of the enzyme glucose-6-phosphate translocase, which transports glucose-6-phosphate into the endoplasmic reticulum for further metabolism. In glycogen storage disease type 1b (GSD-1b), glucose-6-phosphate accumulates intracellularly. Affected neonates present with hypoglycemia, hepatomegaly, growth failure, and neutropenia. Patients with GSD-1b have recurrent bacterial infections, oral ulcers, and inflammatory bowel disease. The gene causing GSD-1b is located on chromosome 11q23.[25] rG-CSF can help patients avoid the recurrent bacterial infections that are otherwise a problematic part of this condition.

Severe Immune-Mediated Neonatal Neutropenia

Most of the very severe and prolonged immune-mediated neutropenias in the neonate are alloimmune.[26-32] However, a few severe and prolonged cases of neonatal neutropenia have been found to be autoimmune neutropenia (maternal autoimmune disease), and a few have been found to be autoimmune neutropenia of infancy (a primary isolated autoimmune phenomenon in neonates).[33-36]

Alloimmune neonatal neutropenia is a relatively common condition in which the mother develops antibodies to antigens present on paternal and fetal neutrophils. Antineutrophil antibodies have been found in the serum of as many as 20% of randomly surveyed pregnant and postpartum women. Most such antibodies cause little problem for the fetus and neonate, but up to 2% of consecutively sampled neonates have neutropenia on this basis. This variety of neutropenia can be severe and prolonged, with a median duration of neutropenia of about 7 weeks, but a range of up to 6 months. Repeated infections can occur in these patients until severe neutropenia remits. Delayed separation of the umbilical cord and skin infections are the most common infectious complications, but serious and life-threatening infections can occur. The mortality rate in this condition, owing to overwhelming infection, is reported to be 5%. Severe cases have been treated successfully with rG-CSF.[29,30,33-35] Unlike in patients with other varieties of SCN, the neutropenia in this condition will remit spontaneously and the rG-CSF treatment can be stopped. Remission occurs when maternal antineutrophil antibody in the neonate has dropped significantly.

Neonatal autoimmune neutropenia occurs when mothers have autoimmune diseases, and their antineutrophil antibodies cross the placenta and bind to fetal neutrophils. Clinical features generally are much milder than in alloimmune neonatal neutropenia, and it is rare that a patient with this variety of neonatal neutropenia needs rG-CSF treatment.[30-32]

Autoimmune neutropenia of infancy is an unusual disorder in which the fetus and subsequently the neonate have a primary isolated autoimmune phenomenon.[33-35] Neutrophil-specific antibodies are found in the neonate's serum, reactive against his/her own neutrophils, but no antibodies are found in the mother's serum. Most cases occur in children between 3 and 30 months of age, with a reported incidence of 1:100,000 children. Affected children present with minor infection. Bux reported 240 cases and reported that 12% presented with severe infection, including pneumonia, sepsis, or meningitis.[34] The neutropenia in this condition persists much longer than cases of alloimmune neutropenia, with a median duration of about 30 months and a range of from 6 to 60 months. This variety of neonatal neutropenia can be severe, with blood neutrophil concentrations often less than $500/\mu L$. rG-CSF administration can increase the neutrophil count and reduce infectious complications.

Neonatal Neutropenia Not Categorized as Severe Chronic Neutropenia

(Table 3-2)

3

Pregnancy-Induced Hypertension (PIH)

Neutropenia due to PIH is the most common variety of neutropenia seen in the neonatal intensive care unit (NICU).[37-41] Perhaps 50% of neonates born to mothers with PIH have this variety of neutropenia. The ANC can be very low, frequently less than $500/\mu L$, but the count generally rises spontaneously within the first days and is almost always greater than $1000/\mu L$ by day 2 or 3. Usually no leukocyte "left shift" is seen, and no toxic granulation, Döhle bodies, or vacuolization is present in the neutrophils. It is not clear whether this variety of neutropenia predisposes neonates to acquire bacterial infection. Usually the condition is so transient that such a predisposition is unlikely. The condition probably is caused by an inhibitor of neutrophil production of placental origin that might function mechanistically by depressing natural G-CSF production.[37-39]

In a multicenter study from Brazil involving more than 900 very low birthweight (VLBW) neonates (300 born after PIH), no increase was observed in early or late neonatal sepsis in the PIH group. Logistic regression indicated that neutropenia significantly increased the odds of early-onset sepsis but not late-onset sepsis. Also, neutropenia was much more common in those who died. It was neutropenia—not PIH—that carried an association with poor outcome; PIH itself was not a risk factor for sepsis or for death.[42] Similarly, in a retrospective analysis by Teng and associates,[43] VLBW neonates with early neutropenia, generally associated with PIH, did not have increased odds of developing late-onset bacterial infection.

Several clinical trials have investigated prophylactic administration of rG-CSF to neonates with neutropenia, most of whom have neutropenia associated with PIH. Kocherlakota found a protective effect of rG-CSF administration toward early infection,[44] and Miura reported a protective effect toward late-onset infection.[45] However, in a large, multicenter, randomized, placebo-controlled trial in France ($n = 200$), rG-CSF recipients had only a transient (2-week) period of fewer infections, but did not have an overall significant improvement in infection-free survival.[46]

Neutropenia Associated With Severe Intrauterine Growth Restriction

This variety of neonatal neutropenia seems to be mechanistically identical to that associated with PIH. In a recent study, we observed no difference in onset, duration, or severity of neutropenia in small for gestational age (SGA) neonates versus neonates

Table 3-2　VARIETIES OF NEUTROPENIA AMONG NEONATES WHO ARE NOT CLASSIFIED AS HAVING SEVERE CHRONIC NEUTROPENIA

Pregnancy-induced hypertension
Severe intrauterine growth restriction
Twin-twin transfusion syndrome
Rh hemolytic disease
Bacterial infection
Fungal infection
Necrotizing enterocolitis
Chronic idiopathic neutropenia of prematurity

born after PIH.[47] Obviously, some neonates born after PIH are also SGA, and it might be true that the most severe neutropenias in this category occur among those with both PIH and SGA. We assume that the neutropenias of PIH and SGA are similar, and that both are transient with few clinical consequences and with no clear benefit of rG-CSF administration.

The Twin-Twin Transfusion Syndrome

The donor in a twin-twin transfusion is generally neutropenic; the recipient can also have neutropenia, although it is usually not as severe.[48] As with the varieties of neutropenia accompanying PIH and SGA, no leukocyte "left shift" is usually noted, nor are neutrophil morphologic abnormalities reported. This condition is transient, with the ANC generally spontaneously rising to greater than 1000/μL by 2 or 3 days; thus no rG-CSF administration is warranted.

Rh Hemolytic Disease

Neonates with anemia from Rh hemolytic disease are almost always neutropenic on the first day of life.[49] This type of neutopenia is similar to that of PIH/SGA and of donors in a twin-twin transfusion; it is likely due to reduced neutrophil production. Neutropenia is transient, generally resolving in a day or two; thus no specific treatment is required.

Bacterial Infection

Two strategies have been proposed for rG-CSF usage during neonatal infection. First, because neutropenia commonly accompanies overwhelming septic shock in neonates, rG-CSF might be a reasonable adjunct to antibiotics and intensive care treatment. Second, because neutrophil function, particularly chemotaxis, is immature among neonates, rG-CSF administration might be a reasonable way to prevent nosocomial infection among high-risk neonatal patients. Animal models for both potential uses of rG-CSF were established and supported these hypotheses. In a Cochrane review, Carr and colleagues examined both potential uses.[50] They located seven studies (involving 257 neonates) in which infected neonates were treated with rG-CSF versus placebo,[45,51-56] and three studies (359 neonates) in which rG-CSF versus placebo was used as prophylaxis against infection.[57-59] Investigators found no evidence that the addition of rG-CSF or rGM-CSF to antibiotic therapy in preterm infants with suspected systemic infection reduces immediate all-cause mortality. No significant survival advantage was seen at 14 days from the start of therapy (typical relative risk [RR], 0.71; 95% confidence interval [CI], 0.38, 1.33; typical risk difference [RD], −0.05; 95% CI, −0.14, 0.04). They conducted a subgroup analysis of 97 infants from three of the studies who, in addition to systemic infection, had a low neutrophil count (<1700/μL) at trial entry. This subgroup did show a significant reduction in mortality by day 14 (RR, 0.34; 95% CI, 0.12, 0.92; RD, −0.18; 95% CI, −0.33, −0.03; number needed to treat [NNT], 6; 95% CI, 3, 33).

The three studies on prophylaxis[57-59] did not show a significant reduction in mortality among neonates receiving rGM-CSF (RR, 0.59; 95% CI, 0.24,1.44; RD, −0.03; 95% CI, −0.08, 0.02). The identification of sepsis as the primary outcome in prophylaxis studies has been hampered by inadequately stringent definitions of systemic infection. However, data from one study suggest that prophylactic rGM-CSF may provide protection against infection when given to preterm infants who are neutropenic.[57] Carr and coworkers concluded that evidence is currently insufficient to support the introduction of rG-CSF or rGM-CSF into neonatal practice, either as treatment for established systemic infection to reduce resulting mortality, or as prophylaxis to prevent systemic infection in high-risk neonates.[50]

Fungal Infection

Thrombocytopenia is known to accompany fungal infection in the NICU, but neutropenia can also accompany such infections. No studies have specifically focused on the use of rG-CSF among neutropenic neonates with fungal infection.

Necrotizing Enterocolitis

Neutropenia is relatively common among severe cases of NEC. Some cases are transient and resemble the neutropenia that follows endotoxin.[60,61] No studies have focused on using rG-CSF among neutropenic neonates with NEC.

Chronic Idiopathic Neutropenia of Prematurity

Certain preterm neonates develop neutropenia when 4 to 10 weeks old. This variety of neutropenia is often associated with a patient's spontaneous recovery from anemia of prematurity. Neutrophil counts are generally less than 1000/μL but rarely less than 500/μL.[62-64] The condition is transient, lasting a few weeks to perhaps a month or longer. It appears to be a hyporegenerative neutropenia because it is not accompanied by a leukocyte "left shift," nor by morphologic abnormalities of the neutrophils. Patients with this condition have an "rG-CSF mobilizable neutrophil reserve," meaning that if rG-CSF is given, neutrophil count increases within hours. This fact has been taken as evidence that patients do not have a significant host-defense deficiency, because in theory they can supply neutrophils to tissues when needed.[63] Thus, although patients are neutropenic, this condition is likely benign and requires no treatment.

Other Proposed Uses for rG-CSF in the NICU

rG-CSF has been tested as a neuroprotectant in a rodent model of neonatal hypoxic-ischemic brain damage.[65] Subcutaneous G-CSF administration, beginning 1 hour after injury, prevented brain atrophy, preserved reflexes, and improved motor coordination and memory. In addition, animals treated with G-CSF had better somatic growth. Clinical studies are planned to test the safety and efficacy of rG-CSF as a neuroprotectant for neonates with hypoxic-ischemic encephalopathy.[65]

G-CSF is found in amniotic fluid, which is swallowed by the fetus in large quantities—up to 200 mL/kg/day. The G-CSF swallowed binds to receptors on enterocytes and conveys antiapoptotic actions.[66] A sterile, isotonic, simulated amniotic fluid containing rG-CSF has been administered to NICU patients who are otherwise NPO (nil per os), with the hypothesis that such will prevent disuse atrophy of the intestinal villi that otherwise occurs during the NPO period. Safety and early efficacy studies of this approach seem promising.[67-69]

Both rG-CSF and rGM-CSF have been examined as means of prophylaxis against nosocomial infection in VLBW neonates. A large, multicenter, randomized trial by Carr, Brockelhurst, and associates[70] involved 280 neonates of 31 weeks' gestation or younger and at less than the 10th percentile for birthweight who were randomized within 72 hours of birth to receive GM-CSF 10 μg/kg/day subcutaneously for 5 days or standard management. The primary outcome was sepsis-free survival 14 days from trial entry. Investigators observed a significant increase in blood neutrophil count among GM-CSF recipients, but no difference in sepsis-free short-term survival. It seems that the current consensus is that rG-CSF and rGM-CSF should not be used routinely in NICUs for prophylaxis against nosocomial infection because evidence for such usage is nil or at best very weak.[70,71]

A Consistent Approach to the Use of rG-CSF in the NICU

The following proposal was introduced as a guideline to serve until sufficient data accumulated for conducting an evidence-based assessment of the risks and benefits associated with the use of rG-CSF in each of the neutropenic conditions in the NICU.[72] Briefly (Fig. 3-3), we propose that if a neonatal patient has neutropenia, and that variety of neutropenia is known to be a variety of SCN, the patient should be enrolled in the SCN International Registry, established in 1994 at the University of Washington, and treatment with rG-CSF initiated. Enrollment in the SCN International Registry can be accomplished at the Website http://depts.washington.edu/registry/, using the entry criteria and exclusion criteria given in Table 3-3.

3

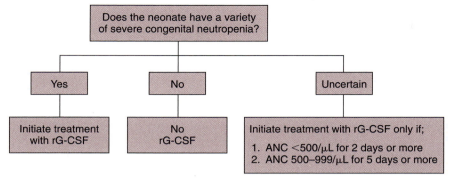

Figure 3-3 Guidelines for assisting in the decision regarding which neutropenic neonatal intensive care unit (NICU) patients should be treated with recombinant granulocyte colony-stimulating factor (rG-CSF), based on the type of neutropenia. *ANC,* Absolute neutrophil count. (Modified from Calhoun DA, Christensen RD, Edstrom CS, et al. Consistent approaches to procedures and practices in neonatal hematology. *Clin Perinatol.* 2000;27:733–753.)

We propose beginning treatment with a dose of 10 μg/kg subcutaneously, once per day for 3 consecutive days. Thereafter, doses are given as needed to titrate the ANC to around 1000/μL. We propose that if a neonatal patient has neutropenia, and the variety of neutropenia is NOT one of the varieties of SCN, rG-CSF treatment should not be used. We propose that if a neonatal patient has neutropenia, and the variety of neutropenia is NOT known (and therefore might be a SCN variety), while the type of neutropenia is evaluated, rG-CSF treatment can be instituted if the ANC was less than 500/μL for 2 or more days, or less than 1000/μL for 5 to 7 days or longer.

We did not include criteria for administering rGM-CSF because we found insufficient evidence for its use in the NICU. If one follows this schema (see Fig. 3-2), rG-CSF will be used very little in any given NICU. However, the schema should focus rG-CSF usage on those patients with the most to gain and the least to lose by its application. As additional pertinent investigative work is published, these guidelines should be modified accordingly.

Table 3-3   SCREENING FOR SEVERE CHRONIC NEUTROPENIA

(http://depts.washington.edu/registry/)

Inclusion Questions
1. Has a blood neutrophil count less than 500/μL been documented on at least three occasions over the past 3 months?
2. Is there a history of recurrent infection? *(specify)*
3. Is the bone marrow evaluation consistent with severe chronic neutropenia? *(date performed)*
4. Has a cytogenetic evaluation been completed?
5. Is the patient now receiving Neupogen (rG-CSF)?

Exclusion Criteria
1. Neutropenia is known to be drug induced.
2. Thrombocytopenia is present (<50,000/μL), except in the case of Shwachman-Diamond syndrome or glycogen storage disease type 1b.
3. Anemia is present (Hgb <8 g/dL), except in the case of Shwachman-Diamond syndrome or glycogen storage disease type 1b.
4. The patient has a myelodysplastic syndrome or aplastic anemia, is HIV positive, has some other hematologic disease or rheumatoid arthritis, or has received previous chemotherapy for cancer.

Hgb, Hemoglobin; *HIV,* human immunodeficiency virus; *rG-CSF,* recombinant granulocyte colony-stimulating factor.

References

1. Borregaard N. Neutrophils, from marrow to microbes. *Immunity*. 2010;24;33:657-670.
2. Bouma G, Ancliff PJ, Thrasher AJ, Burns SO. Recent advances in the understanding of genetic defects of neutrophil number and function. *Br J Haematol*. 2010;151:312-326.
3. Dale DC, Welte K. Cyclic and chronic neutropenia. *Cancer Treat Res*. 2011;157:97-108.
4. Christensen RD, Calhoun DA. Congenital neutropenia. *Clin Perinatol*. 2004;31:29-38.
5. Welte K, Zeidler C. Severe congenital neutropenia. *Hematol Oncol Clin North Am*. 2009;223: 307-320.
6. Zeidler C, Boxer L, Dale DC, Freedman MH, Kinsey S, Welte K. Management of Kostmann syndrome in the G-CSF era. *Br J Haematol*. 2000;109:490-495.
7. Calhoun DA, Christensen RD. The occurrence of Kostmann syndrome in preterm neonates. *Pediatrics*. 1997;99:259-261.
8. Schmutz N, Henry E, Jopling J, Christensen RD. Expected ranges for blood neutrophil concentrations of neonates: The Manroe and Mouzinho charts revisited. *J Perinatol*. 2008;28:275-281.
9. Lambert RM, Baer VL, Wiedmeier SE, Henry E, Burnett J, Christensen RD. Isolated elevated blood neutrophil concentration at altitude does not require NICU admission if appropriate reference ranges are used. *J Perinatol*. 2009;29:822-825.
10. Manroe BL, Weinberg AG, Rosenfeld CR, Browne R. The neonatal blood count in health and disease. I. Reference values for neutrophilic cells. *J Pediatr*. 1979;95:89-98.
11. Mouzinho A, Rosenfeld CR, Sanchez PJ, Risser R. Effect of maternal hypertension on neonatal neutropenia and risk of nosocomial infection. *Pediatrics*. 1992;90:430-435.
12. Watts RG. Neutropenia. In: Greer JP, Foerster J, Rodgers GM, et al, editors. *Wintrobe's Clinical Hematology*. 12th ed. Lippincott: Williams & Wilkins; 2010:1527.
13. Kostmann R. Infantile genetic agranulocytosis; agranulocytosis infantilis hereditaria. *Acta Paediatr*. 1956;45(Suppl 105):1-78.
14. Carlsson G, Fasth A. Infantile genetic agranulocytosis, morbus Kostmann: Presentation of six cases from the original "Kostmann family" and a review. *Acta Paediatr*. 2001;90:757-764.
15. Aprikyan AA, Carlsson G, Stein S, et al. Neutrophil elastase mutations in severe congenital neutropenia patients of the original Kostmann family. *Blood*. 2004;103:389.
16. Zeidler C, Welte K. Kostmann syndrome and severe congenital neutropenia. *Semin Hematol*. 2002; 39:82-88.
17. Zetterstrom R. Kostmann disease–infantile genetic agranulocytosis: Historical views and new aspects. *Acta Paediatr*. 2002;91:1279-1281.
18. Carlsson G, Wahlin YB, Johansson A, et al. Periodontal disease in patients from the original Kostmann family with severe congenital neutropenia. *J Periodontol*. 2006;77:744-751.
19. Ball HL, Zhang B, Riches JJ, et al. Shwachman-Bodian Diamond syndrome is a multi-functional protein implicated in cellular stress responses. *Hum Mol Genet*. 2009;18:3684-3695.
20. Orelio C, Kuijpers TW. Shwachman-Diamond syndrome neutrophils have altered chemoattractant-induced F-actin polymerization and polarization characteristics. *Haematologica*. 2009;94:409-413.
21. Huhta JC, Pomerance HH, Barness EG. Clinicopathologic conference: Barth Syndrome. *Fetal Pediatr Pathol*. 2005;24:239-254.
22. Barth PG, Van den Bogert C, Bolhuis PA, et al. X-linked cardioskeletal myopathy and neutropenia (Barth syndrome): Respiratory-chain abnormalities in cultured fibroblasts. *J Inherit Metab Dis*. 1996; 19:157-160.
23. Barth PG, Valianpour F, Bowen VM, et al. X-linked cardioskeletal myopathy and neutropenia (Barth syndrome): An update. *Am J Med Genet*. 2004;126A:349-353.
24. Ammann RA, Duppenthaler A, Bux J, Aebi C. Granulocyte colony-stimulating factor-responsive chronic neutropenia in cartilage-hair hypoplasia. *J Pediatr Hematol Oncol*. 2004;26:379-381.
25. Pierre G, Chakupurakal G, McKiernan P, Hendriksz C, Lawson S, Chakrapani A. Bone marrow transplantation in glycogen storage disease type 1b. *J Pediatr*. 2008;152:286-288.
26. Lalezari P, Khorshidi M, Petrosova M. Autoimmune neutropenia of infancy. *J Pediatr*. 1986; 109:764-769.
27. Boxer LA. Leukocyte disorders: Quantitative and qualitative disorders of the neutrophil, Part 1. *Pediatr Rev*. 17:19-28. 1996.
28. Boxer LA. Immune neutropenias. Clinical and biological implications. *Am J Pediatr Hematol Oncol*. 1981;3:89-96.
29. Maheshwari A, Christensen RD, Calhoun DA. Immune-mediated neutropenia in the neonate. *Acta Paediatr Suppl*. 2002;91:98-103.
30. Makeshwari A, Christensen RD, Calhoun DA. Immune neutropenia in the neonate. *Adv Pediatri*. 2002;49:317-339.
31. Curtis BR, Reon C, Aster RH. Neonatal alloimmune neutropenia attributed to maternal immunoglobulin G antibodies against the neutrophil alloantigen HNA1c(SH): A report of five cases. *Transfusion*. 2005;45:1308-1313.
32. Davoren A, Saving K, McFarland JG, Aster RH, Curtis BR. Neonatal neutropenia and bacterial sepsis associated with placental transfer of maternal neutrophil-specific autoantibodies. *Transfusion*. 2004; 44:1041-1046.
33. Calhoun DA, Rimsza LM, Burchfield DJ, et al. Congenital autoimmune neutropenia in two premature neonates. *Pediatrics*. 2001;108:181-184.
34. Bux J, Behrens G, Jaeger G, Welte K. Diagnosis and clinical course of autoimmune neutropenia in infancy; analysis of 240 cases. *Blood*. 1998;91:181-186.

3

3

35. Lekjowski M, Maheshwari A., Calhoun, Christensen RD, Skoda-Smith S, Dabrow S. Persistent perianal abscess in early infancy as a presentation of autoimmune neutropenia. *J Perinatol.* 2003:23: 428-430.
36. Conway LT, Clay ME, Kline WE, Ramsay NK, Krivit W, McCullough J. Natural history of primary autoimmune neutropenia in infancy. *Pediatrics.* 1987;79:728-733.
37. Koenig JM, Christensen RD. Incidence, neutrophil kinetics, and natural history of neonatal neutropenia associated with maternal hypertension. *N Engl J Med.* 1989;321:557-562.
38. Koenig JM, Christensen RD. The mechanism responsible for diminished neutrophil production in neonates delivered of women with pregnancy-induced hypertension. *Am J Obstet Gynecol.* 1991;165: 467-473.
39. Tsao PN, Teng RJ, Tang JR, Yau KI. Granulocyte colony-stimulating factor in the cord blood of premature neonates born to mothers with pregnancy-induced hypertension. *J Pediatr.* 1999;135: 56-59.
40. Doron MW, Makhlouf RA, Katz VL, Lawson EE, Stiles AD. Increased incidence of sepsis at birth in neutropenic infants of mothers with preeclampsia. *J Pediatr.* 1994;125:452-458.
41. Paul DA, Kepler J, Leef KH, Siscione A, Palmer C, Stefano JL. Effect of preeclampsia on mortality, intraventricular hemorrhage, and need for mechanical ventilation in very low-birth-weight infants. *Am J Perinatol.* 1998;15:381-386.
42. Procianoy RS, Silveira RC, Mussi-Pinhata MM, et al. Brazilian Network on Neonatal Research. Sepsis and neutropenia in very low birth weight infants delivered of mothers with preeclampsia. *J Pediatr* 2010;157:434-438, 438.e1.
43. Teng RJ, Wu TJ, Garrison RD, Sharma R, Hudak ML. Early neutropenia is not associated with an increased rate of nosocomial infection in very low-birth-weight infants. *J Perinatol.* 2009;29: 219-224.
44. Kocherlakota P, La Gamma EF. Preliminary report: rhG-CSF may reduce the incidence of neonatal sepsis in prolonged preeclampsia-associated neutropenia. *Pediatrics.* 1998;102:1107-1111.
45. Miura E, Procianoy RS, Bittar C, et al. A randomized double-masked, placebo-controlled trial of recombinant granulocyte colony-stimulating factor administration to preterm infants with the clinical diagnosis of early-onset sepsis. *Pediatrics.* 2001;107:30-35.
46. Kuhn P, Messer J, Paupe A, et al. A multicenter, randomized, placebo-controlled trial of prophylactic recombinant granulocyte-colony stimulating factor in preterm neonates with neutropenia. *J Pediatr.* 2009;155:324-330.e1.
47. Christensen RD, Henry E, Wiedmeier SE, Stoddard RA, Lambert DK. Low blood neutrophil concentrations among extremely low birth weight neonates: Data from a multihospital health-care system. *J Perinatol.* 2006;26:682-687.
48. Koenig JM, Hunter DD, Christensen RD. Neutropenia in donor (anemic) twins involved in the twin-twin transfusion syndrome. *J Perinatol.* 1991;11:355-358.
49. Koenig JM, Christensen RD. Neutropenia and thrombocytopenia in infants with Rh hemolytic disease. *J Pediatr.* 1989;114:625-631.
50. Carr R, Modi N, Dore C. G-CSF and GM-CSF for treating or preventing neonatal infections. *Cochrane Database Syst Rev.* 2003;(3):CD003066.
51. Ahmad A, Laborada G, Bussel J, Nesin M. Comparison of recombinant G-CSF, recombinant human GM-CSF and placebo for treatment of septic preterm infants. *Pediatr Infect Dis J.* 2002; 21:1061-1065.
52. Bedford-Russell AR, Emmerson AJB, Wilkinson N, et al. A trial of recombinant human granulocyte colony stimulating factor for the treatment of very low birthweight infants with presumed sepsis and neutropenia. *Arch Dis Child Fetal Neonatal Ed.* 2001;84:F172-F176.
53. Bilgin K, Yaramis A, Haspolat K, Tas A, Gunbey S, Derman O. A randomized trial of granulocyte-macrophage colony-stimulating factor in neonates with sepsis and neutropenia. *Pediatrics.* 2001; 107:36-41.
54. Drossou-Agakidou V, Kanakoudi-Tsakalidou F, Taparkou A, Tzimouli V, Tsandali H, Kremenopoulos G. Administration of recombinant human granulocyte-colony stimulating factor to septic neonates induces neutrophilia and enhances the neutrophil respiratory burst and beta2 integrin expression: Results of a randomized controlled trial. *Eur J Pediatr.* 1998;157:583-588.
55. Schibler KR, Osborne KA, Leung LY, Le TV, Baker SI, Thompson DD. A randomized placebo-controlled trial of granulocyte colony-stimulating factor administration to newborn infants with neutropenia and clinical signs of early-onset sepsis. *Pediatrics.* 1998;102:6-13.
56. Gillan ER, Christensen RD, Suen Y, et al. A randomized, placebo-controlled trial of recombinant human granulocyte colony-stimulating factor administration in newborn infants with presumed sepsis: Significant induction of peripheral and bone marrow neutrophilia. *Blood.* 1994;84: 1427-1433.
57. Cairo MS, Christensen RD, Sender LS, et al. Results of a phase I/II trial of recombinant human granulocyte-macrophage colony-stimulating factor in very low birthweight neonates: Significant induction of circulatory neutrophils, monocytes, platelets, and bone marrow neutrophils. *Blood.* 1995;86:2509-2515.
58. Cairo MS, Agosti J, Ellis R, et al. Randomised double-blind placebo-controlled trial of prophylactic recombinant human GM-CSF to reduce nosocomial infection in very low birthweight neonates. *J Pediatrics.* 1999;134:64-70.
59. Carr R, Modi N, Doré CJ, El-Rifai R, Lindo D. A randomised controlled trial of prophylactic GM-CSF in human newborns less than 32 weeks gestation. *Pediatrics.* 1999;103:796-802.

60. Hutter JJ Jr, Hathaway WE, Wayne ER. Hematologic abnormalities in severe neonatal necrotizing enterocolitis. *J Pediatr*. 1976;88:1026-1031.
61. Kling PJ, Hutter JJ. Hematologic abnormalities in severe neonatal necrotizing enterocolitis: 25 years later. *J Perinatol*. 2003;23:523-530.
62. Juul SE, Calhoun DA, Christensen RD. "Idiopathic neutropenia" in very low birthweight infants. *Acta Paediatr*. 87:963-968. 1998
63. Juul SE, Christensen RD. Effect of recombinant granulocyte colony-stimulating factor on blood neutrophil concentrations among patients with "idiopathic neonatal neutropenia": A randomized, placebo-controlled trial. *J Perinatol*. 2003;23:493-497.
64. Chirico G, Motta M, Villani P, Cavazza A, Cardone ML. Late-onset neutropenia in very low birth-weight infants. *Acta Paediatr Suppl*. 2002;91:104-108.
65. Fathali N, Lekic T, Zhang JH, Tang J. Long-term evaluation of granulocyte-colony stimulating factor on hypoxic-ischemic brain damage in infant rats. *Intensive Care Med*. 2010;36:1602-1608.
66. Gersting JA, Christensen RD, Calhoun DA. Effects of enterally administering granulocyte colony-stimulating factor to suckling mice. *Pediatr Res*. 2004;55:802-806.
67. Sullivan SE, Calhoun DA, Maheshwari A, et al. Tolerance of simulated amniotic fluid in premature neonates. *Ann Pharmacother*. 2002;36:1518-1524.
68. Christensen RD, Havranek T, Gerstmann DR, Calhoun DA. Enteral administration of a simulated amniotic fluid to very low birth weight neonates. *J Perinatol*. 2005;25:380-385.
69. Barney CK, Lambert DK, Alder SC, Scoffield SH, Schmutz N, Christensen RD. Treating feeding intolerance with an enteral solution patterned after human amniotic fluid: A randomized, controlled, masked trial. *J Perinatol*. 2007;27:28-31.
70. Carr R, Brocklehurst P, Doré CJ, Modi N. Granulocyte-macrophage colony stimulating factor administered as prophylaxis for reduction of sepsis in extremely preterm, small for gestational age neonates (the PROGRAMS trial): A single-blind, multicentre, randomised controlled trial. *Lancet*. 2009; 373:226-233.
71. Shann F. Sepsis in babies: Should we stimulate the phagocytes? *Lancet*. 2009;373:188-190.
72. Calhoun DA, Christensen RD, Edstrom CS, et al. Consistent approaches to procedures and practices in neonatal hematology. *Clin Perinatol*. 2000;27:733-753.

3

CHAPTER 4

Nonhematopoietic Effects of Erythropoietin

Christopher Traudt, MD, and Sandra E. Juul, MD, PhD

- **Erythropoietin**
- **Summary**

This chapter will review evidence supporting the neuroprotective properties of erythropoietin (Epo) for the treatment of neonatal brain injury. Background information, in vitro and in vivo data for safety, efficacy, and clinical feasibility, and published clinical studies will be reviewed. Neuroprotective strategies for the treatment of neonatal and adult brain injuries are not known. This chapter will focus primarily on the use of Epo for neonates, given that the mechanisms of brain injury and repair, and the approach to treatment, are distinct for these populations. Two groups of neonates have been the research focus for this neuroprotective treatment: extremely preterm infants and term infants with neonatal encephalopathy due to hypoxia-ischemia. Both of these groups show neurodevelopmental impairment in approximately half of survivors, despite best efforts at prevention and treatment.[1-6] Clearly, new approaches are needed. Epo shows promise as one such approach.

Erythropoietin

Epo is an endogenous growth factor that regulates erythrocyte production.[7] Many randomized controlled trials have been done in adults and children to test its safety and efficacy as an erythropoietic agent, and these studies have been reviewed.[8-11] Neonates require higher doses of Epo, with more frequent dosing to achieve an equivalent hematopoietic response to adults, because of their greater plasma clearance, high volume of distribution, and short fractional elimination time.[12-14] Adverse effects that occur in adults (hypertension, polycythemia, seizures, increased thrombosis, cardiovascular accidents, and death) have not been identified in neonates among the more than 3000 infants studied.

Over the past 15 years, the nonhematopoietic function of Epo as it interacts with Epo receptors (EpoR) has been the subject of extensive investigation. EpoRs are present during embryologic and fetal development.[15] As development proceeds, the distribution of EpoRs becomes increasingly region and cell specific.[16] The function of Epo in the developing brain includes trophic effects on the vascular and nervous systems.[17,18] Brains from EpoR-null mice also have increased neuronal apoptosis and decreased tolerance to hypoxic insults, suggesting other neuroprotective functions.[17] Indeed, Epo has been shown to have neuroprotective properties,[19,20] and the mechanisms by which these effects occur have been studied in a multitude of experimental paradigms ranging from cell cultures to knockout mice to small and large animal models of brain injury.

Epo Analogues

The possibility of developing Epo analogues that express subsets of Epo characteristics has been a topic of great interest, because these molecules might circumvent unwanted clinical effects or might provide improved permeability with the ability to cross the placenta or blood–brain barrier. The neuroprotective functions of Epo can be separated from its stimulatory action on hematopoiesis, as the Epo derivatives asialo-Epo[21] and carbamylated Epo[22,23] have shown. Several structural or functional variants of Epo have now been formulated, as reviewed by Siren and associates.[24] These include Epo-mimetic peptides, which are small peptides that interact with the EpoR despite being structurally distinct from Epo. For example, Epotris is an Epo-mimetic peptide that has neuroprotective properties derived from the C alpha-helix region (amino acid residues 92-111) of human Epo.[25] No studies to date have been done to assess the safety or efficacy of these compounds as prenatal treatments.

In Vitro Epo Effects

EpoRs are present on neural progenitor cells[26] and on select populations of mature neurons,[27] astrocytes,[28] oligodendrocytes,[29] microglia,[30] and endothelial cells[26] within the brain. Epo binds to neuronal cell surface EpoRs, which dimerize to activate antiapoptotic pathways via phosphorylation of Janus kinase 2 (JAK2); phosphorylation and activation of the mitogen-activated protein kinase (MAPK), extracellular signal–regulated kinase (ERK1/2), and phosphatidylinositol 3-kinase (PI3K)/Akt (protein kinase B) pathways; and signal transducer and activator of transcription 5 (STAT5), which are critical in cell survival.[31] Neuronal viability is enhanced by the presence of Epo when neurons are cultured under varied noxious conditions, including hypoxia, glucose deprivation, glutamate toxicity, and nitric oxide toxicity.[31] Increased glutathione production occurs in the presence of Epo and may contribute to enhanced survival of cells in noxious environments.[32] Epo also promotes oligodendrocyte maturation and differentiation in culture,[28] protects these cells from interferon-γ and LPS toxicity,[33] and improves white matter survival in vivo.[34] White matter injury is common among preterm infants and is thought to be due to the vulnerability of developing oligodendrocytes.[35,36] Thus Epo might have protective effects in this population.

In Vivo Epo Effects

Brines and associates demonstrated that high-dose Epo (5000 U/kg IP) penetrates the blood–brain barrier and provides neuroprotection in adult models of brain injury.[37] Further studies in animals and humans have shown that high-dose Epo can be systemically administered, resulting in detectable increases in Epo concentrations in spinal fluid and brain extract, which, based on in vitro work, could be within a neuroprotective range.[38,39] However, the minimum effective dose has not yet been established and may depend on whether the blood–brain barrier is intact. Thus the mechanism of brain injury may dictate the dose of Epo required for neuroprotection, as does the age of the individual.

To date, hundreds of Epo neuroprotection studies have been published using adult and neonatal models of brain injury, including stroke, trauma, kainate-induced seizures, hypoxia-ischemia, and subarachnoid hemorrhage. Epo dosing ranged from 300 U/kg/dose to 30,000 U/kg. The highest doses (20,000 to 30,000 U/kg) lose protective properties, may cause harm, and are not recommended.[40,41] Protective effects important for reducing acute brain injury include decreased excitotoxicity,[42] glutamate toxicity,[43] neuronal apoptosis,[31] and inflammation.[44] Another mechanism that seems to be important in Epo neuroprotection is its stimulation of, and interaction with, other protective factors, such as brain-derived neurotrophic factor (BDNF) and glial cell–derived neurotrophic factor (GDNF).[26,45] Epo actively participates in the prevention of oxidative stress with generation of antioxidant enzymes, inhibition of nitric oxide production, and decreased lipid peroxidation. Epo is also angiogenic, which may be necessary for long-term survival of injured or newly generated cells. Epo, together with vascular endothelial growth factor (VEGF), promotes angiogenesis and repair.[46,47] Epo increases the migration of neural progenitor cells by stimulating the secretion of metalloproteinase-2 and -9 by endothelial cells via PI3K/Akt and ERK1/2 signaling pathways. Thus some protective effects of Epo are the result of direct neuronal receptor–mediated interaction, and others are indirect. In fact, a recent study shows that neuroprotective effects of Epo are seen in the absence of neural EpoR.[48]

Treatment of neuroinflammation and of neurodegeneration with Epo, with mixed success, has been investigated in animal models of multiple sclerosis, autoimmune encephalomyelitis, cerebral malaria, Parkinson's disease, Alzheimer's disease, Huntington's disease, and amyotrophic lateral sclerosis. Neurologic sequelae of cerebral malaria were reduced in rodents given exogenous Epo and in human children with elevated blood levels of Epo.[49,50] A few human clinical trials of Epo for the treatment of adult stroke, schizophrenia, and multiple sclerosis have been published. Reduced stroke lesion size and evolutions, as well as decreased serum markers of glial damage, were seen in adults treated with Epo[51]; however, in a larger follow-up study, increased mortality was noted (16.4% in Epo-treated subject compared with 9.0% in control patients).[52] This excess death may be due to an interaction between advanced age and response to Epo neuroprotection. Tseng and colleagues found that patients younger than 60 years of age responded better to Epo neuroprotection than did older individuals. Sepsis also impaired Epo neuroprotection in this population.[53] In other studies, cognitive improvement was seen in schizophrenic patients treated with Epo, although no changes in psychopathology ratings or psychosocial outcome parameters were noted.[54] High-dose Epo improved motor function and cognition among patients with chronic progressive multiple sclerosis.[55]

Clinical Reports of Epo Neonatal Neuroprotection

The work done in animals has not yet been confirmed in phase III randomized controlled trials of human neonates; however, three reports suggest that Epo might be neuroprotective in this population. In a study designed to test the erythropoietic effects of Epo, infants weighing 1250 g or less at birth were prospectively randomized to Epo or placebo/control from day 4 of life until 35 weeks' corrected gestational age.[56] Infants weighing less than 1000 g with serum Epo concentrations greater than 500 mU/mL had higher Mental Development Index (MDI) scores than infants with Epo concentrations less than 500 mU/mL when tested at 18 to 22 months' corrected age.[57] A retrospective cohort study of 82 infants weighing less than 1500 g at 30 weeks' or less gestation at birth was evaluated at 2 years after neonatal Epo treatment. Higher MDI scores were associated with higher cumulative doses of Epo, among other factors.[58] Another retrospective review of ELBW infants compared 89 Epo-treated versus 57 untreated neonates at 10 to 13 years of age. Epo-treated neonates had better outcomes, with 55% of the Epo group assessed as normal versus 39% untreated ($P < 0.05$). IQ scores were also higher in Epo-treated patients (90.8 vs. 81.3 in untreated infants; $P < 0.005$).[59]

Four clinical trials examining the safety and efficacy of high-dose Epo as a potential therapy for neonatal brain injury have been published: two in preterm infants and two in term infants with HIE.[60-63] For premature infants, pilot studies tested a range of intravenous doses from 500 to 3000 U/kg given daily for the first 3 days of life. No Epo-related adverse events were noted in 60 premature infants in these two studies. Serum concentrations of Epo were greater than 500 mU/L for an average of 18 hours after a single dose of 500 U/kg.[61] A multicenter, randomized, controlled study of Epo neuroprophylaxis in very low birthweight babies is ongoing in Switzerland. Another trial targeting extremely low birthweight infants is in the planning stage in the United States.

Term infants with hypoxia-ischemia were studied in a prospective case-control study of 45 infants, 15 of whom had HIE and received Epo (2500 IU/kg SC daily for 5 days); 15 were HIE controls, and 15 were normal term infants.[63] EEG backgrounds improved ($P = 0.01$) and nitric oxide concentrations decreased ($P < 0.001$) in the HIE-Epo group compared with the HIE-control group. More important, infants in the HIE-Epo group had fewer neurologic ($P < 0.05$) and developmental ($P < 0.05$) abnormalities at 6 months. In the second study of term infants, 167 infants with moderate to severe HIE were randomized to receive Epo ($n = 83$) or conventional treatment ($n = 84$). Epo-treated babies received 300 U/kg ($n = 52$) or 500 U/kg ($n = 31$) every other day for 2 weeks. Death or disability occurred in 43.8%

of controls compared with 24.6% of those in the Epo groups ($P = 0.017$) at 18 months. No discernible differences between Epo doses or adverse effects of Epo were reported.[62] None of the infants in either of these studies received hypothermia as treatment for HIE. Trials in progress include a phase I trial of Epo in HIE patients (**N**eonatal **E**rythropoietin in **A**sphyxiated **T**erm Infants, the NEAT trial) that will provide pharmacokinetic data for term infants with HIE who are receiving hypothermia, and a trial of Epo neuroprotection for neonates requiring surgery for cyanotic cardiac disease.

Dosing

A single Epo dose is not as neuroprotective as multiple Epo doses following brain injury in rodent models.[41,64] The probable mechanisms that explain why multiple dosages are more effective are twofold: (1) Epo decreases the early apoptotic response to injury, as well as the inflammatory response; and (2) Epo decreases late apoptosis and may stimulate processes involved in repair, such as neurogenesis, angiogenesis, and migration of regenerating neurons.[65] Further studies in larger animal models such as sheep[66] and nonhuman primates are ongoing.[67]

Optimal Dose

Although no doses of Epo have been approved by the Food and Drug Administration (FDA) for use in the neonatal population, this medication is used routinely in many NICUs to treat and prevent anemia. The typical Epo dose given to newborns to stimulate erythropoiesis ranges from 200 to 400 U/kg/dose[68,69]; some centers use doses as high as 700 U/kg.[70] Dosing schedules range from daily dosing to three times a week dosing. These doses are well tolerated by neonates for durations ranging from 2 weeks to several months. Only a small percentage of circulating Epo crosses the intact blood–brain barrier[38]; however, penetration is enhanced in the presence of brain injury.[39] Therefore, it is reasonable to predict that 500 U/kg intravenous (IV) will cross the blood–brain barrier if brain injury such as intracranial hemorrhage occurs. An ongoing Swiss study is testing doses as high as 3000 U/kg in preterm infants for neuroprotection, and the results of this randomized controlled trial are pending.[60] Figure 4-1 shows the mean circulating Epo concentrations achieved in ELBW infants given 500 U/kg.[61] Although the Epo concentrations for optimal neuroprotection are not known, this dose provides circulating concentrations above 500 mU/mL (shaded area), associated with improved outcomes on MDI,[57] for an average of 18 hours after a single dose.

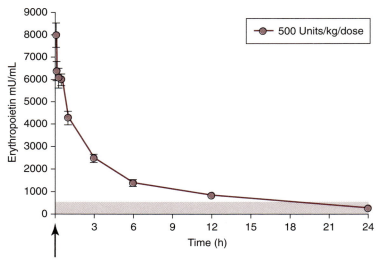

Figure 4-1 Mean circulating erythropoietin (Epo) concentrations achieved in extremely low birthweight (ELBW) infants given 500 U/kg.

Potential Risks of High-Dose Erythropoietin

In adults, complications of Epo treatment for erythropoiesis include polycythemia, rash, seizures, hypertension, shortened time to death, myocardial infarction, congestive heart failure, progression of tumors, and stroke. None of these adverse effects have been reported in randomized controlled studies of Epo-treated neonates receiving up to 2100 U/kg/wk, nor have differences been noted in the incidence of neonatal morbidities, including intraventricular hemorrhage, retinopathy of prematurity (ROP), necrotizing enterocolitis, chronic lung disease, and late-onset sepsis.[68]

Epo is a potent erythropoietic growth factor. Thus, high doses of Epo given for neuroprotective treatment might be expected to increase erythropoiesis, and possibly megakaryocytopoiesis. A transient increase in hematocrit is seen following high-dose Epo in neonatal rats.[71] However, preterm infants given three doses of Epo up to 2500 U/kg showed no change in hematocrit. This is likely due to the phlebotomy losses experienced by these babies.[61] The effects of brief treatments of high-dose Epo on iron balance are not known.

The role of Epo in the development of ROP in preterm infants is controversial. ROP occurs in two phases, the first involving loss of retinal vasculature following birth, and the second involving uncontrolled proliferation of retinal vessels. It is possible that Epo plays a role because EpoRs are present on endothelial cells, and EpoR stimulation by Epo increases their angiogenic expression.[72] High-dose Epo might have a protective effect on the retina during early treatment by ameliorating the first stage of ROP.[73] However, the angiogenic properties of Epo may prevail during late treatment, resulting in an increase in ROP. A Cochrane meta-analysis of prospective studies of Epo (for which ROP was not a primary outcome measure) showed an increased risk of ROP after early Epo exposure.[8] This analysis could not separate out confounders such as effects of anemia or iron treatment. Animal data suggest that timing of Epo exposure might be crucial. Early Epo treatment in mice decreased the development of ROP; late treatment given during the proliferative stage contributed to neovascularization and therefore worsened ROP.[74] However, a rat model of ROP showed no beneficial or harmful effects of repeated high-dose Epo administration (5000 U/kg × 3 doses) on retinal vascularization.[75]

Summary

Epo has great potential as neuroprotective therapy in both preterm and term infants. It has many properties that make it an ideal neuroprotective strategy: it is easy to administer; is FDA approved (although not for neuroprotective indications, and not in neonates), inexpensive, and accessible; and has been safe in all neonatal studies. However, additional data are needed to define the optimal dose, the number of doses, and the timing of treatment. Early apoptosis and inflammation may be best treated with early doses, but stimulation of repair through angiogenesis and neurogenesis might best be accomplished using later doses. A dosing regimen that is optimal for neuroprotection to reduce HIE sequelae may not be ideal for prophylaxis of white matter disease in ELBW preterm infants. Future possibilities include the use of Epo with hypothermia for the treatment of HIE in neonates. Combining hypothermia with Epo is already being investigated in adult populations.[76,77]

References

1. Hack M, Youngstrom EA, Cartar L, et al. Behavioral outcomes and evidence of psychopathology among very low birth weight infants at age 20 years. *Pediatrics.* Oct 2004;114(4):932-940.
2. Taylor HG, Minich NM, Klein N, Hack M. Longitudinal outcomes of very low birth weight: Neuropsychological findings. *J Int Neuropsychol Soc.* Mar 2004;10(2):149-163.
3. Gluckman PD, Wyatt JS, Azzopardi D, et al. Selective head cooling with mild systemic hypothermia after neonatal encephalopathy: Multicentre randomised trial. *Lancet.* Feb 19 2005;365(9460): 663-670.
4. Shankaran S, Laptook AR, Ehrenkranz RA, et al. Whole-body hypothermia for neonates with hypoxic-ischemic encephalopathy. *N Engl J Med.* Oct 13 2005;353(15):1574-1584.
5. Azzopardi DV, Strohm B, Edwards AD, et al. Moderate hypothermia to treat perinatal asphyxial encephalopathy. *N Engl J Med.* Oct 1 2009;361(14):1349-1358.

6. Hintz SR, Kendrick DE, Stoll BJ, et al. Neurodevelopmental and growth outcomes of extremely low birth weight infants after necrotizing enterocolitis. *Pediatrics*. Mar 2005;115(3):696-703.

7. Krantz SB. Erythropoietin. *Blood*. Feb 1 1991;77(3):419-434.

8. Ohlsson A, Aher SM. Early erythropoietin for preventing red blood cell transfusion in preterm and/or low birth weight infants. *Cochrane Database Syst Rev*. 2006;3:CD004863.

9. Aher S, Ohlsson A. Late erythropoietin for preventing red blood cell transfusion in preterm and/or low birth weight infants. *Cochrane Database Syst Rev*. 2006;3:CD004868.

10. Aher SM, Ohlsson A. Early versus late erythropoietin for preventing red blood cell transfusion in preterm and/or low birth weight infants. *Cochrane Database Syst Rev*. 2006;3:CD004865.

11. Garcia MG, Hutson AD, Christensen RD. Effect of recombinant erythropoietin on "late" transfusions in the neonatal intensive care unit: A meta-analysis. *J Perinatol*. Mar 2002;22(2):108-111.

12. Widness JA, Veng-Pedersen P, Peters C, Pereira LM, Schmidt RL, Lowe LS. Erythropoietin pharmacokinetics in premature infants: Developmental, nonlinearity, and treatment effects. *J Appl Physiol*. 1996;80(1):140-148.

13. Brown MS, Jones MA, Ohls RK, Christensen RD. Single-dose pharmacokinetics of recombinant human erythropoietin in preterm infants after intravenous and subcutaneous administration. *J Pediatr*. 1993;122(4):655-657.

14. Krishnan R, Shankaran S, Krishnan M, Kauffman RE, Kumar P, Lucena J. Pharmacokinetics of erythropoietin following single-dose subcutaneous administration in preterm infants. *Biol Neonate*. 1996;70(3):135-140.

15. Juul SE, Anderson DK, Li Y, Christensen RD. Erythropoietin and erythropoietin receptor in the developing human central nervous system. *Pediatr Res*. 1998;43(1):40-49.

16. Juul SE, Yachnis AT, Rojiani AM, Christensen RD. Immunohistochemical localization of erythropoietin and its receptor in the developing human brain. *Pediatr Dev Pathol*. Mar-Apr 1999;2(2):148-158.

17. Yu X, Shacka JJ, Eells JB, et al. Erythropoietin receptor signalling is required for normal brain development. *Development*. Jan 2002;129(2):505-516.

18. Chen ZY, Asavaritikrai P, Prchal JT, Noguchi CT. Endogenous erythropoietin signaling is required for normal neural progenitor cell proliferation. *J Biol Chem*. Aug 31 2007;282(35):25875-25883.

19. Sobh MA, el-Tantawy AE, Said E, et al. Effect of treatment of anaemia with erythropoietin on neuromuscular function in patients on long term haemodialysis. *Scand J Urol Nephrol*. 1992;26(1):65-69.

20. Konishi Y, Chui DH, Hirose H, Kunishita T, Tabira T. Trophic effect of erythropoietin and other hematopoietic factors on central cholinergic neurons in vitro and in vivo. *Brain Res*. Apr 23 1993;609(1-2):29-35.

21. Mennini T, De Paola M, Bigini P, et al. Nonhematopoietic erythropoietin derivatives prevent motoneuron degeneration in vitro and in vivo. *Mol Med*. Jul-Aug 2006;12(7-8):153-160.

22. Sturm B, Helminger M, Steinkellner H, Heidari MM, Goldenberg H, Scheiber-Mojdehkar B. Carbamylated erythropoietin increases frataxin independent from the erythropoietin receptor. *Eur J Clin Invest*. Jun 2010;40(6):561-565.

23. Wang L, Zhang ZG, Gregg SR, et al. The Sonic hedgehog pathway mediates carbamylated erythropoietin-enhanced proliferation and differentiation of adult neural progenitor cells. *J Biol Chem*. Nov 2 2007;282(44):32462-32470.

24. Siren AL, Fasshauer T, Bartels C, Ehrenreich H. Therapeutic potential of erythropoietin and its structural or functional variants in the nervous system. *Neurotherapeutics*. Jan 2009;6(1):108-127.

25. Pankratova S, Kiryushko D, Sonn K, et al. Neuroprotective properties of a novel, non-haematopoietic agonist of the erythropoietin receptor. *Brain*. 2010;133:2281-2294.

26. Wang L, Zhang Z, Wang Y, Zhang R, Chopp M. Treatment of stroke with erythropoietin enhances neurogenesis and angiogenesis and improves neurological function in rats. *Stroke*. Jul 2004;35(7):1732-1737.

27. Wallach I, Zhang J, Hartmann A, et al. Erythropoietin-receptor gene regulation in neuronal cells. *Pediatr Res*. Jun 2009;65(6):619-624.

28. Sugawa M, Sakurai Y, Ishikawa-Ieda Y, Suzuki H, Asou H. Effects of erythropoietin on glial cell development; oligodendrocyte maturation and astrocyte proliferation. *Neurosci Res*. Dec 2002;44(4):391-403.

29. Nagai A, Nakagawa E, Choi HB, Hatori K, Kobayashi S, Kim SU. Erythropoietin and erythropoietin receptors in human CNS neurons, astrocytes, microglia, and oligodendrocytes grown in culture. *J Neuropathol Exp Neurol*. Apr 2001;60(4):386-392.

30. Chong ZZ, Kang JQ, Maiese K. Erythropoietin fosters both intrinsic and extrinsic neuronal protection through modulation of microglia, Akt1, Bad, and caspase-mediated pathways. *Br J Pharmacol*. Mar 2003;138(6):1107-1118.

31. Digicaylioglu M, Lipton SA. Erythropoietin-mediated neuroprotection involves cross-talk between Jak2 and NF-kappaB signalling cascades. *Nature*. Aug 9 2001;412(6847):641-647.

32. Sims B, Clarke M, Njah W, Hopkins ES, Sontheimer H. Erythropoietin-induced neuroprotection requires cystine glutamate exchanger activity. *Brain Res*. Mar 19 2010;1321:88-95.

33. Genc K, Genc S, Baskin H, Semin I. Erythropoietin decreases cytotoxicity and nitric oxide formation induced by inflammatory stimuli in rat oligodendrocytes. *Physiol Res*. 2006;55(1):33-38.

34. Vitellaro-Zuccarello L, Mazzetti S, Madaschi L, Bosisio P, Gorio A, De Biasi S. Erythropoietin-mediated preservation of the white matter in rat spinal cord injury. *Neuroscience*. Feb 9 2007;144(3):865-877.

35. Back SA, Luo NL, Borenstein NS, Levine JM, Volpe JJ, Kinney HC. Late oligodendrocyte progenitors coincide with the developmental window of vulnerability for human perinatal white matter injury. *J Neurosci*. Feb 15 2001;21(4):1302-1312.

36. Back SA, Tuohy TM, Chen H, et al. Hyaluronan accumulates in demyelinated lesions and inhibits oligodendrocyte progenitor maturation. *Nat Med*. Sep 2005;11(9):966-972.

37. Brines ML, Ghezzi P, Keenan S, et al. Erythropoietin crosses the blood-brain barrier to protect against experimental brain injury. *Proc Natl Acad Sci U S A*. 2000;97(19):10526-10531.

38. Juul SE, McPherson RJ, Farrell FX, Jolliffe L, Ness DJ, Gleason CA. Erytropoietin concentrations in cerebrospinal fluid of nonhuman primates and fetal sheep following high-dose recombinant erythropoietin. *Biol Neonate*. 2004;85(2):138-144.

39. Statler PA, McPherson RJ, Bauer LA, Kellert BA, Juul SE. Pharmacokinetics of high-dose recombinant erythropoietin in plasma and brain of neonatal rats. *Pediatr Res*. Jun 2007;61(6):671-675.

40. Weber A, Dzietko M, Berns M, et al. Neuronal damage after moderate hypoxia and erythropoietin. *Neurobiol Dis*. Nov 2005;20(2):594-600.

41. Kellert BA, McPherson RJ, Juul SE. A comparison of high-dose recombinant erythropoietin treatment regimens in brain-injured neonatal rats. *Pediatr Res*. Apr 2007;61(4):451-455.

42. Keller M, Yang J, Griesmaier E, et al. Erythropoietin is neuroprotective against NMDA-receptor-mediated excitotoxic brain injury in newborn mice. *Neurobiol Dis*. 2006;24:357-366.

43. Kawakami M, Sekiguchi M, Sato K, Kozaki S, Takahashi M. Erythropoietin receptor-mediated inhibition of exocytotic glutamate release confers neuroprotection during chemical ischemia. *J Biol Chem*. Oct 19 2001;276(42):39469-39475.

44. Sun Y, Calvert JW, Zhang JH. Neonatal hypoxia/ischemia is associated with decreased inflammatory mediators after erythropoietin administration. *Stroke*. Aug 2005;36(8):1672-1678.

45. Dzietko M, Felderhoff-Mueser U, Sifringer M, et al. Erythropoietin protects the developing brain against N-methyl-D-aspartate receptor antagonist neurotoxicity. *Neurobiol Dis*. Mar 2004;15(2):177-187.

46. Wang L, Chopp M, Gregg SR, et al. Neural progenitor cells treated with EPO induce angiogenesis through the production of VEGF. *J Cereb Blood Flow Metab*. Jul 2008;28(7):1361-1368.

47. Bocker-Meffert S, Rosenstiel P, Rohl C, et al. Erythropoietin and VEGF promote neural outgrowth from retinal explants in postnatal rats. *Invest Ophthalmol Vis Sci*. 2002;43(6):2021-2026.

48. Xiong Y, Mahmood A, Qu C, et al. Erythropoietin improves histological and functional outcomes after traumatic brain injury in mice in the absence of the neural erythropoietin receptor. *J Neurotrauma*. Jan 2010;27(1):205-215.

49. Wiese L, Hempel C, Penkowa M, Kirkby N, Kurtzhals JA. Recombinant human erythropoietin increases survival and reduces neuronal apoptosis in a murine model of cerebral malaria. *Malar J*. 2008;7:3.

50. Casals-Pascual C, Idro R, Picot S, Roberts DJ, Newton CR. Can erythropoietin be used to prevent brain damage in cerebral malaria? *Trends Parasitol*. Jan 2009;25(1):30-36.

51. Ehrenreich H, Hasselblatt M, Dembowski C, et al. Erythropoietin therapy for acute stroke is both safe and beneficial. *Mol Med*. 2002;8(8):495-505.

52. Ehrenreich H, Weissenborn K, Prange H, et al. Recombinant human erythropoietin in the treatment of acute ischemic stroke. *Stroke*. 2009;40:e647-56.

53. Tseng MY, Hutchinson PJ, Kirkpatrick PJ. Interaction of neurovascular protection of erythropoietin with age, sepsis, and statin therapy following aneurysmal subarachnoid hemorrhage. *J Neurosurg*. Jun 2010;112(6):1235-1239.

54. Ehrenreich H, Hinze-Selch D, Stawicki S, et al. Improvement of cognitive functions in chronic schizophrenic patients by recombinant human erythropoietin. *Mol Psychiatry*. Feb 2007;12(2):206-220.

55. Ehrenreich H, Fischer B, Norra C, et al. Exploring recombinant human erythropoietin in chronic progressive multiple sclerosis. *Brain*. Oct 2007;130(Pt 10):2577-2588.

56. Ohls RK, Ehrenkranz RA, Das A, et al. Neurodevelopmental outcome and growth at 18 to 22 months' corrected age in extremely low birth weight infants treated with early erythropoietin and iron. *Pediatrics*. Nov 2004;114(5):1287-1291.

57. Bierer R, Peceny MC, Hartenberger CH, Ohls RK. Erythropoietin concentrations and neurodevelopmental outcome in preterm infants. *Pediatrics*. Sep 2006;118(3):e635-640.

58. Brown MS, Eichorst D, Lala-Black B, Gonzalez R. Higher cumulative doses of erythropoietin and developmental outcomes in preterm infants. *Pediatrics*. Oct 2009;124(4):e681-687.

59. Neubauer AP, Voss W, Wachtendorf M, Jungmann T. Erythropoietin improves neurodevelopmental outcome of extremely preterm infants. *Ann Neurol*. May 2010;67(5):657-666.

60. Fauchere JC, Dame C, Vonthein R, et al. An approach to using recombinant erythropoietin for neuroprotection in very preterm infants. *Pediatrics*. Aug 2008;122(2):375-382.

61. Juul SE, McPherson RJ, Bauer LA, Ledbetter KJ, Gleason CA, Mayock DE. A phase I/II trial of high-dose erythropoietin in extremely low birth weight infants: Pharmacokinetics and safety. *Pediatrics*. Aug 2008;122(2):383-391.

62. Zhu C, Kang W, Xu F, et al. Erythropoietin improved neurologic outcomes in newborns with hypoxic-ischemic encephalopathy. *Pediatrics*. Aug 2009;124(2):e218-226.

63. Elmahdy H, El-Mashad AR, El-Bahrawy H, El-Gohary T, El-Barbary A, Aly H. Human recombinant erythropoietin in asphyxia neonatorum: Pilot trial. *Pediatrics*. May 2010;125(5):e1135-1142.

64. Gonzalez FF, Abel R, Almli CR, Mu D, Wendland M, Ferriero DM. Erythropoietin sustains cognitive function and brain volume after neonatal stroke. *Dev Neurosci*. 2009;31(5):403-411.

4

65. Tsai PT, Ohab JJ, Kertesz N, et al. A critical role of erythropoietin receptor in neurogenesis and post-stroke recovery. *J Neurosci*. Jan 25 2006;26(4):1269-1274.

66. Rees S, Hale N, De Matteo R, et al. Erythropoietin is neuroprotective in a preterm ovine model of endotoxin-induced brain injury. *J Neuropathol Exp Neurol*. Mar 2010;69(3):306-319.

67. Juul SE, Aylward E, Richards T, McPherson RJ, Kuratani J, Burbacher TM. Prenatal cord clamping in newborn Macaca nemestrina: A model of perinatal asphyxia. *Dev Neurosci*. 2007;29(4-5): 311-320.

68. Ohls RK. The use of erythropoietin in neonates. *Clin Perinatol*. 2000;27(3):681-696.

69. Ohls RK, Ehrenkranz RA, Wright LL, et al. Effects of early erythropoietin therapy on the transfusion requirements of preterm infants below 1250 grams birth weight: A multicenter, randomized, controlled trial. *Pediatrics*. 2001;108(4):934-942.

70. Haiden N, Schwindt J, Cardona F, et al. Effects of a combined therapy of erythropoietin, iron, folate, and vitamin B12 on the transfusion requirements of extremely low birth weight infants. *Pediatrics*. Nov 2006;118(5):2004-2013.

71. McPherson RJ, Demers EJ, Juul SE. Safety of high-dose recombinant erythropoietin in a neonatal rat model. *Neonatology*. 2007;91(1):36-43.

72. Ribatti D, Presta M, Vacca A, et al. Human erythropoietin induces a pro-angiogenic phenotype in cultured endothelial cells and stimulates neovascularization in vivo. *Blood*. 1999;93(8):2627-2636.

73. Chen J, Connor KM, Aderman CM, Willett KL, Aspegren OP, Smith LE. Suppression of retinal neovascularization by erythropoietin siRNA in a mouse model of proliferative retinopathy. *Invest Ophthalmol Vis Sci*. Mar 2009;50(3):1329-1335.

74. Chen J, Connor KM, Aderman CM, Smith LE. Erythropoietin deficiency decreases vascular stability in mice. *J Clin Invest*. Feb 2008;118(2):526-533.

75. Slusarski JD, McPherson RJ, Wallace GN, Juul SE. High-dose erythropoietin does not exacerbate retinopathy of prematurity in rats. *Pediatr Res*. 2009;66:625-630.

76. Cariou A, Claessens YE, Pene F, et al. Early high-dose erythropoietin therapy and hypothermia after out-of-hospital cardiac arrest: A matched control study. *Resuscitation*. Mar 2008;76(3):397-404.

77. Tseng MY, Hutchinson PJ, Richards HK, et al. Acute systemic erythropoietin therapy to reduce delayed ischemic deficits following aneurysmal subarachnoid hemorrhage: A Phase II randomized, double-blind, placebo-controlled trial. *J Neurosurg*. Jul 2009;111(1):171-180.

4

CHAPTER 5

Why, When, and How Should We Provide Red Cell Transfusions and Erythropoiesis-Stimulating Agents to Support Red Cell Mass in Neonates?

Robin K. Ohls, MD

Hospitalized neonates, especially preterm infants in the newborn intensive care unit (NICU), receive the greatest number of transfusions of any hospitalized patient group. During the first 2 weeks of life, when blood draws are frequent, approximately 50% of infants weighing less than 1000 g at birth (extremely low birthweight [ELBW]) will receive their first transfusion.[1] By the end of hospitalization, more than 80% of ELBW infants will receive at least one transfusion.[2-4] Although the numbers of transfusions given to preterm infants remain significant, these numbers have decreased over the past 20 years, primarily owing to the institution of restrictive transfusion guidelines.[5,6] This chapter will review the rationale for administering red cell transfusions, will summarize studies evaluating the efficacy of restrictive transfusion guidelines, will provide strategies to decrease red cell transfusions in neonates that include the use of erythropoiesis-stimulating agents (ESAs) such as erythropoietin and darbepoetin, and will propose guidelines for administering red cell transfusions and ESAs.

Oxygen Delivery and Consumption

The primary purpose of a red cell transfusion is to provide an immediate increase in oxygen delivery to the tissues. Oxygen delivery ($\dot{D}O_2$) can be quantified as the product of cardiac output (CO) and arterial oxygen content (CaO_2):

$$CO \, (dL/min) \times CaO_2 \, (mL/dL) = \dot{D}O_2 \, (mL/min)$$

Arterial oxygen content is determined by the hemoglobin concentration, the arterial oxygen saturation (%), the oxygen-carrying capacity of hemoglobin (mL/g × g/dL Hgb), and the solubility of oxygen in plasma (in mL/dL):

$$CaO_2 = (SaO_2 \times 1.34 \times [Hgb]) + (0.0031 \times PaO_2)$$

Improving cardiac output, hemoglobin concentration, or arterial oxygen saturation increases oxygen supply to tissues. If both cardiac output and oxygen saturation are maximized, the only way to deliver more oxygen to tissues is to increase hemoglobin concentrations by increasing red cell mass.

In young, healthy, conscious adults, the critical threshold below which oxygen delivery equals oxygen consumption occurs at less than 7.3 mL of oxygen per kg per minute.[7,8] Any further decrease in oxygen delivery results in a decrease in oxygen consumption and tissue hypoxia. The ratio of oxygen consumption to oxygen delivery, known as the *oxygen extraction ratio,* generally ranges from 0.15 to 0.33, meaning that the body consumes 15% to 33% of the oxygen delivered. As the oxygen extraction ratio reaches or exceeds 0.4, organ and cellular function can begin to deteriorate.[9] Neonates have the added burden of fetal hemoglobin, decreased concentrations of 2,3-diphosphoglycerate (2,3-DPG), and the increased demands of accelerated growth. Despite these added burdens, neonates have an enhanced ability to compensate for a gradual decrease in hemoglobin. For example, neonates born with hemoglobin concentrations less than 4 g/dL as a result of chronic, severe fetomaternal hemorrhage can appear well compensated for this level of hemoglobin, and oxygen delivery appears adequate in that the infant has a normal heart rate, normal perfusion, and no acidosis.[10]

Anemia occurs when the red cell mass is not adequate to meet the oxygen demands of the tissues; the current treatment for anemia is an infusion of red cells. Until the administration of artificial oxygen carriers becomes available,[11] the only way to immediately and significantly increase hemoglobin is by transfusing red cells. The difficulty comes in distinguishing a neonate who is anemic and requires immediate treatment with a red cell transfusion from a neonate with a low hematocrit. Although the risk of transmission of known infectious agents such as human immunodeficiency virus (HIV) and hepatitis B and C is relatively low in the blood supplied to U.S. hospitals, the risk of infectious agents newly identified in transfused blood such as West Nile virus, *Trypanosoma cruzi, Plasmodium* spp., and parvovirus B19, and of newly identified infectious agents such as avian flu, remains to be determined.[12-14] The decision to transfuse therefore should be made with deliberation, and caregivers should consistently (1) obtain consent and (2) document benefit for the neonate following the transfusion.

Development of Transfusion Guidelines

Over the past two decades, increasingly conservative transfusion guidelines have been evaluated and published. The ability of critically ill adult patients to adapt to lower hemoglobin values has been evaluated, and studies in adults and neonates have sought to determine the safety and efficacy of transfusion guidelines.

Adult Transfusion Studies

Studies evaluating transfusion guidelines in critically ill adults have changed transfusion practices significantly over the past decade.[15-19] The most significant of these was the Transfusion Requirements In Critical Care (TRICC) trial, a randomized, controlled clinical trial involving 838 critically ill adults.[15] Investigators sought to determine whether a restrictive approach to transfusions was equivalent to a liberal approach. The 30-day mortality was similar between groups (18.7% restrictive vs. 23.3% liberal); however, mortality rates were significantly lower in the restrictive group among those patients who were less acutely ill (8.7% vs. 16.1%), and in patients younger than 55 years of age. Mortality rates were similar between groups in patients with cardiovascular disease. The mortality rate during hospitalization was significantly lower in the restrictive group (22.2% vs. 28.1%; $P = 0.05$). The authors concluded that a restrictive strategy of red cell transfusion is at least as effective as a liberal transfusion strategy, and is possibly superior. Subsequent studies have reported similar findings,[16-19] resulting in the development of more conservative transfusion guidelines for adult intensive care unit (ICU) patients.

Pediatric Transfusion Studies

Few studies have been performed in the pediatric population, and none published to date were designed as randomized trials. Pediatric ICUs have relied on adult ICU study results, and caregivers have been cautious about implementing more restrictive transfusion guidelines. In one retrospective cohort analysis, children admitted to pediatric intensive care units (PICUs) with Hgb of 9 g/dL or less were evaluated.[20] Of 240 children evaluated, 131 were transfused and 109 were not. Transfusions were associated with increased days of oxygen use, mechanical ventilation, vasopressor infusion, PICU stay, and hospital stay. The authors concluded that red cell transfusions were associated with increased use of resources in critically ill children.

A prospective study was performed in Canada to determine the incidence of red cell transfusions in critically ill children.[21] Among 985 children, at least one transfusion was given in 139 cases (14%). The most common reasons for transfusions in these patients included hemoglobin less than 9.5 g/dL, cardiac disease, increased illness severity, and multiple-organ dysfunction.

Optimal hemoglobin concentrations remain to be determined in PICU patients, especially among those patients with cyanotic heart disease. Marked variability still exists among pediatric intensivists in terms of both hemoglobin thresholds for transfusions and the volume of transfusions ordered.[22] A multicenter study was performed in Canadian PICUs to evaluate the efficacy of restrictive versus liberal transfusion guidelines in critically ill pediatric patients ($n = 59$).[23] Investigators enrolled 637 stable, critically ill children with hemoglobin less than 9.5 g/dL within 7 days of PICU admission. Children were randomized to a transfusion threshold of 7 ($n = 320$) or 9 ($n = 317$) g/dL. Children in the lower hemoglobin threshold maintained hemoglobin 2.1 g/dL lower than the high hemoglobin threshold, with no difference in morbidities or mortality. Fewer children in the low threshold group received transfusions (48% vs. 98% in the higher threshold group). Investigators concluded that in stable, critically ill children, a hemoglobin threshold of 7 g/dL decreased transfusion requirements without increasing adverse outcomes. On the basis of these findings, it is possible that critically ill children and critically ill adults can tolerate hemoglobin ranges similarly.

Neonatal Transfusion Studies

Neonatal transfusion practices have changed significantly during the past three decades. In the 1970s and 1980s, standard transfusion practices in the NICU involved maintaining the infant's hematocrit at or above 40%. Care was taken to monitor the volume of blood removed through phlebotomy, and to replace that blood when losses reached 10 mL/kg. In most units in the United States, it was not until the mid-90s that transfusion practices began to change, in large part after publication of a randomized erythropoietin study performed in the United States by Kevin Shannon and colleagues.[24] These investigators were able to create guidelines for the restrictive use of PRBC transfusions for very low birthweight (VLBW) infants. Infants randomized to Epo treatment received fewer transfusions. The additional significance of this study can be seen in its creation and publication of these guidelines (Table 5-1).

As a result of this and other studies, the number of transfusions given to neonates in the United States, especially ELBW infants, decreased from an average of 10 transfusions per hospitalization to 4 transfusions per hospitalization by the year 2000.[5] Decreases in transfusions administered to preterm infants also occurred to an even greater degree in many countries throughout Europe.[6] The average number of transfusions given to similarly sized infants decreased to three per infant during an entire hospitalization. One reason for the lower number of transfusions was the volume of phlebotomy losses recorded. In numerous multicenter studies in which transfusion guidelines were employed and phlebotomy losses determined, the phlebotomy volume in the United States averaged 80 mL/kg, and losses in European and South American multicenter studies averaged 40 mL/kg.[2-4] Regardless of measures implemented to decrease transfusion needs, there will always be a correlation between blood removed for phlebotomy and blood transfused in critically ill ELBW infants, owing to the significantly small total blood volumes available.[23] This relationship between phlebotomy, transfusions, restrictive transfusion guidelines, and the use of red cell growth factors is graphically represented in Figure 5-1.

Table 5-1   RED CELL TRANSFUSION GUIDELINES FROM THE U.S. EPO TRIAL[24]

Do not transfuse for blood out alone.
Do not transfuse for low hematocrit alone.
Transfuse at Hct ≤35% for infants who are:
• Receiving >35% oxygen
• On CPAP or mechanical ventilation with mean airway pressure of 6–8 cm H_2O

Transfuse at Hct ≤30% for infants who are:
• Receiving any supplemental oxygen
• On CPAP or mechanical ventilation with mean airway pressure <6 cm H_2O
• Having significant apnea and bradycardia (>9 episodes in 12 hours or 2 episodes in 24 hours requiring bagging) while on therapeutic doses of methylxanthines
• Experiencing heart rates >180 beats/min or RR >80 breaths/min for 24 hours
• Experiencing weight gain <10 g/day over at least 4 days while receiving 100 kcal/kg/day
• Undergoing surgery

Transfuse at Hct ≤20% for infants who are:
• Asymptomatic with reticulocytes <100,000/μL

CPAP, Continuous positive airway pressure; *RR,* respiratory rate.

The Canadian Pediatric Society developed transfusion guidelines in 2002 that were more restrictive than the U.S. Epo study guidelines.[25] This occurred in part because of a significant public health scandal in which thousands of patients became infected with human immunodeficiency virus (HIV) and hepatitis C following transfusions distributed by the Canadian Red Cross.[26] Canadian Paediatric Society guidelines are shown in Table 5-2.

Three randomized studies evaluating the impact of restrictive transfusion guidelines for preterm infants have been published. The first, performed by Ellen Bifano and colleagues and published in abstract form,[27,28] evaluated 50 infants with birthweight of 650 to 1000 g. Infants were randomized from week 1 to 36 weeks post menstrual age (PMA) to a "high" hematocrit strategy (hematocrit maintained greater than 32%) or a "low" hematocrit strategy (hematocrit maintained less than or equal to 30%). Hematocrits were maintained in the designated range with transfusions and erythropoietin (Epo) in the high group, and with transfusions alone in the low group. Statistically significant differences in hematocrit were achieved by week 2 of the study and were maintained through 36 weeks PMA (Fig. 5-2).

No differences in baseline characteristics were observed between the two groups, and the average birthweight of all infants enrolled in the study was 805 ± 86 g in the low group and 837 ± 87 g in the high group (mean ± standard deviation [SD]; Table 5-3). At 36 weeks' PMA, comparison of the 22 infants evaluated in the low hematocrit group versus the 21 infants evaluated in the high hematocrit group revealed no difference in weight gain during hospitalization, the number of days

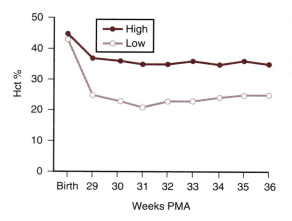

Figure 5-1 Differences in percent hematocrit (Hct) between infants randomized to the high hematocrit strategy *(solid circles)* and infants randomized to the low hematocrit strategy *(open circles)* were achieved by week 2 of the study, and were maintained through 36 weeks post menstrual age (PMA).

Table 5-2 CANADIAN PAEDIATRIC SOCIETY RECOMMENDATIONS FOR RBC TRANSFUSIONS[25]

Red blood cell (RBC) transfusions should be considered in newborn infants in the following specific clinical situations:
- Hypovolemic shock associated with acute blood loss
- Hematocrit between 30% and 35%, or hemoglobin between 10 and 12 g/dL, in extreme illness conditions for which RBC transfusion may improve oxygen delivery to vital organs
- Hematocrit between 20% and 30%, or hemoglobin between 6 and 10 g/dL, with the infant severely ill and/or on mechanical ventilation with compromised oxygen delivery
- Hematocrit falling below 20% or hemoglobin falling below 6 g/dL with absolute reticulocyte count of $100–150 \times 10^3/\mu L$ or less, suggesting low plasma concentration of erythropoietin, with the presence of the following clinical signs: poor weight gain, heart rate >180 beats/min, respiratory distress and increased oxygen needs, and lethargy

5

spent on a ventilator, or the total number of hospital days (see Table 5-3). At 1 year of age, both weight gain and head growth were similar between groups (see Table 5-3). In addition, no differences in neurodevelopmental impairments were noted between the two groups, including a subgroup of infants with hematocrit of 22% or less for longer than 3 weeks (Table 5-4). These investigators concluded that in ELBW infants, treatments aimed at maintaining hematocrit levels above 32% incurred additional cost with no demonstrable benefit. Moreover, restrictive transfusion policies were not associated with adverse outcomes.

In July 2005, Bell and colleagues published their randomized study on liberal versus restrictive guidelines for red cell transfusion in preterm infants.[29] In that study, 100 preterm infants at the University of Iowa with birthweight of 500 to 1300 g were randomized to a liberal or a restrictive transfusion strategy. Infants received transfusions only when their hematocrit dropped below the assigned value, and transfusion thresholds decreased with improving clinical status. The primary outcome was a difference in the number of transfusions. In addition, morbidities associated with prematurity and hospital days were determined.

No differences in baseline characteristics were reported between the two groups, and average birthweight for all enrolled infants was 956 g. Infants randomized to the restrictive strategy received fewer transfusions (an average of 2 fewer transfusions per patient) but had more episodes of apnea. In addition, infants in the restrictive strategy had a greater incidence of intraparenchymal brain hemorrhage or periventricular leukomalacia (PVL). Because of this finding, the authors concluded,

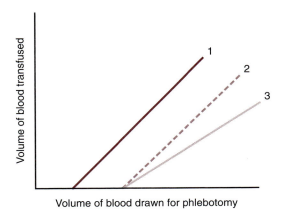

Figure 5-2 Relationship between phlebotomy losses and volume of blood transfused. Despite advances in neonatal transfusion medicine, there will always be a direct relationship between the amount of blood drawn for phlebotomy and the volume of blood returned in the form of a packed red blood cell (PRBC) transfusion. The solid line (line 1) represents the general relationship without the institution of transfusion guidelines. The dashed line (line 2) represents the improvement in decreased blood transfused following instituting restrictive transfusion guidelines. The hatched line (line 3) represents a further decrease in transfused blood volumes through the use of red cell growth factors.

Table 5-3 CHARACTERISTICS OF STUDY INFANTS AT THE START OF THE STUDY, AT 36 CORRECTED WEEKS, AND AT 1 YEAR CORRECTED AGE*[27,28]

	(n = 22)	(n = 21)
Study Entry		
Birth weight, g	805 ± 86	837 ± 8
Gestational age, wk	26 ± 2	26 ± 1
Male/Female	14/8	16/5
Inborn, n (%)	16 (73)	14 (67)
Antenatal steroids, n (%)	18 (82)	14 (67)
36 Weeks		
Weight gain, g/day	22 ± 11	20 ± 4
Linear growth, cm/wk	1.1 ± 0.6	0.9 ± 0.4
Head growth, cm/wk	1.1 ± 0.5	0.8 ± 0.2
Mechanical ventilation, n (%)	32 ± 14	27 ± 13
Supplemental oxygen, n (%)	9 (41)	9 (43)
Postnatal steroids, n (%)	16 (73)	16 (76)
IVH (any), n (%)	3 (14)	4 (19)
Grade III/IV, n (%)	0	1 (5)
One-Year Follow-Up		
Bayley Scales of Infant Development		
MDI	89 ± 16	86 ± 22
PDI	81 ± 19	84 ± 26
MDI or PDI <68, n (%)	6 (27)	6 (29)
Infant Neurologic International Battery		
Normal, n (%)	16 (73)	16 (76)
Suspect, n (%)	2 (9)	2 (10)
Abnormal, n (%)	4 (18)	3 (14)
Early Language Milestones		
Pass, n (%)	19 (86)	17 (81)
Fail, n (%)	3 (14)	4 (19)

IVH, Intraventricular hemorrhage; *MDI,* Mental Developmental Index; *PDI,* Psychomotor Developmental Index.
   *Values are means ± standard deviation (SD).

Table 5-4 OUTCOME OF INFANTS WITH HCT ≤22% FOR >3 WEEKS*[27,28]

	Hematocrit ≤22% (n = 11)	High Hematocrit (n = 21)
Growth		
Weight, percentile	21 ± 23	23 ± 26
Length, percentile	20 ± 19	20 ± 21
Head circumference, percentile	50 ± 22	41 ± 26
Bayley Scales of Infant Development		
Mental Developmental Index	96 ± 12	86 ± 22
Psychomotor Developmental Index	81 ± 19	84 ± 26

*Values are means ± standard deviation (SD).

"Although both transfusion programs were well tolerated, our findings of more frequent major adverse head ultrasound events in the restrictive RBC-transfusion group suggests that the practice of restrictive transfusions may be harmful to preterm infants." These findings were discussed in a series of letters to the editor following publication of the original study.[29-31] All discussions centered on the conclusions reached by the investigators and the need for further study to confirm those conclusions. Bell and colleagues have since that time published developmental follow-up data on 56 (33 liberally transfused infants, 23 restrictively transfused infants) of the original 100 infants, and have reported poorer performance in the liberally transfused group on measures of associative verbal fluency, visual memory, and reading.[33] In addition, magnetic resonance imaging of 44 of the 100 infants revealed reduced brain volumes in neonates randomized to liberal transfusion guidelines, especially among females.[34] The follow-up groups were not balanced in terms of gender, but results lessened some of the original study concerns about neurodevelopmental outcomes in the restrictive guidelines group.

Soon thereafter, Kirpalani and colleagues completed the Premature Infants in Need of Transfusion (PINT) study, which sought to determine whether ELBW infants transfused at lower hemoglobin thresholds versus higher thresholds have different rates of survival or morbidity at discharge.[35] This large, multicenter randomized clinical trial was designed to examine the impact of transfusion strategy on the incidence of a composite outcome—death, retinopathy of prematurity, bronchopulmonary dysplasia, or abnormal brain ultrasound—in ELBW infants. Four hundred fifty-one ELBW infants were randomized to one of two transfusion strategies defined by hemoglobin thresholds for red blood cell (RBC) transfusion. Thresholds varied with age and with the level of respiratory support needed.

No baseline differences were observed between the 223 infants randomized to the low transfusion threshold and the 228 infants randomized to the high transfusion threshold. The average birthweight of study participants was 770 g. Differences in hematocrit between groups were achieved by the first week of the study. The composite primary outcome was similar for both groups: 74% in the low group, 70% in the high group ($P = 0.25$). In particular, the incidence of brain injury detected by ultrasound was 12.6% in the low group and 16% in the high group ($P = 0.53$). The authors concluded that in ELBW infants, maintenance of a higher hemoglobin level caused more infants to receive transfusions but conferred little evidence of benefit. Infants in the PINT study were smaller and sicker, and had a greater risk of mortality and a greater risk of brain injury, than infants enrolled in the Iowa study, yet no difference in morbidities was noted between the two groups. Because the Iowa study was published before the PINT study, controversy arose regarding the benefits and risks of restrictive transfusion guidelines. Table 5-5 summarizes the neurologic findings reported in the three randomized studies reviewed. Follow-up of PINT infants revealed no differences in developmental outcomes

Table 5-5 SUMMARY OF NEUROLOGIC FINDINGS[27-29,35]

Study	Low Hematocrit Strategy	High Hematocrit Strategy
Bifano et al ($n = 50$)	($n = 22$)	($n = 21$)
IVH, n	0	1
Any NDI or growth deficiency, n (%)	12 (55)	10 (48)
Bell et al ($n = 100$)	($n = 28$)	($n = 24$)
IVH, n (%)	5 (10)	8 (16)
PVL, n (%)	4 (14)	0
PINT ($n = 451$)	($n = 175$)	($n = 188$)
"HUS brain injury," n (%)	22 (12.6)	30 (16)

between the two groups; however, post hoc analysis comparing Bayley Scales of Infant Development III (BSID III) cognitive scores revealed an increased number of infants in the restrictive group with cognitive scores lower than 80.[36]

One difficulty associated with interpreting results of transfusion studies in neonates is that those studies measured what infants received, rather than what they actually needed. Neonatal (as well as adult and pediatric) transfusion practices would greatly benefit from studies that generate transfusion guidelines based on need, by identifying a useful transfusion marker. This work remains to be accomplished; however, a few investigators have attempted to define parameters through direct or indirect oxygen delivery,[9] through resolution of signs of anemia,[37-39] or through changes in cardiovascular parameters as seen on echocardiography.[40-42] These studies underscore the difficulty involved in determining which infants should receive PRBCs, and what signs, symptoms, and laboratory measurements should be used to determine that need. In the meantime, implementation of more restrictive transfusion guidelines does serve to limit transfusions. Neonatal investigators with Intermountain Health Care implemented transfusion guidelines in their four largest NICUs, resulting in a decrease in more than 900 transfusions (from 4907 transfusions to 3923 transfusions) with no change in NICU demographics, major morbidities, length of hospital stay, or mortality rate.[43]

The search for an ideal measure or marker for the need for transfusion continues. Work performed by Weiskopf and colleagues evaluated the effects of acute isovolemic hemodilution on neurocognitive functioning in healthy adults, and determined that the P300 latency period reflected changes in oxygen.[44] Near-infrared spectroscopy (NIRS) has been evaluated as a tool that can be used to identify the need for transfusions in preterm infants.[45] Dani and colleagues used NIRS to study the effects of red blood cell (RBC) transfusions in preterm infants with hematocrit less than 25%, to assess whether thresholds for transfusions were appropriate for recognizing a clinical condition, permitting tissue oxygenation improvement.[46] The authors concluded that transfusions administered at chosen thresholds permitted an increase in cerebral, splanchnic, and renal oxygenation. An associated decreased in oxygen tissue extraction might have suggested that the transfusions were well timed for preventing tissue hypoxia,[47] or, alternatively, that they were administered too early and were theoretically pro-oxidant. As with transfusion guidelines, determining the level at which tissue oxygen levels are becoming harmfully low is still an issue, regardless of the sensitivity and specificity of NIRS measurements. Moreover, difficulties in reproducibility among preterm infants[48] and lack of direct measure of cerebral blood flow are some of the concerns preventing the standard use of this technique for NICUs interested in monitoring tissue oxygenation. Arterial spin labeling, or ASL, is a new technique that measures cerebral blood flow during magnetic resonance imaging, but its utility in preterm infants has not been evaluated.

Indications for Red Cell Transfusions

The indications for red cell transfusions in neonates differ primarily according to the rate of fall in hemoglobin, not according to any specific hemoglobin trigger. Neonates with significant acute blood loss require immediate volume resuscitation, but may or may not require a red cell transfusion. Term newborn infants may tolerate perinatal blood losses up to a third of their total blood volume. If acidosis persists in a neonate following volume resuscitation and adequate recirculation of the expanded blood volume, or if hemorrhage is ongoing, the neonate will likely benefit from a red cell transfusion. Infants with Hgb of 10 g/dL or greater following volume expansion may have adequate oxygen delivery to tissues, and may simply require iron supplementation to replace iron stores lost as a result of the hemorrhage.

Determining the volume of PRBCs to transfuse in a neonate with known acute hemorrhage can be performed using the following formula[49]: the volume of PRBCs to transfuse equals the desired rise in hematocrit times 1.6 times the infant's weight. Thus, a term, 3 kg infant with an acute drop in hematocrit at birth to 20% would need 120 mL PRBCs to achieve a desired hematocrit of 45%.

Caution should be taken in determining the transfusion needs of an infant born with a significantly low hematocrit, because it is vitally important to determine whether the infant experienced an acute fall in hematocrit, or a chronic fall in hematocrit. Infants with twin-twin transfusion syndrome or with chronic fetomaternal hemorrhage may be well compensated at birth, despite a hematocrit below 20%. An exchange transfusion should be considered in an infant with a low hematocrit in whom an immediate increase in oxygen delivery to tissues is necessary, because a significant increase in blood volume may result in the development of congestive heart failure.

Chronic Hemorrhage or a Chronic Drop in Hematocrit

All neonates undergo a natural adaptation to the extrauterine environment that allows them to compensate for a gradual drop in hematocrit. Immediately after birth, increased oxygenation results in systemic oxygen delivery that far exceeds the demand of the tissues for oxygen. Lacking the hypoxic stimulus, serum Epo concentrations fall and erythropoiesis rapidly declines. The hemoglobin concentration decreases over the first 2 to 3 months of life as the infant gains weight, remains stable over the next several weeks as erythropoiesis is reinitiated, then rises in the fourth to sixth month of life in response to a greater Epo stimulus.[50] Term infants tolerate these changes in hemoglobin and hematocrit without consequence. Preterm infants experience a drop in hemoglobin lower than that seen in term infants, and the decrease appears proportionate to the degree of prematurity. Hemoglobin concentrations between 7 and 8 g/dL occur commonly in preterm infants who have not undergone significant phlebotomy losses. Epo concentrations in anemic preterm infants are still significantly lower than those found in adults, given the degree of their anemia.[51,52] This normocytic, normochromic anemia, termed *anemia of prematurity*, commonly affects infants at or before 32 weeks' gestation and is the most common anemia seen in the neonatal period. Anemia of prematurity is not specifically responsive to the addition of iron, folate, or vitamin E, although these substrates (as well as B_{12}) are administered to infants receiving erythropoietin to maximize erythropoiesis.[4,53] Some infants may be asymptomatic from their low hematocrit; others demonstrate signs of anemia that are alleviated by transfusion. In preterm infants, determining when to transfuse can be problematic.[54]

Transfusions affect erythropoiesis in newborns, and the decision to transfuse should not be based on hemoglobin concentration alone. For infants who undergo exchange transfusion or multiple transfusions, both Epo concentrations and reticulocyte counts are lower at any given hemoglobin concentration. It is often assumed that oxygen delivery is decreased in newborns because of the presence of high-affinity fetal hemoglobin. In fact, a leftward shift in the hemoglobin-oxygen dissociation curve due to high levels of fetal hemoglobin might actually better maintain oxygen delivery during episodes of severe hypoxemia.[51,52]

When considering a transfusion in a preterm infant with a low hematocrit (not due to acute hemorrhage), the clinician should first determine whether the infant needs an immediate increase in oxygen to tissues (Fig. 5-3). If the answer is yes, then treatment consists of a transfusion of packed red cells. If no evidence suggests that an immediate increase in oxygen delivery is necessary, then treatment with red cell growth factors and appropriate substrates might be considered. Because the process of stimulating erythropoiesis requires at least a week to significantly impact the reticulocyte count, and may not appreciably increase the hemoglobin concentration during that time, the infant should continue to be observed for signs of anemia.

Red Cell Growth Factors to Expand Circulating Erythrocyte Volume

The in vitro response of erythroid progenitors from preterm infants led investigators to begin studies in the early 1990s to evaluate Epo administration to preterm infants. Since that time, numerous studies have been performed to evaluate the use of Epo to prevent and treat anemia of prematurity (reviewed elsewhere).[55] Epo is successful in stimulating erythropoiesis in preterm infants, and transfusion requirements are

5

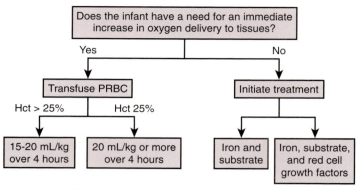

TREATMENT OF AN INFANT WITH A LOW HEMATOCRIT

Figure 5-3 An approach to transfusions in neonates. When evaluating an infant with a low hematocrit (not due to an acute hemorrhage), the clinician should first determine whether the infant is in immediate need of increased oxygen delivery. If this is the case, treatment consists of a packed red blood cell (PRBC) transfusion. If the infant's hematocrit (Hct) is greater than 25% and further phlebotomy losses are estimated to be minimal, a volume of 15 mL/kg can be administered. All other infants receive 20 mL/kg. If it is determined that the infant does not need an immediate increase in oxygen delivery, treatment with red cell growth factors such as erythropoietin and with substrates such as iron, vitamin E, folate, and B_{12} can be instituted.

decreased.[56] Success rates in preventing transfusions in preterm infants are dependent in part on transfusion criteria and the frequency of phlebotomy.[57] Side effects of Epo in published randomized controlled trials (RCTs) have not differed from placebo, although retrospective analyses have suggested a relationship between Epo administration and retinopathy of prematurity (ROP).[58] The development of ROP in preterm infants is likely multifactorial,[59-61] and evidence in some adult studies suggests protective effects of Epo in diabetic retinopathy.[62-64] Prevention of ROP is a significant challenge faced by neonatal caregivers, because more and more babies born ELBW are surviving with morbidities.[65] The relationship between retinal development and elevated vitreal Epo concentrations was first reported by our laboratory,[66] and in vitro investigations continue.

A modified version of Epo, known as darbepoetin alfa (Darbe), was developed by Amgen in 1998.[67,68] Darbe has a longer serum half-life than Epo in adults and preterm infants,[69] allowing increased dosage intervals to be used. Studies using Darbe once a week to once every 3 weeks (as compared with three doses per week of Epo) in adult oncology and end-stage renal failure patients have demonstrated hemoglobin increases equivalent to those of Epo.[70-73] Side effects are similar to Epo, and the production of anti-Epo antibodies has not been reported.[74] Some hospital formularies are moving from one ESA, Epo, to the newer, long-acting ESA, Darbe.

Initial enthusiasm for Epo came from its effect on erythropoiesis in premature infants; however, over the past 10 years, in vitro, animal, and adult clinical studies have suggested that Epo plays a potentially important role in angiogenesis and neurogenesis in the central nervous system.[75,76] It is now known that Epo and Epo receptors are present in nonhematopoietic developing neural tissue in animals and in humans.[76-79] Similar to the mechanism leading to erythropoiesis, Epo binds to its receptor in nonhematopoietic tissues, activating cellular mechanisms that include cell maturation, division, and inhibition of apoptosis.[79,80]

Studies evaluating Epo in adult and neonatal animal models report the prevention of hypoxic-ischemic brain injury, a decrease in infarction volume, reduced vasoconstriction, decreased neuronal apoptosis, and decreased neurologic deterioration in animals treated with high doses of Epo.[80-86] Clinical studies are currently under way to evaluate the long-term neurodevelopment of preterm infants treated with ESAs.

A minimal number of clinical studies evaluating Darbe administration to preterm infants have been published, and randomized trials are ongoing. In contrast,

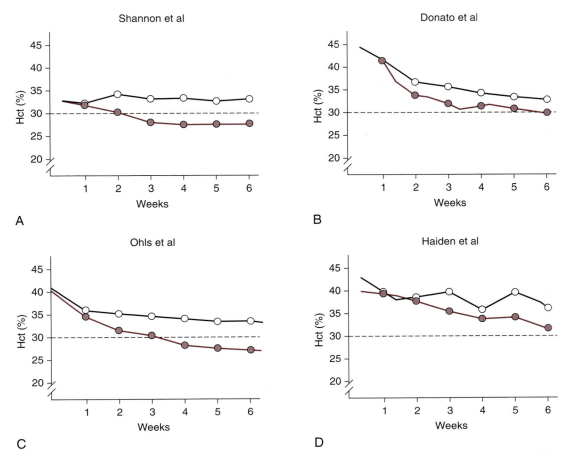

Figure 5-4 Differences in hematocrit between Epo-treated (open circles) and placebo/control (solid circles) infants in four recent randomized, masked studies. In all four studies, hematocrit values averaged 5 percentage points higher among Epo-treated infants, despite restrictive transfusion guidelines and fewer transfusions.

numerous RCTs evaluating Epo administration to preterm infants have consistently shown evidence of increased erythropoiesis and a decrease in transfusions.[55]

A consistent finding in the largest RCTs has been an elevation in hematocrit among Epo-treated infants compared with placebo/controls (Fig. 5-4), despite the implementation of strict transfusion guidelines aimed at maintaining hematocrits in a similar range. For those neonatal practitioners electing to maintain hematocrits at higher levels, the use of Epo can gain a "buffer" of 4% to 6% hematocrit points, decreasing the number of transfusions given. This may benefit preterm infants in a number of ways, given recent studies that have reported associations between RBC transfusions and necrotizing enterocolitis,[87] and between RBC transfusions and intraventricular hemorrhage.[88] Guidelines for Epo administration to preterm infants as part of clinical care are presented in Table 5-6.

Selection of Red Cell Products

Transfusions in neonates should be given as a means to rapidly increase oxygen delivery to tissues. Red cell transfusions may be given under acute settings, such as during resuscitation of an exsanguinated infant at delivery, or under more chronic settings, such as in an infant in the NICU with a hemoglobin concentration that does not deliver adequate oxygen to tissues. In addition, red cell transfusions are used for severe hemolytic disease of the newborn, in the form of a double volume exchange transfusion, and are used to prime extracorporeal membrane oxygenation

Table 5-6 RECOMMENDATIONS FOR EPO AND NUTRITIONAL SUPPLEMENT ADMINISTRATION IN NEONATES

Epo Administration

Recommendations for infants receiving total parenteral nutrition (TPN):
- 200 U/kg/day, added to TPN
- Begin dosing when infant is receiving protein.
- IV administration (if not added to TPN) to run over at least 4 hours; use protein-containing solution to dilute

Recommendations for subcutaneous administration:
- 400 U/kg given three times a week
- Begin dosing at 7–10 days of life, or when IV access is gone
- For preterm infants being discharged, or for infants with late anemia due to Rh or ABO isoimmunization, a dose of 1000 U/kg SC once a week can be used to enhance erythropoiesis.

Recommendations for length of treatment:
- Continue dosing until 34–36 weeks' corrected gestational age.
- Epo is contraindicated in infants with thromboembolic disease, hypertension, or seizures

Iron and Vitamin Supplementation for Infants Receiving Epo

Iron:
- Iron dextran, 3–5 mg/kg once a week added to TPN solution if available (1 mg/kg/day is acceptable; check ferritin after 2 weeks of dosing)
- Ferrous sulfate 4–6 mg/kg/day, depending on formula (4 mg/kg/day) vs. EBM (6 mg/kg/day)

Vitamin E:
- 25 IU/day PO

Folate:
- 50 micrograms/day PO

B_{12} (if available):
- 21 micrograms/wk SC

(ECMO) circuits. Finally, red cell transfusions are often used during neonatal surgery, especially cardiac surgery.

In the setting of severe acute hemorrhage when a red cell transfusion can be lifesaving, O negative "trauma" PRBCs can be used. Type O negative whole blood will contain antibodies directed against the A or B blood group, and will also contain leukocytes. This approach should be used only if the infant's blood type is known to be O negative. Matched whole blood has been used during major neonatal and pediatric cardiac surgery. In early studies, whole blood was shown to be beneficial in decreasing postsurgical bleeding.[89] Recent studies have reported no benefit of whole blood over reconstituted blood.[90,91] Infants receiving reconstituted blood spent less time in intensive care and had a smaller cumulative fluid balance.[92]

Double Volume Exchange Transfusion

For infants requiring a double volume exchange transfusion to treat hemolytic disease of the newborn, whole blood is not recommended. Blood type O Rh negative washed PRBCs should be reconstituted with AB Rh positive plasma to achieve a hematocrit of 45% to 50%. In this way, administration of antibodies directed against the infant's red cells (in the form of remaining plasma associated with O negative blood) is reduced to the greatest degree.

The volume of blood exchanged can be calculated on the basis of a total blood volume of 85 mL/kg body weight. Thus, an infant weighing 2.6 kg would require a total volume as follows:

$$2.6 \text{ kg} \times 85 \text{ mL/kg} = 221 \text{ mL}$$

In many neonatal units, cytomegalovirus (CMV)-negative PRBCs are available for all infants. CMV-negative PRBCs should be used in specific populations, such as infants awaiting or undergoing transplant, immunocompromised infants, infants receiving in utero transfusions, and preterm infants born to CMV-negative mothers.

Leukoreduction, Stored Blood, and Irradiation

Leukoreduced PRBCs should be used in neonates to decrease the spread of infection, and to decrease the possibility of microchimerism,[93] the addition of a small amount of foreign genetic material in addition to the host's genetic material. The shelf life of PRBCs can be as long as 42 days, and there does not appear to be a significant difference in red cells transfused before 7 to 10 days compared with red cells transfused after 21 days.[94,95] Studies comparing potassium concentrations in blood stored for various periods of time show no significant increase in blood stored longer than 21 days compared with blood stored less than 7 days.[95] Many blood banks will also irradiate PRBCs just before neonatal transfusion. Irradiation of RBCs is recommended for fetuses receiving in utero transfusions, for immunocompromised infants, and for infants receiving directed donor blood from a first- or second-degree relative. Irradiation may reduce the rare complication of graft-versus-host disease.

Cord Blood and Delayed Cord Clamping

Cord blood collection has been studied as a form of "autologous" donation, but most NICUs, labor and delivery services, and blood banks are not prepared for collection and storage of neonatal cord blood. An alternative to cord blood collection that reduces erythrocyte transfusions to ill neonates is delayed clamping of the umbilical cord. It is possible to promote placental transfer of blood to preterm infants by delaying clamping of the umbilical cord for 30 seconds. In fact, transfer of 10 to 15 mL/kg body weight can be expected using this method.[96] In a randomized trial by Mercer and colleagues, this maneuver of delayed cord clamping among infants weighing less than 1500 g at birth resulted in less intraventricular hemorrhage and less late-onset sepsis.[97] Even a delay of 30 seconds results in improved iron status,[98] fewer transfusions,[99] and perhaps improved neurodevelopmental outcomes.[97]

Guidelines to Decrease Transfusions in ELBW Infants and Suggested Transfusion Guidelines

When a family has indicated a wish to avoid transfusions in their infant, and a premature birth is anticipated, an action plan can be created to optimize the preterm infant's chances of avoiding transfusion. Without the use of ESAs, a majority (85% to 90%) of ELBW infants receive transfusions. However, the percentage of ELBW infants remaining untransfused can be maximized to near 50%. Successful avoidance of transfusions can be increased through the use of such measures as delayed cord clamping, immediate red cell growth factor and iron therapy, judicious laboratory testing using micro sampling, and a restrictive transfusion policy. Table 5-7 shows suggested guidelines to optimize the ELBW infant's chances of remaining transfusion free. Most important, these measures can be identified and a plan created prenatally with the family. In addition, neonatologists can establish a relationship with the family and can discuss their NICU transfusion thresholds. This is much better done proactively, so that the need for last minute court orders to transfuse can be minimized.

Transfusion guidelines currently used by several NICUs (all located at or above 5000 feet elevation) are provided (Table 5-8). These guidelines have been implemented at the University of New Mexico since 2004. Similar to findings reported by Baer and colleagues,[88] no differences from previous years in ELBW outcomes have been recorded, and the number of transfusions has decreased.

Summary

Previously, limitations in knowledge of the pathophysiology of anemia contributed to unfounded and liberal transfusion practices in preterm infants and to uncertain risk-benefit ratios.[1] Over the past two decades, researchers have explored an array of strategies to minimize transfusions in the most critically ill. Currently, the ideal test for transfusion need does not exist. Studies on the efficacy and outcomes of restrictive transfusion guidelines in adults, children, and neonates should and will

5

Table 5-7 SUGGESTED GUIDELINES TO REDUCE TRANSFUSIONS IN ELBW INFANTS

- Discuss delayed cord clamping with the obstetric team and document the plan in the mother's chart. The infant should be held below the placenta while the cord is intact for 30–45 seconds.
- Initiate erythropoietin (Epo) treatment during the first day of life. This can be achieved by administering a subcutaneous injection of 400 U/kg Epo, or by adding 200 U/kg to a protein-containing intravenous solution (such as a 5% dextrose solution with 2% amino acids), to run over 4–24 hours.
- Administer parenteral iron, 3 mg/kg once a week or 0.5 mg/kg/day (added to TPN or administered IV over 4–6 hours), until the infant is tolerating adequate volume feedings, then administer oral iron at 6 mg/kg/day.
- Use in-line blood sampling or use micro sampling devices such as the I-Stat, to decrease the volume need for each lab.
- Remove central lines as soon as possible
- Order labs judiciously (e.g., no "blood gas q 6 hours" orders), and reconsider the need for "standard" or "routine" labs, such as weekly complete blood counts, daily blood gases, or daily chemistry panels.
- Monitor phlebotomy losses daily.
- Communicate the lowest hemoglobin or hematocrit that will be tolerated for a variety of typical clinical scenarios and days of age, such as (1) infant is on 100% oxygen, significant ventilator support, blood pressure support, and has a metabolic acidosis; (2) infant is on minimal ventilator support or CPAP; (3) infant is receiving enteral feeds and is requiring oxygen; or (4) infant is on full feeds, is growing well, no oxygen support. Consider these scenarios if the infant is younger than 2 weeks of age, is 2–4 weeks of age, or is older than 4 weeks of age.

CPAP, Continuous positive airway pressure; *ELBW,* extremely low birthweight.

Table 5-8 TRANSFUSION GUIDELINES

- A central hematocrit should be obtained on admission. No further hematocrits should be obtained unless specifically ordered.
- Outside of rounds, transfusions generally should be considered only if acute blood loss ≥10% is associated with symptoms of decreased oxygen delivery, or if significant hemorrhage >20% total blood volume occurs.
- In term and preterm infants, a transfusion should be considered if an immediate need for increased oxygen delivery to tissues is clinically suspected.
- Infants should be transfused with 20 mL/kg packed red blood cells (PRBCs) unless Hct is >29%. 20 mL/kg volume could also be used if significant phlebotomy losses are anticipated in smaller infants with Hct >29%.
- For infants receiving Epo, the previous guidelines should be considered regarding the rate of decrease in hemoglobin or hematocrit, the infant's reticulocyte count, the postnatal day of age, the need for supplemental oxygen, and the overall stability of the infant.
- Central measurements of hemoglobin or hematocrit are preferred; alternatively, heel-stick measurements may be obtained after the heel is warmed adequately. An infant meeting the criteria below should not automatically be transfused. Transfusions can be considered for the following:
  1. For infants **requiring moderate or significant mechanical ventilation**, defined as mean airway pressure (MAP) >8 cm H_2O and fraction of inspired oxygen (FiO_2) >0.40 on a conventional ventilator, or MAP >14 and FiO_2 >0.40 on high-frequency ventilator; transfusions *can be considered* if the **hematocrit is ≤30% (Hgb ≥10 g/dL)**.
  2. For infants **requiring minimal mechanical ventilation**, defined as MAP ≤8 cm H_2O and/or FiO_2 ≤0.40, or MAP <14 and/or FiO_2 <0.40 on high frequency; transfusions *can be considered* if the **hematocrit is ≤25% (hemoglobin ≤8 g/dL)**.
  3. For infants on supplemental oxygen who are **not requiring mechanical ventilation**, transfusions *can be considered* if the **hematocrit is ≤20% (hemoglobin ≤7 g/dL)**, and one or more of the following is present:
     - ≥24 hours of tachycardia (heart rate >180) or tachypnea (respiratory rate [RR] >60)
     - Doubling of the oxygen requirement from the previous 48 hours
     - Lactate ≥2.5 mEq/L or an acute metabolic acidosis (pH <7.20)
     - Weight gain <10 g/kg/day over the previous 4 days while receiving ≥120 kcal/kg/day
     - If the infant will undergo major surgery within 72 hours
  4. For infants **without any symptoms**, transfusions *can be considered* if the **hematocrit is ≤18% (hemoglobin ≤6 g/dL)** associated with an absolute reticulocyte count <100,000 cells/μL (<2%).

continue. The use of ESAs in combination with instituting transfusion guidelines acceptable to clinicians offers the greatest promise in utilizing blood products judiciously and wisely, while optimizing the care of critically ill neonates.

Acknowledgment

I wish to thank Erin Austin for her assistance in revising this chapter.

References

1. Bifano EM, Curran TR. Minimizing donor blood exposure in the neonatal intensive care unit. Current trends and future prospects. *Clin Perinatol.* 1995;22:657-669.
2. Maier RF, Obladen M, Muller-Hansen I, et al. Early treatment with erythropoietin beta ameliorates anemia and reduces transfusion requirements in infants with birth weights below 1000 g. *J Pediatr.* 2002;141:8-15.
3. Donato H, Vain N, Rendo P, et al. Effect of early versus late administration of human recombinant erythropoietin on transfusion requirements in premature infants: results of a randomized, placebo-controlled, multicenter trial. *Pediatrics.* 2000;105:1066-1072.
4. Ohls RK, Ehrenkranz RA, Das A, et al; National Institute of Child Health and Human Development Neonatal Research Network. Neurodevelopmental outcome and growth at 18 to 22 months' corrected age in extremely low birth weight infants treated with early erythropoietin and iron. *Pediatrics.* 2004;114:1287-1291.
5. Widness JA, Seward VJ, Kromer IJ, et al. Changing patterns of red blood cell transfusion in very low birth weight infants. *J Pediatr.* 1996;129:680-687.
6. Maier RF, Sonntag J, Walka MM, et al. Changing practices of red blood cell transfusions in infants with birth weights less than 1000 g. *J Pediatr.* 2000;136:220-224.
7. Lieberman JA, Weiskopf RB, Kelley SD, et al. Critical oxygen delivery in conscious humans is less than 7.3 mL O2 × kg(−1) × min(−1). *Anesthesiology.* 2000;92:407-413.
8. Madjdpour C, Spahn DR, Weiskopf RB. Anemia and perioperative red blood cell transfusion: A matter of tolerance. *Crit Care Med.* 2006;34:S102-108.
9. Alverson DC. The physiologic impact of anemia in the neonate. *Clin Perinatol.* 1995;22:609-625.
10. Willis C, Forman Jr CS. Chronic massive fetomaternal hemorrhage: a case report. *Obstet Gynecol.* 1988;71:459-461.
11. Inayat MS, Bernard AC, Gallicchio VS, et al. Oxygen carriers: a selected review. *Transfus Apher Sci.* 2006;34:25-32.
12. Pealer LN, Marfin AA, Petersen LR, et al. Transmission of West Nile virus through blood transfusion in the United States in 2002. *N Engl J Med.* 2003;349:1236-1245.
13. Dodd RY. Emerging infections, transfusion safety, and epidemiology. *N Engl J Med.* 2003;349:1205.
14. Alter HJ, Stamer SL, Dodd RY. Emerging infectious diseases that threaten the blood supply. *Semin Hematol.* 2007;44:32-41.
15. Hebert PC, Wells G, Blajchman MA, et al. A multicenter, randomized, controlled clinical trial of transfusion requirements in critical care. Transfusion Requirements in Critical Care Investigators, Canadian Critical Care Trials Group. *N Engl J Med.* 1999;340:409-417.
16. Napolitano LM, Corwin HL. Efficacy of red blood cell transfusion in the critically ill. *Crit Care Clin.* 2004;20:255-268.
17. Chant C, Wilson G, Friedrich JO. Anemia, transfusion, and phlebotomy practices in critically ill patients with prolonged ICU length of stay: a cohort study. *Crit Care.* 2006;10:R140.
18. Croce MA, Tolley EA, Claridge JA, Fabian TC. Transfusions result in pulmonary morbidity and death after a moderate degree of injury. *J Trauma.* 2005;59:19-23.
19. Malone DL, Dunne J, Tracy JK, et al. Blood transfusion, independent of shock severity, is associated with worse outcome in trauma. *J Trauma.* 2003;54:898-905.
20. Goodman AM, Pollack MM, Patel KM, et al. Pediatric red blood cell transfusions increase resource use. *J Pediatr.* 2003;142:123-127.
21. Armano R, Gauvin F, Ducruet T, et al. Determinants of red blood cell transfusions in a pediatric critical care unit: a prospective, descriptive epidemiological study. *Crit Care Med.* 2005;33:2637-2644.
22. Nahum E, Ben-Ari J, Schonfeld T. Blood transfusion policy among European pediatric intensive care physicians. *J Intensive Care Med.* 2004;19:38-43.
23. Lacroix J, Hébert PC, Hutchison JS, et al. Transfusion strategies for patients in pediatric intensive care units. *N Engl J Med.* 2007;356:1609-1619.
24. Shannon KM, Keith 3rd JF, Mentzer WC, et al. Recombinant human erythropoietin stimulates erythropoiesis and reduces erythrocyte transfusions in very low birth weight preterm infants. *Pediatrics.* 1995;95:1-8.
25. Red blood cell transfusions in newborn infants: Revised guidelines. *Paediatr Child Health.* 2002;7:553-566.
26. Kondro W. Canadian Red Cross found negligent. *Lancet.* 1997;350:1154.
27. Bifano EM. The effect of hematocrit (HCT) level on clinical outcomes in Extremely Low Birthweight (ELBW) infants. *Pediatric Research.* 2001;49:311A.
28. Bifano EM, Bode MM, D'Eugenio DB. Prospective randomized trial of high vs. low hematocrit in Extremely Low Birth Weight (ELBW) infants: one year growth and neurodevelopmental outcome. *Pediatric Research.* 2002;51:325A.

5

29. Bell EF, Strauss RG, Widness JA. Randomized trial of liberal versus restrictive guidelines for red blood cell transfusion in preterm infants. *Pediatrics*. 2005;115:1685-1691.
30. Boedy RF, Mathew OP. Letter to editor: Randomized trial of liberal versus restrictive guidelines for red blood cell transfusion in preterm infants. *Pediatrics*. 2005;116:1048-1049.
31. Murray N, Roberts I, Stanworth S. Letter to editor: Red blood cell transfusion in neonates. *Pediatrics*. 2005;116:1609.
32. Swamy RS, Embleton ND. Letter to editor: Red blood cell transfusions in preterm infants: is there a difference between restrictive and liberal criteria? *Pediatrics*. 2005;115:257-258.
33. McCoy TE, Conrad AL, Richman LC, Lindgren SD, Noupoulos PC, Bell EF. Neurocognitive profiles of preterm infants randomly assigned to lower or higher hematocrit thresholds for transfusion. *Child Neuropsychol*. 2011;17:347-367.
34. Nopoulos PC, Conrad AL, Bell EF, et al. Long-term Outcome of Brain Structure in Premature Infants: Effects of Liberal vs. Restricted Red Blood Cell Transfusions. *Arch Pediatr Adolesc Med*. 2011 May: 165;443-450.
35. Kirpalani H, Whyte RK, Andersen C. The Premature Infants in Need of Transfusion (PINT) study: a randomized, controlled trial of a restrictive (low) versus liberal (high) transfusion threshold for extremely low birth weight infants. *J Pediatr*. 2006;149:301-307.
36. Whyte RK, Kirpalani H, Asztalos EV, et al. Neurodevelopmental outcome of extremely low birth weight infants randomly assigned to restrictive or liberal hemoglobin thresholds for blood transfusion. *Pediatrics*. 2009 Jan:123;207-213.
37. Wardle SP, Garr R, Yoxall CW, Weindling AM. A pilot randomised controlled trial of peripheral fractional oxygen extraction to guide blood transfusions in preterm infants. *Arch Dis Child Fetal Neonatal Ed*. 2002;86:F22-27.
38. Bifano EM, Smith F, Borer J. Relationship between determinants of oxygen delivery and respiratory abnormalities in preterm infants with anemia. *J Pediatr*. 1992;120:292-296.
39. Izraeli S, Ben-Sira L, Harell D, et al. Lactic acid as a predictor for erythrocyte transfusion in healthy preterm infants with anemia of prematurity. *J Pediatr*. 1993;122:629-631.
40. Bard H, Fouron JC, Chessex P, Widness JA. Myocardial, erythropoietic, and metabolic adaptations to anemia of prematurity in infants with bronchopulmonary dysplasia. *J Pediatr*. 1998; 132:630-634.
41. Bohler T, Janecke A, Linderkamp O. Blood transfusion in late anemia of prematurity: effect on oxygen consumption, heart rate, and weight gain in otherwise healthy infants. *Infusionsther Transfusionsmed*. 1994;21:376-679.
42. Alkalay AL, Galvis S, Ferry DA, et al. Hemodynamic changes in anemic premature infants: Are we allowing the hematocrits to fall too low? *Pediatrics*. 2003;112:838-845.
43. Baer VL, Henry E, Lambert DK, et al. Implementing a program to improve compliance with neonatal intensive care unit transfusion guidelines was accompanied by a reduction in transfusion rate: a pre-post analysis within a multihospital health care system. *Transfusion*. 2011;51:264-269.
44. Weiskopf RB, Toy P, Hopf HW, et al. Acute isovolemic anemia impairs central processing as determined by P300 latency. *Clin Neurophysiol*. 2005;116:1028-1032.
45. Soul JS, Taylor GA, Wypij D, Duplessis AJ, et al. Noninvasive detection of changes in cerebral blood flow by near-infrared spectroscopy in a piglet model of hydrocephalus. *Pediatr Res*. 2000; 48:445-449.
46. Dani C, Pratesi S, Fontanelli G, Barp J, Bertini G. Blood transfusions increase cerebral, splanchnic, and renal oxygenation in anemic preterm infants. *Transfusion*. 2010;50;1220-1226. [Epub 2010 Jan 22.]
47. Bailey SM, Hendricks-Munoz KD, Wells JT, Mally P. Packed red blood cell transfusion increases regional cerebral and splanchnic tissue oxygen saturation in anemic symptomatic preterm infants. *Am J Perinatol*. 2010;27:445-453. [Epub 2010 Jan 22].
48. Menke J, Voss U, Moller G, Jorch G. Reproducibility of cerebral near infrared spectroscopy in neonates. *Biol Neonate*. 2003;83:6-11.
49. Morris KP, Naqvi N, Davies P, et al. A new formula for blood transfusion volume in the critically ill. *Arch Dis Child*. 2005;90:724-728.
50. Kling PJ, Schmidt RL, Roberts RA, et al. Serum erythropoietin levels during infancy: associations with erythropoiesis. *J Pediatr*. 1996;128:791-796.
51. Brown MS, Garcia JF, Phibbs RH, et al. Decreased response of plasma immunoreactive erythropoietin to "available oxygen" in anemia of prematurity. *J Pediatr*. 1984;105:793-798.
52. Stockman JA, Graeber JE, Clark DA, et al. Anemia of prematurity: Determinants of the erythropoietin response. *J Pediatr*. 1984;105:786-792.
53. Nadja H, Jens S, Francesco C, et al. Effects of a Combined Therapy of Erythropoietin, Iron, Folate, and Vitamin B12 on the Transfusion Requirements of Extremely Low Birth Weight Infants. *Pediatrics*. 2006;118:2004-2013.
54. Keyes WG, Donohue PK, Spivak JL, et al. Assessing the need for transfusion of premature infants and the role of hematocrit, clinical signs, and erythropoietin level. *Pediatrics*. 1989;84:412-417.
55. Bishara N, Ohls RK. Current Controversies in the Management of Anemia of Prematurity. *Seminars in Perinatology.*, 2009;33:29-34.
56. Ohls RK. Human recombinant erythropoietin in prevention and treatment of anemia of prematurity. *Paediatr Drugs*. 2002;4:111-121.
57. Ohls RK. Erythropoietin treatment in extremely low birth weight infants: blood in versus blood out. *J Pediatr*. 2002;140:3-6.
58. Ohlsson A, Aher SM. Early erythropoietin for preventing red blood cell transfusion in preterm and/or low birth weight infants. *Cochrane Database Syst Rev*. 2006;3:CD004863.

59. Liu PM, Fang PC, Huang CB, et al. 2005. Risk factors of retinopathy of prematurity in premature infants weighing less than 1600 g. *Am J Perinatol*. 2005;22:115-120.
60. Akkoyun I, Oto S, Yilmaz G, et al. Risk Factors in the development of mild and severe retinopathy of prematurity. *J AAPOS*. 2006;10:449-453.
61. Flynn JT, Bacalari E. On supplemental therapeutic oxygen for prethreshold retinopathy of prematurity (STOP-ROP), a randomized, controlled trial. I: Primary outcomes. *J AAPOS*. 2000;4:65-66.
62. Grimm C, Wenzel A, Acar N, Keller S, Seeliger M, Gassmann M. Hypoxic preconditioning and erythropoietin protect retinal neurons from degeneration. *Adv Exp Med Biol*. 2006;588:119-131.
63. Becerra SP, Amaral J. Erythropoietin—an endogenous retinal survival factor. *N Engl J Med*. 2002;347:1968-1970.
64. Fisher JW. Erythropoietin: physiology and pharmacology update. *Exp Biol Med*. 2003;228:1-14.
65. DiBiasie A. Evidence-based review of retinopathy of prematurity prevention in VLBW and ELBW infants. *Neonatal Netw*. 2006;25:393-403.
66. Patel S, Rowe MJ, Winters SA, McConaghy S, Ohls RK. Elevated Erythropoietin mRNA and protein concentrations in the developing human eye. *Pediatr Res*. 2008;63:394-397.
67. Egrie JC, Browne JK. Development and characterization of novel erythropoiesis stimulate protein (NESP). *British J Cancer*. 2001;84(Supplement 1):3-10.
68. Heatherington AC, Schuller J, Mercer AJ. Pharmacokinetics of novel erythropoiesis stimulating protein (NESP) in cancer patients: preliminary report. *British J Cancer*. 2001;84(Supplement 1):11-16.
69. Warwood TL, Ohls RK, Lambert DK, et al. Intravenous administration of Darbepoetin to NICU patients. *J Perinatol*. 2006;26:296-300.
70. Locatelli G, Olivares J, Walker R, et al. Novel erythropoiesis stimulating protein for treatment of anemia in chronic renal insufficiency. *Kidney Intl*. 2001;60:741-747.
71. Glaspy J, Jadeja JS, Justice G, et al. Darbepoetin alpha given every 1 or 2 weeks alleviates anemia associated with cancer chemotherapy. *British J Cancer*. 2002;87:268-276.
72. Allon M, Kleinman K, Walczyk M, et al. Pharmacokinetics and pharmacodynamics of Darbepoetin alpha and epoetin alpha in patients undergoing dialysis. *Clin Pharmacol Ther*. 2002;72:546-555.
73. Ohls RK, Dai A. Long acting erythropoietin: clinical studies and potential uses in neonates. *Clinics Perinatol*. 2004;31:77-89.
74. Bennett CL, Luminari S, Nissenson AR, et al. Pure red-cell aplasia and epoetin therapy. *N Engl J Med*. 2004 Sep 30;351:1403-1408.
75. Carlini RG, Reyes AA, Rothstein M. Recombinant human erythropoietin stimulates angiogenesis in vitro. *Kidney Int*. 1995;47:740-745.
76. Shingo T, Sorokan ST, Shimazaki T, Weiss S. Erythropoietin regulates the in vitro and in vivo production of neuronal progenitors by mammalian forebrain neural stem cells. *J Neurosci*. 2001 Dec 15;21:9733-9743.
77. Dame C, Bartmann P, Wolber E, Fahnenstich H, Hofmann D, Fandrey J. Erythropoietin gene expression in different areas of the developing human central nervous system. *Dev Brain Res*. 2000;125:69-74.
78. Sirén A-L, Knerlich F, Poser W, Gleitner CH, Brück W, Ehrenreich H. Erythropoietin and erythropoietin receptor in human ischemic/hypoxic brain. *Acta Neuropathol*. 2001;101:271-276.
79. Chong ZZ, Kang J-Q, Maiese K. Erythropoietin fosters both intrinsic and extrinsic neuronal protection through modulation of microglia, Akt 1, Bad, and caspase-mediated pathways. *British Journal of Pharmacology*. 2003;138:1107-1118.
80. Wen TC, Sadamoto Y, Tanaka J, et al. Erythropoietin protects neurons against chemical hypoxia and cerebral ischemic injury by upregulating Bcl-xL expression. *J Neurosci Res*. 2002 Mar 15; 67(6):795-803.
81. Erbavraktar S, Grasso G, Sfacteria A, Xie QW, Coleman T, et al. Asialoerythropoietin is a nonerythropoietic cytokine with broad neuroprotective activity in vivo. *Proc Natl Acad Sci U S A*. 2003 May 27; 100(11):6741-6746.
82. Grasso G, Buemi M, Alafaci C, Sfacteria A, Passalacqua M, et al. Beneficial effects of systemic administration of recombinant human erythropoietin in rabbits subjected to subarachnoid hemorrhage. *Proc Natl Acad Sci U S A*. 2002;99:5627-5631.
83. Solaroglu I, Solaroglu A, Kaptanoglu E, Dede S, Haberal A, Beskonakli E, Kilinc K. Erythropoietin prevents ischemia-reperfusion from inducing oxidative damage in fetal rat brain. *Childs Nerv Syst*. 2003 Jan;19:19-22.
84. Sola A, Wen TC, Hamrick SE, Ferrero DM. Potential for protection and repair following injury to the developing brain: a role for erythropoietin? *Pediatr Res*. 2005;57:110R-117R.
85. Chang YS, Mu D, Wendland M, et al. Erythropoietin improves functional and histological outcome in neonatal stroke. *Pediatr Res*. 2005;58:106-111.
86. Siren AL, Fratelli M, Brines M, et al. Erythropoietin prevents neuronal apoptosis after cerebral ischemia and metabolic stress. *Proc Natl Acad Sci U S A*. 2001;98:4044-4049.
87. Blau J, Calo JM, Dozor D, Sutton M, Alpan G, La Gamma EF. Transfusion-related acute gut injury: necrotizing enterocolitis in very low birth weight neonates after packed red blood cell transfusion. *J Pediatr*. 2011 Mar;158(3):403. [Epub 2010 Nov 10].
88. Baer VL, Lambert DK, Henry E, Snow GL, Butler A, Christensen RD. Among very-low-birth-weight neonates is red blood cell transfusion an independent risk factor for subsequently developing a severe intraventricular hemorrhage? *Transfusion*. 2011;51:1170-1178.
89. Manno CS, Hedberg KW, Kim HC, et al. Comparison of the hemostatic effects of fresh whole blood, stored whole blood, and components after open heart surgery in children. *Blood*. 1991;77:930-936.

90. Williams GD, Bratton SL, Ramamoorthy C. Factors associated with blood loss and blood product transfusions: a multivariate analysis in children after open-heart surgery. *Anesth Analg.* 1999;89:57-64.
91. Kwiatkowski JL, Manno CS. Blood transfusion support in pediatric cardiovascular surgery. *Transfus Sci.* 1999;21:63-72.
92. Mou SS, Giroir BP, Molitor-Kirsch EA, Leonard SR, et al. Fresh whole blood versus reconstituted blood for pump priming in heart surgery in infants. *N Engl J Med.* 2004;351:1635-1644.
93. Lee TH, Reed W, Mangawang-Montalvo L, Watson J, Busch MP. Donor WBCs can persist and transiently mediate immunologic function in a murine transfusion model: effects of irradiation, storage, and histocompatibility. *Transfusion.* 2001;41:637-642.
94. Strauss RG, Burmeister LF, Johnson K, et al. Feasibility and safety of AS-3 red blood cells for neonatal transfusions. *J Pediatr.* 2000;136:215-219.
95. Fernandes da Cunha DH, Nunes Dos Santos AM, Kopelman BI, et al. Transfusions of CPDA-1 red blood cells stored for up to 28 days decrease donor exposures in very low-birth-weight premature infants. *Transfus Med.* 2005;15:467-473.
96. Aladangady N, McHugh S, Aitchison TC, et al. Infant's blood volume in a controlled trial of placental transfusion at preterm delivery. *Pediatrics.* 2006;117:93-98.
97. Mercer JS, Vohr BR, McGrath MM, et al. Delayed cord clamping in very preterm infants reduces the incidence of intraventricular hemorrhage and late-onset sepsis: a randomized, controlled trial. *Pediatrics.* 2006;117:1235-1242.
98. Chaparro CM, Neufeld LM, T Alavez G. et al. Effect of timing of umbilical cord clamping on iron status in Mexican infants: a randomized controlled trial. *Lancet.* 2006;367:1997-2004.
99. Philip A. Delayed cord clamping in preterm infants. *Pediatrics.* 2006;117:1235-1242.

CHAPTER 6

Diagnosis and Treatment of Immune-Mediated and Non–Immune-Mediated Hemolytic Disease of the Newborn

Shrena Patel, MD

Introduction

Hemolytic disease of the fetus and newborn (HDFN) describes pathology related to the maternal/fetal or neonatal-driven destruction of red blood cells (RBCs) at a rate that can result in anemia. The hemolysis may or may not be antibody driven, which differentiates HDFN into immune-mediated hemolytic anemia (IMHA) and non–immune-mediated hemolytic anemia (NIMHA). Although numerous causes of HDFN have been postulated, the most common diseases causing pathologies are described in this chapter.

Immune-Mediated Hemolytic Anemia

IMHA describes the allo-sensitization of the maternal immune system to antigens present on fetal red blood cells. When the maternal immune system is exposed to these fetal cells, a cascade of events is initiated, culminating in the formation of immunoglobulin (Ig)G antibodies directed at fetal antigens. Subsequently, the IgG-coated fetal cells are destroyed, resulting in varying intensity of anemia and its possible complications. As many as 50 antigens present on the red blood cell may cause this antibody-mediated response.[1]

HDFN can also be a consequence of non–immune-mediated pathology (NIMHA). In older children and adults, this could be due to trauma, toxin ingestion, or drug sensitivity. In the fetus and neonate, hemolysis is usually a consequence of RBC membrane abnormality, enzyme disorder, or disordered hemoglobin synthesis. Additionally, hemolytic anemia is seen in association with certain infections (TORCH infections [*t*oxoplasmosis, *o*ther agents, *r*ubella, *c*ytomegalovirus, *h*erpes simplex) and drugs (not discussed in this chapter).

Historical Significance

IMHA was first formally described by Wiener in 1946[2]; however, historical significance dates back to 1900, when Landsteiner first described the presence of the ABO blood type systems, categorizing red blood cell surface markers and individuals as type A, B, AB, or O. This led to research on other red cell markers, including work by Haldane in the 1930s utilizing markers for genetic studies.[3]

6

The Rhesus system was simultaneously discovered in the late 1930s and the early 1940s by Levine and Wiener.[2,4] Levine and Stetson discussed a mother whose second pregnancy resulted in a stillbirth. The mother, whose blood type was O, was noted to have intrapartum hemorrhage and was transfused with the father's blood, also type O. She developed a severe transfusion reaction, and her antisera reacted not only with the father's blood, but also with a high proportion of other blood samples against which it was tested. Investigators concluded that another factor (besides the ABO) was present on the cell surface.[4] At the same time, Wiener and Landsteiner described a new antigen upon testing rhesus monkey blood injected into guinea pigs and rabbits. The new factor was thus named Rhesus and includes the C, D, and E system.[5]

Hemolytic disease, hydrops fetalis, and erythroblastosis fetalis have all been described and discussed dating back to the first century and were further delineated in the mid-1930s.[6] Through the mid-19th century, hemolytic anemia affected about 1 in 200 infants.[6] With increased interest in blood group antigens, more laboratories across North America and the United Kingdom began to develop testing (including agglutination and Coombs testing), which subsequently led to the discovery of many of the minor blood group and Kell antigens.[7]

Hemolytic disease associated with Rhesus antigen D results in the greatest severity of hemolysis. Approximately 15% to 20% of the Caucasian population of North America and Europe is RhD negative[8]; therefore, in combination with ABO, Kell, and minor blood group incompatibilities, immune-mediated hemolytic anemia continues to be an issue of interest in fetal and neonatal medicine.

As the diagnosis, treatment, and management of IMHA have progressed and improved, causes of NIMHA have become more prevalent. These causes have been described since the early 1900s, with multiple reports of familial inheritance noted.[9] Initially, the focus was on membrane defects and sickle cell disease; with advancing laboratory and genetic analysis techniques, the enzymatic disorders have come to be understood more completely.

Epidemiology

Before the advent of anti-D immunoglobulin, approximately 95% of all cases of IMHA were associated with anti-D.[10] This equates to 1 in 180 newborn white infants. Approximately 20% of white women are RhD negative, and approximately 1.5% of Asian women and 3% to 5% of black American women are RhD negative.[11] Overall, the Centers for Disease Control and Prevention (CDC) estimates that Rh sensitization currently affects 6.7 newborns per 1000 live births.

An untreated, RhD-negative, nulliparous woman has a 15% to 20% likelihood of becoming sensitized after carrying a D-positive fetus.[11] Although the likelihood of hemolysis usually increases in subsequent pregnancies, a first pregnancy has a small chance of being affected by HDFN. Multiple blood group incompatibilities may protect the fetus, because the red cells are destroyed before the maternal system can develop anti-D. Anti-A and anti-B antibodies are particularly protective. Overall, the incidence of disease can decrease to 2%.[12]

Although 20% of all pregnancies have ABO discrepancies between fetus and mother, only a small number of pregnancies are affected by hemolytic disease.[13] Most cases of ABO incompatibility are noted in blood type O mothers, because they produce enough IgG antibodies against the A and B antigens that cross the placenta. In the United States, 45% of white American and 49% of black Americans are blood type O; most of the remainder have A or B blood type.[14]

After Rhesus and ABO disease, anti-Kell1 antibodies leading to IMHA are the next most common reason for disease. As treatment for Rh disease improves, Kell disease is becoming more prevalent. Ninety-one percent of the white American population is Kell1 negative (K–k+), and 98% of the black American population is Kell1 negative. Of Kell1-positive (K+k+ or K+k–) people, only a small proportion are homozygous for Kell1 (0.2%), leading to delivery of Kell1-positive infants to 4.5% of Kell1-negative mothers.[15] Maternal sensitization is usually due to maternal blood transfusion with Kell1-positive blood, although

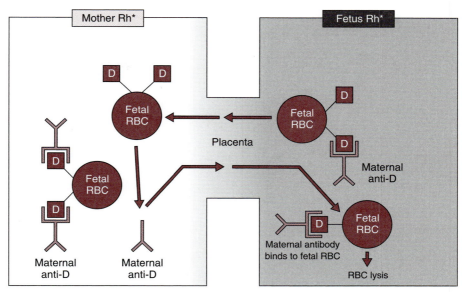

Figure 6-1 Mechanism of Rh isoimmunization secondary to fetal red cells entering into the maternal circulation.

previous pregnancy with a Kell1-positive infant can also lead to an immune response.

Other minor blood group incompatibilities (Duffy system, Kidd, and MNS antibodies) are unusual in clinical practice. No reports have described HDFN associated with Lewis and P system antibodies.[15]

Pathology

The general pathophysiologic mechanism behind IMHA is similar, regardless of the specific blood group incompatibility. The maternal immune system is sensitized to a foreign antigen during exposure to blood with a different antigen profile (Fig. 6-1[16]). This immunization can occur during delivery (most common), amniocentesis/ chorionic villus sampling, cordocentesis, spontaneous or induced abortion, blunt trauma, or any other mechanism that disrupts separation of maternal and fetal circulation.

During the course of an uncomplicated pregnancy, labor, and delivery, less than 0.5 mL of fetal blood enters the maternal circulation. This small amount does not represent a clinically significant source of blood loss for the fetus/neonate; however, it may be enough to trigger an immune response in the mother. Studies have demonstrated that half of women with ABO-compatible, uncomplicated pregnancies have circulating fetal cells, but only 19% of ABO-incompatible, uncomplicated pregnancies have evidence of fetal cells in the maternal circulation.[11] It is estimated that fetomaternal hemorrhage occurs in up to three out of four pregnancies, and the likelihood increases with increasing gestation. Almost one third of pregnancies demonstrate some degree of fetomaternal hemorrhage during the third trimester.[17]

Exposure to the foreign antigen on the fetal red cell activates the production of B lymphocyte clones targeting the foreign antigen. Initial IgM antibodies do not cross to the fetus, because IgM molecules are too large to pass through the placenta. However, IgM antibodies are replaced with IgG antibodies, which do readily cross into the fetal circulation. Subclasses of IgG have been studied in this disease, and it has been shown that most individuals have a combination of IgG1 and IgG3 subclasses. Of note, IgG3 subclass antibodies are able to bind more tightly to reticuloendothelial cells.[18] Consequently, this subclass leads to a greater amount of red cell destruction.

Rhesus

Anti-D–associated disease is the most common and most severe immune-mediated hemolytic disease. The D antigen is highly antigenic (50 times more than the other Rh antigens), and very little is required to stimulate production of antibodies. It is estimated that less than 0.1 mL of fetal blood is needed to immunize the mother and produce a secondary immune response (IgG3 driven). In comparison, the incidence of a primary immune response to the D antigen is 15% after inoculation with 1 mL and 70% to 90% after exposure to 250 mL of fetal blood.[11]

Rhesus c disease is also noted to be potentially severe. Rhesus E disease may present with mild anemia and jaundice. Exposure to the remainder of the Rhesus groups (e and C) uncommonly results in HDFN. The combination of incompatibilities in Rhesus antigens can be severe and potentially fatal.[13]

ABO

Although ABO incompatibility works through a similar pathophysiology, essential differences are evident. For one, most anti-A and anti-B antibodies are IgM in nature and therefore do not cross the placenta. Fetomaternal hemorrhage will lead to an IgG response in subsequent pregnancies. Additionally, many individuals carry IgG antibodies with no clear exposure history.[19] This is likely a result of anti-A and anti-B antibody production stimulated by exposure to environmental toxins and viruses.[19]

ABO incompatibility does not present with the same degree of anemia and complications as are seen with RhD incompatibility. This is thought to be related in part to the presence of the A/B antigen on multiple cell types in the fetus. As a consequence, immune-mediated destruction is more widely dispersed and is not localized to RBCs alone. Additionally, fetal A and B antigens are not fully developed on the red cell surface compared with adult red cells, resulting in availability of fewer antigenic binding sites to the maternally derived antibody. Unlike Rh disease, ABO incompatibility usually does not lead to a more severe phenotype with each subsequent pregnancy.[19] Antibodies to the A and B antigens (termed *isoagglutinins*) are naturally IgM, a subclass that does not cross the placenta and therefore does not lead to a worsened hemolysis with each pregnancy. Occasionally, the antibody is converted to the IgG class, which will cross the placenta, possibly leading to increased hemolysis with subsequent pregnancies.[20]

Kell

Anti-Kell antibodies are usually IgG in class. Kell-associated IMHA works via a different mechanism than is seen with ABO and Rh sensitization. Kell antigens are present on RBC progenitor cells. Anti-K antibodies cause macrophage-driven destruction of these erythroid precursors in the fetal liver. Because progenitor cells lack hemoglobin, a marked increase in bilirubin is not observed in the fetus or newborn.[15]

Minor Incompatibilities

Approximately 50 antigens found on the RBC membrane may cause HDFN (Fig. 6-2[21]). The Duffy antigens (Fy[a] and Fy[b]) have been implicated in transfusion reactions. However, only Fy(a) has been associated with severe HDFN. A recent study reported the presence of anti-Fy(a) antibodies during pregnancy at between 0.01% and 0.54%; this may account for the rarity of Duffy-related HFDN as reported in clinical practice.[22] Of the MNS system (M, N, S, s, U), anti-M, anti-S, anti-s, and anti-U have been associated with severe anemia in the fetus. Anti-N remains IgM in nature and has not been associated with HDFN. As with the Duffy group, incompatibility of the MNS system is unusual in the general population.[23] The Kidd antigens (Jk[a], Jk[b], Jk[3]) are difficult to detect in serum. Antibodies may be IgG or IgM in nature. Although the first description of Kidd-associated HDFN was anti-Jk(a) in nature, antibodies to all three Kidd antigens have been rarely associated with severe HDFN.[24]

NON-RhD ANTIBODIES AND ASSOCIATED HDFN

Antigen system	Specific antigen	Antigen system	Specific antigen	Antigen system	Specific antigen
Frequently associated with severe disease					
Kell	$-K$ (K1)				
Rhesus	$-C$				
Infrequently associated with severe disease					
Colton	$-CO^a$	MNS	$-Mt^a$	Rhesus	$-HOFM$
	$-Co3$		$-MUT$		$-LOCR$
Diego	$-ELO$		$-Mur$		$-Riv$
	$-Di^a$		$-M^v$		$-Rh29$
	$-Di^b$		$-s$		$-Rh32$
	$-Wr^a$		$-s^o$		$-Rh42$
	$-Wr^b$		$-S$		$-Rh46$
	$-Fy^a$		$-U$		$-STEM$
Duffy	$-Js^a$		$-Vw$		$-Tar$
Kell	$-Js^b$	Rhesus	$-Be^a$	Other antigens	$-HJK$
	$-k$ (K2)		$-C$		$-JFV$
	$-Kp^a$		$-Ce$		$-JONES$
	$-Kp^b$		$-C^w$		$-Kg$
	$-K11$		$-C^x$		$-MAM$
	$-K22$		$-ce$		$-REIT$
	$-Ku$		$-D^w$		$-Rd$
	$-Ul^a$		$-E$		
Kidd	$-Jk^a$		$-E^w$		
MNS	$-En^a$		$-Evans$		
	$-Far$		$-e$		
	$-Hil$		$-G$		
	$-Hut$		$-Go^a$		
	$-M$		$-Hr$		
	$-Mi^a$		$-Hr_o$		
	$-Mit$		$-JAL$		
Associated with mild disease					
Dombrock	$-DO^a$	Gerbich	$-Ge^2$	Scianna	$-Sc2$
	$-Gy^a$		$-Ge^3$	Other	$-Vel$
	$-Hy$		$-Ge^4$		$-Lan$
	$-JO^a$		$-Ls^a$		$-At^a$
Duffy	$-Fy^b$	Kidd	$-Jk^b$		$-Jr^a$
	$-Fy3$		$-Jk^3$		

Figure 6-2 Non-RhD antibodies and associated hemolytic disease of the fetus and newborn (HDFN).

Clinical Features

IMHA can present with a wide range of clinical features and severity. Almost half of affected infants do not require treatment. The mildest cases present with minimal anemia, with the potential for mild to moderate tachycardia and slight jaundice. Infants may also have anemia-associated pallor.[19]

With worsening anemia, clinical status may also worsen. Fetuses with profound anemia may present with growth restriction (symmetric or asymmetric), hydrops, or erythroblastosis fetalis. The latter describes the presence of markedly increased numbers of immature RBCs in fetuses and neonates.[25,26] This occurs when RBC destruction outpaces RBC production. As a result, increased immature cells are released into the circulation.[25]

Hydrops fetalis describes increased accumulation of fluid in the subcutaneous tissue, peritoneum, pericardium, and/or pleura. In IMHA, hydrops is associated with anemia, and its presence may be related to placental insufficiency arising from compression of the portal and umbilical venous systems secondary to extramedullary hematopoiesis.[19] Additionally, fetal hypoxia and hypoproteinemia play a role in its development. Hydrops typically is observed when hemoglobin decreases to below 4 to 5 g/dL.[19]

In fetuses with hydrops, the underlying mortality rate is approximately 30%.[8] If a fetus responds to in utero blood transfusions, features of hydrops typically decrease. In contrast, when no response to transfusion occurs, only a quarter survive. A much higher observed rate of hydrops has been reported in male fetuses, with reports suggesting up to a 12-fold increase.[27]

Jaundice is seen in cases of mild (up to 50%) and severe HDFN (98%). In the fetus, bilirubin is cleared by the placenta and therefore becomes apparent in the first hours after birth. Icterus may progress rapidly, with an associated rapid rise in bilirubin levels. Kernicterus is seen in an estimated 7.5% of these infants. Rarely, if fetal anemia is severe and rapid enough, fetal serum bilirubin may be elevated enough (>20 mg/dL) to manifest as jaundice at birth.[8,27,28]

Approximately half of these infants are born preterm or late preterm (up to 34 weeks' gestation) and are noted to have increased rates of asphyxia and/or respiratory distress syndrome. Additionally, a slight increase in the observation of persistent pulmonary hypertension has been reported. Because of extramedullary hematopoiesis, hepatosplenomegaly, portal venous hypertension, and ascites are often observed. Increased islet cell proliferation may occur, leading to potential hypoglycemia.[8,19,27]

Diagnosis

Diagnosis is usually initiated in the prenatal period. Signs of poor growth, decreased growth velocity, hydrops fetalis, or fetal anemia usually prompt investigation. Close monitoring is suggested if the history includes a previous pregnancy affected by IMHA, or if concern about blood type incompatibility arises.[29]

In prenatal visits, it is important to obtain a thorough history, including obstetric history, need for blood transfusions, blood typing, and antibody screening. Anti-D levels can be quantified in the mother and followed serially. Direct Coombs testing detects whether maternal antibodies have already become bound to fetal RBCs. In this testing, a sample of fetal or neonatal RBCs is washed to remove any unbound antibodies. Then, Coombs reagent (antihuman globulin) is added to the sample. Agglutination of RBCs indicates a positive test.[30,31] This testing is useful in determining whether IMHA is present.[29] Of note, however, anti-D immunoglobulin does cross the placenta and therefore may be the cause of a positive result in an unaffected fetus.

Antenatal antibody testing utilizes the indirect Coombs test. This method screens for maternal IgG antibodies in maternal serum. With this method, serum is extracted from the maternal blood sample and incubated with test RBCs of known antigenicity. If antibodies are present, they will bind to the RBCs. The sample is then washed to remove any unbound antibody, and Coombs reagent is added. If maternal antibodies are present and bound to the test RBCs, addition of the Coombs reagent will cause agglutination of the RBCs—a positive indirect Coombs test.[31] Coombs testing is a powerful screening test; however, its main use is in assessing antigenic exposure. It does not seem to predict the need for treatment. It should also be noted that if a mother has received anti-D immunoglobulin, transplacental passage may account for positive testing in the infant.[32]

The Kleihauer-Betke test is performed on maternal blood to determine whether measurable fetomaternal hemorrhage has occurred. This may be used during pregnancy, after an invasive procedure, when concern for trauma arises, or with clinical suspicion. A blood smear from a maternal blood sample is prepared and placed in an acid bath to remove hemoglobin from maternal cells. Fetal hemoglobin is more resistant to acidic conditions and therefore does not elute readily. The remaining (fetal) cells are stained and counted. Fetal cells stain rose, and maternal "ghost" cells appear pale in the background. A ratio is generated and is used to determine the appropriate dose of anti-D globulin to be administered to the mother.[33]

One of the mainstays of diagnosis is ultrasound and Doppler technology. Experienced technicians will be able to evaluate for hydrops, growth discrepancy, and placental thickness. Indeed, many cases of HDFN, particularly non–immune mediated, are found first through ultrasound.[8] Additional evaluation of anemia is done using Doppler monitoring of umbilical vein maximal flow velocity or Doppler estimations of peak systemic blood velocity in the middle cerebral artery. These relatively noninvasive techniques continue to be important in the diagnosis and management of fetal anemia.[11,34] Ultrasound can also be used to guide fetal blood sampling.

In recent years, molecular determination of specific antigenic genes, such as *RHD*, *KEL*, *RHCE*, *FY,* and *JK,* has successfully occurred. DNA can be extracted from fetal cells in amniotic fluid as early as 12 weeks. With the use of primer-specific polymerase chain reaction (PCR), these specific antigens can be tested.[11] This is valuable especially in families affected by severe HDFN and with genetic susceptibility of both partners. Some evidence of functionally inert genes has been found in certain ethnic populations, making PCR alone ineffective in screening and patient counseling.[8] PCR testing can also be performed on cell-free fetal DNA (cffDNA) that can be extracted in the maternal circulation.[8,35]

In the infant with unexplained, persistent, or severe jaundice, Coombs testing is warranted. Evaluation of blood type and a complete blood count looking for anemia, reticulocyte count, and blood smear are useful. Reticulocytosis up to 30% may by noted, and the mean corpuscular volume (MCV) is greater in these infants.[19] However, hemoglobin levels are not always low. Mollison reported that approximately half of infants with HDFN have hemoglobin levels greater than 14.5 g/dL.[11,28]

Management

Because most cases of hemolytic anemia in the fetus continue to be related to RhD antibodies, prophylactic management of RhD-negative mothers with anti-D administration is a mainstay of treatment.[13] The introduction of anti-D dates back to the 1960s, after Chown had demonstrated that fetomaternal hemorrhage was the sensitizing event in this disease.[28] The exact mechanism by which anti-D works is still not clearly understood. It is thought to work by suppressing active immunization stimulation of the antibody-mediated immune response by passive administration of IgG. This administration may induce whole cell destruction (rather than just antigen destruction) before the antigen is presented to dendritic antigen-presenting cells. Alternatively, it may cause an increase in the load of anti-D/D–coated cells presented for destruction and therefore may divert from clonal expansion of B cells.[11,28]

Since its adoption into widespread use, anti-D has been credited with the reduction in Rh disease. Mothers who have had a pregnancy with a previous RhD-positive fetus, or who have a current pregnancy with an RhD-positive fetus, routinely receive Rh anti-D antibody when the pregnancy reaches 28 weeks, and again within 72 hours of delivery.[28] The goal of this treatment is to bind any circulating fetal cells with RhD antigen and avoid maternal production of anti-D antibody. It should be noted that this treatment produces a positive screening result, making differentiation between natural and iatrogenic immune responses difficult.

In women found to be RhD negative and with negative screening, additional testing is performed between 28 and 32 weeks' gestation, and again in the immediate postpartum period.[28] At delivery, cord blood is sent for ABO and Rh typing, as well as for direct Coombs testing. A sample from the maternal circulation is sent to estimate the degree of fetomaternal hemorrhage (Kleihauer-Betke acid elution).

Maternal monitoring during pregnancy includes monthly monitoring of anti-D levels. With anti-D levels less than 5 IU/mL, approximately 4% of affected fetuses require invasive postnatal management. If levels increase above this, closer monitoring for fetal anemia may be warranted. In these cases, amniocentesis becomes the preferred method of testing. Additionally, fetal blood sampling may also be utilized when anti-D levels are very high (> 20 IU/mL).[29]

In conjunction with these levels, serial ultrasound and Doppler studies are used to manage the pregnancy. Ultrasound is targeted at following fetal growth, signs of hydrops or worsening hydrops, and placental appearance. Although studies are still being performed to determine how best to incorporate ultrasound in the management of this disease, it appears to be promising, particularly in the treatment of mild anemia.[8,34] Similarly, serial Doppler estimations of flow gradients and velocity can be used.

Percutaneous umbilical blood sampling (PUBS) is used to directly measure the hemoglobin and/or the hematocrit of the fetus. Under ultrasound guidance, blood is obtained from the umbilical vein. Additional information such as fetal blood type can be obtained from this sampling. However, this technique is available only after approximately 18 weeks of gestation, because the risk for pregnancy loss decreases at that time.[8] The risk of pregnancy loss is greater in the hydropic fetus, with rates approaching 15% before 20 weeks' gestation (compared with 1% in nonhydropic fetuses).[11]

Spectrophotometric measurement of amniotic fluid has been one of the major advances in the treatment of fetal anemia. In cases of severe hemolysis, fetal release of bilirubin becomes a significant indicator of disease. This technique utilizes serial amniocentesis. Serial measurements of optical density deviation at 450 nm (delta OD) from baseline can be used to ascertain which fetuses may benefit from an in utero blood transfusion. The deviation from baseline changes with gestational age, and results are plotted on a curve separating risk into three zones. The initial studies and curve were established by Liley in 1961.[36] Modifications have been attempted since that time. These modified charts (Queenan's modification [Fig. 6-3[37]] and the

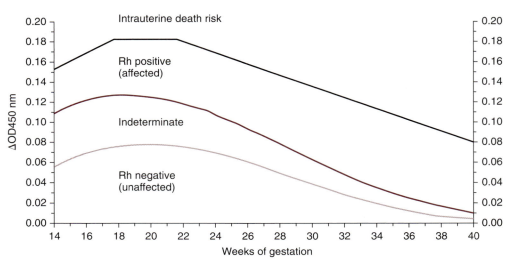

Figure 6-3 Weeks of gestation.

Whitfield action line) represent an attempt to extrapolate data from the first trimester (this was not possible on Liley's curve).[38,39] In general, fetal values plotted in the lower zone are associated with mild disease, and only 10% of infants require exchange transfusion. The middle zone indicates moderate disease. These fetuses may need early delivery and possibly will need exchange transfusions. When values serially plot in the upper zone, severe disease is predicted. The fetus will likely need PUBS and may need blood transfusions.[11]

For the persistently symptomatic anemic fetus, intrauterine blood transfusion continues to be a treatment option. The first transfusions were performed into the peritoneal cavity by Liley in 1963.[36,40] Over the next 20 years, this technique was refined to an intravascular approach (1981),[18] with blood transfused directly into umbilical cord vessels under ultrasound guidance. This approach continues to be used today, with survival rates approaching 90%.[18] However, complications of the procedure are not insignificant and include fetal bradycardia, cord hematoma, and fetal death. Pregnancies significantly affected by hemolytic anemia should be followed by high-risk obstetricians who are comfortable monitoring anemia and performing in utero transfusions. Fetuses requiring multiple invasive procedures, demonstrating significant disease, or exhibiting worsening clinical condition should be delivered when lung maturity safely allows.[11,18]

Infants with HDFN may need treatment for anemia and continued hemolysis. Management of anemia includes the possible need for volume and blood products. Infants with severe hydrops may have a need for mechanical ventilation, pericentesis, pericardiocentesis, or thoracostomy. Infants often require parenteral nutrition and supplemental calories and protein. Infants with hyperbilirubinemia need a range of therapies, from observation and serial bilirubin measurements to phototherapy and intravenous fluids to exchange transfusion. The introduction of the double volume exchange transfusion in Boston in 1946 led to routine treatment for babies with severe IMHA.[41] This intervention is associated with a reduction in mortality associated with Rh disease of 50%.[8,11]

Several pharmaceutical approaches have been considered in these infants and mothers. Of these, the most notable is the use of intravenous immunoglobulin (IVIG). IVIG is used at a dose of up to 1 to 2 g/kg with in utero transfusion or after birth in the neonate. Although the mechanism behind its use is not completely clear, IVIG is thought to bind to the Fc receptor in the reticuloendothelial system, thus reducing hemolysis and decreasing the rapid rise in bilirubin. It should be noted that IVIG is a temporizing measure, because it does not destroy maternal antibodies.[42,43] Additionally, prophylactic use is not necessarily indicated, because it does not seem to reduce the need for exchange transfusions.[44]

Other medications aimed at reducing or temporizing hyperbilirubinemia include heme oxygenase inhibitors. By blocking heme oxygenase, these medications also block the conversion of heme to bilirubin. Phase II/III trials are currently under way, and this medication is available in the United States only for compassionate use.

Outcome

It is no surprise that outcomes for these infants vary with severity and underlying cause. Most infants affected by minor blood group incompatibility alone are very mildly affected and are usually cared for in the well-baby nursery. Infants with maternally derived antibodies directed against D, Kell, and a combination of a minor blood group incompatibility and D or Kell are more severely affected.[5]

In IMHA, antibodies persist in the circulation for up to 6 months. Hemolysis therefore can continue to occur. Some have suggested weekly monitoring of hematocrit and/or recombinant human erythropoietin administration for persistent anemia[45]; however, most centers practice observation, with close follow-up with pediatrics. This late anemia is particularly present among infants who have received in utero transfusions.

Although follow-up studies on these infants are scarce, information on those with immune-mediated hemolysis has been reported. Overall, affected children have good developmental outcomes, with 10% showing evidence of neurodevelopmental impairment. This is the same percentage as is found in the general population. A relationship between disease severity and chance of impairment is not evident.[41,46] A fivefold to tenfold increase in hearing loss occurs in children who required in utero transfusions.[46]

Non–Immune-Mediated Hemolytic Anemia

Epidemiology

Hemolysis can also occur with inherited disorders of the RBC membrane. Of these, hereditary spherocytosis (HS) is the most common. HS is usually inherited in an autosomal dominant fashion, although a 25% rate of spontaneous mutation has been reported, and rarely, the disease can be autosomal recessive.[47] Overall, the incidence is 1:5000.[9] Hemolysis is most common among Northern Europeans and Japanese, with an incidence of 1:2000 in Northern Europeans.[48]

The RBC can be elliptoid in shape, as happens with hereditary elliptocytosis (HE). The true incidence of this disease is unknown, primarily because clinical manifestations can range from asymptomatic to severely anemic.[9] Therefore, individuals with this disease may not be symptomatic (an estimated 90%). However, the presence of disease-associated mutations is not rare in the general population, especially because a certain subset of elliptoid cells may be protective against malarial infection.[9] It also is possible for an infant to inherit multiple mutations. The resulting phenotype has the potential to be more severe. Overall incidence in the United States is thought to be 3 to 5/10,000, and up to 1/3000 worldwide, with numbers approaching 1% to 2% in parts of Africa.[49]

Infantile pyknocytosis appears to be a form of abnormal morphology as well, although little is known about the disease. It was first described in a case series in 1959, and very few reports have been published since then. It is thought to be transmitted in an autosomal recessive fashion and has a male predominance (2:1). Its true incidence is unknown.[50]

Anemia can result from biochemical defects of the RBC. The most common of these is glucose-6-phoshate dehydrogenase (G6PD) deficiency. This disease is inherited usually in an X-linked recessive fashion; females are thought to be affected secondary to the Lyon hypothesis. It is more common among people of South Asian, Mediterranean, and African descent. This is likely due in part to the protection it offers against malaria. Individuals with A-negative blood type are also seen to have G6PD deficiency.[51]

Pyruvate kinase deficiency is the second most common RBC enzymatic defect. It is usually inherited in an autosomal recessive fashion, but autosomal dominant inheritance has also been observed. It is common among individuals of Northern European descent.[52]

Pathology

In HS, cell membrane proteins integral in maintaining the biconcave disc shape of the RBC are ineffective or absent. Included in this group are spectrin, ankyrin, band 4.2, and band 3 protein (Fig. 6-4[53]).[54,55] The resulting RBC is therefore structurally unstable and is targeted for destruction by the splenic system. Increased clinical symptoms of jaundice are associated when the neonate has polymorphism at *UDPGT1*.[56]

The next most common membrane defect is HE. Similar to HS, HE affects the stability and integrity of the RBC wall. Assumed passage of RBCs of elliptical shape through narrow capillaries or tortuous vessels is not reversed. These elliptical cells are removed by the spleen. Similar proteins are involved in the pathogenesis of HS and HE, including spectrin and band 4.1 (see Fig. 6-4).[53,56]

Infantile Pyknocytosis (IP) is thought to be the result of an extracorpuscular agent which causes morphologic changes in the RBC membrane. The resulting cells are small and fragmented, with spicules. Little is known, and infants achieve resolution by 4 months of age.[50]

HETEROGENEITY OF HEREDITARY SPHEROCYTOSIS			
Protein defect	**Hemolysis**	**Inheritance pattern**	**Frequency**
Spectrin α chain	Severe	Autosomal recessive	Rare
Spectrin β chain	Mild to moderate	Autosomal dominant	Common, often associated ankyrin deficiency; ~20% of cases
Ankyrin deficiency	Mild to severe	Autosomal dominant	Common; ~60% of cases
AE₁ (band 3) deficiency	Mild to moderate	Autosomal dominant	Common; ~20% of cases
Protein 4.1 deficiency	Mild	Autosomal dominant	Most common in North Africa
Protein 4.2 deficiency	Moderate to severe (not responsive to splenectomy)	Autosomal recessive	Most common in Japan; rare in European populations
AE, Anion exchanger.			

Figure 6-4 Heterogeneity of hereditary spherocytosis.

Enzymatic defects cause hemolysis of the RBC as well. For example, the body utilizes G6PD in the pentose phosphate pathway to make NADPH, which can be used to make energy for the RBC. NADPH is also responsible for reducing glutathione, the source of antioxidant used by the RBC. Without G6PD, RBCs are unable to make glucose and relieve oxidative stress, thus shortening their life span. Similarly, pyruvate kinase is used in the last step of glycolysis in the RBC, resulting in RBCs with less adenosine triphosphate (ATP) availability.[9,54] This affects energy-driven pumps in the cell membrane, eventually affecting the shape of the membrane and targeting the cell for destruction. Other deficiencies in enzymatic pathways (such as hexokinase deficiency) can also cause hemolytic anemia. However, they occur rarely.[19]

Finally, disordered or inappropriate composition of hemoglobin may result in excessive hemolysis. After the first 10 to 12 weeks of embryonic development, hemoglobin consists of one heme molecule and a tetramer of two dimers, including an alpha globin chain with a non-alpha chain (four globin chains in total).[19] In the fetus, the non-alpha chains are gamma globin. Near the end of gestation, production of gamma chains decreases while that of beta chains increases. Fetal hemoglobin reflects the presence of two alpha chains and two gamma chains (HbF); adult hemoglobin refers to two alpha chains and two beta chains (HbA).[19] HbF remains detectable for the first several months of life and provides certain advantages, most notably a higher affinity to bind oxygen in a relevantly hypoxic in utero environment.[19] Defective production of hemoglobin is seen in diseases such as sickle cell disease.[57] Sickle cell disease is manifested when a valine is present for glutamic acid substitution at position 6 on the gene for the beta-globin chain of hemoglobin. The resultant HgS is prone to cause the RBC to sickle under oxidative stress. This sickling reduces the elasticity of the RBC, and it is targeted for destruction.[57] Sickle cell disease is not usually a cause of HDFN, likely owing to the protective presence of HbF.

The thalassemias are a group of diseases that cause decreased or absent production of the alpha or beta chains through deletion or mutation of globin genes. One of the most severe subtypes is thalassemia major, in which complete absence of the beta chains causes an excessive quantity of unpaired alpha chains, which bind to the red cell membrane and destroy them. With the exception of thalassemia major, the disease usually is not manifested in the neonatal period.

Clinical Features

NIMHA has some similar characteristics to IMHA. Infants usually present with unexplained or prolonged jaundice in the neonatal period. Infants also have varying

6

degrees of anemia and reticulocytosis. However, the degrees of hyperbilirubinemia, anemia, and reticulocytosis are usually not as severe. Splenomegaly can also be seen, in particular with HS and HE.[9]

Diagnosis

With the advancement and expansion of neonatal screening programs, many of these disorders are found before symptoms manifest. Because these disorders usually have a known genetic basis, family history also plays a role. Additionally, microscopic evaluation of the RBCs may uncover increased hemolysis (macrocytosis, anisocytosis, poikilocytosis) or abnormal red cell morphology (spherocytes, elliptocytes, sickle-shaped cells).

HS can be diagnosed with the aid of the osmotic fragility test. Defective RBCs are more permeable to water/salt and rupture at a lower osmolality. Sickle cell is diagnosed on Hb gel electrophoresis, and the enzymatic disorders are diagnosed using enzymatic activity testing.[9,19]

Management

Cell membrane disorders, including HS, HE, and IP, are managed conservatively. In severe cases, splenectomy may be warranted. Special attention must be paid to vaccination against encapsulated organisms and penicillin prophylaxis in these cases.[9,19]

RBC biochemical defects may have worsened disease during times of oxidative stress. Therefore the mainstay of treatment is counseling families to avoid substances that promote oxidative stress, including certain medications (sulfa drugs, antimalarials) and hypoglycemia.[19]

Outcome

Nonimmune hemolytic anemia has a generally good prognosis. The largest risk seems to be the need for possible splenectomy and vigilance for infection following surgery. In sickle cell, crisis management and pain management continue to be important areas of consideration and research.

Future Directions

Research continues to be targeted at improving clinical monitoring for fetuses affected by anemia. Ultrasound and Doppler data continue to be gathered to noninvasively identify fetuses at greater risk. Additionally, the routine use of cffDNA data may prove to be a promising avenue of research. The timing of in utero interventions continues to be studied. Emerging research indicates that chorionic villus sampling may permit typing on fetal blood in the first trimester. However, fetal loss continues to be an issue with these methods. Finally, there is a growing focus on refining anti-D immunoglobulin to better target and modulate the immune response in susceptible people.

Summary

The mechanisms behind HDFN remain relatively common in the general population. However, in the last 75 years, significant advances have been made in the diagnosis, management, and treatment of affected fetuses and neonates. As a result, severely affected fetuses and neonates present for care earlier and show increased survival. Unfortunately, treatment for many causes of HDFN continues to be invasive in nature. Current and future research is aimed at enhancing our ability to extract information in a less invasive (and therefore risky) manner, while intervening at an early and optimal time.

References

1. Bowman JM. Hemolytic disease (erythroblastosis fetalis). In: Creasy RK, Resnik R, eds. *Maternal-fetal medicine.* 4th ed. Philadelphia: WB Saunders; 1999:736-767.
2. Wiener AS. Congenital hemolytic disease and erythroblastosis fetalis; two disease syndromes. *Journal of Parenteral Therapy.* 1946;2(2):12.

3. Owen R. Karl Landsteiner and the first human marker locus. *Genetics*. 2000;155:995-998.
4. Levine P, Stetson R. An unusual case of intra-group agglutination. *Journal of the American Medical Association*. 1939;113:126-127.
5. Wiener AS, Landsteiner K. History of Rh-blood group system. *New York State Journal of Medicine*. 1969;69:2915-2935.
6. Clarke CA, Mollison PL. Deaths from Rh haemolytic disease of the fetus and newborn 1977–87. *Journal of the Royal College of Physicians*. 1989;23:181-184.
7. Moise KJ. Hemolytic disease of the fetus and newborn. In: Creasy RK, Resnik R, eds. *Maternal-fetal Medicine: Principles and Practice*. 6th ed. Philadelphia: WB Saunders; 2008:477-503.
8. Illanes S, Soothill P. Management of red cell alloimmunisation in pregnancy: The non-invasive monitoring of the disease. *Prenat Diagn*. 2010;30:668-673.
9. Gallagher P. Red cell membrane disorders. Hematology/ the Education Program of the American Society of Hematology. *American Society of Hematology. Education Program*. 2005:13-18.
10. The Rhesus factor and disease prevention. In: Zallen DT, Christie DA, Tansey EM, eds. Witness Seminar. Vol 2, London, UK: Wellcome Trust Centre for the History of Medicine at UCL; 2004.
11. Urbaniak SJ, Greiss MA. RhD haemolytic disease of the fetus and the newborn. *Blood reviews*. 2000;14:44-61.
12. Fung K, Eason E, Crane J, et al. Prevention of Rh alloimmunization. *J Obstet Gynaecol Can*. 2003; 25(9):765-773.
13. Letsky EA, Leck I, Bowman JM. Rhesus and other haemolytic diseases. In: Wald D, Leck I, eds. *Antenatal and Neonatal Screening*, 2nd ed. Oxford, UK: Oxford University Press; 2000.
14. Blood types in the U.S. Bloodcenter. Stanford, Calif: Stanford University; 2008.
15. Dean L. The Kell blood group. In: *Blood groups and Red Cell Antigens*. Bethesda, Md: National Center for Biotechnology Information; 2005:1-5.
16. Perkins S. Hematopoietic system. In: Gilbert-Barness E, Kapur R, Oligny L, et al., eds. *Potter's Pathology of the Fetus, Infant and Child*. 2nd ed. Philadelphia: Elsevier; 2007:1462.
17. Bowman JM, Pollock JM, Pensto LO. Fetomaternal transplacental hemorrhage during pregnancy and after delivery. *Vox Sang*. 1986;51:117-121.
18. Zimring J. Blood banking. In: Anderson KC, Ness PM, eds. *Scientific Basis of Transfusion Medicine: Implication for Clinical Practice*. 2nd ed. Philadelphia: WB Saunders; 2000:43-67.
19. Perkins S. Hematopoietic System. In: Gilbert-Barness E, Kapur R, Oligny L, et al., eds. *Potter's Pathology of the Fetus, Infant and Child*. 2nd ed. Philadelphia: Elsevier; 2007:1453-1515.
20. Bakkeheim E, Bergerud U, Schmidt-Melbye AC, et al. Maternal IgG anti-A and anti-B titres predict outcome in ABO-incompatibility in the neonate. *Acta Paediatr*. 2009;98(12): 1896-1901.
21. Moise KJ. Hemolytic disease of the fetus and newborn. In: Creasy RK, Resnik R, Iams JD, et al., eds. *Maternal-Fetal Medicine Principles and Practices*. 6th ed. Philadelphia, Pa: Saunders; 2009:545.
22. Hughes LA, Rossi KQ, Krugh D, et al. Management of pregnancies complicated by anti-Fy^a alloimmunization. *Transfusion*. 2007;47(10):1858-1861.
23. De Young-Owens A, Kennedy M, Rose RL, et al. Anti-M isoimmunization: Management and outcome at the Ohio State University from 1969 to 1995. *Obstet Gynecol*. 1997;90(6): 962-966.
24. Dean L. The Kidd blood group. In: *Blood groups and Red Cell Antigens*. Bethesda, Md: National Center for Biotechnology Information;2005:1-5.
25. Koenig JM. Evaluation and treatment of erythroblastosis fetalis in the neonate. In: Christensen RD, ed. *Hematologic Problems of the Neonate*. Philadelphia: WB Saunders; 2000:185-207.
26. Diamond LK, Blackfan KD, Daty JM. Erythroblastosis fetalis and its association with universal edema of the fetus, icterus gravis neonatorum and anemia of the newborn. *J. Pediatr*. 1932;1(3):269-309.
27. Eder AF. Update on HDFN: New information on long-standing controversies. *Immunohematology*. 2006;22(4):188-195.
28. Urbaniak SJ. Proceedings of the Joint Royal College of Physicians of Edinburgh and the Royal College of Obstetricians and Gynaecologists Consensus Conference on anti-D prophylaxis. *Br. J Obstet Gynaecol*. 1998;105: s18.
29. Moise Jr KJ. Red blood cell alloimmunization in pregnancy. *Seminars in Hematology*. 2005;42: 169-178.
30. Coombs FHC, Mourant A, Race RR. Detection of weak and 'incomplete' Rh agglutinins: A new test. *Lancet*. 1945a;2:15.
31. Coombs FHC, Mourant A, Race RR. A new test for the detection of weak and 'incomplete Rh agglutinins. *British Journal of Experimental Pathology*. 1945b;26:255-266.
32. Murray NA, Roberts IA. Haemolytic disease of the newborn. *Arch Dis Child Fetal Neonatal Ed*. 2007; 92:F83-F88.
33. Katiyar R, Kriplani A, Agarwal N, et al. Detection of fetomaternal hemorrhage following chorionic villus sampling by Kleihauer Betke test and rise in maternal serum alpha feto protein. *Prenat Diagn*. 2007;27(2):139-142.
34. Mari G, Deter RL, Carpenter RL, et al. Non-invasive diagnosis by Doppler ultrasonography of fetal anemia due to maternal red-cell alloimmunization. *N Engl J Med*. 2000;342:9-14.
35. Lo YM. Fetal DNA in maternal plasma: Application to non-invasive blood group genotyping of the fetus. *Transfusion Clinique et Biologique*. 2001;8:306-310.
36. Liley AW. Liquor amnii analysis in the management of the pregnancy complicated by rhesus sensitization. *Am J Obstet and Gynecol*. 1961;82:1359-1370.
37. Queenan JT, Tomai TP, Ural SH, et al. Deviation in amniotic fluid optical density at a wavelength of 45 nm in Ph-immunzed pregnanices from 14-40 weeks' gestation: A proposal for clinical management. *Am J Obstet Gynecol*. 1993;168(5);1374.

38. Nicolaides KH, Rodeck CH, Mibashan RS, et al. Have Liley charts outlived their usefulness? *Am J Obstet Gynecol*. 1986;155(1):90-94.

39. Queenan JT, Tomai TP, Ural SH, et al. Deviation in amniotic fluid optical density at a wavelength of 450 nm in Rh-immunized pregnancies from 14 to 40 weeks' gestation: A proposal for clinical management. *Am J Obstet Gynecol*. 1993;168(5):1370-1376.

40. Liley AW. 1963. Intrauterine transfusion of fetus in haemolytic disease. *BMJ*. 1963;2:1107-1109.

41. Steiner LA, Bizzarro MJ, Ehrenkranz RA, et al. A decline in the frequency of neonatal exchange transfusions and its effect on exchange-related morbidity and mortality. *Pediatrics*. 2007;120(1):27-32.

42. Gottstein R, Cooke RW. Systematic review of intravenous immunoglobulin in haemolytic disease of the newborn. *Arch Dis Child Fetal Neonatal Ed*. 2003 Jan;88(1):F6-10.

43. Kappas A. A method for interdicting the development of severe jaundice in newborns by inhibiting the production of bilirubin. *Pediatrics*. 2004;113:119-123.

44. Smits-Wintjens VE, Walther FJ, Rath ME, et al. Intravenous immunoglobulin in neonates with Rhesus hemolytic disease: A randomized controlled trial. *Pediatrics*. 2011;127(4):680-686.

45. Ohls RK, Wirkus PE, Christensen RD. Recombinant erythropoietin as treatment for the late hyporegenerative anemia of Rh hemolytic disease. *Pediatrics*. 1992;90:678-680.

46. Hudon L, Moise KJ, Hegemier SE, et al. Long-term neurodevelopmental outcome after intrauterine transfusion for the treatment of fetal hemolytic disease. *Am J Obstet Gynecol*. 1998;179(4):858-863.

47. Eber S, Lux SE. Hereditary spherocytosis—defects in proteins that connect the membrane skeleton to the lipid bilayer. *Semin Hematol*. 2004;41(2):118-141.

48. Perrotta S, Gallagher PG, Mohandas N. Hereditary spherocytosis. *Lancet*. 2008;372:1411-1426.

49. Hoffman R, Benz E, Shattil V, et al. *Hoffman Hematology: Basic Principles and Practice*. 4th ed. Philadelphia: Churchill Livingstone; 2005:631-640.

50. Kraus D, Yacobovich J, Hoffer V, et al. Infantile pyknocytosis: A rare form of neonatal anemia. *Isr Med Assoc J*. 2010;12:188-189.

51. Frank JE. Diagnosis and management of G6PD deficiency. *Am Fam Physician*. 2005;72 (7): 1277-1282.

52. Pyruvate kinase deficiency of red cells. www.Ncbi.nlm.nih.gov/omim/266200.

53. Perkins S. Hematopoietic system. In: Gilber-Barness E, Kapur R, Oligny L, et al., eds. *Potter's Pathology of the Fetus, Infant and Child*. 2nd ed. Philadelphia: Elsevier; 2007:1469.

54. Gallagher PG, Forget BG. Hematologically important mutations: Spectrin and ankyrin variants in hereditary spherocytosis. *Blood Cell Mol Dis*. 1998;24(4):539-543.

55. Bolton-Maggs PH, Stevens RF, Dodd NJ, et al. Guidelines for the diagnosis and management of hereditary spherocytosis. *Br J Haematol*. 2004;126 (4):455-474.

56. McMullin MF. The molecular basis of disorders of the red cell membrane. *J Clin Pathol*. 1999;52(4): 245-248.

57. Desai DV, Dhanani H. Sickle cell disease: History and origin. *The Internet Journal of Haematology*. 2004;1(2).

CHAPTER 7

Hematology and Immunology: Coagulation Disorders

Jennifer L. Armstrong-Wells, MD,
and Marilyn J. Manco-Johnson, MD

7

- ● **Introduction**
- ● **Etiology and Pathogenesis**
- ● **Mutations in Genes Involved in Inflammation**
- ● **Maternal Inflammation and Predictors of Fetal/Neonatal Thrombosis**
- ● **Cytokines**
- ● **Inflammation and Systemic Neonatal Thrombosis**
- ● **Summary/Conclusion**

Introduction

With a 15-fold increase in rate compared with infants and children, thrombosis is an important problem in the neonate. Most neonatal thromboses are diagnosed in the intensive care nursery in association with myriad underlying disorders, many of which are inflammatory. Clinically, most cases of neonatal thrombosis occur in two discrete situations: spontaneous perinatal events (primarily stroke and renal vein thrombosis), and catheter-related thrombosis related to neonatal intensive supportive care. The relationship of inflammation to these two categories of thrombosis is currently unknown.

A bidirectional cross-talk between inflammation and thrombosis has been elucidated in recent years.[1] Inflammatory cytokines activate coagulation via stimulation of tissue factor expression on endothelial and monocyte cell surfaces, decrease natural anticoagulant mechanisms, and impair fibrinolysis.[1] The procoagulant enzyme thrombin activates the acute inflammatory response via intracellular signal transduction initiated through protease-activated receptors (PARs) of endothelial cells.[2] The link between inflammation and arterial thrombosis and atherosclerosis has been clearly established in adults.[3] Data implicating inflammation and venous thrombosis have been less clear.[4] Although the inflammatory marker C-reactive protein (CRP) performs similarly to d-dimer as a predictor in the diagnosis of venous thromboembolism (VTE) in adults, the use of CRP as a biomarker predicting the development of new VTE was not significant after correcting for the effect of body mass index (BMI); however, this risk factor is not clinically relevant in the newborn infant.[4] This chapter will explore evidence for the association of inflammation and thrombosis in perinatal arterial and venous events.

Etiology and Pathogenesis

Placental Inflammation, Thrombi, and Infarcts

A role for inflammation, coagulation activation, and thrombosis in diverse fetal and perinatal pathologies was suggested by the finding of placental thromboses and infarcts in cases of fetal growth restriction or demise. Histologic evidence of chronic inflammation of the distal placental villous tree is found in 76 to 136/1000 live births; evidence for an infectious origin of this placental inflammation, known as villitis of unknown etiology (VUE), has been lacking.[5] At the more extreme end of this pathologic spectrum, a true fetal large vessel vasculitis develops with vessel wall damage, occlusion, and, potentially, release of inflammatory cytokines into the fetal circulation.[5] Fetal thrombotic vasculopathy is significantly more frequent in the placentas of term infants with neurologic impairment.[6] A systematic review of inflammatory biomarkers in term infants with neonatal encephalopathy determined that elevated levels of interleukin (IL)-6 in cord blood were positive predictors of adverse neurologic outcomes.[7] Whether neurologic damage in fetal thrombotic vasculopathy is mediated by thrombotic ischemia or by direct inflammatory damage to neurons is currently unresolved.

Mutations in Genes Involved in Inflammation

Reports of vascular impairment in infants found to carry genetic mutations affecting proteins involved in inflammation have provided rare clues into the physiologic gestational and perinatal interactions between inflammation and coagulation. A polymorphism in the promoter region of the cyclooxygenase-2 gene (−765 G>C), conveying 30% reduction in the expression of COX-2 levels with GC or CC polymorphisms compared with GG, was associated with a threefold reduction in histopathologic evidence of placental ischemia and malperfusion, and a fourfold reduction in the rate of intrauterine growth restriction.[8] Reduced levels of COX-2 have been associated with decreased levels of CRP and thromboxane A2 and with increased levels of prostaglandin E2.[9-11] Conversely, an autoinflammatory disease caused by a 175-kb homozygous deletion at chromosome 2q13, which encompasses several IL-1 family members, including the IL-1-receptor antagonist, was associated with marked elevations in markers of inflammation, including CRP, and extensive systemic thrombosis during the neonatal period.[12]

In a study of more than 1000 very low birthweight infants, no increase in adverse outcomes, including sepsis, bronchopulmonary dysplasia, intraventricular hemorrhage, or periventricular leukomalacia, was noted among carriers of a thrombophilia mutation, such as Factor V Leiden or prothrombin 20210.[13] It is interesting to note that the Factor XIII-Val34Leu mutation, which results in thinner fibrin fibrils that are more resistant to fibrinolysis, was associated with increased risk of sepsis. Additionally, the Factor VII-323del/ins (323 A1/A2) promoter polymorphism, which is associated with a 20% decrease in plasma Factor VII activity, was associated with a reduced risk of bronchopulmonary dysplasia. The tissue factor/Factor VII complex promotes inflammation through activation of PARs; lower levels of Factor VII activity could result in decreased inflammatory signaling. In both of these examples, mutations in coagulation genes exerted effects on neonatal outcomes through interactions with inflammatory pathways, rather than by direct effects on hemostasis and thrombosis.

Maternal Inflammation and Predictors of Fetal/Neonatal Thrombosis

Most investigations of neonatal inflammation and thrombosis have been performed in the context of arterial ischemic stroke. Perinatal stroke can be seen in a variety of systemic disturbances and manifests as perinatal arterial ischemic stroke (PAS), perinatal hemorrhagic stroke (PHS), or cerebral sinovenous thrombosis (CSVT). Although birth trauma and delivery-related anoxia were previously thought to be major causes of perinatal stroke, new studies now invoke other pathogeneses, including inflammation. Maternal factors, such as infertility, diabetes, preeclampsia, and chorioamnionitis, have been associated with PAS.[14-16] Chorioamnionitis has also been associated with neonatal CSVT.[17] Further, fetal distress and postmaturity are strong predictors for intracerebral hemorrhage in term and late-preterm newborns.[18] Inflammatory risk factors for perinatal stroke are identifiable before birth, allowing the unique opportunity for early screening and intervention for newborns identified as at risk.

Antiphospholipid Antibodies in Pregnancy

Maternal inflammatory factors may play a pivotal role in neonatal thrombosis, including stroke, because pregnant women with antiphospholipid antibodies (APAs) have a higher rate of placental thrombosis.[19] APAs can be acquired and transiently observed with infection, tissue injury, and certain drugs, or can be part of an autoimmune syndrome. The diagnosis of obstetric antiphospholipid syndrome (APS) requires at least one clinical and one laboratory criterion. Clinical criteria include objectively confirmed vascular thrombosis or pregnancy morbidity. Qualifying obstetric complications include three or more unexplained consecutive spontaneous abortions before the 10th week of gestation; one or more unexplained deaths of a morphologically normal fetus beyond the 10th week of gestation, with morphology confirmed by direct examination or ultrasound; or one or more births of a morphologically normal premature infant of less than 34 weeks' gestation due to eclampsia, severe preeclampsia, or recognized features of placental insufficiency.[20] It has been speculated but not proven that the syndrome of hemolytic anemia, elevated liver enzymes, and low platelets (HELLP) of pregnancy is induced or exacerbated by APS in pregnancy. Laboratory criteria required for the diagnosis of APS include medium- to high-titer immunoglobulin (Ig)G and/or IgM anticardiolipin antibodies (ACA) or anti-β_2 glycoprotein I (anti-β_2GPI) antibodies detected in an enzyme-linked immunosorbent assay (ELISA), or the presence of the lupus anticoagulant (LA). Diagnosis of the LA requires prolongation of a phospholipid-based clotting assay, failure to correct the prolongation with addition of normal plasma, and correction with the addition of excess phospholipid.

The mechanisms of adverse pregnancy outcomes in obstetric APS include direct fetal resorption and placental insufficiency; abnormal development of spiral arteries of the placenta; damage to placental trophoblasts; interference with activation of protein C; interference in fibrinolysis; alterations in the structure and function of annexin V; increases in proinflammatory cytokines; and increases in complement activation.[20] Obstetric morbidity and fetal loss are increased with the number of positive APA tests.[21] Transplacentally derived maternal APA may be a risk factor for perinatal stroke or thrombosis.[16,22,23]

Cytokines

Cytokines are small, soluble polypeptides that bind to cell surface receptors, instigating myriad responses by changing the behavior of target cells. Cytokines mediate inflammation and are elicited as part of an immune response.[24] Individual cytokines rarely work in isolation, but rather act with other cytokines, whether it be by inhibition, synergism, or other unpredictable effects; they also may induce release of other cytokines, the so-called cytokine cascade.[24]

Cytokines have been recognized recently as integral in endothelial cell maintenance. Cytokines can promote expression of adhesion molecules while activating the endothelium, leading to procoagulant activity. Specifically, IL-1 has been shown to cause endothelial cells to generate and express tissue factor on their cell surface, which allows binding of Factor VIIa and therefore initiates the extrinsic clotting pathway. IL-1 and tumor necrosis factor (TNF)-α also inhibit anticoagulant activated protein C (APC) by decreasing thrombomodulin expression. Both IL-1 and TNF-α increase plasminogen activator inhibitor type 1 (PAI-1), which inhibits the intrinsic fibrinolytic system of the endothelial cell. Therefore, IL-1 and TNF-α are thought to work in an additive fashion as procoagulant cytokines. Further, they are also classified as inflammatory cytokines, with ultimate induction of leukocyte activation and adhesion by the cytokine cascade (IL-1), as well as direct endothelial action and lymphocytic inflammation (TNF-α). Other cytokines, including IL-2, IL-6, and IL-8, have also been classified as proinflammatory. Additionally, IL-18 (formally known as IL-1γ because of its homology to IL-1β) has been implicated in ongoing inflammatory brain injury.[25,26]

Because of the similarity between endothelial damage caused by inflammatory cytokines and damage that occurs in preeclampsia, levels of circulating cytokines in preeclamptic women have been studied. Increased levels of TNF-α and IL-6 have been found in women with preeclampsia.[27,28] It has been shown that in infants with neonatal hypoxia, encephalopathy, or subsequent cerebral palsy, elevated serum levels of IL-1β, IL-6, or IL-8; cerebrospinal fluid levels of IL-1β or neuron-specific enolase; or brain concentrations of IL-1β or TNF-α have been determined.[29,30] These proinflammatory cytokines, triggered by infection or hypoxia, are involved in a final common pathway within a molecular cascade that may lead to perinatal brain damage.[31,32] Consequently, this inflammatory reaction is suggested to arise from the fetus itself—the so-called fetal inflammatory response—and has been postulated as a mechanism for perinatal brain injury.[31] Studies conducted to date demonstrate that the fetal inflammatory response and cytokine activation—with possible underlying genetic susceptibility—are associated with cerebral palsy in the term/late-preterm newborn, and therefore may also be associated in the pathophysiology of perinatal stroke.[29-31]

Inflammation and Systemic Neonatal Thrombosis

Few data are available regarding the relationship of inflammation to thrombosis in other syndromes of neonatal thrombosis. In one study of newborn infants undergoing palliative surgery for single-ventricle congenital heart disease, preoperative elevations in CRP predicted postoperative venous thrombosis.[32] Thornburg and colleagues reported a positive association between thromboses and infections in newborn infants who did not have lines removed for infection and described a subset of catheter-related thromboses in newborn infants characterized by onset late in the presence of catheter-associated bloodstream infection.[33] They hypothesized that catheter-related thrombosis in the newborn infant may be caused by inflammation induced by infection. Other systemic thrombi that occur in the perinatal period, particularly renal vein thrombosis, could be hypothesized to occur through similar mechanisms of placental inflammation with systemic emboli through the umbilical vein; however, no objective evidence currently supports this.

Clinical Aspects

To date, there is almost no clinical application of existing data on the contributions of inflammation to the prediction, prevention, or management of thrombosis in the newborn infant. The only exception is obstetric APS, in which clinical testing and management of the newborn infant by a skilled perinatal team can be facilitated by known APA positivity in the mother. Some intriguing data suggest that neonatal inflammation may be predicted by maternal obstetric conditions, and that adverse consequences of fetal and neonatal inflammation, primarily effects on perinatal brain development, may be ameliorated by interventions targeted to antagonize neonatal proinflammatory cytokines and to promote anti-inflammatory cytokines.[31]

Differential Diagnosis

There is no direct application of emerging knowledge regarding placental and fetal inflammation on the differential diagnosis of neonatal thrombosis. However, neonatologists caring for infants born to mothers with the obstetric conditions discussed previously, which are characterized by the inflammatory response, may be alerted to a potentially increased risk for thrombosis in these infants, facilitating prompt recognition and diagnosis of clinical thrombosis.

Prognosis

Evidence from preliminary studies suggests that serum and cerebrospinal fluid IL-1β, serum IL-6, and cerebrospinal fluid neuron-specific enolase predict poor neonatal outcomes.[29] However, none of the research in cytokine biomarkers has been developed to clinical usage. The prognosis for neonatal thrombosis related to maternal or fetal/neonatal inflammatory conditions, such as chorioamnionitis or obstetric APS, is related to the site, extent, and response to therapy of the thrombus itself.

Table 7-1   DOSING FOR ANTITHROMBOTIC THERAPY IN CHILDREN

	Unfractionated Heparin Continuous IV	Enoxaparin Every 12 Hours Subcutaneous	Tissue Plasminogen Activator Continuous IV
Loading dose	Newborn <37 weeks: 50 U/kg Newborn ≥37 weeks: 100 U/kg	None	None
Initial maintenance dose	Newborn <37 weeks: 20–25 U/kg/hr	1.5 mg/kg/dose	0.06–0.12 mg/kg/hr
	Newborn ≥37 weeks: 28 U/kg/hr (may need up to 50 U/kg/hr to achieve therapeutic anti-Xa level)	1.5 mg/kg/dose (may require up to 2.0 mg/kg/dose)	0.06–0.12 mg/kg/hr
Monitoring	Anti-Xa activity following 4–6 hours of infusion; target range: 0.3–0.7 U/mL	Anti-Xa activity 4 hours following first or second dose; target range: 0.5–1.0 U/mL	

Therapy and Treatments

Currently, the only neonatal antithrombotic therapy specifically influenced by inflammation is given for neonatal thrombosis in an infant with APA. In addition to standard anticoagulant and thrombolytic agents, some affected infants have been treated with isovolemic exchange transfusion and low-dose aspirin.[23]

Recommendations for antithrombotic therapy in the newborn infant with thrombosis (excluding PAS) are given in Table 7-1.[34] The risk of thrombus progression and recurrence in the newborn infant appears to be low. This may be true because most perinatal inflammation promoting thrombosis appears to derive from placental and maternal inflammatory conditions that are resolved once the infant is born. For this reason, antithrombotic therapy generally is not indicated in PAS. Peripheral arterial thrombi may be treated until blood flow is restored for a brief period (e.g., 48 hours); thereafter, the entire course is often 10 to 14 days. Chest guidelines for antithrombotic therapy suggest a standard duration of anticoagulation of 3 months for the neonate, equal to that recommended for older children and adults.[35] However, resolution of venous thrombi in the newborn infant is often rapid and thrombus recurrence risk is low. If an underlying trigger for thromboembolism is reversed, extracranial venous thrombi may be treated until thrombus resolution, which often occurs within 10 to 30 days. Neonatal renal vein thrombosis has been a particularly challenging lesion, with no therapeutic regimen particularly effective and with most affected infants suffering sequelae of partial or complete renal infarction or hypertension.[36,37] Although some advocate for the use of heparin-based therapy in neonatal CSVT, most clinicians agree that treatment is determined on a case-by-case basis; treatment may be withheld unless the thrombus is progressive.

Tissue plasminogen activator (TPA), interventional thrombolysis, and mechanical thrombectomy are useful in selected cases of extracranial thrombosis, provided contraindications are strictly followed as outlined in Table 7-2. Thrombolysis is indicated chiefly when life- or limb-threatening ischemia is present, and should be considered for completely occlusive thrombi of the aorta, superior or inferior vena cava, abdominal thrombi, and arterial occlusion of the limb. There is no role at this time for TPA, interventional thrombolysis, or mechanical thrombectomy for cerebral thrombosis (PAS or CSVT) in the neonate.

Summary/Conclusion

Evidence for inflammation as a cause of neonatal thrombosis can be found mainly in studies of placental pathology and perinatal arterial ischemic stroke, but data relating catheter thrombosis to infection and inflammation are intriguing. Future

Table 7-2 CONTRAINDICATIONS TO SPECIFIC ANTITHROMBOTIC THERAPIES IN NEWBORN INFANTS AND CHILDREN

Unfractionated Heparin	Low Molecular Weight Heparin	Systemic TPA	Thrombolysis by Interventional Radiology
Known allergy	Known allergy	Known allergy	Known allergy
History of heparin-induced thrombocytopenia (thrombosis) (HIT(T))	Invasive procedure <24 hours	Active bleeding Central nervous system ischemia/surgery ≤10 days (includes birth asphyxia) Surgery ≤7 days Invasive procedure ≤3 days Seizures ≤48 hours	In cases where needed, inability to place a Greenfield filter Limitations: size of involved vessels and experience of interventionists
*Fibrinogen <100 mg/dL Platelet count <50,000/μL	*Fibrinogen <100 mg/dL Platelet count <50,000/μL	*Fibrinogen <100 mg/dL Platelet count <50,000/μL INR >2	*Fibrinogen <100 mg/dL Platelet count <50,000/μL INR >2

INR, International normalized ratio; *TPA,* tissue plasminogen activator.
  *With transfusion support, if necessary.

research directed at determination of biomarkers for maternal inflammation may allow us to predict and prevent thrombosis in the developing fetus and the newborn infant. Anti-inflammatory therapies directed at activation of cytokines, complement proteins, and inflammatory cells applied to decrease cellular dysfunction and tissue infarction consequent to inflammation and thrombosis are in early stages. Anti-inflammatory therapies offer the hope of substantial advancement of therapy, particularly for perinatal arterial ischemic stroke.

References

1. Esmon CT. The interactions between inflammation and coagulation. *Br J Haematol.* 2005;131: 417-430.
2. Martorell L, Martínez-González J, Rodríguez C, et al. Thrombin and protease-activated receptors. PARs; in atherothrombosis. *Thromb Haemost.* 2008;99:305-315.
3. Ridker PM, Cushman M, Stampfer MJ, et al. Inflammation, aspirin, and the risk of cardiovascular disease in apparently healthy men. *N Engl J Med.* 1997;336:973-979.
4. Fox EA, Kahn SR. The relationship between inflammation and venous thrombosis. A systematic review of clinical studies. *Thromb Haemost.* 2005;94:362-365.
5. Redline RW. Inflammatory responses in the placenta and umbilical cord. *Semin Fetal Neonatal Med.* 2006;11:296-301.
6. Redline RW. Severe fetal placental vascular lesions in term infants with neurologic impairment. *Am J Obstet Gynecol.* 2005;192:452-457.
7. Ramaswamy V, Horton J, Vandermeer B, et al. Systematic review of biomarkers of brain injury in term neonatal encephalopathy. *Pediatr Neurol.* 2009;40:215-226.
8. Polydorides AD, Kalish RB, Witkin SS, et al. A fetal cyclooxygenase-2 gene polymorphism is associated with placental malperfusion. *Int J Gynecol Pathol.* 2007;26:284-290.
9. Hausman N, Beharry K, Nishihara K, et al. Antenatal administration of celecoxib, a selective cyclooxygenase (COX)-2 inhibitor, appears to improve placental perfusion in the pregnant rabbit. *Prostaglandins Other Lipid Mediat.* 2003;70:303-315.
10. Papafili A, Hill MR, Brull DJ, et al. Common promoter variant in cyclooxygenase-2 represses gene expression: Evidence of role in acute-phase inflammatory response. *Arterioscler Thromb Vasc Biol.* 2002;22:1631-1636.
11. Cipollone F, Toniato E, Martinotti S, et al. A polymorphism in the cyclooxygenase 2 gene as an inherited protective factor against myocardial infarction and stroke. *JAMA.* 2004;291:2221-2228.
12. Reddy S, Jia S, Geoffrey R. An autoinflammatory disease due to homozygous deletion of the IL1RN locus. *N Engl J Med.* 2009;360:2438-2444.
13. Härtel C, König I, Köster S, et al. Genetic polymorphisms of hemostasis genes and primary outcome of very low birth weight infants. *Pediatrics.* 2006;118:683-689.

14. Lee J, Croen LA, Backstrand KH, et al. Maternal and infant characteristics associated with perinatal arterial stroke in the infant. *JAMA.*, 2005;293: 723-729.
15. Wu YW, Escobar GJ, Grether JK, et al. Chorioamnionitis and cerebral palsy in term and near-term infants. *JAMA.* 2003;290:2677-2684.
16. Golomb MR. The contribution of prothrombotic disorders to peri- and neonatal ischemic stroke. *Semin Thromb Hemost.* 2003;29:415-424.
17. Armstrong-Wells J, Johnston SC, Wu YW. Prevalence and predictors of perinatal hemorrhagic stroke. *Pediatrics.* 2009;123:823-828.
18. Wu YW. Systematic review of chorioamnionitis and cerebral palsy. *Ment Retard Dev Disabil Res Rev.* 2002;8:25-29.
19. Nelson KB. Thrombophilias, perinatal stroke, and cerebral palsy. *Clin Obstet Gynecol.* 2006;49: 875-884.
20. Tincani A, Bazzani C, Zingarelli S, et al. Lupus and the antiphospholipid antibody syndrome in pregnancy and obstetrics: Clinical characteristics, diagnosis, pathogenesis and treatment. *Semin Thromb Hemost.* 2008;34:267-272.
21. Ruffatti A, Tonello M, Cavazzana A, et al. Laboratory classification categories and pregnancy outcome in patients with primary antiphospholipid syndrome prescribed antithrombotic therapy. *Thromb Res.* 2009;123:482-487.
22. Silver RK, MacGregor SN, Pasternak JF, Neely SE. Fetal stroke associated with elevated maternal anticardiolipin antibodies. *Obstet Gynecol.* 1992;80:497-499.
23. Boffa M-C, Lachassinne E. Infant perinatal thrombosis and antiphospholipid antibodies: A review. *Lupus.* 2007;16:634-641.
24. Pober JS, Cotran RS. Cytokines and endothelial cell biology. *Physiol Rev.* 1990;70:427-451.
25. Wheeler RD, Boutin H, Touzani O, et al. No role for interleukin-18 in acute murine stroke-induced brain injury. *J Cereb Blood Flow Metab.* 2003;23:531-535.
26. Wheeler RD, Brough D, LeFeuvre RA, et al. Interleukin-18 induces expression and release of cytokines from murine glial cells: Interactions with interleukin-1 beta. *J Neurochem.* 2003;85: 1412-1420.
27. Conrad KP, Benyo DF. Placental cytokines and the pathogenesis of preeclampsia. *Am J Reprod Immunol.* 1997;37:240-249.
28. Conrad KP, Miles TM, Benyo DF. Circulating levels of immunoreactive cytokines in women with preeclampsia. *Am J Reprod Immunol.* 1998;40:102-111.
29. Ramaswamy V, Horton J, Vendermeer B, et al. Systematic review of biomarkers of brain injury in term neonatal encephalopathy. *Pediatr Neurol.* 2009;40:215-226.
30. Girard S, Kadhim H, Roy M, et al. Role of perinatal inflammation in cerebral palsy. *Pediatr Neurol.* 2009;40:168-174.
31. Dammann O, O'Shea TM. Cytokines and perinatal brain damage. *Clin Perinatol.* 2008;35:643-663.
32. Cholette JM, Ruberstein JS, Alfieris GM, et al. Elevated risk of thrombosis in neonates undergoing initial palliative cardiac surgery. *Ann Thorac Surg.* 2007;84:1320-1325.
33. Thornburg CD, Smith PB, Smithwick ML, et al. Association between thrombosis and bloodstream infection in neonates with peripherally inserted catheters. *Thromb Res.* 2008;122:782-785.
34. Manco-Johnson MJ. How I treat venous thrombosis in children. *Blood.* 2006;107:1-9.
35. Monagle P, Chalmers E, Chan A, et al. Antithrombotic therapy in neonates and children. *Chest.* 2008;133:887S-968S.
36. Kosch A, Kuwertz-Bröking E, Heller C, et al. Renal venous thrombosis in neonates: Prothrombotic risk factors and long-term follow-up. *Blood.* 2004;104:1356-1360.
37. Nuss R, Hays T, Manco-Johnson M. Efficacy and safety of heparin anticoagulation for neonatal renal vein thrombosis. *Am J Pediatr Hematol Oncol.* 1994;16:127-131.

7

CHAPTER 8

A Practical Approach to the Neutropenic Neonate

Akhil Maheshwari, MD, and L. Vandy Black, MD

- ● **Definition of Neonatal Neutropenia**
- ● **Clinical Evaluation of Neutropenia in Neonates**
- ● **Clinical Management of a Neonate with Neutropenia**

Neutropenia is a commonly detected problem in the neonatal period, affecting 6% to 8% of all patients in neonatal intensive care units (NICUs).[1-5] Of the 600,000 or so neonates admitted annually to NICUs in the United States, as many as 48,000 infants may be recognized as neutropenic. The incidence of neutropenia is highest among preterm infants, with estimates ranging between 6% and 58%, depending on the definition of *neutropenia*.[6] The frequency of neutropenia also rises with decreasing birth weight; it is seen in 3% of term infants weighing more than 2500 g, in 13% infants of weighing less than 2500 g, and in up to 38% of those weighing less than 1000 g.[1,7] Although neutropenia usually is transient and limited in most infants to the first few days after birth, it may be severe and prolonged in some cases to constitute a serious deficiency in innate immunity.

Definition of Neonatal Neutropenia

The diagnosis of neutropenia is based on a low blood neutrophil concentration. An absolute neutrophil count (ANC) can be calculated from a routine complete blood count as follows:

$$\text{Absolute neutrophil count} = \text{White cell count } (/\mu L) \times \text{Neutrophil percentage}$$

where the neutrophil percentage is calculated as the sum of the percentage figures for segmented and band neutrophils on the differential count.

Interpretation of an ANC value in a neonate usually involves comparison with available reference ranges. In a statistical sense, *neutropenia* is defined as an ANC two standard deviations below the mean value for age,[8] or, alternatively, as an ANC below the lower limits of normal for an age-defined population.[9,10] The reference ranges used most commonly were provided by Manroe and associates,[11] who obtained their data set from a cohort of 434 neonates born at 38.9 ± 2.4 weeks' gestation. Neutrophil counts peaked at 12 to 24 hours with 95% confidence limits of 7800 to 14,500/μL and then decreased to achieve a stable lower value of 1750/μL by 72 hours of life (Fig. 8-1). A stable upper limit was achieved at 6.6 days of age.

The reference ranges reported by Manroe and colleagues are widely accepted for term and near-term infants but are less appropriate for very low birthweight (VLBW) infants.[12-15] Mouzinho and coworkers[10] revised the reference ranges for blood neutrophil concentrations in VLBW infants (see Fig. 8-1). Serial counts (N = 1788) were obtained prospectively between birth and 28 days of age from 63 normal infants of 29.9 ± 2.3 weeks' gestation. No difference in the upper limit of normal was observed between those VLBW infants and their more mature counterparts as reported in 1979. However, greater variation was noted at the lower end of the ranges, and neutropenia was defined as a concentration less than 2000/μL at

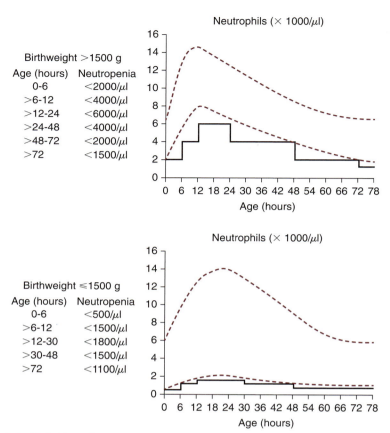

Neutrophils (× 1000/μl)

Birthweight >1500 g

Age (hours)	Neutropenia
0-6	<2000/μl
>6-12	<4000/μl
>12-24	<6000/μl
>24-48	<4000/μl
>48-72	<2000/μl
>72	<1500/μl

Age (hours)

Neutrophils (× 1000/μl)

Birthweight ≤1500 g

Age (hours)	Neutropenia
0-6	<500/μl
>6-12	<1500/μl
>12-30	<1800/μl
>30-48	<1500/μl
>72	<1100/μl

Age (hours)

Figure 8-1 Definition of neutropenia. The upper panel gives the normal reference range for neutrophils *(in between dashed lines)* as established by Manroe.[11] Values below the solid line were considered neutropenic for neonates with a birth weight greater than 1500 g. The lower panel gives the normal reference range for neutrophils *(in between dashed lines)* as established by Mouzinho[10] for neonates with a birth weight of 1500 g or less. Values below the solid line were considered neutropenic. (To be reproduced with permission from Funke A, Berner R, Traichel B, et al. Frequency, natural course, and outcome of neonatal neutropenia. *Pediatrics.* 2000;106:45-51.)

12 hours of life and less than 1000/μL after 48 hours. In a follow-up study[16] comparing reference ranges in septic VLBW infants, the figures from Manroe and associates were observed to provide greater sensitivity, but the ranges reported by Mouzinho and colleagues were more specific when neonates with early-onset group B streptococcal infection were compared with a matched control group.

In a recent report,[5] Schmutz and coworkers re-examined the reference ranges for neutrophil counts by compiling data from 30,354 blood counts performed on neonates of 23 to 42 weeks' gestation. The strengths of this data set are its large sample size and the use of automated blood counting instrumentation, which allows the enumeration of larger, consistent numbers of cells for each report and eliminates interobserver variability in visual identification of neutrophils.[17] In the interval between 72 and 240 hours, neonates born at greater than 36 weeks' gestation had an ANC in the range of 2700 to 13,000/μL (5th to 95th percentile), and those born at 28 to 36 weeks between 1000 and 12,500/μL, whereas neonates born at less than 28 weeks' gestation had an ANC in the range of 1300 to 23,000/μL. The upper limits of neutrophil counts in this data set were higher than in the Manroe and Mouzhino charts; this may be due to differences in methods of enumeration of neutrophils or, alternatively, an effect of the high altitude at which the hospitals participating in this study were located.[18,19]

Reference ranges are useful for accurate interpretation and follow-up of neutrophil counts. The definition of *neutropenia,* that is, the lower limit of normal for blood neutrophil concentrations, has been variously reported as 1500/μL (Xanthou), 1800/μL (Manroe), and 1100/μL (Mouzinho).[10,11,20] These "cutoff" values are aimed at providing the clinician with a critical threshold to initiate investigation and, if indicated, treatment. However, the relationship between blood neutrophil concentrations and the risk of developing an infection is not well established in neonates. Extrapolating from the chronic severe neutropenia registry and chemotherapy studies in children, neonates with neutrophil counts above 1000/μL are not likely to be at increased risk. Neonates with blood neutrophil concentrations less than 500/μL probably are at increased risk, particularly if the neutropenia persists for several days or weeks.[21-23] Neonates with blood neutrophil counts between 500/μL and 1000/μL may be at some intermediate risk.

Clinical Evaluation of Neutropenia in Neonates

Neutropenia can occur secondary to decreased production of neutrophils, excessive neutrophil margination, increased neutrophil destruction, or combinations of these three mechanisms (Table 8-1). The most commonly encountered causes of neonatal neutropenia are those related to maternal hypertension, sepsis, twin-twin transfusion, alloimmunization, and Rh hemolytic disease of the newborn.[24] When considering the origin of neutropenia, it is imperative to pay close attention to the other cell lineages. The presence of concomitant anemia or thrombocytopenia may suggest a more global production defect in the bone marrow.

Evaluation for Etiology

1. Perinatal information: maternal history of hypertension with fetal growth retardation, multiple gestation with disparity between twins, or an infectious illness during pregnancy can be diagnostic. Similarly, the presence of high-risk factors for early-onset sepsis, such as prolonged rupture of membranes or chorioamnionitis, can provide useful clues.
2. In a well-appearing infant with persistent neutropenia, the diagnosis of an immune-mediated neutropenia may be considered.[25-29] This group of disorders comprises three distinct entities that involve a low neutrophil count resulting from increased destruction of neutrophils by antibodies directed against cell membrane antigens.[30] These include alloimmune neonatal neutropenia (ANN), neonatal autoimmune neutropenia, and a third relatively less well-defined category, autoimmune neutropenia of infancy (AINI). Alloimmune neonatal neutropenia (ANN) is the neutrophil counterpart of the erythrocyte disorder known as *hemolytic disease of the newborn.* It occurs when a mother becomes sensitized to a foreign antigen present on the neutrophils of her infant that was inherited from the father. This leads to the maternal production of specific immunoglobulin G (IgG) antibodies directed against the fetal neutrophil antigen. Transplacental passage of these maternally derived antibodies into the fetal circulation produces neutropenia.[26] Neonatal autoimmune neutropenia, on the other hand, is related to the passage of maternal autoantibodies formed against antigens on the mother's own neutrophils. The presence of neutropenia or autoimmune disease in the mother can suggest the presence of transplacental transfer of antineutrophil autoantibodies.[26,27] In autoimmune neutropenia of infancy (AINI), unlike the previous two entities of transplacental origin, the antineutrophil antibodies are produced by the infant.[29]
3. Concurrent illnesses, such as necrotizing enterocolitis, bacterial or fungal sepsis, immunodeficiency, cardiomyopathy (Barth syndrome), intractable metabolic acidosis or other electrolyte derangements, or the presence of anemia and/or thrombocytopenia, can provide useful information.
4. Physical examination: characteristic dysmorphic features, such as skeletal dysplasia, radial or thumb hypoplasia (congenital bone marrow failure

Table 8-1   CAUSES OF NEONATAL NEUTROPENIA

Decreased Neutrophil Production

Infants of hypertensive mothers (unknown; possible causes include presence of a placenta-derived inhibitor of neutrophil production and decreased responsiveness of precursors to G-CSF)

Donors of twin-twin transfusions

Neonates with Rh hemolytic disease (progenitor "steal" whereby precursors are diverted toward erythroid differentiation; "wash-out" effect of exchange transfusions)

Congenital neutropenias

Bone Marrow Failure Syndromes
- Kostmann syndrome (maturation arrest and increased apoptosis of precursors; neutrophil elastase mutations that lead to exclusive membrane localization of the enzyme)
- Reticular dysgenesis (inherited form of severe combined immunodeficiency with impairment of both myeloid and lymphoid production)
- Barth syndrome (organic aciduria, dilated cardiomyopathy, and neutropenia; neutropenia presumably due to a neutrophil membrane defect)
- Shwachman-Diamond syndrome (exocrine pancreatic insufficiency, failure to thrive, skeletal abnormalities, and neutropenia; defect in SBDS protein, which may be involved in ribosomal biogenesis)
- Cartilage-hair hypoplasia (short-limbed dwarfism; impairment of proliferation in neutrophil precursors)
- Cyclic neutropenia (cyclic hematopoiesis with nadirs at 3-week intervals; neutrophil elastase mutations that prevent membrane localization of the enzyme)

Inborn Errors of Metabolism
- Organic acidemias (metabolic intermediates inhibit proliferation of neutrophil precursors)
- Glycogen storage disease type 1b (increased neutrophil apoptosis)

Viral Infections (infection of neutrophil progenitors, hypersplenism)
- Rubella
- Cytomegalovirus

Copper Deficiency

Alloimmune Neutropenia Associated With Anti-NB1 Antibodies (NB1 antigen is present on neutrophil precursors)

Increased Neutrophil Destruction

Bacterial or fungal sepsis (increased tissue migration; marrow suppression in overwhelming sepsis)

Necrotizing enterocolitis (circulating neutrophil pool depleted owing to increased migration into the intestines and peritoneum; increased demargination)

Alloimmune neonatal neutropenia (analogous to Rh-hemolytic disease of the newborn, where the mother produces an antibody against an antigen present on fetal neutrophils that has been inherited from the father)

Neonatal autoimmune neutropenia (passively acquired antineutrophil antibodies from the mother, who has autoimmune neutropenia)

Autoimmune neutropenia of infancy (infant becomes sensitized to self-antigens present on neutrophils and produces antibodies against own neutrophils)

Other Causes

Idiopathic neutropenia of prematurity (a diagnosis of exclusion; readily reversible with G-CSF therapy)

Drug-induced neutropenia (can occur with a large number of drugs; those commonly incriminated in the NICU include β-lactam antibiotics, thiazide diuretics, ranitidine, and acyclovir)

Pseudoneutropenia (a benign condition in which the circulating neutrophil pool is smaller than the vascular demarginated pool)

Artifactual neutropenia (a benign condition in which neutrophils agglutinate upon exposure to EDTA, an anticoagulant used in blood collection tubes)

EDTA, Ethylenediaminetetraacetic acid; *G-CSF,* granulocyte colony-stimulating factor; *NICU,* neonatal intensive care unit.

syndromes), hepatosplenomegaly (TORCH infections, storage disorders), or skin/hair pigmentary abnormalities (Chédiak-Higashi syndrome), can be helpful.

5. Chronological age: several disorders are associated with specific time periods. Neutropenia associated with maternal hypertension is usually observed in the first week, and persistence beyond 5 to 7 days should trigger further work-up. Congenital bone marrow failure syndromes also can present early. Inborn errors of metabolism usually present late in the first week and

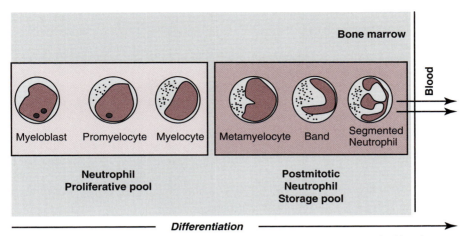

Figure 8-2   Mature segmented neutrophils are released from the bone marrow into the bloodstream in a series of differentiation-dependent events. The appearance of earlier, less mature forms (such as bands) suggests that the postmitotic storage pool of mature neutrophils has been depleted. Such depletion can be assessed by calculating the "immature to total neutrophil (I/T) ratio."

beyond. Copper deficiency may be seen rarely in growing premature infants dependent on parenteral nutrition. Idiopathic neutropenia of prematurity also occurs late in the hospital course of growing VLBW infants and resolves spontaneously.

Evaluation of Neutrophil Kinetics

In the bone marrow, the neutrophil population comprises a neutrophil proliferative pool (consisting of myeloblasts, promyelocytes, and myelocytes) and a postmitotic neutrophil storage pool (consisting of metamyelocytes, band neutrophils, and segmented neutrophils). The release of mature segmented neutrophils is tightly regulated in a differentiation-dependent manner.[31] Thus, the appearance of bands and other immature neutrophil precursors in the circulation indicates that the bone marrow pool of mature neutrophils has already been depleted (Fig. 8-2). In neonatal neutropenias, an approximate kinetic evaluation can be performed by calculating the immature-to-total neutrophil ratio (I/T) from the differential white blood cell count:

$$\frac{(\text{Bands} + \text{Metamyelocytes} + \text{Myelocytes})}{(\text{Segmented neutrophils} + \text{Bands} + \text{Metamyelocytes} + \text{Myelocytes})}$$

Schelonka and associates reported that normal I/T ratios in term neonates have a mean value of 0.16 (standard deviation [SD] 0.10), with a 10th to 90th percentile range extending from 0.05 to 0.27.[32] An elevated I/T ratio (≥0.3) in the presence of neutropenia reflects (1) depletion of the postmitotic neutrophil storage pool in the bone marrow due to increased peripheral destruction/tissue recruitment of neutrophils, and (2) in most instances, an increase in the marrow production of neutrophils. A normal or low I/T ratio in the presence of severe neutropenia suggests that the neutropenia results from decreased production, just as would be inferred for erythrocytes in an anemic patient with a low reticulocyte count.

The I/T neutrophil ratio is best known for its value in screening tests for sepsis in neonates, even though elevated ratios can be seen in many other conditions. Unlike the ANC, which shows a wider spread, the I/T ratio retains its discriminatory value for sepsis, even in VLBW infants, and can be successfully employed in conjunction with other screening tests, such as C-reactive protein concentrations.[33-35]

A bone marrow biopsy can be useful in cases of prolonged (>2 weeks), unusual, or refractory neutropenia. The procedure usually is performed in the tibial marrow using an Osgood needle.[36] The marrow is evaluated for proliferative and postmitotic storage pools of neutrophils. Reduction in both cellular populations suggests decreased marrow production, and increased numbers of proliferative precursors with a depleted storage pool are consistent with increased peripheral destruction of neutrophils. The combination of an expanded proliferative pool with a normal storage pool generally is seen during marrow recovery and is relatively nonspecific.[37,38] However, it should be noted that although marrow findings can provide vital kinetic information, the observations are rarely of diagnostic value. For instance, marrow findings can be very similar between a person in a hyporegenerative state as disparate as Kostmann syndrome and an infant born to a hypertensive mother, even when the clinical conditions are completely different in terms of origin and outcome.

Evaluation of Clinical Severity

Risks of infection and mortality in neutropenic neonates correlate with the following:
1. Severity of neutropenia (risk related inversely to the ANC).[39]
2. Overall severity of sickness/concurrent illnesses, because it increases the probability of invasive monitoring and lower tissue resistance.[29] In VLBW infants, the risk of infection secondary to neutropenia and the mortality attributable to infection in the setting of neutropenia are significantly higher than in term newborns.[39]
3. Duration of neutropenia: the risk of infection increases with duration, and persistent neutropenia should trigger evaluation and/or treatment even if it is moderate in severity.[23]

Clinical Management of a Neonate with Neutropenia

The clinical approach to the neonate with neutropenia should depend on the severity, duration, and cause of the disorder. In an ill neutropenic neonate, sepsis should always be considered as a possibility, and antibiotic therapy should be started pending culture maturation. If the neutropenia is severe and prolonged, reverse isolation procedures may be considered.

The role of prophylactic antibiotics in neonatal neutropenia is unclear. In children with chronic idiopathic or chemotherapy-associated neutropenia, antibiotics sometimes are recommended until neutrophil counts reach $1000/\mu L$.[40-42] Because most causes of neonatal neutropenia are transient, and in view of the concern for emerging multidrug-resistant bacterial strains, routine antibiotic prophylaxis is not recommended in newborn infants at this time.

Hematopoietic Growth Factors

Granulocyte-colony stimulating factor (G-CSF) and granulocyte-macrophage colony-stimulating factor (GM-CSF) are naturally occurring cytokines that are in routine clinical use in adults and children to accelerate neutrophil recovery following anticancer therapy. G-CSF increases the number of circulating neutrophils by stimulating the release of neutrophils from bone marrow, inducing myeloid proliferation, and reducing neutrophil apoptosis.[43] GM-CSF was initially defined by its ability to generate both granulocyte and macrophage colonies from precursor cells as a result of proliferation and differentiation.[44] Under physiologic conditions, G-CSF is the primary systemic regulator of the circulating concentrations of neutrophils.[43] GM-CSF, on the contrary, does not play a major role in steady state conditions but is upregulated at tissue sites of inflammation to enhance neutrophil and macrophage maturation.[45]

Recombinant G-CSF and GM-CSF have been evaluated in neonates with neutropenia. Both agents hold promise in correction of circulating neutrophil concentrations, although the efficacy varies with the cause. The effects of these growth factors on clinical outcomes remain unresolved.

Role in Neonatal Sepsis

Recombinant G-CSF has been evaluated in neonatal sepsis and neutropenia in several trials. Gillan and associates reported a dose-dependent biologic effect of G-CSF.[46] They studied 42 neonates with presumed bacterial infection during their first 3 days of life. Infants were randomized to receive placebo or 1, 5, 10, or 20 μg/kg/day of G-CSF for 3 consecutive days. A dose-dependent increase in blood neutrophil concentrations was observed. Since then, the efficacy of G-CSF in neonatal sepsis has been examined by Schibler,[47] Bedford-Russell,[48] Miura,[49] Barak,[50] and Kocherlakota.[51] In a meta-analysis based on these studies, Bernstein and colleagues[42] reported that 73 G-CSF recipients had a lower mortality rate than 82 infants in a control arm. However, when the nonrandomized studies were excluded, results did not remain statistically significant.

Recombinant GM-CSF therapy has also been tried in neonatal sepsis. Cairo and associates observed dose-dependent increases in circulating neutrophil and monocyte concentrations within 48 hours of GM-CSF administration (5 or 10 μg/kg/day). Tibial marrow aspirates revealed an increase in neutrophil reserves, and neutrophil C3bi receptor expression was increased within 24 hours of the start of treatment.[52] Bilgin and colleagues, in a prospective, randomized study, administered GM-CSF to 30 patients for 7 consecutive days. Twenty-five patients from the GM-CSF group and 24 from the conventionally treated group had early-onset sepsis; the remaining 11 patients had late-onset sepsis. The GM-CSF–treated group showed significantly higher absolute neutrophil counts and a lower mortality rate.[53]

GM-CSF therapy has been evaluated in VLBW infants as prophylaxis against nosocomial infections. Both neutrophils and mononuclear phagocytes are known to be functionally immature in neonates, and hence prophylactic use of GM-CSF was well supported by pathophysiologic considerations. Carr and colleagues initiated a 5-day course of prophylactic GM-CSF therapy (10 μg/kg) in 75 noninfected VLBW neonates within the first 72 hours of life. GM-CSF therapy abolished neutropenia in treated infants, including those with and without sepsis, during a 4-week period following study entry. Although GM-CSF recipients had fewer symptomatic, blood culture–positive septic episodes than controls, the difference did not reach statistical significance.[54] In another large, randomized, placebo-controlled trial in 264 extremely low birthweight (ELBW) neonates, prophylactic GM-CSF administration at 8 μg/kg for the first 7 days and then every other day for 21 days led to higher ANCs but did not change the incidence of confirmed nosocomial infections.[55] Similar findings were reported in a recent multicenter, randomized controlled trial of 280 neonates from 26 centers, suggesting that although GM-CSF corrects neutropenia, it does not lead to lower rates of sepsis or improved survival.[56]

Recombinant G-CSF may be more efficacious in raising neutrophil counts than GM-CSF. When cord blood neutrophils are treated with these agents in vitro, only G-CSF delays apoptosis.[57] In a small study, Ahmad and coworkers[58] compared the relative efficacy of G-CSF versus GM-CSF in correcting sepsis-induced neutropenia. Twenty-eight patients were randomized: 10 received G-CSF (10 μg/kg/day), 10 received GM-CSF (8 μg/kg/day), and 8 received placebo for a maximum of 7 days, or until an ANC of 10,000/μL was reached. The neutrophil count in the G-CSF–treated group increased more rapidly than in the GM-CSF–treated group.

Carr and associates reviewed existing evidence for the use of G-CSF/GM-CSF in neonatal sepsis.[59] In preterm infants with suspected systemic infection, G-CSF or GM-CSF did not provide additional survival advantage beyond antibiotic therapy (typical relative risk of death, 0.71 [95% confidence interval {CI}, 0.38 to 1.33]). However, in a subgroup analysis of 97 infants who, in addition to systemic infection, had clinically significant neutropenia at trial entry (ANC <1700/μL), investigators did find a significant reduction in mortality by day 14 (relative risk, 0.34 [95% CI, 0.12 to 0.92]; risk difference, −0.18 [95% CI, −0.33 to −0.03]; number needed to treat, 6 [95% CI, 3 to 33]). In prophylactic studies, recombinant GM-CSF did not reduce mortality (relative risk, 0.59 [95% CI, 0.24 to 1.44]; risk difference, −0.03 [95% CI, −0.08 to 0.02]).

Role in Neonatal Immune-Mediated Neutropenias

Recombinant G-CSF has been successfully used in correcting immune-mediated neutropenias in infants. Besides its effects on neutrophil production and delayed apoptosis, G-CSF provides beneficial effects on immune-mediated neutropenias by downregulating antigen expression, thus rendering the neutrophils less vulnerable to circulating antibodies.[60] This effect may be most pronounced with antigens located on the FcγIIIb, such as HNA-1a and HNA-1b. G-CSF activates neutrophils and might also correct some of the functional impairments induced in neutrophils by antineutrophil antibodies.[61] It is notable that in patients with immune-mediated neutropenias, serum G-CSF levels may not rise appropriately unless they have an infection, providing further justification for recombinant therapy.[62] A review of immune-mediated neutropenias in neonates can be found elsewhere.[25]

G-CSF may have to be used with caution in patients with immune-mediated neutropenias secondary to antibodies against the neutrophil antigen HNA-2a (NB1). Stroncek and associates demonstrated that unlike its downregulating effects on HNA-1a and -1b antibodies, G-CSF increased expression of HNA-2a antibodies in healthy adult volunteers.[63] Neonates with alloimmune neutropenia secondary to anti-HNA-2a antibodies may have severe, prolonged neutropenia and may require unusually high doses of G-CSF.[28,64]

Role in Congenital Neutropenias

G-CSF is highly effective in patients with congenital neutropenias.[65] This group of disorders broadly includes various inherited forms of neutropenia such as Kostmann syndrome (severe congenital neutropenia), cyclic neutropenia, Shwachman-Diamond syndrome, and inborn errors of metabolism (e.g., glycogen storage disease 1b, organic acidemias). These conditions can be associated with ANCs below 500/μL and increased susceptibility to bacterial infection.[65-67]

Kostmann syndrome is marked by severe neutropenia presenting in early infancy with ANCs of less than 200/μl and recurrent bacterial infections. Most patients have mutations in the neutrophil elastase (ELA2/ELANE) gene, although mutations in GFI1, HAX1, G6PC3, and WAS genes have also been reported.[66,68] G-CSF therapy is highly effective in patients with Kostmann syndrome. Data on more than 1100 patients collected by the Severe Chronic Neutropenia International Registry (SCNIR) since 1994 have shown that recombinant G-CSF therapy was effective in more than 90% of patients in maintaining the ANC at or above approximately 1000/μL.[69] All responding patients required significantly fewer antibiotics and days of hospitalization.[70] Over the past two decades, recombinant G-CSF therapy has significantly improved the survival of these patients.[71]

Human cyclic neutropenia is a rare hematologic disorder characterized by regular fluctuations in the serial counts of blood neutrophils.[72] Oscillations occur at approximately 3-week intervals, when neutrophil counts often fall to less than 250/μL for 3 to 5 days. Bone marrow examination reveals a variable morphology, which appears normal during periods of higher neutrophil counts, along with a "maturation arrest" of neutrophilic production during or just before the onset of severe neutropenia. Other blood cells, such as platelets and reticulocytes, often vary in a cyclic pattern. G-CSF is considered in these infants if infections occur during periods of severe neutropenia. Continuous G-CSF therapy can elevate blood neutrophil counts to a safe level with lower risk of infection. Although the characteristic cycles are not eliminated by G-CSF, the period of severe neutropenia is shortened.[73] In contrast to G-CSF, patients respond very poorly to GM-CSF.[74]

Shwachman-Diamond syndrome (SDS) is characterized by exocrine pancreatic insufficiency, neutropenia, poor growth, and skeletal abnormalities. Neutropenia might be seen in the neonatal period[75] and is the most common hematologic abnormality, occurring in 88% to 100% of patients.[76] The neutropenia is usually intermittent, fluctuating from severely low to normal levels, but it can also be chronic. G-CSF therapy is effective in inducing a clinically beneficial neutrophil response. GM-CSF has been used but with inconsistent results.[77]

Glycogen storage disease type 1b is a rare metabolic disorder that affects the transport system of glucose-6-phosphatase metabolism. Patients present with hepatomegaly, failure to thrive, renal dysfunction, and recurrent infections. Chronic neutropenia in these patients is accompanied by functional defects in chemotaxis and phagocytosis. G-CSF therapy corrects neutropenia in these patients and restores some of the functional activity of these cells.[78]

Role in Neutropenia Related to Maternal Pregnancy-Induced Hypertension (PIH)

G-CSF has been used successfully in the neutropenia of PIH. Makhlouf and associates treated nine neutropenic infants born to mothers with preeclampsia with G-CSF (10 µg/kg/day), starting within 24 hours of birth, and for a maximum of three doses if neutropenia persisted. The ANC increased significantly in eight of the nine infants within 6 hours, and neutrophilia was sustained for at least 72 hours after administration of a single dose of G-CSF.[79] Similar results were reported by La Gamma and associates, who treated four infants with G-CSF for up to 3 days. ANCs increased nearly fourfold within 48 hours, reaching their maximum values 9 days after initiation of therapy. Total leukocyte counts subsequently decreased but remained in the normal range.[80]

Conflicting reports have discussed whether neonates with neutropenia related to maternal PIH are at higher risk of infection.[81-84] G-CSF therapy may reduce the incidence of infection in some of these infants.[85] However, infants born to preeclamptic mothers may have a slower neutrophilic response with G-CSF when compared with their counterparts born to normotensive mothers.[86] It remains unclear which neonates with neutropenia of PIH would be well served by G-CSF treatment.

Role in "Idiopathic" Neutropenia

Juul and Christensen reported a severe, prolonged, idiopathic, but self-resolving variety of neutropenia among preterm neonates.[87] These infants were neutropenic at or shortly following delivery and remained neutropenic (generally <500/µL) for 1 to 9 weeks. Blood and bone marrow studies indicated that the neutropenia was (1) the kinetic result of diminished neutrophil production; (2) not alloimmune; (3) not cyclic; and (4) not associated with recognized inborn errors of metabolism, bacterial or viral infection, or medications. Treatment with G-CSF in these patients led to an immediate, marked increase in blood neutrophil concentrations. This effect persisted to day 5, but counts were not different from those of five placebo recipients on days 12 and 15. These patients apparently have a substantial G-CSF–mobilizable marrow neutrophil reserve, and on this basis, the authors speculated that idiopathic neonatal neutropenia may not constitute a significant deficiency in antibacterial defense.[88] The decision to treat these well infants may have to be individualized, depending on the duration and severity of neutropenia. The diagnosis of idiopathic neutropenia remains one of exclusion and is often considered in retrospect following a dramatic resolution of neutropenia with G-CSF therapy.

Dosing and Safety of G-CSF Therapy

The usual dose of G-CSF is 5 to 10 µg/kg/day administered by intravenous or subcutaneous injection. In most situations, the response is evident within 24 to 48 hours. In well neutropenic infants, treatment should be considered only if neutropenia persists for longer than 2 to 3 days, because many of these babies will recover spontaneously, and the overall risk of sepsis in otherwise healthy neonates has been reported to be about 8.5%. G-CSF therapy is not used routinely in sepsis-induced neutropenia because it is often a transient phenomenon, endogenous G-CSF levels are often high in these patients, and definite evidence of its benefit is lacking. In patients with neutropenia related to maternal hypertension, treatment is considered if ANCs are fewer than 500/µL and persist at this level

8

8

for many days. Neonates with immune-mediated neutropenia usually respond promptly to G-CSF but often need continued treatment for 2 to 3 weeks.

In an occasional patient, G-CSF therapy will not raise blood neutrophil counts. In these apparently refractory cases, a bone marrow examination should be considered. G-CSF doses may be increased in increments of 10 μg/kg at 7- to 14-day intervals if the ANC remains below 1000/μL.[25] Doses can be reduced or withheld once ANCs reach 5000/μL or above, and attempts should be made to use the lowest dose necessary to maintain a "safe" neutrophil count that is high enough to overcome infection.

The adverse effects of short term G-CSF administration to neutropenic neonates are minimal, although Gilmore and associates noted that one of their infants with alloimmune neutropenia was irritable after the first two doses.[89] These authors considered the possibility of bone pain, because it is often seen in older children receiving G-CSF for other indications. However, this did not necessitate cessation of therapy and quickly resolved after completion of treatment. Moderate thrombocytopenia has been reported in infants receiving higher doses or prolonged courses of therapy.[90] With long-term G-CSF therapy, as in congenital neutropenias, mild splenomegaly, osteoporosis, myeloid hypoplasia, malignant transformation into myelodysplastic syndrome/leukemia, and anti-GCSF antibodies have been described.[91,92] The risk of malignant transformation with long-term G-CSF therapy in patients with Kostmann syndrome has been estimated to be about 2 to 3 cases per 100 patients per year after 10 years of treatment.[93]

Intravenous Immunoglobulins

Intravenous immunoglobulins (IVIGs) have been used with success in alloimmune and autoimmune neutropenia, with a response rate of about 50%.[29,94,95] The elevation in neutrophil counts is often transient, lasting for about a week, although long-term remissions have been reported.[29,96,97] Muscarin and Ventura used anti-Rh (D) immunoglobulin in a 7-month-old infant with autoimmune neutropenia and achieved an improvement in neutrophil counts, but the effect again lasted for only about 10 days.[98] In view of logistic difficulties in outpatient administration of IVIG, lack of a titratable dose-response effect, and the fact that IVIG can rarely induce neutropenia as a side effect, it has been used less often than G-CSF in patients with immune-mediated neutropenia.[99] However, it may be a viable second-line option.[96]

IVIG has been used with moderate success in neonatal sepsis. Administration of IVIG can successfully mobilize neutrophils from the marrow storage pool into the circulation, thereby helping, at least transiently, to ameliorate neutropenia.[100,101]

Corticosteroids

Steroids have been tried in the management of immune-mediated neutropenias and in congenital bone marrow failure syndromes. In alloimmune neutropenia, steroids are not very effective. Of five infants reported independently by Lalezari and Buckwold, only one showed a partial response.[102,103] The response has been slightly better in autoimmune neutropenia of infancy but is still inconsistent. Bux and colleagues treated seven patients and documented a sustained rise in neutrophil counts in four during the treatment period.[29,104]

Steroids have been used in conjunction with G-CSF in a patient with Kostmann syndrome who was refractory to treatment with G-CSF alone.[105] Activation of the glucocorticoid receptor can synergize G-CSF signals to promote proliferation of myeloid cells.

Other Modalities

Exchange transfusions have not been successful in treating immune-mediated neutropenia.[106] Granulocyte transfusions with cells negative for the incriminated antigen can be helpful acutely,[107] but the effect often lasts for only a few hours. Current evidence does not show a clear beneficial effect for their use.[108]

References

1. Baley JE, Stork EK, Warkentin PI, et al. Neonatal neutropenia. Clinical manifestations, cause, and outcome. *Am J Dis Child*. 1988;142:1161-1166.
2. Aladjidi N, Casanova JL, Canioni D, et al. Severe aplastic anemia of neonatal onset: A single-center retrospective study of six children. *J Pediatr*. 1998;132:600-605.
3. Christensen RD, Rothstein G. Exhaustion of mature marrow neutrophils in neonates with sepsis. *J Pediatr*. 1980;96:316-318.
4. Gessler P, Luders R, Konig S, et al. Neonatal neutropenia in low birthweight premature infants. *Am J Perinatol*. 1995;12:34-38.
5. Schmutz N, Henry E, Jopling J, et al. Expected ranges for blood neutrophil concentrations of neonates: The Manroe and Mouzinho charts revisited. *J Perinatol*. 2008;28:275-281.
6. al-Mulla ZS, Christensen RD. Neutropenia in the neonate. *Clin Perinatol*. 1995;22:711-739.
7. Christensen RD, Henry E, Wiedmeier SE, et al. Low blood neutrophil concentrations among extremely low birth weight neonates: Data from a multihospital health-care system. *J Perinatol*. 2006;26:682-687.
8. Athens JW. Disorders of neutrophil proliferation and circulations: A pathophysiological view. *Clin Haematol*. 1975;4:553-566.
9. Manroe BL, Rosenfeld CR, Weinberg AG, et al. The differential leukocyte count in the assessment and outcome of early-onset neonatal group B streptococcal disease. *J Pediatr*. 1977;91:632-637.
10. Mouzinho A, Rosenfeld CR, Sanchez PJ, et al. Revised reference ranges for circulating neutrophils in very-low-birth-weight neonates. *Pediatrics*. 1994;94:76-82.
11. Manroe BL, Weinberg AG, Rosenfeld CR, et al. The neonatal blood count in health and disease. I. Reference values for neutrophilic cells. *J Pediatr*. 1979;95:89-98.
12. Coulombel L, Dehan M, Tchernia G, et al. The number of polymorphonuclear leukocytes in relation to gestational age in the newborn. *Acta Paediatr Scand*. 1979;68:709-711.
13. Lloyd BW, Oto A. Normal values for mature and immature neutrophils in very preterm babies. *Arch Dis Child*. 1982;57:233-235.
14. Faix RG, Hric JJ, Naglie RA. Neutropenia and intraventricular hemorrhage among very low birth weight (less than 1500 grams) premature infants. *J Pediatr*. 1989;114:1035-1038.
15. Prober CG, Stevenson DK, Neu J, et al. The white cell ratio in the very low birth weight infant. *Clin Pediatr (Phila)*. 1979;18:481-486.
16. Engle WD, Rosenfeld CR, Mouzinho A, et al. Circulating neutrophils in septic preterm neonates: Comparison of two reference ranges. *Pediatrics*. 1997;99:E10.
17. Bourner G, Dhaliwal J, Sumner J. Performance evaluation of the latest fully automated hematology analyzers in a large, commercial laboratory setting: A 4-way, side-by-side study. *Lab Hematol*. 2005;11:285-297.
18. Carballo C, Foucar K, Swanson P, et al. Effect of high altitude on neutrophil counts in newborn infants. *J Pediatr*. 1991;119:464-466.
19. Maynard EC, Reed C, Kircher T. Neutrophil counts in newborn infants at high altitude. *J Pediatr*. 1993;122:990-991.
20. Xanthou M. Leucocyte blood picture in healthy full-term and premature babies during neonatal period. *Arch Dis Child*. 1970;45:242-249.
21. Cartron J, Tchernia G, Celton JL, et al. Alloimmune neonatal neutropenia. *Am J Pediatr Hematol Oncol*. 1991;13:21-25.
22. Dale DC. Immune and idiopathic neutropenia. *Curr Opin Hematol*. 1998;5:33-36.
23. Gray PH, Rodwell RL. Neonatal neutropenia associated with maternal hypertension poses a risk for nosocomial infection. *Eur J Pediatr*. 1999;158:71-73.
24. Christensen RD, Calhoun DA, Rimsza LM. A practical approach to evaluating and treating neutropenia in the neonatal intensive care unit. *Clin Perinatol*. 2000;27:577-601.
25. Black LV, Maheshwari A. Immune-mediated neutropenia in the neonate. *Neoreviews*. 2009;10:446-453.
26. Maheshwari A, Christensen RD, Calhoun DA. Immune-mediated neutropenia in the neonate. *Acta Paediatr Suppl*. 2002;91:98-103.
27. Maheshwari A, Christensen RD, Calhoun DA. Immune neutropenia in the neonate. *Adv Pediatr*. 2002;49:317-339.
28. Maheshwari A, Christensen RD, Calhoun DA. Resistance to recombinant human granulocyte colony-stimulating factor in neonatal alloimmune neutropenia associated with anti-human neutrophil antigen-2a (NB1) antibodies. *Pediatrics*. 2002;109:e64.
29. Bux J, Behrens G, Jaeger G, et al. Diagnosis and clinical course of autoimmune neutropenia in infancy: Analysis of 240 cases. *Blood*. 1998;91:181-186.
30. Clay ME, Schuller RM, Bachowski GJ. Granulocyte serology: Current concepts and clinical significance. *Immunohematology*. 2010;26:11-21.
31. van Eeden SF, Miyagashima R, Haley L, et al. A possible role for L-selectin in the release of polymorphonuclear leukocytes from bone marrow. *Am J Physiol*. 1997;272:H1717-H1724.
32. Schelonka RL, Yoder BA, desJardins SE, et al. Peripheral leukocyte count and leukocyte indexes in healthy newborn term infants. *J Pediatr*. 1994;125:603-606.
33. Rodwell RL, Leslie AL, Tudehope DI. Early diagnosis of neonatal sepsis using a hematologic scoring system. *J Pediatr*. 1988;112:761-767.
34. Spector SA, Ticknor W, Grossman M. Study of the usefulness of clinical and hematologic findings in the diagnosis of neonatal bacterial infections. *Clin Pediatr (Phila)*. 1981;20:385-392.

8

35. Christensen RD, Bradley PP, Rothstein G. The leukocyte left shift in clinical and experimental neonatal sepsis. *J Pediatr.* 1981;98:101-105.
36. Sola MC, Rimsza LM, Christensen RD. A bone marrow biopsy technique suitable for use in neonates. *Br J Haematol.* 1999;107:458-460.
37. Christensen RD. Granulocytopoiesis in the fetus and neonate. *Transfus Med Rev.* 1990;4:8-13.
38. Christensen RD. Neutrophil kinetics in the fetus and neonate. *Am J Pediatr Hematol Oncol.* 1989; 11:215-223.
39. Funke A, Berner R, Traichel B, et al. Frequency, natural course, and outcome of neonatal neutropenia. *Pediatrics.* 2000;106:45-51.
40. Trifilio S, Verma A, Mehta J. Antimicrobial prophylaxis in hematopoietic stem cell transplant recipients: Heterogeneity of current clinical practice. *Bone Marrow Transplant.* 2004;33:735-739.
41. Bernini JC, Wooley R, Buchanan GR. Low-dose recombinant human granulocyte colony-stimulating factor therapy in children with symptomatic chronic idiopathic neutropenia. *J Pediatr.* 1996;129: 551-558.
42. Calhoun DA, Christensen RD, Edstrom CS, et al. Consistent approaches to procedures and practices in neonatal hematology. *Clin Perinatol.* 2000;27:733-753.
43. Calhoun DA, Christensen RD. Human developmental biology of granulocyte colony-stimulating factor. *Clin Perinatol.* 2000;27:559-576, vi.
44. Burgess AW, Metcalf D. The nature and action of granulocyte-macrophage colony stimulating factors. *Blood.* 1980;56:947-958.
45. Hamilton JA, Anderson GP. GM-CSF Biology. *Growth Factors.* 2004;22:225-231.
46. Gillan ER, Christensen RD, Suen Y, et al. A randomized, placebo-controlled trial of recombinant human granulocyte colony-stimulating factor administration in newborn infants with presumed sepsis: Significant induction of peripheral and bone marrow neutrophilia. *Blood.* 1994;84: 1427-1433.
47. Schibler KR, Osborne KA, Leung LY, et al. A randomized, placebo-controlled trial of granulocyte colony-stimulating factor administration to newborn infants with neutropenia and clinical signs of early-onset sepsis. *Pediatrics.* 1998;102:6-13.
48. Bedford Russell AR, Emmerson AJ, Wilkinson N, et al. A trial of recombinant human granulocyte colony stimulating factor for the treatment of very low birthweight infants with presumed sepsis and neutropenia. *Arch Dis Child Fetal Neonatal Ed.* 2001;84:F172-F176.
49. Miura E, Procianoy RS, Bittar C, et al. A randomized, double-masked, placebo-controlled trial of recombinant granulocyte colony-stimulating factor administration to preterm infants with the clinical diagnosis of early-onset sepsis. *Pediatrics.* 2001;107:30-35.
50. Barak Y, Leibovitz E, Mogilner B, et al. The in vivo effect of recombinant human granulocyte-colony stimulating factor in neutropenic neonates with sepsis. *Eur J Pediatr.* 1997;156:643-646.
51. Kocherlakota P, La Gamma EF. Human granulocyte colony-stimulating factor may improve outcome attributable to neonatal sepsis complicated by neutropenia. *Pediatrics.* 1997;100:E6.
52. Cairo MS, Christensen R, Sender LS, et al. Results of a phase I/II trial of recombinant human granulocyte-macrophage colony-stimulating factor in very low birthweight neonates: Significant induction of circulatory neutrophils, monocytes, platelets, and bone marrow neutrophils. *Blood.* 1995;86:2509-2515.
53. Bilgin K, Yaramis A, Haspolat K, et al. A randomized trial of granulocyte-macrophage colony-stimulating factor in neonates with sepsis and neutropenia. *Pediatrics.* 2001;107: 36-41.
54. Carr R, Modi N, Dore CJ, et al. A randomized, controlled trial of prophylactic granulocyte-macrophage colony-stimulating factor in human newborns less than 32 weeks gestation. *Pediatrics.* 1999;103:796-802.
55. Cairo MS, Agosti J, Ellis R, et al. A randomized, double-blind, placebo-controlled trial of prophylactic recombinant human granulocyte-macrophage colony-stimulating factor to reduce nosocomial infections in very low birth weight neonates. *J Pediatr.* 1999;134:64-70.
56. Carr R, Brocklehurst P, Dore CJ, et al. Granulocyte-macrophage colony stimulating factor administered as prophylaxis for reduction of sepsis in extremely preterm, small for gestational age neonates (the PROGRAMS trial): A single-blind, multicentre, randomised controlled trial. *Lancet.* 2009; 373:226-233.
57. Molloy EJ, O'Neill AJ, Grantham JJ, et al. Granulocyte colony-stimulating factor and granulocyte-macrophage colony-stimulating factor have differential effects on neonatal and adult neutrophil survival and function. *Pediatr Res.* 2005;57:806-812.
58. Ahmad A, Laborada G, Bussel J, et al. Comparison of recombinant granulocyte colony-stimulating factor, recombinant human granulocyte-macrophage colony-stimulating factor and placebo for treatment of septic preterm infants. *Pediatr Infect Dis J.* 2002;21:1061-1065.
59. Carr R, Modi N, Dore C. G-CSF and GM-CSF for treating or preventing neonatal infections. *Cochrane Database Syst Rev.* 2003:CD003066.
60. Rodwell RL, Gray PH, Taylor KM, et al. Granulocyte colony stimulating factor treatment for alloimmune neonatal neutropenia. *Arch Dis Child Fetal Neonatal Ed.* 1996;75:F57-F58.
61. Kerst JM, de Haas M, van der Schoot CE, et al. Recombinant granulocyte colony-stimulating factor administration to healthy volunteers: Induction of immunophenotypically and functionally altered neutrophils via an effect on myeloid progenitor cells. *Blood.* 1993;82:3265-3272.
62. de Haas M, Kerst JM, van der Schoot CE, et al. Granulocyte colony-stimulating factor administration to healthy volunteers: Analysis of the immediate activating effects on circulating neutrophils. *Blood.* 1994;84:3885-3894.

8

63. Stroncek DF, Jaszcz W, Herr GP, et al. Expression of neutrophil antigens after 10 days of granulocyte-colony-stimulating factor. *Transfusion*. 1998;38:663-668.
64. Tomicic M, Starcevic M, Zach V, et al. Alloimmune neonatal neutropenia due to anti-HNA-2a allo-immunization with severe and prolonged neutropenia but mild clinical course: Two case reports. *Arch Med Res*. 2007;38:792-796.
65. Christensen RD, Calhoun DA. Congenital neutropenia. *Clin Perinatol*. 2004;31:29-38.
66. Dale DC, Person RE, Bolyard AA, et al. Mutations in the gene encoding neutrophil elastase in congenital and cyclic neutropenia. *Blood*. 2000;96:2317-2322.
67. Zeidler C. Congenital neutropenias. *Hematology*. 2005;10(Suppl 1):306-311.
68. Boztug K, Klein C. Genetic etiologies of severe congenital neutropenia. *Curr Opin Pediatr*. 2011;23:21-26.
69. Dale DC, Bolyard AA, Schwinzer BG, et al. The Severe Chronic Neutropenia International Registry: 10-year follow-up report. *Support Cancer Ther*. 2006;3:220-231.
70. Zeidler C, Boxer L, Dale DC, et al. Management of Kostmann syndrome in the G-CSF era. *Br J Haematol*. 2000;109:490-495.
71. Freedman MH. Safety of long-term administration of granulocyte colony-stimulating factor for severe chronic neutropenia. *Curr Opin Hematol*. 1997;4:217-224.
72. Dale DC, Hammond WPT. Cyclic neutropenia: A clinical review. *Blood Rev*. 1988;2:178-185.
73. Schmitz S, Franke H, Wichmann HE, et al. The effect of continuous G-CSF application in human cyclic neutropenia: A model analysis. *Br J Haematol*. 1995;90:41-47.
74. Schmitz S, Franke H, Loeffler M, et al. Model analysis of the contrasting effects of GM-CSF and G-CSF treatment on peripheral blood neutrophils observed in three patients with childhood-onset cyclic neutropenia. *Br J Haematol*. 1996;95:616-625.
75. Black LV, Soltau T, Kelly DR, et al. Shwachman-Diamond syndrome presenting in a premature infant as pancytopenia. *Pediatr Blood Cancer*. 2008;51:123-124.
76. Dror Y. Shwachman-Diamond syndrome. *Pediatr Blood Cancer*. 2005;45:892-901.
77. van der Sande FM, Hillen HF. Correction of neutropenia following treatment with granulocyte colony-stimulating factor results in a decreased frequency of infections in Shwachman's syndrome. *Neth J Med*. 1996;48:92-95.
78. Lesma E, Riva E, Giovannini M, et al. Amelioration of neutrophil membrane function underlies granulocyte-colony stimulating factor action in glycogen storage disease 1b. *Int J Immunopathol Pharmacol*. 2005;18:297-307.
79. Makhlouf RA, Doron MW, Bose CL, et al. Administration of granulocyte colony-stimulating factor to neutropenic low birth weight infants of mothers with preeclampsia. *J Pediatr*. 1995;126:454-456.
80. La Gamma EF, Alpan O, Kocherlakota P. Effect of granulocyte colony-stimulating factor on preeclampsia-associated neonatal neutropenia. *J Pediatr*. 1995;126:457-459.
81. Procianoy RS, Silveira RC, Mussi-Pinhata MM, et al. Sepsis and neutropenia in very low birth weight infants delivered of mothers with preeclampsia. *J Pediatr*. 2010;157:434-438.
82. Sharma G, Nesin M, Feuerstein M, et al. Maternal and neonatal characteristics associated with neonatal neutropenia in hypertensive pregnancies. *Am J Perinatol*. 2009;26:683-689.
83. Doron MW, Makhlouf RA, Katz VL, et al. Increased incidence of sepsis at birth in neutropenic infants of mothers with preeclampsia. *J Pediatr*. 1994;125:452-458.
84. Paul DA, Leef KH, Sciscione A, et al. Preeclampsia does not increase the risk for culture proven sepsis in very low birth weight infants. *Am J Perinatol*. 1999;16:365-372.
85. Kocherlakota P, La Gamma EF. Preliminary report: rhG-CSF may reduce the incidence of neonatal sepsis in prolonged preeclampsia-associated neutropenia. *Pediatrics*. 1998;102:1107-1111.
86. Zuppa AA, Girlando P, Florio MG, et al. Influence of maternal preeclampsia on recombinant human granulocyte colony-stimulating factor effect in neutropenic neonates with suspected sepsis. *Eur J Obstet Gynecol Reprod Biol*. 2002;102:131-136.
87. Juul SE, Calhoun DA, Christensen RD. "Idiopathic neutropenia" in very low birthweight infants. *Acta Paediatr*. 1998;87:963-968.
88. Juul SE, Christensen RD. Effect of recombinant granulocyte colony-stimulating factor on blood neutrophil concentrations among patients with "idiopathic neonatal neutropenia": A randomized, placebo-controlled trial. *J Perinatol*. 2003;23:493-497.
89. Gilmore MM, Stroncek DF, Korones DN. Treatment of alloimmune neonatal neutropenia with granulocyte colony-stimulating factor. *J Pediatr*. 1994;125:948-951.
90. Wiedl C, Walter AW. Granulocyte colony stimulating factor in neonatal alloimmune neutropenia: A possible association with induced thrombocytopenia. *Pediatr Blood Cancer*. 2010;54:1014-1016.
91. Yakisan E, Schirg E, Zeidler C, et al. High incidence of significant bone loss in patients with severe congenital neutropenia (Kostmann's syndrome). *J Pediatr*. 1997;131:592-597.
92. Taniguchi S, Shibuya T, Harada M, et al. Decreased levels of myeloid progenitor cells associated with long-term administration of recombinant human granulocyte colony-stimulating factor in patients with autoimmune neutropenia. *Br J Haematol*. 1993;83:384-387.
93. Rosenberg PS, Zeidler C, Bolyard AA, et al. Stable long-term risk of leukaemia in patients with severe congenital neutropenia maintained on G-CSF therapy. *Br J Haematol*. 2010;150:196-199.
94. Yoshida N, Shikata T, Sudo S, et al. Alloimmune neonatal neutropenia in monozygous twins. High-dose intravenous gammaglobulin therapy. *Acta Paediatr Scand*. 1991;80:62-65.
95. Kemp AS, Lubitz L. Delayed umbilical cord separation in alloimmune neutropenia. *Arch Dis Child*. 1993;68:52-53.

8

96. Desenfants A, Jeziorski E, Plan O, et al. Intravenous immunoglobulins for neonatal alloimmune neutropenia refractory to recombinant human granulocyte colony-stimulating factor. *Am J Perinatol.* 2011;28:461-466.

97. Bussel J, Lalezari P, Fikrig S. Intravenous treatment with gamma-globulin of autoimmune neutropenia of infancy. *J Pediatr.* 1988;112:298-301.

98. Mascarin M, Ventura A. Anti-Rh(D) immunoglobulin for autoimmune neutropenia of infancy. *Acta Paediatr.* 1993;82:142-144.

99. Lassiter HA, Bibb KW, Bertolone SJ, et al. Neonatal immune neutropenia following the administration of intravenous immune globulin. *Am J Pediatr Hematol Oncol.* 1993;15:120-123.

100. Christensen RD, Brown MS, Hall DC, et al. Effect on neutrophil kinetics and serum opsonic capacity of intravenous administration of immune globulin to neonates with clinical signs of early-onset sepsis. *J Pediatr.* 1991;118:606-614.

101. Lamari F, Anastassiou ED, Stamokosta E, et al. Determination of slime-producing S. epidermidis specific antibodies in human immunoglobulin preparations and blood sera by an enzyme immunoassay: Correlation of antibody titers with opsonic activity and application to preterm neonates. *J Pharm Biomed Anal.* 2000;23:363-374.

102. Buckwold AE, Emson HE. Acute neonatal neutropenia in siblings. *Can Med Assoc J.* 1959;80:116-119.

103. Lalezari P. Alloimmune neonatal neutropenia and neutrophil-specific antigens. *Vox Sang.* 1984;46:415-417.

104. Bux J, Hartmann C, Mueller-Eckhardt C. Alloimmune neonatal neutropenia resulting from immunization to a high-frequency antigen on the granulocyte Fc gamma receptor III. *Transfusion.* 1994;34:608-611.

105. Dror Y, Ward AC, Touw IP, et al. Combined corticosteroid/granulocyte colony-stimulating factor (G-CSF) therapy in the treatment of severe congenital neutropenia unresponsive to G-CSF: Activated glucocorticoid receptors synergize with G-CSF signals. *Exp Hematol.* 2000;28:1381-1389.

106. Hinkel GK, Schneider I, Gebhardt B, et al. Alloimmune neonatal neutropenia: Clinical observations and therapeutic consequences. *Acta Paediatr Hung.* 1986;27:31-41.

107. Vrielink H, Meijer B, van't Ende E, et al. Granulocyte transfusions for pediatric patients and the establishment of national treatment guidelines and donor registry. *Transfus Apher Sci.* 2009;41:73-76.

108. Mohan P, Brocklehurst P. Granulocyte transfusions for neonates with confirmed or suspected sepsis and neutropaenia. *Cochrane Database Syst Rev.* 2003:CD003956.

8

CHAPTER 9

What Evidence Supports Dietary Interventions to Prevent Infant Food Hypersensitivity and Allergy?

David A. Osborn, MBBS, MMed (Clin Epi), FRACP, PhD, and
John K.H. Sinn, MBBS, FRACP, MMed (Clin Epi)

- Nomenclature
- Allergy and Food Hypersensitivity
- Prevention
- Future Directions
- Conclusions

Food hypersensitivity and allergy are a prevalent and substantial health problem that may be increasing in developed countries.[1,2] A major focus has been placed on the mechanisms for development of immune tolerance and allergen sensitization in the fetus and newborn, and on primary prevention strategies. This chapter focuses on evidence for the use of dietary interventions in pregnant and breast-feeding women, and on feed-related interventions in infants for the prevention of food hypersensitivity and allergy. Mechanisms for the in utero development of immune tolerance and allergy, consensus nomenclature for food hypersensitivity and allergy, and mechanisms, epidemiology, and risk factors for the development of food hypersensitivity and allergy are addressed.

Nomenclature

The terminology used to describe allergy and allergy-like reactions is confusing. As a result, the World Allergy Organization in 2003 reported an update of standardized nomenclature for allergy.[3] Briefly, the term *hypersensitivity* has been advocated to describe "objectively reproducible symptoms or signs initiated by exposure to a defined stimulus at a dose tolerated by a normal person." *Allergy* is a "hypersensitivity reaction initiated by immunologic mechanisms." *Atopy* is a "personal and/or familial tendency to become sensitized and produce immunoglobulin (Ig)E antibodies in response to ordinary exposures to allergens, usually proteins. As a consequence, these infants can develop typical symptoms of asthma, rhinoconjunctivitis, or eczema." Therefore, eczema may be atopic, which is IgE mediated, or non-atopic, which more commonly presents as chronic eczema associated with a lymphocytic infiltrate on skin biopsy. The presence of allergen-specific IgE is established by allergen skin-prick tests or by in vitro allergen-specific IgE measurements (e.g., radioallergosorbent test [RAST]). In infants with food hypersensitivity, food-specific IgG antibodies are not clinically important but indicate previous exposure to the food. If IgE is involved, the term *IgE-mediated food allergy* is used.

Allergy and Food Hypersensitivity

Several population-based studies using identical methods of ascertainment at intervals of 10 to 15 years have shown significant increases in the prevalence of allergic disease in children over the past 30 years in developed countries.[2,4,5] The manifestations of allergic disease are age dependent. Infants commonly present with

9

symptoms and signs of atopic eczema, gastrointestinal symptoms, and recurrent wheezing. Asthma and rhinoconjunctivitis become prevalent in later childhood. Sensitization to allergens tends to follow a characteristic pattern, with sensitization to food allergens in the first 2 to 3 years of life, then to indoor allergens (e.g., house dust mites, pets), and subsequently to outdoor allergens (e.g., rye, Timothy grass). The cumulative prevalence of allergic disease in childhood is high, with up to 7% to 8% developing a food allergy, 15% to 20% atopic eczema, and 31% to 34% asthma or recurrent wheezing. Of these, 7% to 10% will continue to have asthma symptoms beyond 5 years of age.[2]

Food hypersensitivities affect around 6% of infants younger than 3 years of age, with prevalence decreasing over the first decade.[6,7] Despite the vast array of food allergens that we are exposed to, relatively few account for the majority of food reactions. Cow's milk, soy, egg, and peanuts account for most cases of food hypersensitivity in children, whereas peanuts, tree nuts, fish, and shellfish are the most common food allergies in adults. A majority of infants who develop cow's milk reactions do so in the first year. Between 40% and 60% of these infants will have IgE-mediated reactions to proteins, including casein, β-lactoglobulin, bovine serum albumin, IgG heavy chains, and lactoferrin.[8] Many children outgrow their food hypersensitivity, although around 25% retain sensitivities in the second decade, and around 35% develop sensitizations to other foods. Clinical tolerance for most food allergens develops over time, with the exceptions of peanuts, nuts, and seafood.[2,6,7,9] However, prospective studies have reported that early sensitization to cow's milk, egg, and house dust mites is highly predictive of subsequent clinical allergic disease, including persistent atopic eczema and asthma, particularly in high-risk infants.

The Fetus: Immune Tolerance versus Sensitization

The fetus is capable of mounting sophisticated immune responses.[10] Circulating B lymphocytes can be detected with IgM surface immunoglobulin from as early as 19 to 20 weeks, implying that the full sensitization process, from antigen presentation to T cell proliferation to B cell stimulation and antibody production, has occurred. Almost universal priming to environmental antigens occurs in utero, with most infants subsequently being tolerant to exposure to the same antigens. However, the balance is altered toward sensitization in infants destined to have allergic disease. A minority of all infants will already have raised cord blood total IgE and specific IgE. IgE is reasonably specific but is not very sensitive for predicting later allergic disease.

Studies to date suggest that infants who develop allergies have a disturbance in the balance between cytokines that suppress an allergic response, as characterized by T helper-1 (Th-1) phenotypic responses, and allergy-promoting Th-2 responses. This balance appears to be affected by factors such as maternal atopy (risk), maternal IgG responses (protective), and potentially maternal and fetal nutritional factors. Two potential routes of fetal antigen exposure are from ingested antigens in the amniotic fluid and transplacental exposure. Although antigen-presenting cells are present in the fetal gut, they are not found in the skin or airways. It is thought that sensitization is more likely to occur in the gut, where mature active immune cells are found.[11] The second major route is via the placenta. Antigen is mostly complexed with maternal IgG, and this occurs maximally in the third trimester of pregnancy. However, transplacental passage of dietary antigens, including cow's milk β-lactoglobulin and egg ovalbumin, occurs as early as 26 weeks' gestation. The passage of antigens is enhanced across the preterm placenta and is increased by dose of exposure and decreasing molecular weight.[12] However, for immunologic priming to occur, the antigen must have access to sites where it can be taken up by dendritic cells for processing and presentation to naïve T cells. The specifics of these interactions, and how they are affected by genetic and environmental factors, are likely to be important in the understanding of fetal sensitization to allergens.

The Infant: Food Tolerance versus Sensitization

Food allergy is a manifestation of an abnormal mucosal immune response to ingested dietary antigens.[6] The gastrointestinal barrier is a complex physiochemical and cellular barrier. Innate (natural killer cells, neutrophils, macrophages, epithelial cells) and adaptive (intraepithelial and lamina propria lymphocytes, Peyer's patches, secretory IgA, cytokines) immune responses provide an active barrier to antigens. Even so, around 2% of ingested food antigens are absorbed. The efficiency of this gut barrier is reduced in the newborn period. Perinatal risk factors reported for asthma and/or allergy have included prematurity[13-15] and fetal growth restriction,[13] both of which are associated with an immature and potentially injured gut mucosal barrier. Maternal smoking may explain some of these effects.[14]

Mechanisms and Risk Factors for Development of Childhood Allergy and Food Hypersensitivity

A substantial proportion of children with clinical allergic disease are non-atopic, although this differs with the phenotypic expression of the disease.[2] In the Isle of Wight study,[16] among infants with a diagnosed allergic phenotype, only 32% were found to be atopic (identified by skin-prick test and serum-specific IgE). Of these, 14% had early transient sensitization at 4 years, 52% had persistent sensitization at 4 and 10 years, and 35% had delayed sensitization at 10 years. These atopic phenotypes had different risk factors, with sibling food allergy being the only heredity risk factor in regression analysis for delayed childhood atopy. Chronically atopic children were much more likely to have diagnosed asthma, eczema, and rhinoconjunctivitis. Their symptoms were more likely to be persistent and to be diagnosable as clinical allergy. The development of atopic disease is likely to be dependent on the complex interaction between genetic and environmental factors. Genetic factors are estimated to account for more than 50% of cases of asthma and allergy[2,17] but are unlikely to explain increasing prevalence over the past 30 years.[2] Dietary and environmental exposures to allergens, as well as modifying factors such as immaturity at birth,[13,15] high head-to-weight ratios,[13] infection,[18,19] intestinal miroflora, tobacco smoke,[14,18,20-22] dietary factors,[23] and pollution,[24] may well contribute to the development of asthma and allergy. Peat and Li[24] have developed a useful classification of risk factors for childhood asthma, which assists in the identification of high-risk children and serves as a guide to primary prevention.

Identifying Infants at High Risk of Food Sensitization or Allergy

Less than half of those who develop childhood allergic disease have a first-degree family history of allergy. However, the risk of development of allergic disease increases substantially with family heredity. Around 10% of children without a first-degree allergic relative develop allergic disease, compared with 20% to 30% with single allergic heredity (parent or sibling) and 40% to 50% with double allergic heredity.[18,25-27] Maternal and sibling allergy is a stronger predictor of childhood allergic disorders than is paternal allergy,[23] although paternal allergy is a stronger predictor of atopic sensitization.[21]

The use of cord blood IgE levels results in improved predictive ability for subsequent allergy. Although the combination of atopic family heredity and cord blood IgE levels has frequently been used in dietary preventive studies in infants, they still are not seen as sufficiently predictive for routine clinical use.[2] Defining a high-risk group as having double parental allergic predisposition or severe single parent allergy, combined with an infant cord blood IgE of 0.3 kU/L, results in the high-risk group constituting 8% to 10% of the total birth cohort, compared with 16% to 20% if cord blood IgE is not used, and 30% to 40% if all those with at least single atopic predisposition are included.[26] Studies of dietary interventions for the prevention of food hypersensitivity and allergy have variably defined high risk as a single first-degree relative with allergy, dual first-degree heredity, or a combination of first-degree heredity and cord blood IgE of 0.3 kU/L or 0.5 kU/L.[27,28] Clearly, there is a balance between achieving a high positive predictive value and having adequate sensitivity for allergy. To date, no highly accurate method is available for predicting food hypersensitivity and allergy in children. Current recommendations generally define high-risk infants in terms of atopic heredity.[29,30]

9

Prevention

By consensus,[30] prevention of allergy is divided into (1) primary prevention: the prevention of immunologic sensitization (development of IgE antibodies); (2) secondary prevention: preventing the onset of allergic disease following sensitization, such as the progression from eczema and rhinoconjunctivitis to more severe disease such as asthma; and (3) tertiary prevention: the treatment of allergic disease so as to prevent complications. The focus on the newborn is on primary prevention. Use of primary prevention measures requires meeting the following criteria[30]:

1. Measures have the potential to benefit a major proportion of the population.
2. Measures cause no known harm to anyone.
3. Measures do not involve unreasonable costs.

Factors facilitating primary prevention include the finding that infants with a family history of allergy are at increased risk of IgE sensitization, and the risk of developing IgE-mediated disease is related to family history for a specific allergic phenotype. Genetic factors are thought to contribute in excess of 50% of the development of IgE sensitization and IgE-mediated allergic disease. However, specific genes allowing identification of high-risk infants are yet to be adequately described. In addition, although sensitization to foods and other allergens precedes the development of allergy, exposure to dietary and environmental allergens is a ubiquitous and usually harmless phenomenon associated with tolerance.[31] In many infants, early sensitization to dietary allergens, although predictive of allergic disease, is followed by loss of sensitization. Therefore, the aim of primary prevention is to prevent not just sensitization, but also allergic disease. Primary prevention measures include those aimed at reducing or changing exposures to antigens and modifying adjuvant risk factors and exposures. This review focuses on evidence for dietary and adjuvant treatments that have the potential to be used for the primary prevention of clinical allergic disease, not just sensitization.

Maternal Dietary Allergen Avoidance in Pregnancy

A systematic review[32] identified three randomized trials enrolling 334 pregnant women that examined the effects of maternal dietary allergen avoidance in pregnancy for the prevention of infant allergy. All studies enrolled pregnant women with a first-degree family history of allergy (Table 9-1). Dietary interventions included a cow's milk and egg avoidance diet from 28 weeks' gestation,[33] a low milk and low egg diet during the third trimester,[34] and a milk-free diet from 36 weeks' gestation and during lactation.[35] No significant effect was reported for fetal or infant sensitization as indicated by cord blood IgE and infant skin-prick testing. Meta-analysis of the three trials[32] found no evidence of a protective effect of maternal dietary antigen avoidance during pregnancy for atopic eczema, asthma, urticarial, or any atopic

Table 9-1 RANDOMIZED TRIALS OF MATERNAL DIETARY ALLERGEN AVOIDANCE DURING PREGNANCY FOR PREVENTION OF ALLERGY IN INFANTS

Trial	N	Participants	Maternal Allergen Avoidance	Control
Falth-Magnusson et al, 1987, 1988, 1992[91-93]	212	Pregnant women with history of allergy in self, husband, or previous children	Cow's milk and egg avoidance diet from 28 weeks' gestation	Normal diet
Lilja et al, 1989, 1991[94,95]	171	Pregnant women with history of respiratory allergy to pollen and/or dander	Low milk and low egg diet during third trimester	High milk and high egg diet during third trimester
Lovegrove et al, 1994[35]	44	Pregnant women with atopic history in self or partner	Milk-free diet from 36 weeks' gestation and during lactation	Normal diet

Table 9-2 META-ANALYSES OF RANDOMIZED TRIALS OF MATERNAL DIETARY ALLERGEN AVOIDANCE DURING PREGNANCY FOR PREVENTION OF ALLERGY IN INFANTS[32]

Outcome	Studies/Participants	RR	95% CI
Atopic eczema (first 18 months)	2/334	1.01	0.57-1.79
Asthma (first 18 months)	2/334	2.22	0.39-12.67
Any atopic condition (first 18 months)	1/163	0.76	0.42-1.38
Urticaria (first 18 months)	1/163	1.01	0.21-4.87
Preterm birth	2/236	10.06	0.53-192.2
Pregnancy weight gain (%)	1/164	−3.00	−5.21-0.79
Birth weight (g)	2/236	−83.45	221.87-54.97

CI, Confidence interval; *RR,* relative risk.

condition in the first 18 months (Table 9-2). A restricted diet during pregnancy was associated with a slight but statistically significant lower maternal mean gestational weight gain and nonsignificant trends toward higher risks of preterm birth and reduced mean infant birthweight.

Maternal dietary allergen avoidance during pregnancy has been a component of the intervention strategies used in other randomized trials.[18,36-38] However, because those trials examined the effects of allergen avoidance during both pregnancy and lactation, with the use of other allergen avoidance strategies for the infant, no conclusions can be drawn pertaining to allergen avoidance during pregnancy. Larger trials of maternal dietary antigen avoidance during pregnancy are required to detect even modest reductions in risk of allergy among infants and children. Adverse effects of maternal antigen avoidance on gestational weight gain, fetal growth, and preterm birth should be reported. A better understanding of mechanisms for the development of food tolerance and sensitization will facilitate efforts to develop effective allergy prevention strategies.

Breast-feeding

Breast-feeding is the natural and recommended method of infant nutrition for the first months after birth. Few data are available from randomized controlled trials to determine the effects of breast-feeding on prevention of food intolerance and allergy in children. Lucas and associates[39] randomized preterm infants weighing less than 1850 g to expressed human milk versus sole or supplemental preterm cow's milk formula feeds, up until hospital discharge. At 18 months, no significant differences in incidence of eczema (human milk 20% vs. preterm formula 20%), reactions to cow's milk (4% vs. 3%), all food reactions (10% vs. 11%), and asthma and/or wheezing (23% vs. 23%) were noted. In subgroup analysis restricted to a small number of infants with a family history of allergy, a significant reduction in the incidence of eczema (relative risk [RR], 0.3; 95% confidence interval [CI], 0.1 to 0.8) was observed in infants fed human milk. In a cluster randomized trial of an intervention modeled on the Baby Friendly Hospital Initiative of the World Health Organization and the United Nations Children's Fund,[40] infants from intervention sites were significantly more likely to be breast-fed and had a significantly reduced incidence of atopic eczema at 1 year (3.3% vs. 6.3%; adjusted odds ratio [OR], 0.54; 95% CI, 0.31 to 0.95).

Two trials[41,42] have compared the use of human milk versus cow's milk formula for early supplemental or sole feeding of infants before hospital discharge. Both trials used inadequate methods of infant allocation to feeds over alternate periods. Juvonen and colleagues[41] enrolled 92 infants and reported no significant differences in any childhood allergy or specific allergy, including asthma, eczema, and food allergy. Saarinen and coworkers,[42] who allocated 3602 infants to treatment, reported no significant difference in cow's milk allergy (RR, 0.80; 95% CI, 0.51 to 1.53) among infants fed human milk compared with cow's milk formula. Both trials also enrolled a group fed a hydrolyzed infant formula. Systematic review[43] of these two trials found no significant difference between the use of a hydrolyzed infant formula and human milk. Again, Juvonen and associates[41] reported no significant difference in any childhood allergy or any specific allergy, including asthma, eczema, and food allergy. Saarinen and colleagues[42] reported no significant difference in cow's milk allergy (RR, 0.71; 95% CI, 0.45 to 1.12) among infants given a hydrolyzed formula compared with human milk.

In observational studies, conflicting results have been reported for the association between breast-feeding and the development of clinical allergy, even to adulthood. Several studies[44-50] have reported an increase in allergy in association with breast-feeding but have been criticized methodologically,[51] especially regarding the potential for recall bias and lack of a dose-response relationship. It is likely that some of these findings may be the result of "reverse causality"; high-risk infants are more likely to be breast-fed and are more likely to develop allergy. Several reviews[52-56] have attempted to meta-analyze study data associating breast-feeding with clinical allergy. Considerable difficulty in appraising the results of these reviews given the lack of comparable groups has resulted from inclusion of observational studies in all reviews. However, attempts have been made to determine whether results were sensitive to study quality, with conclusions robust to the exclusion of studies with greatest methodologic concern.[53,54] Overall, among high-risk infants, meta-analyses have reported benefits in infancy from exclusive breast-feeding for the first few months in terms of reduced atopic dermatitis (OR, 0.58; 95% CI, 0.41 to 0.92)[53] and asthma (OR, 0.52; 95% CI, 0.35 to 0.79),[54] but not allergic rhinitis.[53] In low-risk infants, no evidence of benefit was reported for any manifestation of allergy.[52-54]

Several studies have reported that longer, rather than shorter, duration of exclusive breast-feeding offers additional protective effects against allergy. Results of several of these studies[57-60] have led the American Academy of Pediatrics (AAP)[29] and the European Society for Pediatric Allergy and Clinical Immunology Committee on Hypoallergenic Formulas/European Society for Paediatric Gastroenterology, Hepatology, and Nutrition (ESPACI/ESPGHAN)[61] to recommend at least 6 months and 4 to 6 months of exclusive breast-feeding, respectively. In contrast, in a systematic review conducted to determine the optimal duration of breast-feeding, Kramer and Kakuma[56] reported no significant reduction in risk of atopic eczema, asthma, or other atopic outcomes in infants exclusively breast-fed for 6 months compared with a shorter duration. However, the data from this review were mainly accrued from observational studies, including the use of nonrandomized groups from the Belarus cluster randomized trial of the Baby Friendly Hospital Initiative.[40] A reduction in clinical but not food challenge–confirmed allergy at 1 year was reported by one included cohort study.[57]

In summary, evidence from observational studies suggests that exclusive breast-feeding may prevent infant allergy, particularly eczema and possibly asthma. However, evidence from observational studies is heterogeneous, with not all population-based studies finding a significant beneficial effect.[44-50] Observational studies are unable to account for all confounding through bias in study design, measurement error, or failure to measure potential confounders. Meta-analysis of observational studies does not account for this bias, but merely increases the power of the analysis to detect a biased outcome. Most evidence supportive of exclusive breast-feeding for allergy prevention suggests durations of at least 4 to 6 months before other foods are introduced.[56-60] It is difficult to see whether this question will ever be adequately answered given the other potential benefits of breast-feeding, particularly reduced infectious morbidity,[56] and, in preterm infants, necrotizing enterocolitis.[62] Currently, the AAP[29] recommends exclusive breast-feeding for 6 months and the ESPACI/ESPGHAN[61] and the Australasian Society of Clinical Immunology and Allergy (ASCIA)[1] for 4 to 6 months for prevention of cow's milk hypersensitivity and infant allergy.

Maternal Dietary Allergy Avoidance During Lactation

A systematic review found insufficient data from controlled trials to determine the role of allergen avoidance in lactating women.[32] One trial of antigen avoidance during lactation enrolled only 26 lactating women.[35] No significant protective effect of maternal antigen avoidance on the incidence of atopic eczema up to 18 months (RR, 0.73; 95% CI, 0.32 to 1.64) was reported. Two trials[63,64] included in previous versions of the review were excluded owing to data validity concerns.

For infants with a family history of food-related anaphylaxis (e.g., peanuts, nuts, seafood), data were insufficient to recommend any specific maternal dietary interventions to prevent infant sensitization. Currently, for high-risk infants, only the AAP[29] makes a recommendation for maternal allergen avoidance, recommending the elimination of peanuts and nuts from the diets of lactating (and possibly pregnant) women. Both the AAP[29] and the ASCIA[1] recommend considering avoidance of peanuts, nuts, and shellfish from the infant's diet until 3 years of age, although no evidence has been found to support this recommendation.

Infant Formula

A substantial proportion of the world's infants are not exclusively breast-fed.[65] Until health interventions redress this issue, humanized infant formulas are available to provide for infants not exclusively breast-fed owing to maternal or infant illness, maternal or infant inability, or parental preference. Formulas prescribed to infants with the intention of preventing allergy and food intolerance have included hydrolyzed cow's milk, elemental and adapted soy, and hydrolyzed soy formulas. Hydrolyzed formulas are designed to change the allergenic milk protein with the aim of preventing sensitization. They may be produced from cow's milk or soy, may be derived from predominantly whey or casein proteins, and may be partially or extensively hydrolyzed. The process of producing a hydrolyzed formula is individual to the formula, and in general the methods are commercially protected. They involve processes of enzyme-induced cleavage of protein and subsequent purification. Extensively hydrolyzed infant formulas have a majority of milk proteins of less than 1500 kDa and require clinical testing in infants with demonstrated cow's milk or cow's milk–based formula hypersensitivity.[29] The extensively hydrolyzed formula should be tolerated by a minimum of 90% of infants in double-blind placebo-controlled conditions, with 95% confidence. Extensively hydrolyzed formulas, or elemental equivalents with amino acid–only protein fractions, are used for the treatment of infants with cow's milk hypersensitivity. In Australia, prescription requires documented cow's milk hypersensitivity. Formulas based on partially hydrolyzed cow's milk protein have 10^3 to 10^5 times the concentrations of intact cow's milk protein compared with extensively hydrolyzed formulas, and are not used for the treatment of hypersensitive infants. This review summarizes the evidence for extensive and partially hydrolyzed infant formulas, as well as the role of soy formula. Systematic reviews of hydrolyzed formulas were performed using Cochrane Collaboration methods and included only controlled clinical trials with 20% losses and no allergy-preventing co-interventions that were performed differently in treatment and control groups. Treatment groups were analyzed as "intention to treat," that is, in the group of initial patient allocation. For outcomes, infants are defined as up to 2 years of age and children as 2 to 10 years of age.

Early Short-Term Use of a Hydrolyzed Infant Formula

A systematic review of controlled trials[43] found two studies[41,42] that compared a short duration of early supplemental or sole hydrolyzed formula versus donor human milk feeds or cow's milk formula in infants who were subsequently encouraged to breast-feed. Both used inadequate methods of treatment allocation. Both studies enrolled unselected infants, not infants selected on the basis of allergic heredity. Neither study reported significant benefit from the use of hydrolyzed compared with donor human milk. One study[42] reported a reduction in infant cow's milk allergy of borderline significance (RR, 0.62; 95% CI, 0.38 to 1.00) from the use of an extensively hydrolyzed formula compared with a cow's milk formula, with subgroup analysis suggesting that the benefit was seen only in infants at high risk of allergy. The role of early short-term use of a hydrolyzed infant formula for prevention of food hypersensitivity and allergy remains unclear. No evidence of benefit suggests that a hydrolyzed formula should be advised in preference to exclusive breast-feeding. Where exclusive breast-feeding is not possible, additional large trials are required to define the role of hydrolyzed formula in early short-term infant feeding.

Prolonged Feeding With a Hydrolyzed Infant Formula

A systematic review of controlled trials[43] found 10 eligible studies that compared prolonged feeding with hydrolyzed (extensively or partially hydrolyzed) formula versus cow's milk formula (Table 9-3). Almost all trials enrolled infants at high risk

Table 9-3   STUDIES INCLUDED IN META-ANALYSIS OF TRIALS OF HYDROLYZED INFANT FORMULA VERSUS COW'S MILK FORMULA FOR PREVENTION OF FOOD HYPERSENSITIVITY AND ALLERGY[43]

Reference	Infants	Indication	Methods	Treatment
Chiroco et al[96]	Infants of mothers with atopy	Prolonged supplemental or sole formula feeds	Random; blinding not reported; losses, unclear	PHWF vs. CMF
De Seta et al[97]	Infants with one or more first-degree relatives with allergy	Prolonged supplemental or sole formula feeds	Random; method not reported; blinding not reported; losses, not reported	PHWF vs. CMF
Halken et al[68]	Infants with biparental atopy or uniparental atopy and cord IgE ≥0.3 kU/L	Prolonged supplemental or sole formula feeds	Quasi-random; blinded treatment; losses, 20%	EHCF vs. EHWF vs. PHWF
Juvonen et al[41]	Healthy infants; 62% had family history of atopy	Early, short-term (first 3 days) sole formula feeds in hospital	Quasi-random; blinding not reported; losses, 10%	HM vs. EHCF vs. CMF
Lam et al[98]	High-risk: criteria not reported	Prolonged supplemental or sole formula feeds	Random; method not reported; blinding not reported; losses, 8%	PHW vs. CMF
Maggio et al[99]	Preterm infants, birth weight ≤1750 g and ≤34 weeks	Prolonged supplemental or sole formula feeds identical in calories and nitrogen	Random; blinded; no losses	Preterm HWF vs. preterm CMF
Mallett et al[100]	Infants with first-degree family history of allergy	Prolonged supplemental or sole formula feeds	Random; method not reported; not blinded; losses 7% at 4 months; >20% later	EHWF vs. CMF
Marini et al[101]	Infants with definite family history of allergy	Prolonged supplemental or sole formula feeds	Random; method not reported; unblinded; losses 19% at 3 years	PHWF vs. CMF
Nentwich et al[70]	Infants with family history of atopy in first-degree relative	Prolonged supplemental or sole formula feeds	Quasi-random; unblended; losses 1% (further 18% not reported in allocated group)	PHWF vs. EHWF

CMF, Cow's milk formula; *EHCF,* extensively hydrolyzed casein formula; *EHWCF,* extensively hydrolyzed whey casein formula; *EHWF,* extensively hydrolyzed whey formula; *HM,* human milk; *HWF,* Hydrolyzed whey formula; *PHW,* Partially hydrolyzed whey; *PHWCF,* partially hydrolyzed whey casein formula; *PHWF,* partially hydrolyzed whey formula.

Table 9-3 STUDIES INCLUDED IN META-ANALYSIS OF TRIALS OF HYDROLYZED INFANT FORMULA VERSUS COW'S MILK FORMULA FOR PREVENTION OF FOOD HYPERSENSITIVITY AND ALLERGY—cont'd

Reference	Infants	Indication	Methods	Treatment
Oldaeus et al[69]	Infants with two allergic family members or one allergic family member and cord IgE ≥0.5 kU/L	Infants weaning from breast	Random; blinded; losses 9%	EHCF vs. PHWF vs. CMF
Picaud et al[102]	Low birth weight infants <1500 g	Preterm infants with prolonged sole formula feeds	Random; method not reported; blinded; losses 11%	Preterm PHWF vs. preterm CMF
Saarinen et al[42]	Term infants	Early short-term (4 days) supplemental formula feeding in hospital	Quasi-random; blinded; losses unclear	HM vs. EHWF vs. CMF
Szajewska et al[103]	Low birth weight <2000 g, appropriate for gestational age	Prolonged sole formula feeds	Random; method not reported; blinded; no losses	Preterm EHWCF vs. preterm CMF
Tsai et al[104]	Infants enrolled according to Family History of Allergy Score	Prolonged supplemental or sole formula feeds	Random; method not reported; unblended; losses unclear	PHWF vs. CMF
Vandenplas et al[66]	Infants with two or more first-degree allergic relatives	Prolonged sole formula feeds	Random; method not reported; blinded; losses 11%	PHWF vs. CMF
Vandenplas et al[105]	Term newborn infants with no family history of atopy	Prolonged sole formula feeds	Random; method not reported; blinded; losses 9%	PHWF vs. CMF
von Berg et al[67]	Infants with family history of atopy in first-degree relative	Prolonged supplemental or sole formula feeds	Random; blinded; losses in "intention to treat" analysis: 1 year, 14.7%; 3 years, 19%	PHWF vs. EHWF vs. EHCF vs. CMF
Willems et al[106]	Infants with family history allergy and cord IgE ≥0.5 kU/L	Prolonged sole formula feeds	Quasi-random; unblended; losses 13%	PHWF vs. CMF

of allergy based on first-degree heredity, and some studies included additional screening with cord blood IgE levels. Meta-analysis (Table 9-4) found a significant reduction in infant allergy (seven studies; 2514 infants; typical RR, 0.79; 95% CI, 0.66 to 0.94), but not allergy in later childhood (two studies; 950 infants; typical RR, 0.85; 95% CI, 0.69 to 1.05). No significant difference in any specific allergy, including eczema, asthma, rhinitis, or food allergy, was reported. However, the significant reduction in infant allergy did not persist when analysis was restricted to trials that blinded investigators and participants to formula type, or to trials that used adequate methods of infant allocation with less than 10% losses to follow-up. In addition, no eligible trial examined the effects of prolonged hydrolyzed formula feeding on allergy beyond early childhood. Meta-analysis of three trials found that preterm or low birth weight infants fed a hydrolyzed preterm formula versus a

Table 9-4   META-ANALYSIS OF TRIALS OF HYDROLYZED FORMULA VERSUS COW'S MILK FORMULA FOR PREVENTION OF FOOD HYPERSENSITIVITY AND ALLERGY[43]

Outcome	Studies/Participants	RR	95% CI
Infant allergy	7/2514	0.79	0.66-0.94
Childhood allergy	2/950	0.85	0.69-1.05
Infant asthma	4/318	0.57	0.31-1.04
Childhood asthma incidence	1/78	0.38	0.08-1.84
Childhood asthma prevalence	1/872	1.06	0.70-1.61
Infant eczema	8/2558	0.84	0.68-1.04
Childhood eczema incidence	2/950	0.83	0.63-1.10
Childhood eczema prevalence	1/872	0.66	0.43-1.02
Infant rhinitis	2/256	0.52	0.14-1.85
Food allergy	1/141	1.82	0.64-5.16
Cow's milk allergy	1/67	0.36	0.15-0.89

CI, Confidence interval; *RR*, relative risk.

preterm cow's milk formula had significantly reduced weight gain, but not reduced growth in head circumference or length. Studies in term infants report no adverse effects on growth.

Prolonged Feeding With Partially Hydrolyzed Formula versus Extensively Hydrolyzed Formula

Three sets of analyses contribute to this comparison in a systematic review[43]: those comparing partially hydrolyzed and extensively hydrolyzed formula versus cow's milk formula, and trials comparing partially hydrolyzed versus extensively hydrolyzed formulas. In studies of partially hydrolyzed formula versus cow's milk formula, meta-analysis (seven studies; 1482 infants) found a significant reduction in infant allergy (seven studies; 1482 infants; RR, 0.79; 95% CI, 0.65 to 0.97), which did not persist to childhood. For specific allergies, no significant differences were reported in infant or childhood asthma, eczema, or rhinitis. Data from one small study[66] show that use of a partially hydrolyzed whey formula resulted in a significant reduction in cow's milk allergy, confirmed by testing for atopy (RR, 0.36; 95% CI, 0.15 to 0.89). Studies demonstrating benefit used a partially hydrolyzed 100% whey formula, with meta-analysis of six studies including 1391 infants finding a significant reduction in infant allergy (RR, 0.73; 95% CI, 0.59 to 0.90), but not allergy into childhood or for any specific allergy or food hypersensitivity.

Four studies compared extensively hydrolyzed formula versus cow's milk formula. No individual study reported a significant reduction in allergy or in any specific allergy or food hypersensitivity from the use of extensively hydrolyzed formula. Meta-analysis found no significant differences in infant allergy (two studies; 1561 infants; RR, 0.87; 95% CI, 0.68 to 1.13) or childhood allergy (one study; 651 infants; RR, 0.89; 95% CI, 0.71 to 1.13). No significant difference was found in infant or childhood asthma, eczema, or rhinitis or food allergy. Upon comparing extensively hydrolyzed casein–containing formula versus cow's milk formula, the German Infant Nutritional Intervention (GINI) Study[67] of 431 infants reported (intention to treat data obtained from authors) a significant reduction in childhood allergy (RR, 0.72; 95% CI, 0.53 to 0.97). Meta-analysis of three studies including 1237 infants found a significant reduction in infant eczema (RR, 0.71; 95% CI, 0.51 to 0.97), with the GINI study reporting a significant reduction in the incidence of childhood eczema (RR, 0.66; 95% CI, 0.44 to 0.98) and prevalence (RR, 0.50; 95% CI, 0.27 to 0.92) at 3 years.

Four studies[67-70] compared prolonged feeding with extensively hydrolyzed formula versus partially hydrolyzed formula in infants at high risk of allergy. No individual study reported any significant differences in allergy or food hypersensitivity. Meta-analysis (three studies; 1806 infants) found no significant difference in infant allergy (RR, 0.93; 95% CI, 0.75 to 1.16). Von Berg[67] reported no significant difference in the incidence of childhood allergy (RR, 0.93; 95% CI, 0.74 to 1.18). Meta-analysis of two studies[68,69] found a significant reduction in infant food allergy (RR, 0.43; 95% CI, 0.19 to 0.99), although one of these studies reported no significant difference in infant cow's milk allergy.[68]

In summary, evidence for benefit from the use of hydrolyzed infant formula for the prevention of food hypersensitivity and allergy is inconclusive. Some evidence has been found for the use of both a partially hydrolyzed 100% whey formula and an extensively hydrolyzed casein formula in infants at high risk of allergy. Extensively hydrolyzed formula may be better than partially hydrolyzed formula in preventing food allergy. No evidence suggests that hydrolyzed formulas should be used in preference to exclusive breast-feeding, and no evidence of benefit has been found for use in infants without a first-degree family history of allergy. Concerns have been raised about the adequacy of growth of preterm or low birth weight infants fed hydrolyzed preterm infant formula. Additional large, rigorous trials are needed to compare partially hydrolyzed whey and extensively hydrolyzed casein versus cow's milk formulas in infants at high risk of allergy. All hydrolyzed formulas should have the ability to support adequate nutrition and growth as assessed in appropriately designed controlled clinical trials.

Soy-Based Infant Formula (SBIF)

Current SBIFs are derived from soy protein isolate (SPI) or purified modified soy protein isolate with lower levels of phytoestrogens than soy flour, and are iodine supplemented. Nutritional modifications include methionine fortification, reduction of phytate content, and improved mineral suspension resulting in increased absorption of micronutrients.[71,72] A review[73] of the effects of SBIF on growth and development, including both randomized and observational studies, reported that modern SBIFs support normal growth and nutritional status in healthy full-term infants in the first year, and current data do not suggest effects on sexual or reproductive development. However, insufficient long-term data have been reported regarding reproductive development, immune function, visual acuity, cognitive development, and thyroid function.

A systematic review of studies of SBIF[74] found three eligible studies enrolling high-risk infants with a history of allergy in a first-degree relative (Table 9-5). No

Table 9-5 CHARACTERISTICS OF INCLUDED STUDIES COMPARING SOY-BASED INFANT FORMULAS VERSUS COW'S MILK AND HYDROLYZED FORMULAS FOR INFANT FEEDING

Study	Population	Methods	Formulas	Criteria for Diagnosis
Johnstone et al[107]	Infants not breast-fed with history of allergy in first-degree relative	Random; method not reported; unblinded; lost, 19.5%	SBIF versus evaporated CMF for at least 7 months	Unblinded pediatrician assessment
Kjellman et al[75]	Infants weaning from breast with history of allergy in both parents	Random; method not reported; unblinded; lost, 4%	SBIF versus CMF for at least 9 months	Unblinded pediatrician assessment
Miskelly et al[108]	Breast-fed infants with supplemental feeds if required; history of allergy in first-degree relative	Random; unblinded; lost: 1 year, 9%; 7 years, 16%	Supplemental SBIF versus "normal diet" (99% cow's milk exposed) for at least 4 months	Blinded physician assessment; skin-prick tests 6, 12 months; specific and total IgE 3, 12 months

CMF, Cow's milk formula; *SBIF,* soy-based infant formula.

Table 9-6   META-ANALYSIS OF TRIALS OF SOY-BASED INFANT FORMULA
VERSUS COW'S MILK FORMULA FOR PREVENTION OF FOOD
HYPERSENSITIVITY AND ALLERGY[74]

Outcome	Studies/Participants	RR	95% CI
All allergy up to childhood	2/283	0.67	0.18-2.46
Infant asthma	1/474	1.10	0.86-1.40
Childhood asthma	3/729	0.71	0.26-1.92
Infant eczema	1/461	1.20	0.95-1.52
Childhood eczema	2/283	1.57	0.90-2.75
Infant rhinitis	1/460	0.94	0.76-1.16
Childhood rhinitis	1/283	0.69	0.06-8.00
Cow's milk allergy	1/48	1.09	0.24-4.86
Soy allergy	1/48	3.26	0.36-29.17

CI, Confidence interval; RR, relative risk.

eligible study enrolled infants fed human milk. No study examined the effect of early, short-term soy formula feeding. All compared prolonged soy formula versus cow's milk formula feeding. One study[75] used adequate methods and no unbalanced allergy-preventing cointerventions in treatment groups. Meta-analysis (Table 9-6) found no significant difference in childhood allergy (two studies; typical RR, 0.73; 95% CI, 0.37 to 1.44) or specific allergy, including asthma, eczema, and rhinitis. No significant difference in cow's milk hypersensitivity or allergy was reported. No study compared soy formula versus hydrolyzed protein formula. Feeding with a soy formula cannot be recommended for prevention of allergy or food hypersensitivity in high-risk infants. Given the lack of high-quality studies, further research may be warranted to determine the role of soy formula in the prevention of allergy or food hypersensitivity in infants unable to be breast-fed who have a strong family history of allergy or cow's milk protein hypersensitivity.

Prebiotics and Probiotics

Differences in intestinal microflora have been found in infants delivered by cesarean section compared with those delivered vaginally, and in breast-fed versus formula-fed infants.[76] Colonizing bifidobacteria and lactobacilli inhibit the growth of pathogenic microorganisms through production of lactic, acetic, and other organic acids, with a consequent decrease in intraluminal pH that inhibits the growth of some bacterial pathogens. The composition of the intestinal microflora may be different in those with atopic eczema, and such differences may precede the development of eczema. The most consistent finding in such studies is a reduced proportion of bifidobacteria species in the feces of infants with eczema[77,78] and atopic sensitization,[79] but not of wheezy children.[78] Recognition of the importance of intestinal flora has led to the development of strategies aimed at manipulating bacterial colonization in formula-fed infants, including the use of prebiotics and probiotics. Prebiotics are nondigestible food components that beneficially affect the host by selectively stimulating the growth or activity of bacteria in the colon. They have frequently been added to infant formula. To be effective, prebiotics should escape digestion and absorption in the upper gastrointestinal tract, reach the large bowel, and be used selectively by microorganisms that have been identified to have health-promoting properties. Studies to date in infants have demonstrated significant increases in fecal bifidobacteria in response to formula supplementation with oligosaccharides[80-84]; one study also demonstrated an increase in lactobacilli,[81] but none demonstrated an effect on potentially pathogenic bacteria. In a recent randomized trial, 259 infants at high risk of allergy (parental history of asthma, eczema, or rhinitis) were randomized to galacto- and long-chain fructo-oligosaccharides or placebo added to an extensively hydrolyzed whey formula. Losses in excess of 20% were reported by the trial, and in a subgroup of infants with fecal bacterial counts, differences at baseline in lactobacilli counts were noted between groups. Fecal bifidobacteria counts increased significantly in the prebiotic group. Among 206 infants followed for up to 6 months, those receiving oligosaccharide supplementation had significantly reduced clinical eczema (RR, 0.42; 95% CI, 0.21 to 0.84), although eczema severity scores were not significantly different. No adverse effects were reported. Further research is required to determine whether prebiotics are effective in preventing eczema.

Probiotics are live bacteria that colonize the gut and provide a health benefit to the host. Benefits from the use of probiotic bacteria have been found in a systematic review of randomized trials[85] for the treatment of infectious diarrhea, with the use of probiotics reducing diarrhea at 3 days (RR, 0.66; 95% CI, 0.55 to 0.77) and mean duration of diarrhea by 30 hours (95% CI, 18 to 42 hours). Several randomized studies have demonstrated the efficacy of the use of probiotics in infants with active eczema,[86-89] although not all studies have shown conclusive benefits.[89] For prevention of allergy, one randomized, placebo-controlled trial[90] reported that supplementation with *Lactobacillus* given prenatally to mothers who had at least one first-degree relative with atopic eczema, rhinitis, or asthma, and postnatally for 6 months to their infants, reduced the incidence of atopic eczema by up to 2 years (from 46% to 23%; RR, 0.51; 95% CI, 0.32 to 0.84). No significant effect on total or specific serum IgE or skin-prick tests over this period was reported. Excessive (17%) postrandomization losses prevent strong conclusions from being drawn from this study. Additional studies are needed before probiotics can be recommended in high-risk infants for the prevention of allergy. To date, the most promising data for both prebiotics[84] and probiotics[90] have been reported for infants with or at risk of atopic eczema.

Future Directions

To date, dietary primary prevention strategies for food hypersensitivity and allergy have yielded largely unconvincing results. Greater understanding of genetic, physiologic, and environmental factors resulting in immune tolerance and sensitization no doubt would facilitate future efforts, particularly how the fetus and the immature newborn are exposed to and process antigens, and which genetic and immune developmental mechanisms program sensitization and tolerance. Identification of genetic markers for allergic sensitization will facilitate the identification of infants likely to benefit from primary prevention strategies.

Low rates of exclusive breast-feeding have the potential to contribute substantially to the burden of infant allergy and early food hypersensitivity. In the government and public health domain, greater efforts are required, including in developed countries, to facilitate and encourage exclusive breast-feeding. A reasonable goal of all maternity and infant health care providers is implementation of the Baby Friendly Hospital Initiative.[40]

For specific approaches to infant feeding designed to reduce the incidences of allergy and early food hypersensitivity, adequately powered and rigorous trials of prebiotics and probiotics in high-risk infants are needed, particularly those undertaken with the goal of preventing infant atopic eczema. Although some evidence has been found for the use of both partially and extensively hydrolyzed formulas, in view of methodologic concerns and inconsistent findings, additional large, well-designed trials comparing partially hydrolyzed whey and extensively hydrolyzed casein versus cow's milk formula are needed.

It should be noted that although sensitization is common, clinical reactions to foods are relatively uncommon, and inclusion of substantial numbers of infants will be required to detect benefits in terms of reduced cow's milk allergy or food allergy in the context of randomized controlled trials. Therefore, other, more prevalent clinical allergic manifestations, particularly infant eczema and wheezing, and subsequent childhood asthma and rhinitis, become appropriate goals for primary prevention, especially in view of their potential public health benefit. It is important that trials focused on prevention address the clinical manifestations of allergy, not just sensitization.

Conclusions

For primary prevention of allergy and early food hypersensitivity, current data support the implementation of public health policies designed to facilitate exclusive breast-feeding in all infants up to the first 6 months. Evidence of benefit for other specific maternal and infant dietary recommendations is found only in infants at high risk of allergy. As yet, no consensus has been reached regarding the definition of high-risk infants, although the addition of cord blood IgE testing is not adequately predictive to warrant use outside of clinical trials. The predictive value of family history for clinical allergy is greatest for allergy in first-degree relatives and maternal or sibling allergy as opposed to paternal allergy, and double as opposed to single allergic heredity. Despite identification of allergic heredity, only around half of infants who subsequently develop clinical allergies are identified at birth.

Where exclusive breast-feeding is not possible in the first 6 months, evidence has been found for the use of hydrolyzed formula for the prevention of allergy in high-risk infants. For specific types of hydrolyzed formula, evidence supports the use of both partially hydrolyzed 100% whey formula and extensively hydrolyzed casein formula in infants at high risk of allergy. An extensively hydrolyzed formula may be better than a partially hydrolyzed formula in preventing food hypersensitivity, but it is likely to have higher costs. Additional rigorous, adequately powered trials are needed to confirm these findings. Concern has been raised regarding the nutritional adequacy of specialized preterm hydrolyzed formula in terms of adequacy of weight gain in low birth weight infants.

No evidence supports the use of maternal dietary avoidance measures during lactation and/or breast-feeding, and concerns regarding the nutritional impact of these measures, particularly during pregnancy, have been expressed. No evidence supports recommending soy formulas in preference to cow's milk formulas for prevention of allergy and food hypersensitivity. Further trials of prebiotics and probiotics are needed before their use can be recommended in high-risk infants for the prevention of atopic eczema.

References

1. Prescott SL, Tang ML. The Australasian Society of Clinical Immunology and Allergy position statement: Summary of allergy prevention in children. *Med J Aust.* 2005;182:464-467.
2. Halken S. Prevention of allergic disease in childhood: Clinical and epidemiological aspects of primary and secondary allergy prevention. *Pediatr Allergy Immunol.* 2004;15(Suppl 16):4-5.
3. Johansson SG, Bieber T, Dahl R, et al. Revised nomenclature for allergy for global use: Report of the Nomenclature Review Committee of the World Allergy Organization, October 2003. *J Allergy Clin Immunol.* 2004;113:832-836.
4. Burr ML, Butland BK, King S, et al. Changes in asthma prevalence: Two surveys 15 years apart. *Arch Dis Child.* 1989;64:1452-1456.
5. Schultz Larsen F. Atopic dermatitis: An increasing problem. *Pediatr Allergy Immunol.* 1996;7:51-53.
6. Sampson HA. Update on food allergy. *J Allergy Clin Immunol.* 2004;113:805-819, quiz 20.
7. Osterballe M, Hansen TK, Mortz CG, et al. The prevalence of food hypersensitivity in an unselected population of children and adults. *Pediatr Allergy Immunol.* 2005;16:567-573.
8. Natale M, Bisson C, Monti G, et al. Cow's milk allergens identification by two-dimensional immunoblotting and mass spectrometry. *Mol Nutr Food Res.* 2004;48:363-369.
9. Skolnick HS, Conover-Walker MK, Koerner CB, et al. The natural history of peanut allergy. *J Allergy Clin Immunol.* 2001;107:367-374.
10. Warner JO. The early life origins of asthma and related allergic disorders. *Arch Dis Child.* 2004;89:97-102.
11. Jones CA, Vance GH, Power LL, et al. Costimulatory molecules in the developing human gastrointestinal tract: A pathway for fetal allergen priming. *J Allergy Clin Immunol.* 2001;108:235-241.
12. Thornton CA, Vance GH. The placenta: A portal of fetal allergen exposure. *Clin Exp Allergy.* 2002;32:1537-1539.
13. Bernsen RM, de Jongste JC, Koes BW, et al. Perinatal characteristics and obstetric complications as risk factors for asthma, allergy and eczema at the age of 6 years. *Clin Exp Allergy.* 2005;35:1135-1140.
14. Jaakkola JJ, Gissler M. Maternal smoking in pregnancy, fetal development, and childhood asthma. *Am J Public Health.* 2004;94:136-140.
15. Raby BA, Celedon JC, Litonjua AA, et al. Low-normal gestational age as a predictor of asthma at 6 years of age. *Pediatrics.* 2004;114:e327-e332.

16. Kurukulaaratchy RJ, Matthews S, Arshad SH. Defining childhood atopic phenotypes to investigate the association of atopic sensitization with allergic disease. *Allergy.* 2005;60:1280-1286.
17. Moffatt MF, Cookson WO. Gene identification in asthma and allergy. *Int Arch Allergy Immunol.* 1998; 116:247-252.
18. Arshad SH, Kurukulaaratchy RJ, Fenn M, et al. Early life risk factors for current wheeze, asthma, and bronchial hyperresponsiveness at 10 years of age. *Chest.* 2005;127:502-508.
19. Sunyer J, Mendendez C, Ventura PJ, et al. Prenatal risk factors of wheezing at the age of four years in Tanzania. *Thorax.* 2001;56:290-295.
20. Devereux G, Barker RN, Seaton A. Antenatal determinants of neonatal immune responses to allergens. *Clin Exp Allergy.* 2002;32:43-50.
21. Tariq SM, Matthews SM, Hakim EA, et al. The prevalence of and risk factors for atopy in early childhood: A whole population birth cohort study. *J Allergy Clin Immunol.* 1998;101:587-593.
22. Dunstan JA, Mori TA, Barden A, et al. Fish oil supplementation in pregnancy modifies neonatal allergen-specific immune responses and clinical outcomes in infants at high risk of atopy: A randomized, controlled trial. *J Allergy Clin Immunol.* 2003;112:1178-1184.
23. Arshad SH, Stevens M, Hide DW. The effect of genetic and environmental factors on the prevalence of allergic disorders at the age of two years. *Clin Exp Allergy.* 1993;23:504-511.
24. Peat JK, Li J. Reversing the trend: Reducing the prevalence of asthma. *J Allergy Clin Immunol.* 1999; 103:1-10.
25. Bergmann RL, Edenharter G, Bergmann KE, et al. Predctability of early atopy by cord blood-IgE and parental history. *Clin Exp Allergy.* 1997;27:752-760.
26. Hansen LG, Halken S, Host A, et al. Prediction of allergy from family history and cord blood IgE levels. A follow-up at the age of 5 years. Cord blood IgE. IV. *Pediatr Allergy Immunol.* 1993;4: 34-40.
27. Kjellman NI. Atopic disease in seven-year-old children. Incidence in relation to family history. *Acta Paediatr Scand.* 1977;66:465-471.
28. Croner S. Prediction and detection of allergy development: Influence of genetic and environmental factors. *J Pediatr.* 1992;121:S58-S63.
29. AAP. American Academy of Pediatrics: Committee on Nutrition. Hypoallergenic infant formulas. *Pediatrics.* 2000;106:346-349.
30. Asher I, Baena-Cagnani C, Boner A, et al. World Allergy Organization guidelines for prevention of allergy and allergic asthma. *Int Arch Allergy Immunol.* 2004;135:83-92.
31. Host A, Halken S. Primary prevention of food allergy in infants who are at risk. *Curr Opin Allergy Clin Immunol.* 2005;5:255-259.
32. Kramer MS, Kakuma R. Maternal dietary antigen avoidance during pregnancy or lactation, or both, for preventing or treating atopic disease in the child. *Cochrane Database Syst Rev.* 2006;3:CD000133.
33. Falth-Magnusson K, Kjellman NI. Development of atopic disease in babies whose mothers were receiving exclusion diet during pregnancy—a randomized study. *J Allergy Clin Immunol.* 1987;80: 868-875.
34. Lilja G, Dannaeus A, Falth-Magnusson K, et al. Immune response of the atopic woman and foetus: Effects of high- and low-dose food allergen intake during late pregnancy. *Clin Allergy.* 1988;18:131-142.
35. Lovegrove JA, Hampton SM, Morgan JB. The immunological and long-term atopic outcome of infants born to women following a milk-free diet during late pregnancy and lactation: A pilot study. *Brit J Nutr.* 1994;71:223-238.
36. Appelt GK, Chan-Yeung M, Watson WTA, et al. Breastfeeding and food avoidance are ineffective in preventing sensitization in high risk children. *J Allergy Clin Immunol.* 2004;113:S99.
37. Hide DW, Matthews S, Tariq S, et al. Allergen avoidance in infancy and allergy at 4 years of age. *Allergy.* 1996;51:89-93.
38. Zeiger RS. Food allergen avoidance in the prevention of food allergy in infants and children. *Pediatrics.* 2003;111:1662-1671.
39. Lucas A, Brooke OG, Morley R, et al. Early diet of preterm infants and development of allergic or atopic disease: Randomised prospective study. *BMJ.* 1990;300:837-840.
40. Kramer MS, Chalmers B, Hodnett ED, et al. Promotion of Breastfeeding Intervention Trial (PROBIT): a randomized trial in the Republic of Belarus. *JAMA.* 2001;285:413-420.
41. Juvonen P, Mansson M, Andersson C, et al. Allergy development and macromolecular absorption in infants with different feeding regimens during the first three days of life. A three-year prospective follow-up. *Acta Paediatr.* 1996;85:1047-1052.
42. Saarinen KM, Juntunen-Backman K, Jarvenpaa AL, et al. Supplementary feeding in maternity hospitals and the risk of cow's milk allergy: A prospective study of 6209 infants. *J Allergy Clin Immunol.* 1999;104:457-461.
43. Osborn DA, Sinn J. Formulas containing hydrolysed protein for prevention of allergy and food intolerance in infants. *Cochrane Database Syst Rev.* (2) CD003664, 2006
44. Taylor B, Wadsworth J, Golding J, et al. Breast feeding, eczema, asthma, and hayfever. *J Epidemiol Community Health.* 1983;37:95-99.
45. Kaplan BA, Mascie-Taylor CG. Biosocial factors in the epidemiology of childhood asthma in a British national sample. *J Epidemiol Community Health.* 1985;39:152-156.
46. Rusconi F, Galassi C, Corbo GM, et al. Risk factors for early, persistent, and late-onset wheezing in young children. SIDRIA Collaborative Group. *Am J Respir Crit Care Med.* 1999;160:1617-1622.
47. Wright AL, Holberg CJ, Taussig LM, et al. Factors influencing the relation of infant feeding to asthma and recurrent wheeze in childhood. *Thorax.* 2001;56:192-197.
48. Bergmann RL, Diepgen TL, Kuss O, et al. Breastfeeding duration is a risk factor for atopic eczema. *Clin Exp Allergy.* 2002;32:205-209.

9

49. Miyake Y, Yura A, Iki M. Breastfeeding and the prevalence of symptoms of allergic disorders in Japanese adolescents. *Clin Exp Allergy.* 2003;33:312-316.

50. Sears MR, Greene JM, Willan AR, et al. Long-term relation between breastfeeding and development of atopy and asthma in children and young adults: A longitudinal study. *Lancet.* 2002;360:901-907.

51. Friedman NJ, Zeiger RS. The role of breast-feeding in the development of allergies and asthma. *J Allergy Clin Immunol.* 2005;115:1238-1248.

52. Mimouni Bloch A, Mimouni D, Mimouni M, et al. Does breastfeeding protect against allergic rhinitis during childhood? A meta-analysis of prospective studies. *Acta Paediatr.* 2002;91:275-279.

53. Gdalevich M, Mimouni D, David M, et al. Breast-feeding and the onset of atopic dermatitis in childhood: A systematic review and meta-analysis of prospective studies. *J Am Acad Dermatol.* 2001;45:520-527.

54. Gdalevich M, Mimouni D, Mimouni M. Breast-feeding and the risk of bronchial asthma in childhood: A systematic review with meta-analysis of prospective studies. *J Pediatr.* 2001;139:261-266.

55. van Odijk J, Kull I, Borres MP, et al. Breastfeeding and allergic disease: A multidisciplinary review of the literature (1966–2001) on the mode of early feeding in infancy and its impact on later atopic manifestations. *Allergy.* 2003;58:833-843.

56. Kramer MS, Kakuma R. Optimal duration of exclusive breastfeeding. *Cochrane Database Syst Rev.* (2):CD003517, 2002

57. Kajosaari M, Saarinen UM. Prophylaxis of atopic disease by six months' total solid food elimination. Evaluation of 135 exclusively breast-fed infants of atopic families. *Acta Paediatr Scand.* 1983;72:411-414.

58. Kull I, Almqvist C, Lilja G, et al. Breast-feeding reduces the risk of asthma during the first 4 years of life. *J Allergy Clin Immunol.* 2004;114:755-760.

59. Kull I, Wickman M, Lilja G, et al. Breast feeding and allergic diseases in infants—a prospective birth cohort study. *Arch Dis Child.* 2002;87:478-481.

60. Oddy WH, Holt PG, Sly PD, et al. Association between breast feeding and asthma in 6 year old children: Findings of a prospective birth cohort study. *BMJ.* 1999;319:815-819.

61. Host A, Koletzko B, Dreborg S, et al. Dietary products used in infants for treatment and prevention of food allergy. Joint Statement of the European Society for Pediatric Allergy and Clinical Immunology (ESPACI) Committee on Hypoallergenic Formulas and the European Society for Pediatric Gastroenterology, Hepatology and Nutrition (ESPGHAN) Committee on Nutrition. *Arch Dis Child.* 1999;81:80-84.

62. McGuire W, Anthony MY. Donor human milk versus formula for preventing necrotising enterocolitis in preterm infants: Systematic review. *Arch Dis Child Fetal Neonatal Ed.* 2003;88:F11-F14.

63. Chandra RK, Puri S, Suraiya C, et al. Influence of maternal food antigen avoidance during pregnancy and lactation on incidence of atopic eczema in infants. *Clin Allergy.* 1986;16:563-569.

64. Chandra RK, Puri S, Hamed A. Influence of maternal diet during lactation and use of formula feeds on development of atopic eczema in high risk infants. *BMJ.* 1989;299:228-230.

65. UNICEF. *Progress for Children: A Report Card on Nutrition (No. 4).* New York: UNICEF; 2006.

66. Vandenplas Y, Hauser B, Van den Borre C, et al. Effect of a whey hydrolysate prophylaxis of atopic disease. *Ann Allergy.* 1992;68:419-424.

67. von Berg A, Koletzko S, Grubl A, et al. The effect of hydrolyzed cow's milk formula for allergy prevention in the first year of life: The German Infant Nutritional Intervention Study, a randomized double-blind trial. *J Allergy Clin Immunol.* 2003;111:533-540.

68. Halken S, Hansen KS, Jacobsen HP, et al. Comparison of a partially hydrolyzed infant formula with two extensively hydrolyzed formulas for allergy prevention: A prospective, randomized study. *Pediatr Allergy Immunol.* 2000;11:149-161.

69. Oldaeus G, Anjou K, Bjorksten B, et al. Extensively and partially hydrolysed infant formulas for allergy prophylaxis. *Arch Dis Child.* 1997;77:4-10.

70. Nentwich I, Michkova E, Nevoral J, et al. Cow's milk-specific cellular and humoral immune responses and atopy skin symptoms in infants from atopic families fed a partially (pHF) or extensively (eHF) hydrolyzed infant formula. *Allergy.* 2001;56:1144-1156.

71. Merritt RJ, Jenks BH. Safety of soy-based infant formulas containing isoflavones: The clinical evidence. *J Nutr.* 2004;134:1220S-1224S.

72. AAP. Committee on Nutrition: Soy protein-based formulas: Recommendations for use in infant feeding. *Pediatrics.* 1998;101:148-153.

73. Mendez MA, Anthony MS, Arab L. Soy-based formulae and infant growth and development: A review. *J Nutr.* 2002;132:2127-2130.

74. Osborn DA, Sinn J. Soy formula for prevention of allergy and food intolerance in infants. *Cochrane Database Syst Rev.* 2006;(3):CD003741.

75. Kjellman NI, Johansson SG. Soy versus cow's milk in infants with a biparental history of atopic disease: Development of atopic disease and immunoglobulins from birth to 4 years of age. *Clin Allergy.* 1979;9:347-358.

76. Agostoni C, Axelsson I, Goulet O, et al. Prebiotic oligosaccharides in dietetic products for infants: A commentary by the ESPGHAN Committee on Nutrition. *J Pediatr Gastroenterol Nutr.* 2004;39:465-473.

77. Bjorksten B, Sepp E, Julge K, et al. Allergy development and the intestinal microflora during the first year of life. *J Allergy Clin Immunol.* 2001;108:516-520.

78. Murray CS, Tannock GW, Simon MA, et al. Fecal microbiota in sensitized wheezy and non-sensitized non-wheezy children: A nested case-control study. *Clin Exp Allergy.* 2005;35:741-745.

79. Kalliomaki M, Kirjavainen P, Eerola E, et al. Distinct patterns of neonatal gut microflora in infants in whom atopy was and was not developing. *J Allergy Clin Immunol*. 2001;107:129-134.
80. Boehm G, Lidestri M, Casetta P, et al. Supplementation of a bovine milk formula with an oligosaccharide mixture increases counts of faecal bifidobacteria in preterm infants. *Arch Dis Child Fetal Neonatal Ed*. 2002;86:F178-F181.
81. Moro G, Minoli I, Mosca M, et al. Dosage-related bifidogenic effects of galacto- and fructooligosaccharides in formula-fed term infants. *J Pediatr Gastroenterol Nutr*. 2002;34:291-295.
82. Schmelzle H, Wirth S, Skopnik H, et al. Randomized double-blind study of the nutritional efficacy and bifidogenicity of a new infant formula containing partially hydrolyzed protein, a high beta-palmitic acid level, and nondigestible oligosaccharides. *J Pediatr Gastroenterol Nutr*. 2003;36: 343-351.
83. Decsi T, Arato A, Balogh M, et al. Prebiotikus hatasu oligoszacharidok egeszseges csecsemok szekletflorajara gyakorolt hatasanak randomizalt, placeboval kontrollalt vizsgalata. *Orvosi Hetilap*. 2005;146:2445-2450.
84. Moro G, Arslanoglu S, Stahl B, et al. A mixture of prebiotic oligosaccharides reduces the incidence of atopic dermatitis during the first six months of age. *Arch Dis Child*. 2006;91:814-819.
85. Allen SJ, Okoko B, Martinez E, et al. Probiotics for treating infectious diarrhoea. *Cochrane Database Syst Rev*. (1):CD003048, 2004
86. Majamaa H, Isolauri E. Probiotics: A novel approach in the management of food allergy. *J Allergy Clin Immunol*. 1997;99:179-185.
87. Isolauri E, Arvola T, Sutas Y, et al. Probiotics in the management of atopic eczema. *Clin Exp Allergy*. 2000;30:1604-1610.
88. Rosenfeldt V, Benfeldt E, Nielsen SD, et al. Effect of probiotic Lactobacillus strains in children with atopic dermatitis. *J Allergy Clin Immunol*. 2003;111:389-395.
89. Viljanen M, Savilahti E, Haahtela T, et al. Probiotics in the treatment of atopic eczema/dermatitis syndrome in infants: A double-blind placebo-controlled trial. *Allergy*. 2005;60:494-500.
90. Kalliomaki M, Salminen S, Arvilommi H, et al. Probiotics in primary prevention of atopic disease: A randomised placebo-controlled trial. *Lancet*. 2001;357:1076-1079.
91. Falth-Magnusson K, Kjellman NI. Allergy prevention by maternal elimination diet during late pregnancy—a 5-year follow-up of a randomized study. *J Allergy Clin Immunol*. 1992;89:709-713.
92. Falth-Magnusson K, Oman H, Kjellman NI. Maternal abstention from cow milk and egg in allergy risk pregnancies. Effect on antibody production in the mother and the newborn. *Allergy*. 1987;42: 64-73.
93. Kjellman NI, Bjorksten B, Hattevig G, et al. Natural history of food allergy. *Ann Allergy*. 1988;61: 83-87.
94. Lilja G, Dannaeus A, Foucard T, et al. Effects of maternal diet during late pregnancy and lactation on the development of atopic diseases in infants up to 18 months of age—in-vivo results. *Clin Exp Allergy*. 1989;19:473-479.
95. Lilja G, Dannaeus A, Foucard T, et al. Effects of maternal diet during late pregnancy and lactation on the development of IgE and egg- and milk-specific IgE and IgG antibodies in infants. *Clin Exp Allergy*. 1991;21:195-202.
96. Chirico G, Gasparoni A, Ciardelli L, et al. Immunogenicity and antigenicity of a partially hydrolyzed cow's milk infant formula. *Allergy*. 1997;52:82-88.
97. de Seta L, Siani P, Cirillo G, et al. La prevenzione delle malattie allergiche con formula H.A.: Follow-up a 24 mesi. *Pediatr Med Chir*. 1994;16:251-254.
98. Lam BC, Yeung CY. The effect of breast milk, infant formula and hypoallergenic formula on incidence of atopic manifestation in high risk infants. Nestle Internal Report, Fremont, Mich, 1992.
99. Maggio L, Zuppa AA, Sawatzki G, et al. Higher urinary excretion of essential amino acids in preterm infants fed protein hydrolysates. *Acta Paediatr*. 2005;94:75-84.
100. Mallet E, Henocq A. Long-term prevention of allergic diseases by using protein hydrolysate formula in at-risk infants. *J Pediatr*. 1992;121:S95-S100.
101. Marini A, Agosti M, Motta G, et al. Effects of a dietary and environmental prevention programme on the incidence of allergic symptoms in high atopic risk infants: Three years' follow-up. *Acta Paediatr Suppl*. 1996;414:1-21.
102. Picaud JC, Rigo J, Normand SL, et al. Nutritional efficacy of preterm formula with a partially hydrolyzed protein source: A randomized pilot study. *J Pediatr Gastroenterol Nutr*. 2001;32:555-561.
103. Szajewska H, Albrecht P, Stoitiska BP, et al. Extensive and partial protein hydrolysate preterm formulas: The effect on growth rate, protein metabolism indices, and plasma amino acid concentrations. *J Pediatr Gastroenterol Nutr*. 2001;32:303-309.
104. Tsai YT, Chou CC, Hsieh KH. The effect of hypoallergenic formula on the occurrence of allergic diseases in high risk infants. *Zhonghua Min Guo Xiao Er Ke Yi Xue Hui Za Zhi*. 1991;32:137-144.
105. Vandenplas Y, Hauser B, Blecker U, et al. The nutritional value of a whey hydrolysate formula compared with a whey-predominant formula in healthy infants. *J Pediatr Gastroenterol Nutr*. 1993; 17:92-96.
106. Willems R, Duchateau J, Magrez P, et al. Influence of hypoallergenic milk formula on the incidence of early allergic manifestations in infants predisposed to atopic diseases. *Ann Allergy*. 1993;71: 147-150.
107. Johnstone DE, Dutton AM. Dietary prophylaxis of allergic disease in children. *N Engl J Med*. 1966; 274:715-719.
108. Miskelly FG, Burr ML, Vaughan-Williams E, et al. Infant feeding and allergy. *Arch Dis Child*. 1988;63: 388-393.

CHAPTER 10

Maternally Mediated Neonatal Autoimmunity

Neelufar Mozaffarian, MD, PhD; Elizabeth A. Shaw, DO;
and Anne M. Stevens, MD, PhD

10

Transplacental passage of maternal antibodies was first described in 1895 with the finding of anti-diphtheria toxin antibodies in fetal blood by Fischl and Von Wundscheim.[1] Over the past century, the role of maternally derived antibodies in passive neonatal immunity has been extensively studied, but this protection against infection comes with a price: self-reactive antibodies transferred to the fetus may result in neonatal autoimmunity. The resultant antibody-mediated disease phenotype depends not only on the antigen specificity, titer, and affinity of the antibody transferred, but on the gestational age and underlying health of the newborn, because these factors can influence the transplacental and gastrointestinal acquisition of immunoglobulins from the mother.[2-4]

In addition to maternal–fetal antibody transfer, transplacental acquisition and retention of whole maternal cells by the human fetus can occur[5-7]—a phenomenon previously believed to be impossible. These maternal cells persist and are detectable in healthy individuals for years after birth,[8] signifying a chronic chimeric state termed maternal microchimerism (MMc).

In the first half of this chapter, we will review examples of maternal antibody–mediated autoimmunity in the neonate (Table 10-1) and will speculate on hypothetical roles for maternal antibodies in modulating the risk of autoimmune disease. In the second half, we will describe the relationship between MMc and neonatal autoimmune disease, and the role of T regulatory cells in controlling neonatal autoimmunity.

Table 10-1 SOME OF THE TRANSPLACENTALLY ACQUIRED MATERNAL AUTOANTIBODIES AND ASSOCIATED DISEASE IN THE FETUS/INFANT

Maternal Antibodies	Associated Disease
	Collagen Vascular Diseases
Anti-SSA/Ro, anti-SSB/La, and anti-RNP antibodies	Neonatal lupus syndrome/heart block
Anti-neutrophil cytoplasmic antibodies (ANCA)	Neonatal vasculitis
Monoclonal IgG	Type I cryoglobulinemia
Monoclonal IgG	Glomerulonephritis
	Hematologic Diseases
Anti-erythrocyte	Neonatal anemia
Anti-platelet	Neonatal thrombocytopenia
Anti-neutrophil	Neonatal neutropenia
Anti-lymphocyte	Neonatal lymphopenia
	Endocrine Diseases
Anti-thyroid antibodies	Neonatal hyper/hypothyroidism
Diabetes-related antibodies	Unknown
Anti-adrenal antibodies	Unknown
	Neuromuscular Junction Diseases
Anti-acetylcholine receptor (ACh R) antibodies	Neonatal myasthenia gravis
Unknown	Neonatal Guillain-Barré
Anti-ganglioside GM-1 antibodies	Neonatal lower motor neuron disease
	Cardiac Diseases
Anti-β-adrenoceptor/cholinergic receptor antibodies	Neonatal cardiac disease
Anti-myolemmal antibodies	Fetal arrhythmias
	Skin Diseases
Anti-desmoglein antibodies	Neonatal pemphigus
	Nutritional deficiencies
Anti-folate receptor antibodies	Neural tube defects
Anti-intrinsic factor antibodies	Neonatal B_{12} deficiency
	Complications of Pregnancy
Anti-angiotensin II receptor antibodies	Preeclampsia
Anti-phospholipid antibodies	Preeclampsia, IUGR, fetal loss
Anti-laminin-1 antibodies	Spontaneous abortion
Anti-tissue transglutaminase antibodies	Spontaneous abortion, IUGR
Anti-AChR antibodies	Complications of labor
	Liver Diseases
Anti-nuclear antibodies (ANA)	Neonatal liver diseases
Antibodies to unknown target(s)	Neonatal hemochromatosis

MATERNAL ANTIBODIES AND NEONATAL AUTOIMMUNITY

Normal Physiology

Humans begin to receive immunoglobulin (Ig) from their mothers during fetal development. Transfer of maternal IgG to the fetus involves initiation of antibody transport shortly after the first trimester through term, with most antibody acquisition occurring in the third trimester.[9] Transplacental transfer of maternal antibodies is effected by the interaction of annexin II with neonatal Fc receptors (FcRn) on placental syncytiotrophoblasts.[10,11] These FcRn actively transport IgG in a subclass-specific fashion; for example, IgG_1 and IgG_4 are transferred to the fetus more efficiently than IgG_2 or IgG_3.[9,12,13] Although placental cells regulate the isotype, amount, and timing of antibody transfer, transfer is inherently dependent on circulating antibody levels in the pregnant mother. Alterations in maternal immunoglobulin titers or infusion of exogenous immunoglobulins to the pregnant woman will directly affect fetal antibody acquisition. These are important considerations because maternally derived antibodies do not merely play a passive role in neonatal immunity but can direct the development of the immune system of the newborn.[14,15] At birth, the infant's IgG levels are similar to or higher than those of the mother,[13] providing early protection against infection, because the half-life of maternal IgG in the infant is approximately 30 to 50 days.[16] Postnatally, levels of maternal IgG in the infant steadily decline, until more than half of the maternal IgG load is lost after 3 months, and virtually all of it is catabolized by 6 to 9 months of age.

In addition to IgG, evidence for prenatal IgE uptake has been found. Fetal gut lymphoid follicles express IgE receptors after week 16 of gestation, and human amniotic fluid samples from 16 to 18 weeks' gestation contain intact IgE, probably derived from the maternal circulation.[17] Therefore, maternal IgE may be acquired by the fetus via ingestion of amniotic fluid, possibly to protect from parasitic infection in endemic areas. Additionally, the interaction of maternal IgG and IgE may modulate neonatal autoimmunity. IgE levels at birth correlate with the infant's risk of developing atopic disease, but protection from atopy is seen in newborns with high titers of IgG anti-IgE, acquired from the maternal circulation.[18]

To further enhance the immunoglobulin repertoire, the newborn receives additional maternal antibodies via ingestion of breast milk, which provides substantial amounts of IgA (mostly dimeric), some IgM, and some subtypes of IgG.[19] The initial colostrum contains the highest titers of IgA, putatively to coat the newborn's unprotected mucosal surfaces. Gastrointestinal passage of breast milk does not result in proteolysis of immunoglobulins in the neonate. For example, protective anti-enteropathogenic *Escherichia coli* IgA antibodies acquired via colostrum can be found intact in the feces of breast-fed neonates.[20] In addition to providing mucosal protection, breast milk immunoglobulins may be transferred to the neonatal circulation. Human intestinal cells have been found to express the neonatal Fc receptor, suggesting a mechanism for IgG acquisition from gastrointestinal sources.[21]

The importance of acquired antibody in protection against infection and its effects on infant vaccination have been previously described.[22-24] But antibody acquisition can also lead to fetal or neonatal disease. Potential pathogenic mechanisms for maternal antibodies in neonatal disease include antibody-mediated depletion of specific cell types (via complement- or cell-mediated lysis, reticuloendothelial clearance, or initiation of apoptosis), interference with normal cellular/metabolic processes, immune complex (IC) formation and deposition, and/or initiation of a T cell–mediated immune response. Although some disease-related maternal autoantibodies can be routinely screened for in the neonate, it is likely that other, as yet unknown antibodies remain to be identified.

Developmental Differences Between the Fetus and the Newborn

Several developmentally regulated proteins are expressed only in the fetal or neonatal period, or are expressed in a "fetal" or "neonatal" form, which later transitions to the "adult" form (e.g., fetal acetylcholinesterase receptor, fetal hemoglobin), indicating that some of the disorders we currently refer to as "congenital" or "idiopathic" actually result from maternally derived antibodies that bind fetal/neonatal antigens but cause little or no disease in the mother. If the mother is asymptomatic, an underlying antibody disorder is not suspected, and the infant would not be tested. Therefore, the true prevalence of maternal antibody–mediated disease in neonates may be underestimated. Conversely, neonates may be protected from antibody-mediated diseases owing to differences in antigen expression or presentation. For example, infants are resistant to the development of anti-glomerular basement membrane (anti-GBM)-mediated glomerulonephritis owing to decreased antigen accessibility in fetal and neonatal renal tissues[25,26] and to antibody-mediated pemphigus foliaceus owing to redundant expression of cell adhesion proteins.[27]

Special Physiologic Aspects of Preterm Infants

Because most transplacental antibody transfer occurs in the third trimester, preterm birth can result in diminished antibody acquisition. However, full gestation does not necessarily ensure normal antibody levels in the neonate. Umbilical cord serum samples from low birth weight infants born at term revealed reduced IgG levels, similar to those seen in preterm infants of adequate weight ($\geq$2.5 kg).[28] Low birth weight and preterm infants have qualitative differences in maternal IgG acquisition, with disproportionately reduced concentrations of IgG_1 and IgG_2 subclasses. After birth, immune development may be further altered in preterm or low birth weight infants owing to decreased intake of breast milk.[29] It is not known whether gastrointestinal antibody uptake in these neonates is also qualitatively different. The role of altered antibody transfer in preterm infants in the development of neonatal autoimmunity is not known.

The Role of Breast Milk in Neonatal Autoimmunity

The role of milk-borne antibodies in neonatal autoimmunity is uncertain. For example, lupus-associated autoantibodies may cause fetal or neonatal lupus syndrome when acquired transplacentally. However, breast-fed infants of women with these autoantibodies have not been found to be at increased risk of disease, even though breast milk samples contain these autoantibodies in both IgA and IgG isotypes.[30] Ingestion of breast milk from asthmatic women has been linked to increased risk of allergy in human infants,[31] but this was not confirmed in other studies.[32-34] To test whether substances transferred in breast milk could promote atopy, an experimental mouse model was created whereby pups born to asthmatic and non-asthmatic mice were switched at birth and adoptively nursed.[35] After ingestion of breast milk from asthmatic mothers, the healthy pups also developed airway hyperreactivity. Whether this is related to transfer of IgE, IgG anti-IgE, or other breast milk components is not known. Additional studies are needed to investigate this phenomenon in preclinical and clinical settings.

Relevance of Physiologic Differences to the Disease Process

The transfer of maternal autoantibody is necessary but is not sufficient to cause autoimmune disease in the fetus/neonate. Additional factors, such as variability in transfer of maternal antibody, function of the endogenous immune system, and expression of target antigens (due to developmental, nutritional, and environmental factors), likely play a role. For example, some neonates born to mothers with lupus-associated autoantibodies develop cutaneous inflammation when exposed to sunlight, whereas other infants may show evidence of cutaneous inflammation at delivery, indicating that additional environmental or other factors are involved in pathogenesis.[36] The importance of factors other than maternally derived antibody in neonatal autoimmune disease is also demonstrated by reports of discordance in autoimmune disease in sets of twins and triplets.

Potential Mechanisms of Antibody-Mediated Autoimmune Disease

Acquired maternal antibodies can cause fetal or neonatal disease via multiple pathogenic mechanisms. Some autoantibodies cause disease by binding to antigen targets normally sequestered within the plasma and/or nuclear membranes of individual cells. Exposure of these antigens to the immune system may occur during apoptosis—a type of programmed cell death initiated by cellular insults such as infection, and also invoked in regulated waves during developmental remodeling.[37] The apoptotic program results in the processing of several intracellular and intranuclear proteins and their presentation at the cell surface. Antibodies to these antigens have been implicated in the pathogenesis of systemic lupus erythematosus and other autoimmune diseases, such as the anti-SSA/Ro and anti-SSB/La antibodies.

Other maternally derived antibodies cause neonatal disease by binding cell surface molecules, resulting in loss of the targeted cell from the circulation or tissues via complement-mediated lysis, antibody-mediated cellular cytotoxicity, reticuloendothelial clearance, or induction of apoptosis. Neonatal cytopenias are often caused by these types of antibodies. Rarely, antibodies are true maternal autoantibodies, causing disease in the mother and in the fetus, but more typically, they are *allo*antibodies, reacting against paternal antigens expressed by the fetus. Alloantibodies do not cause symptoms in the mother because her cells do not express the antigenic targets. Antibody-mediated neonatal cytopenias can be severe and may lead to death of the affected neonate if not aggressively treated. Examples of these antibodies include anti-erythrocyte, anti-platelet, anti-neutrophil, and anti-lymphocyte antibodies.

Maternal anti-receptor antibodies bind endogenous cell surface molecules and act as receptor agonists or antagonists. Anti-receptor antibodies can bind their targets at the normal ligand binding site or at another location, and may alter receptor interaction with endogenous ligand, depending on whether the antibody causes steric hindrance or a conformational change in the receptor. These autoantibodies may also alter receptor turnover or expression at the cell surface, or may bind to and clear a soluble receptor from the circulation or tissues. As noted previously, cell surface–bound antibodies may also lead to destruction of the targeted cell. In general, agonistic antireceptor antibodies cause active cell signaling, with the problem that the antibodies are not cleared, degraded, or regulated as endogenous ligand would be by the normal feedback pathways, resulting in signaling that can be tonic, mistimed, in aberrant locations, and/or at abnormal levels. These antibodies may act as partial agonists, full agonists, or supraphysiologic agonists at the targeted receptor. An example of this type of antibody is the agonistic anti-thyroid-stimulating hormone receptor (TSH-R) antibody.[38] In contrast, antagonistic anti-receptor antibodies typically reduce normal cell signaling. Examples of antagonistic anti-receptor antibodies include the anti-β_1-adrenoceptor and anti-acetylcholine receptor antibodies.

Antibodies to cell adhesion molecules are similar to the anti-receptor antibodies in that their targets are endogenous surface proteins, but in this case they disrupt cell–cell interactions important in signaling and/or maintaining tissue integrity, for example, anti-desmoglein antibodies.[39]

Another type of anti-receptor antibody is the anti-nutrient antibody. These maternal autoantibodies bind to endogenous receptors and interfere with fetal or neonatal nutrient acquisition. Antibody-mediated nutritional deficiency can result in a neonatal phenotype indistinguishable from true nutritional deficiency or congenital absence of the relevant receptor. However, it is important to make the distinction between these types of neonatal disease, so that appropriate treatment and/or preventive measures can be initiated. Examples of these types of antibodies include the anti-folate receptor and anti-intrinsic factor receptor antibodies.[40,41]

Anti-ligand antibodies bind to and limit the amount of endogenous ligand available for signaling. The affected individual must then increase production of the targeted protein or suffer the consequences of diminished signaling, or both. Similar to other autoantibodies, these may cross-react with more than one target, causing pleiotropic effects in the fetus or neonate. An example is the anti-insulin antibody.[42,43]

Some maternal antibodies cause disease by binding target antigens to form immune complexes. These immune complexes can be acquired by the fetus and may circulate at very high titers. In addition to altering blood viscosity, immune complexes may deposit in organs or vessel walls. Alternatively, transplacentally transferred maternal antibodies may form immune complexes directly in situ, in fetal tissues that contain their target antigen. In either case, these antibody–antigen complexes cause disease by inciting an intense, localized inflammatory response. Cryoglobulinemia is one example of maternal immune complex–mediated neonatal disease.

Interaction of Maternally Derived Antibodies with the Neonatal Immune System

Autoimmune disease initiated by maternally derived antibodies may depend on the presence of other factors, including an intact adaptive immune system. In murine studies, acquisition of maternal autoantibodies against a specific ovarian protein resulted in neonatal autoimmune ovarian disease (AOD) and premature ovarian failure, but only if T cells were also present.[44] Passive transfer of T cells from mice with AOD resulted in disease in the recipients, demonstrating that once the process was initiated by autoantibodies, antigen-specific effector T cells could mediate disease independently. These findings have important implications for the human neonate because maternal antibodies could prime an autoimmune T cell response, which would continue even after loss of transiently acquired maternal antibodies.

Maternal Alloimmunization due to Genetic Mutations

Although maternal antibodies against specific targets such as blood group antigens often develop because the woman lacks these alleles as a result of normal variation, descriptions of maternal alloimmunization related to idiosyncratic genetic mutations have been put forth. Absence of a normal gene may cause the encoded protein to appear foreign to the mother's immune system, leading to antibody production. For example, the gene for CD36 encodes a protein normally expressed on platelets, monocytes, and endothelial cells; a woman lacking CD36 expression owing to genetic mutation developed anti-CD36 IgG, and normal transplacental antibody transfer resulted in hydrops fetalis in her infants.[45] In another case, neonatal disease was caused by maternal antibodies to neutral endopeptidase (NEP), a protein normally expressed on renal podocytes.[46] Women with mutations in the gene for NEP become alloimmunized to this protein during pregnancy, when it is produced by placental syncytiotrophoblasts. Transplacental transfer of anti-NEP IgG antibodies results in antenatal membranous glomerulonephritis.

These examples raise the possibility that other neonatal diseases may be a result of alloimmunization in women with unusual genetic mutations. Typically, women with these types of genetic mutations have no antibody-related symptoms because they lack the target antigens. These maternal antibodies are not suspected; therefore, first pregnancies are at greatest risk for complications. Subsequent fetuses have an improved prognosis because they are more likely to be closely monitored. To protect the fetus from maternal antibody–mediated disease, pregnant women with known genetic mutations should be monitored for antibody titer and isotype, and possibly treated with intravenous immunoglobulin (IVIG) and/or plasma exchange, although no clinical trials have investigated these types of syndromes. Neutralizing agents such as the anti-D antibodies used in women at risk for alloimmunization to erythrocyte antigens may be developed for other alloimmunization.

Specific Maternal Antibody–Mediated Neonatal Autoimmune Diseases

Neonatal Cardiac Diseases

The passage of anti-cardiac autoantibodies and/or immune complexes from the mother may lead to neonatal cardiac disease, resulting in a myriad of inflammatory changes in the heart such as myositis, fibrosis, and even myocyte apoptosis.[47] The best studied are the lupus-associated anti-Ro/SSA and anti-La/SSB autoantibodies, which can lead to severe congenital heart block (CHB). However, CHB and cardiac arrhythmias have also been associated with antibodies to cardiac adrenoceptors, muscarinic cholinergic receptors, and myolemmal antigens.[48]

In most cases, autoantibodies implicated in cardiac conduction disorders may actually play a protective role, in that they also bind antigens derived from infectious agents; antibodies to the bundle of His, SSB/La, cardiac myosin heavy chain, or the laminin B1 chain cross-react with antigens from *Streptococcus pyogenes,* and antibodies to sarcolemmal epitopes cross-react with antigens from Coxsackie viruses.[49] The factors that turn a protective antibody into a pathogenic one remain unclear. The affinity, isotype, and titer of the autoantibody; characteristics of the target antigens; major histocompatibility complex (MHC) alleles; and the cellular immune system likely play a role.

Neonatal Lupus Syndrome and Congenital Heart Block

Neonatal lupus syndrome (NLS), not to be confused with systemic lupus erythematosus (SLE), is an autoimmune disease initiated during gestation by transplacental passage of maternal autoantibodies to intranuclear antigens, typically anti-SSA/Ro, anti-SSB/La, and/or anti-U1-ribonuclear protein (anti-RNP). Mothers with these autoantibodies classically have Sjögren's syndrome or SLE but may be clinically asymptomatic, although this latter group often develops autoimmune disease in the years following delivery.[50] NLS has also been associated with maternal leukocytoclastic vasculitis.[51,52] Fetal acquisition of lupus-related autoantibodies may lead to systemic or limited syndromes, including cardiac disease, cutaneous lesions, nephritis, cytopenias, pneumonitis, central nervous system disorders, and/or hepatobiliary disease.[53] Infants with NLS do not appear to have an increased risk of developing SLE[54] but may be at risk for developing other connective tissue disorders.[55,56] Siblings of neonates with NLS have been reported to have an elevated risk of developing SLE, even if healthy at birth, supporting the idea that these families have an underlying genetic susceptibility for lupus. Like SLE, NLS has a gender predilection. Females are more likely to be affected than males, with a 2 : 1 ratio for cardiac disease and a 3 : 1 ratio for skin lesions.[57] However, in contrast to SLE, NLS does not appear to preferentially affect a particular racial group.

NLS occurs in approximately 1 in 12,500 to 20,000 live births and is believed to represent a combination of pathogenic antibody acquisition and genetic/environmental factors.[57] Only 2% to 5% of infants who acquire these maternal autoantibodies manifest signs and symptoms of NLS, supporting the idea that other factors are required for disease pathogenesis.[58,59] In fact, discordant clinical expression of NLS has been reported in sets of twins where both infants were positive for maternally derived autoantibodies.[60-62] Discordant expression of NLS has also been reported in a set of triplets carried by a mother with anti-SSA/Ro and anti-SSB/La autoantibodies.[63] Specific MHC class I and II alleles in the mothers have been associated with the development of NLS in their infants.[64] However, there appears to be no correlation between the development of NLS and the human leukocyte antigen (HLA) alleles of the infants themselves,[65] suggesting that maternal cells acquired by the fetus may play a role in the pathogenesis of NLS. A recent case of NLS with congenital heart block was diagnosed in a neonate born to a surrogate mother via ovodonation (biologic mother and father genes).[66] The surrogate mother had no known autoimmune disease at the time of implantation but was later found to have anti-nuclear antibodies (1 : 640 titer) and anti-SSA/Ro and SB/La antibodies. The authors observed that CHB may develop in a genetically unrelated child who was exposed to anti-SSA/Ro antibodies in utero. The role of maternal genes and their potential contribution to the development of NLS are still under investigation.

NLS can manifest in a variety of ways: approximately half of all cases have congenital heart block, 25% develop cutaneous lesions, and 10% occur with concurrent skin and cardiac disease.[53] Similar to SLE, NLS can cause life-threatening nephritis; however, unlike SLE, this manifestation is extremely rare. The skin lesions of NLS typically consist of scaly, annular erythematous plaques at sun-exposed areas (often the head and neck), but other variations have been described.[36] Exposure to sunlight causes ultraviolet (UV) radiation–induced apoptosis of skin cells, with presentation of normally sequestered intranuclear antigens. This process becomes problematic in the context of acquired maternal autoantibodies, which bind apoptotic targets and incite a perivascular inflammatory infiltrate. Of note, sunlight is not absolutely required for the development of skin disease because some antibody-positive infants exhibit cutaneous NLS at birth.[36] Infants with NLS-related skin inflammation can be treated with topical corticosteroids and prevention of sun exposure. The skin lesions generally resolve over several months without residual effects, although they can result in permanent scarring in severe cases. In general, neonates with only skin, hematologic, or hepatic involvement have a better prognosis than those with cardiac disease; affected infants typically improve clinically with decline of maternal autoantibodies in the infant's circulation.[67]

10

The most significant problem in NLS is the development of congenital heart block (CHB), which carries high morbidity and mortality.[68] CHB was reported as early as 1901 but was not linked to maternal autoantibodies until the 1980s.[69,70] We now know that antibody-mediated NLS is responsible for most cases of CHB.[57] More than 85% of fetuses who have conduction defects in the setting of a structurally normal heart have mothers with these autoantibodies,[71,72] but only approximately 2% of women who have these pathogenic autoantibodies will have a child with CHB.[73,74] NLS-related CHB is associated with inflammatory fibrosis of the cardiac conducting system, endocardial fibroelastosis, endocardial hyperplasia, and other cardiomyopathies.[75-77] Unlike other manifestations of NLS, CHB is irreversible, even after loss of maternal autoantibodies from the infant's circulation. This may be due to the fact that antibody-mediated cardiac damage occurs in utero, as evidenced by detectable conduction abnormalities before the third trimester of gestation. Infants with CHB who survive often require pacemaker insertion and can develop left ventricular cardiomyopathy even with adequate treatment.[78]

Cardiomyocyte apoptosis is required for the development of NLS, to allow exposure of target antigens at the lipid membrane of dying cells.[79] Injection of human anti-SSB/La antibodies into pregnant mice resulted in antibody binding to apoptotic cells in selected organs, including fetal heart, skin, liver, and bone,[80] supporting the role of these autoantibodies in the pathogenesis of NLS. Antibody-coated apoptotic blebs may promote tissue scarring by stimulating local macrophages to produce transforming growth factor-β (TGF-β), a pro-fibrotic cytokine.[81] Genetic polymorphisms linked to high TGF-β production have been associated with increased risk for CHB.[82]

In fetuses at risk for acquiring lupus-related autoantibodies, careful prenatal monitoring is warranted, including measurement of maternal autoantibody titers and Doppler evaluation to detect cardiac conduction defects in utero, because fetal CHB carries a 50% death rate.[68,75,83] Women with these antibodies and a history of an affected fetus have a two- to threefold higher risk of fetal CHB in subsequent pregnancies.[68] Maternal plasmapheresis or immunoabsorption with and without dexamethasone may be beneficial during pregnancy,[84-87] and in some cases dexamethasone has been associated with reversal of fetal conduction abnormalities and increased survival at 1 year.[75,88] However, in cases that respond to corticosteroid administration, heart block may progress over time, even after maternal antibodies have been degraded (Research Registry for Neonatal Lupus [RRNL] data appear in papers by Saleeb and Buyon[89,90]). IVIG at replacement dosages does not appear to prevent the recurrence of CHB in neonates born to mothers with a previously affected neonate with CHB.[91,92]

Treatment of affected neonates is largely symptomatic. Most infants with CHB will require pacemaker insertion and long-term monitoring because CHB-related morbidity is high, and neonatal mortality approximates 10%.

Congenital Heart Block and Anti-Adrenoceptor/Cholinergic Receptor Antibodies

An antibody that binds both the cardiac β_1-adrenoceptor and the muscarinic acetylcholine receptor has been found in patients with "idiopathic" dilated cardiomyopathy (DCM),[93] DCM-associated atrial fibrillation,[94] and congestive heart failure.[95] Binding of this antibody to a ribosomal protein of *Trypanosoma cruzi* has also suggested a role for it in Chagas disease–associated cardiomyopathy, and implies an infectious cause for its existence.[96-99] Although it does not cause DCM in neonates, this autoantibody has been identified in infants with CHB.[48,100] Using rat heart tissue samples, anti-adrenoceptor and anti-muscarinic cholinergic receptor IgG was found in infants with CHB and in their mothers, but not in controls. These autoantibodies could bind to and activate cardiac receptors, block ligand binding, and alter myocardial contractility, but only in neonatal rat tissues, suggesting a fetal antigen as the pathogenic target.

Although normally receptor agonists, these IgG antibodies act as receptor inhibitors when enzymatically cleaved to form monovalent antigen-binding fragments (Fab) by removal of the antibody constant region.[101] In laboratory studies, monovalent Fab fragments derived from a stimulatory anti-β_2-adrenoceptor IgG antibody acted as receptor antagonists, inducing conformational changes in the adrenoceptor and preventing ligand binding. The Fab fragments reacquired agonist activity when they were cross-linked to form divalent antibody. These findings are potentially relevant to neonatal disease because high-affinity IgG-derived Fab fragments constitute the major form of immunoglobulin in meconium, even in babies who have not been breast-fed, suggesting a transplacental source.[102] Thus, the effect of maternal autoantibodies in the neonate may depend not only on antigen specificity, affinity, and antibody isotype, but also on whether the antibody is in a dimeric state. Because the role of these anti-neurotransmitter antibodies in CHB is not yet well understood, affected neonates should receive standard cardiac care. Comparison of fetal outcomes with measurement of antibody titers in women with previously affected infants or with a history of Chagas disease may provide a rationale for prenatal treatment in the future.

Fetal Arrhythmias and Anti-Myolemmal Antibodies

Anti-myolemmal antibodies (AMLA) cause lysis of cardiomyocytes in vitro and have been implicated in adult cardiac diseases such as DCM and viral myocarditis. Transplacental transfer of AMLA from women with myocarditis may be responsible for fetal cardiac arrhythmia.[103] The cord blood of infants born to mothers with and without myocarditis revealed that in 18 cases of fetal arrhythmia of unknown origin, 13 mothers were positive for AMLA, as were 5 infants. Among 19 healthy women, only 3 were found to have AMLA, and unaffected infants did not have these autoantibodies. Management of fetal arrhythmias has been previously discussed,[104] but no guidelines are currently available for prenatal treatment of AMLA-exposed fetuses.

Hematopoietic Cell Diseases

Hemolytic Disease of the Newborn/Neonatal Anemia

Hemolytic disease of the newborn (HDN) has been well described[105] and will only briefly be summarized here. Nearly all autoimmune HDN is caused by antibodies to Rhesus group antigen D (RhD), produced by women who lack the gene for this protein and thus do not express RhD on their own erythrocytes. The incidence of anti-RhD-related HDN is currently 1 to 6 per 1000 live births.[105] First pregnancies usually are not affected. Women typically develop anti-RhD antibodies after delivery or loss of an RhD-positive infant, placing their subsequent pregnancies at risk for transplacental antibody transfer and disease. The anti-RhD antibodies are usually of IgG_1 or IgG_3 isotypes, and IgG_1 is more pathogenic to the fetus than IgG_3.[106]

For prevention of anti-RhD disease, administration of anti-D antibodies to RhD-negative women has greatly improved neonatal outcomes by inhibiting maternal alloimmunization.[107] Fortunately, injection of anti-D immunoglobulin in pregnant women at risk for developing anti-RhD antibodies has not been found to result in fetal or neonatal hemolysis.[108] For women who already have anti-RhD antibodies, anti-D infusion is not useful; various maneuvers have been attempted to reduce fetal morbidity and mortality, including maternal plasmapheresis, high-dose IVIG, and neonatal exchange transfusion, with variable success.[109-112] In infants at risk of HDN, the occurrence of hydrops fetalis and other complications has been greatly reduced by fetal blood sampling and in utero erythrocyte transfusions.[113] In affected neonates, early serum bilirubin measurements are helpful in predicting whether an infant will develop severe hemolysis and significant hyperbilirubinemia.[114,115] The use of exchange transfusion in infants with ABO-incompatible HDN was found to have significant risks, including mortality.[116] One randomized clinical trial of single versus double volume exchange transfusion for HDN showed that single volume exchange transfusion was as effective as double volume, and it introduced less risk.[117]

Although antibodies to RhD are the most common, transplacental transfer of maternal antibodies to other erythrocyte antigens may lead to fetal anemia, including anti-other Rh antigens (c, C, e, E), anti-ABO, anti-MNS, anti-Kell (K, k), anti-Duffy (Fya, Fyb), anti-Kidd (Jka, Jkb), anti-Lewis, anti-Lutheran, anti-Diego, and

10

others.[118-121] Moreover, the mechanism of action of these antibodies may involve more than just hemolysis. For example, anti-Kell antibodies have been found to cause fetal anemia in part by inhibiting bone marrow erythropoiesis.[122] In these cases, measurement of maternal antibody titers or amniotic bilirubin levels is less useful for monitoring, and direct fetal blood sampling is required.[123] Postnatal injections of erythropoietin have been used successfully to treat infants with anti-Kell-related anemia.[124]

The use of cell-free fetal DNA (cffDNA) genotype testing in maternal blood to aid in identification of the fetal D type has been studied.[125] When maternal blood is used, the fetal D type can be genotyped from cffDNA, thus identifying fetuses who are D-negative and are not at risk for HDN, or who are D-positive and would need intervention and monitoring.[126,127] Use of this new genotyping test on a large scale is controversial from a cost and benefit standpoint, and further analysis as to its role in the work-up of HDN is required.[128]

Neonatal Thrombocytopenia

Neonatal thrombocytopenia can be caused by the transplacental transfer of anti-platelet antibodies from the mother to the fetus. Rarely, these antibodies are autore-active and cause thrombocytopenia in the mother as well as in the fetus, as in cases of maternal idiopathic thrombocytopenic purpura (ITP). More commonly, however, the maternal antibodies are a result of feto-maternal incompatibility for human platelet-specific antigens (HPA)[129] and cause neonatal alloimmune thrombocytopenia (NAIT). NAIT is the primary cause of severe neonatal thrombocytopenia, occurring in approximately 1 in 1500 to 5000 live births.[130]

Unlike maternal antibody–related hemolytic anemia, which requires sensitization to erythrocyte antigens in a prior pregnancy, most cases of NAIT occur during the first pregnancy because the woman is sensitized to fetally expressed paternal antigens during gestation. Although many maternal antibody–mediated cytopenias resolve over time with loss of the offending maternal antibody, fetal thrombocyto-penias can be severe enough in utero to cause life-threatening intracranial hemorrhage. Even if the fetus survives, intracranial hemorrhage may result in significant sequelae, including neonatal spasticity/hypotonia, seizures, developmental delay, or cortical blindness.[131] In NAIT, the incidence of intracranial hemorrhage has been estimated at 20% to 30%, and neonatal death at approximately 10%.[130,132] In reality, the overall complication rate is even higher because these numbers included closely monitored second pregnancies in women with a history of NAIT. When only first-born infants are taken into account, incidence and fatality rates increase to 47% and 24%, respectively.[132]

Management of NAIT has been recently reviewed.[131] Prevention of NAIT-related complications includes fetal blood sampling to measure platelet counts as early as the 20th week of gestation. Women with currently affected fetuses or with a history of severely affected fetuses may benefit from weekly IVIG, with the addition of corticosteroids if the fetal platelet count does not respond. In fetuses with significant thrombocytopenia just before delivery, intrauterine platelet transfusions or delivery by cesarean section has been beneficial.[132] Postnatally, infants may require IVIG or platelet transfusions. Platelet levels should be followed for at least 1 month after birth, until maternal antibodies have diminished.[131]

Neonatal Neutropenia

Anti-neutrophil IgG transmitted to the fetus across the placenta may result in profound neutropenia. Neutropenia becomes a significant problem shortly after birth because these neonates are susceptible to severe bacterial infections, which can lead to death or permanent disability.[133] As with neonatal thrombocytopenia, neonatal neutropenia may be caused by maternal autoantibodies, which also cause neutropenia in the mother, or, more commonly, by maternal alloantibodies, which cause disease only in the fetus.[134] The incidence of neonatal alloimmune neutropenia is approximately 1 in 2000 live births,[135] and true autoimmune neutropenia is rare.

Most of the maternal anti-neutrophil antibodies target human neutrophil-specific antigens (HNA),[136,137] but several reports have described antibodies against neutrophil targets other than HNA,[133,138-140] and neonatal lupus syndrome may also cause neutropenia.[141,142] Prenatal management of IgG-mediated neutropenia involves monitoring of maternal anti-neutrophil antibody titers (and maternal neutrophil counts, in cases of autoimmune neutropenia). After delivery, the infant's neutrophil count can be followed, and neonates treated with antibiotics as needed. Prenatal and postnatal administration of recombinant human granulocyte colony-stimulating factor has also been shown to be beneficial in the treatment of both autoimmune and alloimmune neonatal neutropenia.[136,143]

Neonatal Lymphocytopenia

Maternal antibody–mediated neonatal lymphocytopenia is rare. Two infants with severe antibody-mediated lymphocytopenia and thrombocytopenia were born to a woman who had been sensitized to fetally expressed paternal antigens during her five previous pregnancies.[144] Antibody transfer resulted in congenital immunodeficiency in both infants. One of the affected neonates died 16 days after birth owing to severe graft-versus-host disease (GVHD), caused by transplacental acquisition of maternal lymphocytes. The other infant was diagnosed with sepsis and treated with exchange transfusion, which resulted in reversal of the antibody-mediated cytopenias and recovery. IgG from the mother was found to react with non-HLA paternal antigens expressed on neonatal lymphocytes, and serial testing after her last pregnancy revealed a steady decline in her anti-paternal IgG titers.

Neonatal Endocrine Diseases

Neonatal Hypothyroidism and Antagonistic Anti-Thyroid Antibodies

Circulating autoantibodies in pregnant women with autoimmune thyroid disease may cross the placenta and cause aberrant thyroid function in the fetus and neonate.[145] Autoantibodies associated with autoimmune hypothyroidism include anti-thyroid-stimulating hormone (anti-TSH) antibodies, antagonistic TSH receptor (TSH-R) antibodies, and anti-thyroid peroxidase antibodies. As with other maternal antibody–mediated diseases, neonatal manifestations usually resolve with catabolism of the relevant autoantibodies. However, cases of congenital malformation have been described in neonates born to mothers with autoimmune thyroiditis,[146] and severe cases of maternal antibody–mediated gestational hypothyroidism can lead to permanent damage, including abnormal brain development or fetal loss.[147] The long-term effects of transient exposure to maternal anti-thyroid autoantibodies are not known, although the presence of anti-thyroid peroxidase antibodies in cord blood has been associated with increased risk of future autoimmune thyroiditis[148] and with lower scores on cognitive testing, even in offspring of mothers who were euthyroid.[149]

Fetuses of women with autoimmune thyroiditis are at risk for acquiring other maternal autoantibodies as well, owing to the association of autoimmune thyroid disease with connective tissue disorders such as Sjögren's syndrome or SLE.[150-152] In addition, fetal disease caused by other maternally derived autoantibodies can be exacerbated in the context of maternal hypothyroidism. Infants of women with lupus-associated anti-SSA/La or anti-SSB/Ro antibodies had a ninefold increased risk of developing complete CHB if the mother was also hypothyroid.[153] The mechanism of this synergy is not clear.

Management of neonatal hypothyroidism involves laboratory monitoring of the mother throughout pregnancy, with exogenous thyroxine administration as needed, taking into account her gestational requirements.[154] After birth, the neonate can be followed with serial evaluations of thyroid function and maternal autoantibody titers, and can be treated with thyroxine until thyroid function has normalized. In a series of neonates with transient hyperthyroxinemia whose mothers had autoimmune thyroid disease, 21% of neonates had severe hyperbilirubinemia, suggesting that clinical examination and additional blood testing for hyperbilirubinemia should be performed in neonates exposed to anti-thyroid peroxidase (TPO) antibodies.[155]

Neonatal Hyperthyroidism and Agonistic Anti-TSH Receptor Antibodies

Neonatal hyperthyroidism is less common than neonatal hypothyroidism. The prevalence of Graves' disease among pregnant women is estimated to be 0.2%, and clinically apparent hyperthyroidism due to transplacental transmission of stimulatory anti-TSH-R antibodies occurs in less than 1% of these pregnancies.[38] As with other maternal antibody–mediated diseases, neonatal hyperthyroidism typically resolves with loss of maternal antibodies in the first 4 months of life.[156] However, if untreated, fetal and neonatal thyrotoxicosis may lead to death.

Although the anti-TSH-R antibodies produced in Graves' disease are typically agonistic, antagonistic antibodies are often produced as well. In a study of pregnant women over time, the ratio of these antibody types was found to change during pregnancy, such that the antibody specificity became predominantly one of TSH-R blockade.[157] Although maternal autoantibody–mediated effects on the developing fetus were not evaluated in this particular study, it is clear that there are potential dangers for induction of both neonatal hyperthyroidism and hypothyroidism during pregnancies complicated by Graves' disease.

Management of neonatal thyroid disease involves laboratory evaluation of the mother throughout pregnancy, as well as monitoring of fetal growth and heart rate. Prenatal thyroid status can be followed using ultrasonography to measure fetal thyroid gland size and progression of skeletal maturation.[158] In selected cases, umbilical cord blood sampling can be used to directly measure thyroid hormone levels.[159] Fetal hyperthyroidism can be treated by administration of medications to the pregnant woman. After birth, the infant should undergo serial laboratory evaluations of thyroid function, and pharmacotherapy until thyroid function has normalized.[156,160]

Neonatal Exposure to Diabetes-Related Autoantibodies

Type 1 diabetes mellitus (DM 1) is caused by the autoimmune destruction of pancreatic β-cells and is associated with the presence of specific autoantibodies against insulin, the insulin receptor, and various islet cell antigens. These diabetes-associated autoantibodies can be transferred to the fetus.

Anti-insulin Autoantibodies

Transplacental acquisition of anti-insulin autoantibodies (AIA) or insulin–AIA complexes has been documented in infants of women with these IgGs.[42,43,161,162] Individuals with AIA also often produce its anti-idiotypic antibody.[150] The anti-idiotypes not only bind AIA, but can block the insulin receptor, leading to neonatal fatality in some cases. However, if both AIA and anti-idiotype are present at high levels, they will bind to and neutralize each other, preventing interference with insulin signaling (Fig. 10-1). About a third of the polyclonal AIA from diabetic patients cross-reacts

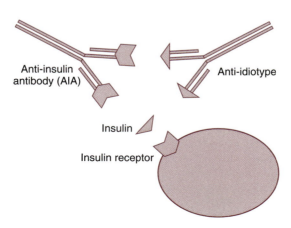

Anti-insulin antibody (AIA)

Anti-idiotype

Insulin

Insulin receptor

Figure 10-1 Anti-insulin and anti-idiotype autoantibodies. Anti-insulin antibody (AIA) can bind insulin or anti-idiotype antibodies. The anti-idiotype antibody can bind AIA or the insulin receptor. If both antibodies are present in adequate concentrations, they can bind and neutralize each other.

with nerve growth factor (NGF)[163]; this may explain the occurrence of neuropathy in children born to mothers with AIA.

In genetically susceptible nonobese diabetic (NOD) mice, the risk of neonatal diabetes does not correlate with maternally derived AIA,[164] although maternal AIA likely plays a central role in neonatal disease in many other models.[165,166] In human neonates, the transient presence of AIA has not been associated with the future development of diabetes,[167,168] although the presence of autoantibodies after 9 months of age, by which time the maternally derived antibodies should have cleared, is associated with increased risk.[167] Because the pathogenetic role of AIA in neonatal disease is unknown, specific preventive or therapeutic measures are not recommended at this time. Infants who manifest signs of hyperglycemia should receive standard diabetes management.

Anti-Islet Cell, Anti-Glutamic Acid Decarboxylase, and Anti-IA-2 Protein Autoantibodies

Other maternal autoantibodies associated with DM 1 include anti-islet cell antibodies (ICA), anti-glutamic acid decarboxylase (anti-GAD) antibodies, and anti-protein tyrosine phosphatase IA-2 (anti-IA-2) antibodies, which are also transferred across the placenta. Levels of these autoantibodies in the serum of pregnant women were compared with those in their infants' cord blood after birth.[169] Among women with DM 1, almost 40% had ICA, 55% had anti-GAD, and 54% had anti-IA-2. Of infants born to diabetic mothers, 33% had ICA, 50% had anti-GAD, and 51% had anti-IA-2. In nondiabetic mothers, 5.2% had ICA, 5.2% had anti-GAD, and 3% had anti-IA-2. Of infants born to nondiabetic mothers, 6% had ICA, 2.2% had anti-GAD, and none had anti-IA-2. The effect of prenatal exposure to autoantibodies on the risk of developing DM 1 is not known; infants with anti-GAD, anti-IA-2, or AIA in their cord blood were not found to have significantly altered birth weights or insulin concentrations when compared with controls.[170,171]

Anti-Adrenal Autoantibodies

Little is known regarding the fetal effects of maternal autoantibodies in relation to other autoimmune endocrine diseases. Transplacental transfer of anti-adrenal autoantibodies has been reported in rare cases. One infant born to a mother with Addison disease and gestational DM was found to have anti-adrenal cortex and anti-islet cell antibodies at birth, but no signs or symptoms of disease.[172] Another infant born to a woman with autoimmune polyendocrine syndrome type II (Addison disease, DM 1, and autoimmune thyroiditis) had anti-adrenal cortex and anti-steroid-21-hydroxylase autoantibodies at birth, but also remained clinically asymptomatic.[173] Although these cases suggest that anti-adrenal autoantibodies do not cause fetal pathology, establishing treatment recommendations will require screening a larger number of selected infants for subclinical adrenal disease.

Neuromuscular Diseases

Neonatal Myasthenia Gravis and Anti-Acetylcholine Receptor (AChR) Antibodies

Neonatal myasthenia gravis (NMG) is caused by transplacentally acquired maternal anti-AChR antibodies or muscle-specific kinase (MuSK) antibodies, typically presenting with muscle weakness within the first 72 hours of life.[174] As in other types of maternal antibody–mediated syndromes, the severity of disease does not necessarily correlate with the antibody titer in the mother or infant. Reports have described neonates with acquired anti-AChR antibodies who remain clinically asymptomatic[175] and cases of NMG in which only one fetus of a twin gestation is affected,[176,177] suggesting that antibody acquisition alone may not be enough to cause clinical manifestations.[178]

Some maternal anti-AChR antibodies are specific for the *fetal* form of AChR and cause NMG only in the fetus, while the mother remains asymptomatic.[179,180] Examination of human skeletal muscle revealed that the fetal form of AChR is present until 31 weeks' gestation,[181] suggesting that antibody-mediated damage may take place early in development. Clinical disease generally is more severe in cases with anti-fetal AChR antibodies, and the risk of NMG in subsequent pregnancies of these women is estimated to be 100%. Although the absolute autoantibody levels in women vary greatly, the ratio of anti-fetal/anti-adult AChR remains fairly constant in individual mothers over time, and is a much better predictor of the development of NMG.[182] The risk for NMG in neonates born to women with MuSK-myasthenia gravis may be lower than in AChR-myasthenia gravis perhaps owing to the transport of IgG subclasses across the placenta. Anti-AChR antibodies are mostly IgG_1, and anti-MuSK antibodies are mainly IgG_4.[183] NMG usually resolves as maternal antibody is lost from the neonatal circulation between 1 and 6 months of age.[184] However, if the disease is severe enough during gestation, long-term, irreversible sequelae may occur. For example, anti-AChR antibody-mediated major fetal akinesia may lead to arthrogryposis multiplex congenita (congenital polyarticular contractures), abnormal pulmonary development, velopharyngeal incompetence, and even death.[179,180,185,186]

No preventive measures for NMG are known. Maternal myasthenia gravis is not a contraindication to pregnancy, and successful pregnancy can be achieved with appropriate prenatal and postnatal care.[177,187] Prevention of NMG involves identifying women with myasthenia gravis, but this is complicated by the fact that some women with anti-AChR antibodies are completely asymptomatic.[188] If the fetus is affected by NMG, ultrasonography may reveal reduced fetal movement or polyhydramnios due to decreased swallowing, and the pregnant woman may note a change in fetal activity. An oxytocin challenge can be used to evaluate fetal health, and continuous fetal monitoring may be beneficial in selected cases. After delivery, infants suspected of having NMG can be tested using neostigmine or other cholinesterase inhibitors.

Management of NMG consists of supportive treatment. Neonatal autoantibody levels can be monitored with the expectation that clinical manifestations of NMG will regress within the first 2 months as antibody levels decline. Some have tried using neonatal plasmapheresis or IVIG to speed the recovery process.[189,190] However, unlike in adults, treatment with IVIG has not been proved effective in NMG,[190] and IVIG use in any patient is associated with serious risks, including anaphylactic reactions, aseptic meningitis, acute renal failure, cardiovascular thromboses, transmission of viral pathogens, and other complications.[191,192]

Neonatal Guillain-Barré

Campylobacter jejuni enteritis is associated with the development of Guillain-Barré syndrome in 1 in 1000 cases.[193,194] In susceptible individuals, production of an anti-*Campylobacter* antibody cross-reactive with a human peripheral nerve antigen may lead to Guillain-Barré syndrome. Infants of women with Guillain-Barré syndrome can develop a transient version of this neuromuscular disease, called *neonatal Guillain-Barre (NGB)*. Cases of NGB have also been described in infants born to women with active ulcerative colitis during pregnancy.[195,196] This is interesting in that inflammatory bowel disease has also been linked to a history of bacterial enteritis. However, the responsible antibody and antigenic target(s) have not been identified.

One infant born to a woman with active Guillain-Barré syndrome developed NGB 12 days after birth, characterized by flaccid paralysis and respiratory distress.[197] Because he had not been breast-fed, his disease was attributed to transplacental transfer of maternal autoantibodies. In laboratory testing, IgG from the mother or infant blocked neuromuscular transmission in murine diaphragmatic muscle explants. However, IgG-mediated neuromuscular blockade did not require interaction with complement components or leukocyte Fc receptors because monovalent antigen-binding fragments (Fab) of this antibody had the same effect. Diaphragmatic muscles from mice younger than 5 days of age were not affected by this antibody, and no clinical signs were observed in the infant until nearly 2 weeks after birth, suggesting that the target antigen is not expressed, active, or accessible in fetal tissues. Thus, acquisition of maternal autoantibody against a developmentally regulated protein spared the fetus from disease but caused neuromuscular pathology in the neonate.

As with many of the rare maternal antibody–mediated neonatal diseases, prevention and treatment of NGB have not been systematically studied. In the case of maternally derived NGB described earlier, the infant was treated with IVIG and recovered quickly. He had no further sequelae, and subsequent laboratory testing showed loss of pathogenic IgG from his circulation by 3 months of age.[197]

Neonatal Lower Motor Neuropathy and Anti-Ganglioside Antibody

Maternal autoantibodies associated with other neuropathies can also be transferred during gestation. For example, anti-ganglioside GM-1 antibodies were transplacentally acquired by the fetus of a woman with multifocal motor neuropathy, although she had been treated with monthly IVIG throughout pregnancy.[198] Monoclonal IgG was detectable in neonatal serum for 4 months after birth, and distal muscle atrophy and weakness were present both prenatally and postnatally. Although the infant's distal motor function improved over time, he suffered long-term sequelae, revealed by abnormal nerve conduction studies in childhood.

Collagen Vascular Diseases

Anti-Neutrophil Cytoplasmic Antibody

Anti-neutrophil cytoplasmic antibodies (ANCA) directed at neutrophil-derived myeloperoxidase (MPO) are associated with systemic small vessel vasculitides. Transmission of maternal MPO-ANCA to the fetus can result in neonatal vasculitis. A pregnant woman with MPO-ANCA gave birth at 33 weeks' gestation to an infant who developed life-threatening pulmonary hemorrhage and renal disease on day 2 of life.[199] Anti-MPO antibody was present in the infant's cord blood at birth. The neonate was treated with high-dose corticosteroids on day 2 and with exchange transfusion on day 5, resulting in undetectable antibody by day 25 and no further recurrence of the disease. However, another pregnant woman with MPO-ANCA (treated with oral steroids and azathioprine during pregnancy) gave birth at 38 weeks to a healthy infant who had documented elevated levels of anti-MPO antibody but no clinical signs of disease.[200]

Women with ANCA-associated diseases should be carefully monitored and antibody levels well controlled at the time of pregnancy. It is unknown whether corticosteroid treatment during pregnancy would improve neonatal outcome, but extrapolation from other maternal antibody–mediated diseases suggests that this may be beneficial. However, the benefits of prenatal and postnatal corticosteroid administration must be weighed against its potential adverse effects, which include perinatal death, cardiovascular disease, neurologic abnormalities,[201-203] and, possibly, increased risk of future autoimmunity.[204]

Monoclonal Gammopathies

Neonatal connective tissue diseases may result from the transfer of monoclonal maternal antibodies or immune complexes. A neonate born to a woman with monoclonal IgG-λ developed glomerulonephritis and acute renal failure within the first week after delivery.[205] This infant was found to have an antibody that was electrophoretically identical to that found in her mother. Treatment with neonatal exchange transfusion was successful in resolving her clinical symptoms. In another case, a woman with a diagnosis of essential type I cryoglobulinemia gave birth to a set of twins who developed cyanotic macules when exposed to cold.[206] Both had the same monoclonal IgG as their mother, and their clinical manifestations resolved after 6 months, supporting a direct role for maternal antibodies as the cause of this neonatal disease. Finally, a preterm infant was incidentally found to have a monoclonal gammopathy identical to that of his mother,[207] suggesting that the incidence of neonatal monoclonal gammopathies may be higher than expected because these antibodies do not always cause clinically apparent disease. Owing to the heterogeneity of this

10

rare syndrome, infants with monoclonal gammopathies can be managed only on a case-by-case basis.

Nutritional Deficiencies

Neural Tube Defects and Anti-Folate Receptor Antibodies

Folate deficiency during gestation results in neural tube defects, fetal loss, preterm birth, and intrauterine growth restriction (IUGR).[208] Although folate supplementation in pregnant women greatly reduces the risk of neural tube defects, most women with affected fetuses do not have clinical folate deficiency during pregnancy, suggesting that additional folate is needed to overcome a block to folate uptake by the developing fetus.[40] In support of this hypothesis, autoantibodies to the folate receptor were found in 9 of 12 women with a pregnancy complicated by neural tube defects, and in 2 of 20 controls (although these antibodies were of lower affinity).[40] These maternal autoantibodies were found to bind folate receptors isolated from human placenta, suggesting a mechanism of action for fetal pathogenesis. Most of the affected fetuses in this study were the result of a first pregnancy, making it difficult to ascertain whether the maternal autoantibodies had been generated as a result of alloimmunization during pregnancy or in response to an unrelated antigen. Owing to the high rate of disease in first-born infants and lack of clinical signs in their mothers, screening for anti-folate receptor autoantibodies is not feasible, nor is it cost-effective. Rather, all women should receive folate supplementation throughout conception, gestation, and breast-feeding because supplementation appears to be able to overcome the effects of these maternal autoantibodies.[40]

Neonatal Pernicious Anemia and Anti-Intrinsic Factor Antibodies

Transplacental transfer of maternal autoantibodies, which bind intrinsic factor, may lead to cobalamin (vitamin B_{12}) deficiency. In adults, these autoantibodies interfere with intrinsic factor–mediated uptake of cobalamin from the gut, leading to pernicious anemia, neuropathy, and atrophic gastritis in severely affected cases.[209] Anti-intrinsic factor autoantibodies acquired during gestation can cause fetal cobalamin deficiency with cytopenias, failure to thrive, and neurologic deficits.[41] Similar to many autoantibodies, the presence of anti-intrinsic factor antibodies indicates an increased risk of other maternal autoimmune diseases, including autoimmune thyroiditis, DM 1, and SLE, because these syndromes often coexist.[210-212] Therefore, the finding of anti-intrinsic factor antibodies in the neonate should prompt consideration of other maternal autoantibody–mediated diseases, and vice versa. To prevent fetal pathology, pregnant women with anti-intrinsic factor autoantibodies should receive cobalamin supplementation to ensure adequate serum levels. Neonates can be supplemented with cobalamin until loss of maternal autoantibody has been verified.

Skin Disease

Neonatal Pemphigus and Anti-Desmoglein Antibodies

Desmoglein (Dsg) is a cadherin-like adhesion molecule that functions to maintain tissue integrity and facilitates cell–cell communication. These proteins are the target antigens in epidermal blistering diseases such as pemphigus, caused by autoantibody-mediated acantholysis (disruption of keratinocyte adhesion).[213] To date, four isoforms of desmogleins (Dsg1-4) have been identified in humans.[214] These isoforms are differentially expressed in various epithelial tissues, so that antibody specificity plays a significant role in determining the clinical outcome. For example, autoantibodies to Dsg-1 cause pemphigus foliaceus (PF) in adults, with prominent skin blistering in the upper layers of the epidermis, and anti-Dsg-3 antibodies cause pemphigus vulgaris (PV), with blistering in the suprabasal layer of the skin and in the mucous membranes.[213] Transplacental transfer of autoantibodies from women with PF only rarely causes clinical symptoms in infants[27] because the Dsg target isoforms have a different distribution (Table 10-2). The neonatal epidermal Dsg

Table 10-2 CORRELATION OF AUTOANTIBODIES WITH ADULT AND NEONATAL SKIN DISEASE

	Anti-Dsg-1 Antibodies	Anti-Dsg-3 Antibodies
Adult disease	Pemphigus foliaceus	Pemphigus vulgaris
Neonatal disease	Rare effects	Pemphigus vulgaris

pattern more closely resembles that of adult mucous membranes, suggesting that high levels of Dsg-3 can compensate for antibody-mediated loss of Dsg-1.[215] Functional studies using transgenic mice engineered to express human Dsg-3 in their epidermis confirmed protection from human anti-Dsg-1 antibodies. The importance of Dsg-3 in neonatal disease is further exemplified by case reports of infants with extensive PV following acquisition of maternal anti-Dsg-3,[216,217] including one case in which the mother's PV was in remission.[218]

Adult PV is endemic in Brazil, and a correlation has been noted between individuals with anti-Dsg-1 and a history of infectious disease, notably onchocerciasis and Chagas disease.[219] It is interesting to speculate that transplacental transfer of anti-Dsg-1 in endemic areas may be meant to protect the offspring from infection without causing pemphigus, owing to the skewed fetal expression of desmogleial isoforms as outlined previously. The heterogeneity of the anti-epidermal antibodies makes prediction of neonatal disease difficult; investigators found that a subset of antibodies to Dsg-1 could cross-react with the Dsg-4 isoform,[220] revealing that the pathogenic profile of anti-Dsg antibodies varies based not only on the distribution of Dsg isoforms in the affected individual, but on antigen specificity of the auto-antibody. Autoantibody production in these diseases is typically polyclonal, with IgG$_4$ produced early in the disease, and IgG$_1$ later; both of these IgG isotypes may cross the placenta.[213] Other important factors may be involved in mediating pemphigus as well. Anti-Dsg serum antibody titers were found to correlate with dermal dendritic cell numbers in lesioned skin, suggesting that cellular immune factors may play a role,[221] but currently no data are available regarding dermal dendritic cells in neonatal pemphigus.

Not only is clinical disease painful, but it subjects the neonate to risks of infection, fluid loss, and weight loss due to diminished feeding.[213] No preventive measures are known. In women with active or historical blistering skin disease, serial measurements of autoantibody titers can guide treatment, which may include plasma exchange and/or corticosteroids.[222,223] Infants of these women are monitored for disease and treated symptomatically. In animal models, cholinergic agonists block antibody-induced acantholysis,[224] and application of wheat germ agglutinin can interfere with autoantibody binding to Dsg-1,[225] but these approaches have not yet been tried in humans.

Neonatal Liver Diseases

Neonatal Liver Disease and Anti-Nuclear Antibody

Mothers of infants with idiopathic neonatal cholestasis, biliary atresia, or other liver diseases were found to have a higher than expected frequency of serum anti-nuclear antibodies (ANA), suggesting a link between maternal autoimmunity and neonatal liver disease.[226] However, no specific role for ANA has been elucidated, and it is unclear whether ANA are directly pathogenic or merely markers of disease.

Neonatal Hemochromatosis

Neonatal hemochromatosis (NH) is a rare disease manifested by cirrhosis, liver fibrosis, and intrahepatic and extrahepatic siderosis.[227] Fetuses with NH often suffer with IUGR and can die during gestation. Those who survive until delivery may have oligohydramnios or renal dysgenesis, and may develop fulminant hepatic failure necessitating transplantation. Although twins and triplets discordant for NH have been described, their apparently healthy siblings also have abnormal measures of hepatic function on laboratory testing, suggesting an underestimation of the true incidence of NH.[228,229]

10

Transmission of NH is unusual; no genetic mutation for this disease has been identified, and after a woman has one infant with NH, her chance of having a subsequently affected pregnancy is approximately 80%.[230] Based on this information, maternal alloimmunization to an unidentified fetal liver antigen has been considered a possibility. In a prospective study, 48 women with a history of a previous pregnancy affected by NH were treated with IVIG weekly from week 18 until the end of gestation. Healthy infants were born to 45 women in the treatment group, compared with historical control gestations, of which 2 had good outcomes (with medical therapy) and 46 had poor outcomes (fetal or neonatal death or liver failure necessitating liver transplantation). The authors concluded that gestational therapy with IVIG improved the outcomes of infants at risk of being affected by NH.[231] In another clinical trial, 15 women with a history of NH in a previous pregnancy received weekly IVIG starting at week 18 of gestation until delivery[232]; all 16 neonates born to these women survived without surgical treatment, although 12 had signs of NH. In contrast to previous pregnancies, no cases of IUGR, fetal distress, or oligohydramnios occurred, suggesting that this treatment was safe and beneficial. Postnatal management of NH includes use of magnetic resonance imaging (MRI) for detection of siderosis in neonatal tissues, and measurement of serum α-fetoprotein (AFP) and ferritin as sensitive markers of disease.[229] Chelation therapies and antioxidant cocktails administered to newborns with NH have had only limited success, with high morbidity and mortality.[233,234] Treatment of 16 neonates born with NH using exchange transfusion (ET) and IVIG was recently reported, with 12 neonates having good outcomes (defined as survival without orthotopic liver transplantation [OLT]).[235] ET/IVIG treatment was initiated on day 1 of life through day 30; the 131 historical control subjects received a combination of chelation-antioxidants and/or coagulation support. Compared with the historical controls, therapy with ET/IVIG significantly improved outcomes (P <0.001).

Complications of Pregnancy

Several maternal autoantibodies have been linked to decreased fertility and/or pregnancy complications.[236] Although some of these antibodies cause maternal autoimmune disease, which can be directly associated with decreased fertility, these autoantibodies may also bind fetal-placental antigens and cause gestational disease in a manner unrelated to their primary mode of action.

Anti-Angiotensin II Receptor Antibody

Anti-angiotensin II receptor (anti-AT-1) autoantibodies in the serum of pregnant women have been associated with preeclampsia. Antibody-mediated receptor stimulation upregulates production of tissue factor by vascular smooth muscle cells and expression of plasminogen activator inhibitor-1 and interleukin-6 by trophoblasts and mesangial cells, and increases the rate of cardiomyocyte contraction.[237-239] In an experimental animal model, rats with anti-AT-1 autoantibodies also developed a preeclampsia-like syndrome,[240] supporting a pathogenic role for these antibodies in vivo.

Although these autoantibodies have been linked to preeclampsia, it is not known whether their transplacental transfer causes autoimmune disease in the neonate. Recent studies reveal the presence of these autoantibodies in patients with renal allograft rejection and malignant hypertension,[241] suggesting that transfer of these antibodies to the fetus may cause renovascular disease.

Anti-Phospholipid Antibody

Anti-phospholipid antibodies (APLA) are found in nearly 40% of women with SLE and in approximately 5% of the child-bearing population.[242] The presence of maternal APLA has been associated with spontaneous abortion, fetal death, IUGR, and preeclampsia.[243] APLA may interfere with normal trophoblast function in early and late gestation and may create a hypercoagulable state (by inhibition of endogenous anticoagulants, activation of platelets and endothelial cells, and disruption of vascular endothelium), leading to spontaneous abortion and/or placental thrombosis and infarction.[244]

APLA can be transplacentally acquired, and neonatal APLA antibody titers, isotypes, and specificities correlate with maternal levels.[245,246] These autoantibodies generally are not associated with disease in the neonate,[245] but fetal stroke has been reported in pregnant women with high APLA titers.[247] In the neonate, APLA levels decline over time, becoming undetectable at 6 months, consistent with transplacental acquisition of maternal autoantibodies. Long-term effects of perinatal exposure to APLA, including the future development of SLE, are not known.

Many interventions have been attempted for the prevention of fetal disease in women with symptomatic APLA syndrome; however, the most promising treatment involves the use of heparin.[243] Many APLA effects are related to excessive antibody-mediated complement activation, which is blocked by heparin.[248,249] Current recommendations for pregnant women include treatment with heparin or heparin-derived compounds in conjunction with low-dose aspirin.[243,244] Cases refractory to pharmacotherapy can be treated with high-dose IVIG.

Anti-Laminin-1 Antibody

The laminin-1 glycoproteins in uterine and fetal tissues play an integral role in normal implantation and are required for maintenance of placental integrity.[250-252] Maternal anti-laminin-1 autoantibodies have been linked to recurrent spontaneous abortion,[252,253] and pathogenicity of these antibodies was demonstrated in an animal model that revealed increased fetal resorption rates in mice immunized with laminin-1.[250] Pregnant mice with anti-laminin-1 autoantibodies also had underweight fetuses and placentas compared with controls. No data are available regarding the effects of transplacental acquisition of anti-laminin-1 autoantibodies on infants who survive to term.

Anti-Tissue Transglutaminase Antibody

Autoantibodies to tissue transglutaminase (anti-tTg) are classically associated with celiac disease and dermatitis herpetiformis because its target protein is expressed in both the gastrointestinal tract and the skin.[254] However, women with celiac disease also have decreased fertility, higher rates of spontaneous abortion, IUGR, and low birth weight infants, all of which are vastly improved by adherence to a gluten-free diet.[255] These observations have led to the hypothesis that anti-tTg antibodies are directly detrimental to the fetus. In support of this idea, human tissue transglutaminase has been found to be temporally and compartmentally expressed in placental stromal cells, trophoblasts, and decidual cells, and was shown to be functionally active in fibroblast extracellular matrix and syncytial microvillous membranes.[256,257] Additionally, circulating anti-tTg antibodies were able to bind to trophoblast cells and affect invasiveness, induce apoptosis, and increase DNA fragmentation.[258]

These data suggest an important role for tissue transglutaminase in normal placental development and function. It is not known whether maternal autoantibodies traverse the placenta and cause disease in the fetus itself, but maternal anti-tTg antibodies are detectable in cord blood.[254] Anti-tTg antibodies in the neonate do not appear to increase the risk of developing future celiac disease.

Anti-AChR Antibody

Women with myasthenia gravis have increased rates of premature rupture of membranes, major congenital anomalies, necessity for cesarean section, and other complications, all of which significantly increase fetal morbidity and mortality.[259] These effects are not merely due to maternal disease because women with asymptomatic myasthenia gravis—in remission or before initial diagnosis—also have higher rates of protracted labor, induced labor, and perinatal mortality.[260]

Anti-Thyroid Antibody

Anti-thyroid autoantibodies may cause gestational complications such as preterm birth and spontaneous abortion, even if the mother is euthyroid.[261,262] Maternal

10

*hypo*thyroidism–related autoantibodies have been linked to spontaneous abortion, preterm delivery, and neuropsychiatric abnormalities. Maternal *hyper*thyroidism–related autoantibodies have been linked to spontaneous abortion, preterm delivery, placenta abruptio, congestive heart failure, preeclampsia, and fetal thyrotoxicosis.[263] The mechanisms of autoantibody action in some of these complications are not known.

Anti-U1-RNP Antibody

Chondrodysplasia punctata (CDP) is a heterogeneous disorder that results in abnormal development of the fetal skeleton. It has been associated with single gene disorders, chromosomal and biochemical abnormalities, and teratogenic exposures. Clinically, affected neonates have a characteristic facial appearance, cataracts, shortening of the limbs, and stippling in regions of endochondral bone formation. Other features include ichthyosis, growth failure, decreased survival, and psychomotor retardation.[264]

Women with mixed connective tissue disease (MCTD) often harbor anti-RNP antibodies at high titer. Several cases have described fetuses with chondrodysplasia punctata born to women with high-titer anti-RNP antibodies and SLE or MCTD who lacked any identifiable genetic or biochemical abnormality or exposure to teratogen.[264-267] A few cases described women who had no autoimmune disease before the time of birth but developed SLE postnatally.[264,266] The authors propose that transplacental crossing of anti-RNP (or perhaps another autoantibody) may mediate the pathogenesis of CDP, but the exact mechanism has yet to be determined.[265]

Maternally Derived Antibodies and the Development of Future Autoimmunity

Although autoantibody-mediated diseases in the newborn often resolve upon the loss of maternal antibodies, autoimmunity that develops later in life may have its origins in the perinatal period, making even the transient presence of maternally derived antibodies a critical factor. In fact, rather than autoantigens, most maternal antibodies are directed against infectious agents. However, these anti-pathogen antibodies could also play a role in promotion or prevention of autoimmunity. For example, transfer of maternal antibodies against a virus or bacterium may alter the fetal or neonatal immune response and/or level of infection, thereby changing the role of this pathogen in the development of autoimmunity. Conversely, the antibody may promote transplacental transfer of a virus or other pathogen that could infect the fetus and influence future autoimmunity.

Maternal antibodies may transfer noninfectious proteins, which could trigger a cross-reactive autoimmune response in the fetus, or alter cytokine and chemokine expression via interaction with fetal/neonatal leukocyte Fc receptors. Theoretically, environmental toxins could also cross the placenta via binding to maternal antibodies, resulting in vertical transmission of mutagens, which may play a role in autoimmunity. Food or other environmental antigens/allergens in the fetus may also be targets of maternal antibodies, with the resultant immune complexes playing a role in the development of autoimmunity.

One example of the link between early antibody transfer and future autoimmunity is seen in relation to the development of type 1 diabetes mellitus (DM 1). The prevalence of DM 1 in a population is inversely correlated with maternal anti-enterovirus antibody levels, suggesting that maternal anti-pathogen antibodies may protect against the development of DM 1.[268] Moreover, the production of diabetes-associated autoantibodies (anti-insulin, anti-ICA, anti-GAD, or anti-IA-2) in susceptible children has been associated with antecedent enteroviral infection, with 13% of the infections in this study occurring before 6 months of age.[269] In another study, enterovirus infections led to the production of antibodies that were cross-reactive with IA-2 in 7% of patients, supporting the idea that these infections lead to production of antibodies against DM 1-associated antigens.[270] Whether maternal anti-enterovirus antibodies mediate protection from autoimmunity by preventing viral propagation and immune stimulation, by blocking pathogenic antigens cross-reactive with host proteins, or by interacting with other antibodies or viruses unrelated to the primary infection is unknown.

MATERNAL MICROCHIMERISM (MMC) AND NEONATAL AUTOIMMUNITY

Normal Physiology

Two-way cellular traffic between the fetus and the mother during pregnancy was first described in the 1960s.[271,272] The small number of maternal cells living within a child is termed *maternal microchimerism* (MMc)[8] to signify the origin of the allogeneic cells in the chimeric offspring. Maternal DNA can be detected in the healthy human fetus as early as the 13th week of gestation,[273] and in the mouse, maternal cell transfer begins between 9 and 12 days' gestation, when the placental circulation develops and fetal hematopoiesis begins.[274] In contrast to maternal antibody titer, which is low in preterm infants and increases with gestational age, the level of MMc in the blood does not seem to be affected by gestational age.[273,275] However, the levels of MMc in developing organs have yet to be quantitated.

A major challenge in the study of MMc is its accurate quantification. Previous methods used semi-quantitative polymerase chain reaction (PCR) or tedious cell counting of female cells identified in male subjects. To quantitate low levels of MMc in patients and controls, a panel of quantitative PCR assays has been developed to target nonshared maternal HLA genes.[276] With 14 specific HLA sequences, the assay panel is informative for 90% of patient–mother pairs, with a sensitivity of 1 in 100,000. It is important to note that these assays have been validated in 47 cell lines expressing different HLA alleles to demonstrate that there is no cross-reactivity. In an initial study of MMc, maternal DNA was detected in genomic DNA isolated from peripheral blood mononuclear cells in 22% of healthy adults, with levels ranging from 0 to 68.6 genome equivalents per million host cells, suggesting that MMc is a normal and not infrequent occurrence in the general population.[276]

MMc is commonly detected in cord blood. Early studies used labeled maternal blood re-transfused into the mother shortly before delivery to track transfer of maternal cells into cord blood during parturition.[272,277] More recently, the presence of maternal DNA in 40% to 100% of human umbilical cord blood samples was revealed using the high-sensitivity quantitative polymerase chain reaction (Q-PCR).[275,278-280] However, it is known that cell-free DNA may circulate between mother and fetus, and thus detection of DNA alone does not prove cell trafficking. In fact, when mother-to-fetus cell transfer was examined, the fractional concentration of maternal DNA in cord plasma samples was more than 10-fold greater than maternal nucleated cells detected.[281] With the use of fluorescence in situ hybridization (FISH) for X- and Y-chromosome sequences in whole cells, 20% of male cord blood samples were found to contain female cells, presumably maternal.[5]

It is not known how maternal cells transfer to the fetus, or what regulates the transfer. After birth, maternal cells may also be acquired by infants during breast-feeding. MMc has been found in multiple peripheral blood cell types, including macrophages, B cells, natural killer cells, and natural killer T cells,[282] and maternal T lymphocytes have been identified in cases of childhood disease.[283,284] That maternal T lymphocytes are active after transfer is evidenced by the finding of cells retaining their original antigen specificity. For example, approximately 15% of neonates born to women with antituberculin immunity had lymphocytes reactive to purified protein derivative (PPD) 4 to 6 weeks after birth, although none of the infants born to nonimmune women did.[285] These data support the idea that not only had the infants acquired maternal T lymphocytes, but that these cells were functional after transfer. Of note, the anti-PPD response waned by 3 months of age, suggesting death of maternal cells and/or activation of infant regulatory cells to control the maternal anti-PPD response postnatally.

MMc in the newborn may also transmit malignancy. Almost 50 years ago, Hodgkin disease was hypothesized to be derived from unregulated maternal cells in children[271]; since that time, case reports have described infants with monocytic leukemia, natural killer cell lymphoma, and malignant melanomas derived from maternal blood.[286-289]

Maternally derived cells have been found not only as circulating leukocytes in the offspring,[5] but as differentiated tissue cells in every human organ examined to date, including skin, thymus, heart, lung, pancreas, liver, spleen, kidney, muscle, and bone marrow.[6,290-292] These findings support the idea that an undifferentiated maternal stem cell engrafts into the fetal bone marrow and provides a continuous source of allogeneic precursors. These maternal stem cells may normally be recruited into fetal tissues during early development to participate in organogenesis along with fetal cells, and may provide a source of cells for tissue repair and regeneration in areas of injury. Although the role of MMc in these processes remains speculative, recent data from a mouse model of renal disease demonstrate that bone marrow transplant–derived stem cells were recruited to damaged glomeruli, where they participated in healing.[293] Alternatively, maternal cells that express antigens not inherited by the fetus could act as targets for the fetal/neonatal immune system, or even for neonatally acquired maternal autoantibodies.

Regulation of MMc Levels in Infants

If it is assumed that the PCR-based DNA detection and FISH methods are reproducible and sensitive enough to omit large variation by chance, it is not clear why MMc is found in the circulation of some healthy persons, but not others. One explanation is that MMc is transferred with higher frequency in some pregnancies or deliveries. Factors regulating the transplacental transfer of maternal cells to the fetus are not fully understood, but high-risk deliveries with antepartum problems such as fetal anomalies, preeclampsia, placental insufficiency, and chorioamnionitis have been associated with increased maternal–fetal cell transfer.[294-298] However, a direct comparison of MMc levels in normal vaginal delivery, complicated delivery with excess bleeding, and cesarean section has not been performed. After birth, breast-feeding may affect levels of MMc. Some breast milk may contain a greater number of maternal cells or may have cell subsets with different survival advantages in the neonate. Maternal alloantigens may induce antigen-specific tolerance in the neonatal immune system; this may be dependent on the genes of both the mother and the fetus. In a mouse study, levels of MMc were influenced by maternal–fetal histocompatibility, where MHC homozygous progeny had slightly higher levels of MMc than heterozygous progeny.[299] MHC alleles may also affect the transfer, survival, or expansion of chimeric cells in humans. Data reveal that the level of MMc in human peripheral blood correlates with maternal–fetal compatibility at MHC class II molecules DRB1 and DQB1, and with specific DQA1*0501 and DQB1*0301 alleles.[275,283,300] It is not known how specific HLA molecules contribute to higher levels of microchimerism in the blood.

The fact that any "foreign" maternal cells are tolerated by the neonatal immune system suggests that maternally derived cells and/or antigens may play a role in thymic education. In support of this hypothesis, studies reveal the presence of maternal DNA in human and murine thymuses.[299,301] Regulatory T cells educated in the thymus may also play a role in mediating tolerance to MMc, but this has not yet been demonstrated.

Although a role for maternal cells in autoimmunity has been suggested, they probably play a beneficial role in most individuals. MMc may assist with protection against infection, autoimmunity, and even cancer, and may play a role in normal pregnancy and fetal/neonatal development. Maternal cells expressing allogeneic antigens may also provide a source of constant stimulation to host T lymphocytes to maintain the T cell receptor repertoire.[302]

Other Sources of Microchimerism

In addition to maternal and fetal microchimerism, foreign cells may be derived from other potential sources during pregnancy, including from a twin, an unrecognized vanished twin (estimated to occur in 5% of pregnancies), or siblings in a multiplex pregnancy.[303-306] One case report describes a fertile, healthy woman, who was found to have near-complete replacement of her hematopoietic system with male cells (99% of cells examined), although her somatic karyotype was female. She had a twin brother who died shortly after birth, suggesting that successful, naturally occurring feto–fetal transfusion had occurred during gestation.[307]

Fetal cells can be detected for decades in a woman after delivery, or even after an early spontaneous abortion,[308-310] suggesting that a subsequent fetus theoretically could receive not only his mother's cells, but also cells from any prior pregnancies carried by his mother. Because his mother may also be carrying cells acquired during her own gestation, the fetus could receive cells from his maternal grandmother and maternal aunts, uncles, and so forth. In this sense, each infant is potentially a multichimeric organism composed of cells from not just multiple individuals, but multiple generations. In samples from females too young to have been pregnant, male microchimerism has been detected in five of six girls and seven of eleven fetuses, supporting the idea that cells from older siblings may also be transferred via the transplacental route.[311]

Developmental Differences Between Fetus and Newborn

The stage of development at which a foreign (i.e., maternal or transfused) cell is transferred to the fetus may influence the outcome. MMc has been detected as early as 13 weeks' gestation, and NLS-related heart block is usually detected at 17 weeks' gestation, supporting the idea that maternal cells may play a role in the pathogenesis of atrioventricular (AV) node inflammation.[290,312] MMc may also alter the effects of transplacentally acquired maternal antibodies, depending on whether maternal cells carry the target antigens and/or are integrated into host tissues.

The fate of allogeneic maternal cells transferred to the fetus may be hypothesized to parallel the fate of donor cells transplanted during gestation. In some cases, in utero transplantation leads to long-lasting tolerance in the recipient.[313-317] In immunocompetent mice, in utero hematopoietic stem cell transplantation with MHC-mismatched bone marrow cells resulted in durable low-level engraftment beyond 20 weeks of age (well into adulthood).[315] However, in other cases, cells acquired during gestation do not induce tolerance and may even be pathogenic. Transfusion of spleen cell subsets to mice in utero was found to result in persistent microchimerism but did not improve acceptance of skin grafts placed 6 months after birth.[318] Rather, accelerated rejection of donor tissues was observed in the previously transfused mice. In some murine studies, early postnatal infusion of homozygous parental cells to heterozygous offspring caused GVHD with many features of SLE.[319] GVHD has also been observed in immunocompetent human infants after intrauterine and exchange transfusions for hemolytic disease.[320] Thus, the outcome of maternal cell acquisition by the neonate depends on the route of transfer, the age of the recipient, the developmental stage, genetic profiles of donor and recipient, and the cell type transferred.[318,321,322]

The Role of Breast Milk in Acquisition and Function of MMc

Studies in mice have suggested that persistence of maternal cells in blood and tissues derived in utero is dependent on oral tolerance induced by breast milk antigens ingested by the neonate.[323] Maternal HLA molecules may play a role in this process because they are found as both soluble and cell membrane–associated proteins in breast milk.[324] The protective effect of breast-feeding on the future development of autoimmune disease suggests that maternal cells, antibodies, and antigens contained in breast milk may interact with the neonatal immune system in a beneficial way.[325]

Maternal cells in breast milk are believed to pass into the infant's circulation, although evidence for this is indirect. Cell types in breast milk are varied, but a vast majority are granulocytes, macrophages, and other antigen-presenting cells, along with 1% to 7% lymphocytes.[326-329] A majority of T lymphocytes in human milk are activated or memory cells, thus the infant may benefit from his mother's immunologic experience.[327,328] The role of maternal immune cells in the infant is not well understood, but maternal B cells appear to become antibody-secreting mucosal plasma cells that can protect the newborn against gastrointestinal and respiratory pathogens, while the infant's intrinsic immune system is still developing.[330] Immunocompetent mouse pups nursed by lymphopenic mothers were found to have reduced antibody production, suggesting that maternal lymphocytes and/or immunoglobulins in breast milk normally contribute to the neonatal immune response.[331]

Exposure to maternal antigens during gestation may regulate neonatal B cell development. Female mice expressing specific MHC I antigens were bred to male mice with high or moderate affinity germline B cell receptors against these proteins.[332] Pups that did not inherit the genes for these antigens but were presumed to have been exposed to maternal antigens during gestation and breast-feeding showed changes in their antigen-specific B cell populations. Their high-affinity antigen-specific B cells were deleted, and their moderate-affinity B cells showed an activated phenotype. These results demonstrate that B cell development may be affected by neonatal exposure to maternal antigens, as well as by the affinity of the B cell receptor for its antigen.

Exposure to maternal milk may alter the host T lymphocyte response to MMc and other antigens. Newborn calves fed whole colostrum exhibited increased T cell responses in a mixed leukocyte reaction within 24 hours of feeding, but this did not occur in calves fed cell-free colostrum until 2 or more weeks after birth.[333] Moreover, calves that ingested whole colostrum developed reduced reactivity to maternal alloantigens, which may lead to tolerance and persistence of MMc, preventing a chronic inflammatory response against HLA-mismatched maternal cells.

Whole maternal cells in bovine colostrum are not digested in the gut but are traceable in the circulation between 12 and 36 hours after ingestion.[334] Of note, ingestion of maternal cells without colostrum resulted in diminished entry into the circulation. Although normal maternal lymphoid cells in colostrum are absorbed from the gastrointestinal tract, heat-treated lymphoid cells and those isolated from peripheral blood are not,[335] suggesting that a heat-labile surface molecule is required for survival and/or transfer of maternal cells across the epithelial barrier.

Relevance of Physiologic Differences to the Disease Process

MMc in Immunodeficient Infants

Observations in infants with severe combined immunodeficiency (SCID) have provided evidence that host immune tolerance plays a role in the level of maternal cell acquisition. Infants with immunodeficiencies have long been known to harbor high levels of maternal hematopoietic cells,[336,337] suggesting that the immunocompetent host limits the amount of MMc normally accepted. However, MMc does not reconstitute a functional immune system in these infants, although engrafted infants may have a survival advantage over those without maternal cells. Maternal T cells that are transferred do not respond normally to in vitro stimulation and express a limited T cell receptor repertoire,[338,339] suggesting that a few T cells may be transferred to immunocompromised offspring and may expand in response to specific antigenic stimuli, or that only small T cell subsets are allowed to transfer or persist in allogeneic individuals.

In immunodeficient infants, engraftment with maternal cells leads to GVHD in 60% of cases.[340] The T cells transferred may already be expanded in the mother, as evidenced by the case of a 5-month-old male with SCID and chronic GVHD with skin and hepatic manifestations.[341] He had aberrant peripheral T cell subsets, which included rare CD4+ T cells and a CD8+ γ/δ^+ population, of which more than 50%

were maternally derived clonal T cells. The clonal CD8$^+$ γ/δ^+ T cell population constituted 10% of the mother's peripheral blood mononuclear cells; this decreased over time after delivery. These cells may have been stimulated by paternal antigens carried by the fetus, with transplacental transfer of these maternal anti-paternal T cells to the immunodeficient fetus. In support of this hypothesis, studies in transgenic mice reveal a threefold increase in anti-fetal CD8$^+$ T cells specific for inherited paternal MHC class I antigens, especially in lymph nodes draining the uterus.[342] The fact that major immunodeficiency can lead to high levels of MMc raises the question of whether more subtle immune defects, such as those seen in common variable immunodeficiency, chronic granulomatous disease, and hyper IgM syndrome, could also lead to increased maternal engraftment. Whether the autoimmune diseases that occur in these patients are related to MMc remains to be examined.

MMc in Neonatal Autoimmunity

Just as maternal cells in immunodeficient infants can cause GVHD, maternal cells in immunocompetent individuals sometimes may be involved in the initiation or perpetuation of autoimmune disease.[276]

Neonatal Scleroderma

Systemic sclerosis is a rare autoimmune disease resembling GVHD. MMc has been detected in adult scleroderma patients,[343] and a role for MMc (and/or maternal autoantibodies) in neonatal scleroderma is suggested by rare case reports of affected infants born to mothers with connective tissue disease.[344-347] Infants affected by systemic sclerosis can present with diffuse cutaneous involvement (tight, shiny skin) at birth, with or without visceral involvement. In one reported case, the neonate's condition gradually improved over time,[345] consistent with the idea that a large initial load of MMc may have played a role in disease pathogenesis. Neonates with autoimmune disease are currently treated with immunosuppression as needed for skin, vascular, and musculoskeletal manifestations. With recent findings of MMc in affected infants, it is hoped that more targeted therapy will be developed.

Neonatal Lupus Syndrome

MMc has been investigated in the context of neonatal lupus syndrome (NLS)-associated congenital heart block.[54] Although maternally derived autoantibodies are necessary, but not sufficient, for the development of NLS-related heart block, more than 95% of infants born to women with anti-SSA and/or anti-SSB antibodies are healthy.[54,348] One factor implicated in the pathogenesis of CHB has been the presence of allogeneic cells in the child that may interact with the host immune system. With the use of quantitative PCR, both maternal and sibling microchimerism has been demonstrated in the peripheral blood of twins and triplets discordant for CHB.[306] In one set of triplets, microchimerism was present in the blood of two infants affected with CHB, but not in their sibling, who had only a transient hepatitis. Moreover, evolution of the disease in these two siblings correlated with measurements of microchimerism in serial peripheral blood samples. In contrast, in a pair of discordantly affected twins, microchimerism was detected in the healthy infant, not in the twin with CHB.

To further investigate the role of MMc in CHB, heart tissues from male infants with and without NLS were analyzed for female (maternal) cells using FISH to identify X and Y chromosome–specific sequences.[290] Maternal cells were found in all 15 sections of heart tissue from four NLS patients, accounting for 0.025% to 2.2% of myocardial cells. Maternal cells were also found in two of eight control cardiac sections, but at lower levels (0.05% to 0.1%). A minority of maternal cells expressed CD45, suggesting that these were maternally derived leukocytes, but a majority expressed sarcomeric α-actin, a marker specific for cardiac myocytes. The finding of maternal cardiomyocytes at the site of disease has important implications for autoimmunity because maternal cells may be the pathogenic target of transplacentally acquired maternal autoantibodies, or they may be beneficial to the neonate by contributing to the process of tissue repair.

MMc and the Risk of Future Autoimmune Disease

Although many autoimmune diseases become apparent only years after birth, their origins may be inherently dependent on the acquisition of MMc during the fetal and neonatal periods. MMc has been implicated in the pathogenesis of several autoimmune diseases affecting children and adults, including systemic sclerosis,[276] myositis,[283,284,349] *pityriasis lichenoides*,[292] rheumatoid arthritis,[350] and a case of chronic idiopathic GVHD-type syndrome.[351] With FISH used to identify X and Y chromosomes, MMc was found in ten of ten skin and muscle biopsies from boys with juvenile idiopathic inflammatory myopathy.[284] Only two of ten biopsies from children with noninflammatory muscle disorders were positive for MMc. In eight of nine children with autoimmune myositis, MMc was also noted in peripheral blood T cells.[284] Rare cases of inflammatory myopathy have been described in neonates,[352,353] suggesting that MMc may be involved in myositis early in life.

Inherited and Noninherited Maternal Genes in the Risk for Neonatal Disease

Human leukocyte antigen (HLA) alleles have been associated with many autoimmune diseases, although the mechanisms for how they contribute to disease are not known.[354] It has been shown that HLA compatibility of mother and fetus at MHC class II loci increases the risk for both neonatal and future autoimmunity.[65] Males who develop lupus are more likely to be HLA-identical with their mothers at the HLA DRB1 locus,[355] suggesting a mechanism whereby they could tolerate greater MMc acquisition during gestation and breast-feeding.

Other studies have shown that noninherited maternal alleles can also be associated with increased risk of developing autoimmune disease, although this is controversial.[350,356-359] First explored in adult-onset rheumatoid arthritis, noninherited maternal alleles (NIMA) have been implicated in the risk of development of disease in some but not all populations.[295,298,299,360] Additionally, several studies have demonstrated correlation between the mother's HLA alleles and the neonate's development of CHB, but no correlation between fetal HLA alleles and CHB,[361-365] suggesting that maternal cells are transferred to the fetus and play a direct role in the pathogenesis of heart block. Therefore, immunologic studies in neonates should include the contribution of antigens inherited via microchimerism, as well as those inherited genetically.

The mechanisms whereby noninherited maternal alleles affect the immune system of the offspring are not known. One possibility is that MMc can tolerize the neonatal immune system to maternal cells. For example, in experimental murine studies, bone marrow transplants from offspring to half-matched adults resulted in lower GVHD if the donor's mother matched the recipient, suggesting that the donor had been exposed perinatally to the noninherited allele.[366] Reduced GVHD in this study was found to be dependent on the presence of donor T regulatory cells, possibly generated as a result of exposure to maternal cells in utero. Support for the idea of perinatal tolerization in humans comes from studies of RhD-negative women, who typically are susceptible to alloimmunization following pregnancy with an RhD-positive fetus. These women were found to be less likely to develop an anti-RhD antibody response if their own mothers were RhD positive, suggesting that they had become tolerant of this antigen during exposure in utero.[367] Another example of tolerance to noninherited maternal antigens involves the anti-HLA response generated in recipients of multiple blood transfusions. Fifty percent of these transfusion recipients were found to lack antibodies to noninherited maternal HLA, suggesting that they had been tolerized to these antigens perinatally.[368] More evidence comes from retrospective evaluation of renal and hematopoietic stem cell transplants, which revealed better outcomes in cases where a donor–recipient HLA mismatch was compensated for by HLA alleles of the donor's mother.[369] However, in contrast, a review of 5000 renal transplants did not find that offspring were more tolerant of maternal antigens, because there was no apparent advantage of maternal-to-child over paternal-to-child renal donations.[370] It should be noted that findings in humans are confounded by the issue of compliance with immunosuppressive regimens and whether the patient was breast-fed as an infant, because this may be a necessary factor for full tolerization to maternal cells acquired in utero.[323] Overall, the evidence for perinatal tolerization to noninherited maternal alleles is strong, implying that MMc acquired early in life may play a significant role in immune development.

Role of T Regulatory Cells in Neonatal Autoimmunity

Much has been learned regarding the role of T regulatory cells (Treg) in human autoimmunity, but less is known with respect to their function in fetal/neonatal disease. Several types of Treg have been described to date, but we will use the term Treg here to mean the "classic" CD4[+], CD25[+] Foxp3[+] T regulatory cells, found to be pivotal in the prevention and amelioration of multiple forms of human and animal autoimmunity.[371-373] After positive selection in the thymus, Treg enter the circulation to monitor ongoing immune responses and to mediate their suppressive effects. In mice, Treg do not appear in the circulation until approximately 3 days after birth, so thymectomy before this time leads to widespread autoimmune disease. However, in humans, Treg enter the circulation before birth, so that neonatal thymectomy does not usually result in overt autoimmunity.[374] In both mice and humans, not only are circulating Treg found very early in life, they are also functional at these stages.[17,375] For example, in an animal model of neonatal autoimmune ovarian disease (AOD), mice were susceptible to autoantibody-initiated, T cell–dependent AOD, but only before 7 days of age.[44] Resistance to disease gained after 7 days of life correlated with the presence of and response to CD4[+]/CD25[+] Treg.

Although human maternal Treg increase in the circulation during pregnancy, are found in the early decidua, and contribute to maternal tolerance of the fetus,[376,377] it is not clear whether maternal Treg can be acquired transplacentally. It is known that Treg are present and functional in human cord blood,[378] and a recent study demonstrated that cord blood Treg were more potent inhibitors of an in vitro anti-myelin oligodendrocyte glycoprotein (MOG) thymocyte response than Treg derived from neonatal thymus.[379] Cord blood Treg inhibited both T effector interferon-γ production and cell proliferation, and Treg derived from thymic tissue suppressed only cytokine production. This discordance in Treg function may be a result of further Treg development after thymic egress, but it would be interesting to determine whether any of the cord blood Treg were maternally derived.

Treg may be a major factor mediating the offspring's tolerance of maternal cells. To evaluate the role of Treg in tolerance to noninherited maternal antigens, an experimental mouse model was created by breeding a female mouse heterozygous for class I histocompatibility alleles with a male mouse homozygous at this locus. Pups that lacked the maternal antigen were examined for their immune response to the noninherited allele. Testing of CD4[+] splenic T cells from these offspring revealed a reduced in vitro immune response to maternal cells compared with control mice, and injection of their splenic CD4[+] T cells into lethally irradiated recipients with the same noninherited allele resulted in less T cell expansion and GVHD compared with donors whose mothers lacked this allele.[366] Of note, the donor's tolerance of noninherited maternal alleles was lost if CD4[+]CD25[+] T cells were depleted before infusion, supporting the idea that in utero exposure to noninherited maternal alleles had resulted in induction of antigen-specific Treg. However, this study did not examine the level of MMc in these offspring, nor did it explore whether any maternal Treg were present among the CD4[+]CD25[+] Treg population; this may have played a role in tolerance to noninherited maternal alleles.

The effects of MMc (and maternal antibody acquisition) on the development and function of Treg in the human fetus and neonate are not known. Cord blood–derived mononuclear cells from babies born to atopic mothers have decreased expression of Treg-related genes upon stimulation with peptidoglycans in vitro.[376] However, it is not clear whether these differences are intrinsic to the newborn or are maternally mediated, and the implications of these findings are not yet fully understood. Thus, the importance of Treg in maternally derived neonatal autoimmunity is an exciting area that remains to be explored.

Conclusions

We are just beginning to understand the complex short- and long-term immune interactions between the maternal and fetal immune systems. These signals are composed not only of transplacentally and orally acquired immunoglobulins, lymphocytes, antigen-presenting cells, and immature precursor cells, but also of numerous protein- and nucleic acid–based signaling molecules, such as growth factors, cytokines, chemokines, and free-floating DNA. Fetal–maternal interaction can result in protection of the neonate from infection but can also promote autoimmune disease, depending on the antigen specificity of the antibodies or leukocytes involved, variations in maternal–fetal HLA composition, genetic and environmental factors, and physiologic maturity of the host. Studies in these areas may lead to improved diagnostic and therapeutic maneuvers not only in neonatal autoimmunity, but also in infection, pregnancy, and transplantation biology.

Acknowledgments

The authors would like to thank Dr. Kristina Adams for her critical review of the manuscript, and Ms. Debra George, IBCLC, for her input regarding the role of breast milk.

Abbreviations

AChR	acetylcholine receptor
AIA	anti-insulin antibodies
AMLA	anti-myolemmal antibodies
ANA	anti-nuclear antibodies
ANCA	anti-neutrophil cytoplasmic antibodies
AOD	autoimmune ovarian disease
APLA	anti-phospholipid antibodies
AT-1	angiotensin II receptor
AV	atrioventricular
CHB	congenital heart block
DCM	dilated cardiomyopathy
DM	diabetes mellitus
DNA	deoxyribonucleic acid
Dsg	desmoglein
Fab	fragment, antigen binding (monovalent antibody)
FISH	fluorescence in situ hybridization
GAD	glutamic acid decarboxylase
GVHD	graft-versus-host disease
HLA	human leukocyte antigen
HDN	hemolytic disease of the newborn
IA-2	protein tyrosine phosphatase IA-2
ICA	islet cell antibodies
Ig	immunoglobulin
IUGR	intrauterine growth restriction
IVIG	intravenous immunoglobulin
MHC	major histocompatibility complex

MMc	maternal microchimerism
MPO	myeloperoxidase
NAIT	neonatal alloimmune thrombocytopenia
NEP	neutral endopeptidase
NGB	neonatal Guillain-Barré
NH	neonatal hemochromatosis
NLS	neonatal lupus syndrome
NMG	neonatal myasthenia gravis
NOD	nonobese-diabetic (mouse strain)
PF	pemphigus foliaceus
PPD	purified protein derivative
PV	pemphigus vulgaris
Q-PCR	quantitative PCR
Rh	Rhesus group antigen
RNP	ribonuclear protein
SCID	severe combined immunodeficiency
SLE	systemic lupus erythematosus
Treg	T regulatory cells
TSH	thyroid-stimulating hormone
TSH-R	thyroid-stimulating hormone receptor
tTg	tissue transglutaminase

10

References

1. Kaul A, Smith GF. Immunobiology of the fetus and newborn—historical perspectives and recent advances. In: Smith GF, Vidyagasar D, eds. *Historical review and recent advances in neonatal and perinatal medicine*. Jakarta, Indonesia: Mead Johnson Nutritional Division; 1980.
2. Linder N, Waintraub I, Smetana Z, et al. Placental transfer and decay of varicella-zoster virus antibodies in preterm infants. *J Pediatr*. 2000 Jul;137(1):85-89.
3. Wesumperuma HL, Perera AJ, Pharoah PO, et al. The influence of prematurity and low birthweight on transplacental antibody transfer in Sri Lanka. *Ann Trop Med Parasitol*. 1999 Mar;93(2): 169-177.
4. Hanson LA, Korotkova M, Lundin S, et al. The transfer of immunity from mother to child. *Ann N Y Acad Sci*. 2003 Apr;987:199-206.
5. Hall JM, Lingenfelter P, Adams SL, et al. Detection of maternal cells in human umbilical cord blood using fluorescence in situ hybridization. *Blood*. 1995;86(7):2829-2832.
6. Srivatsa B, Srivatsa S, Johnson KL, et al. Maternal cell microchimerism in newborn tissues. *J Pediatr*. 2003;142(1):31-35.
7. Stevens AM, Hermes HM, Rutledge JC, et al. Myocardial-tissue-specific phenotype of maternal microchimerism in neonatal lupus congenital heart block. *Lancet*. 2003;362(9396):1617-1623.
8. Maloney S, Smith A, Furst DE, et al. Microchimerism of maternal origin persists into adult life. *JClin Invest*. 1999;104(1):41-47.
9. Simister NE. Placental transport of immunoglobulin G. *Vaccine*. 2003 Jul 28;21(24):3365-3369.
10. Saji F, Samejima Y, Kamiura S, et al. Dynamics of immunoglobulins at the feto-maternal interface. *Rev Reprod*. 1999 May;4(2):81-89.
11. Kristoffersen EK, Matre R. Co-localization of the neonatal Fc gamma receptor and IgG in human placental term syncytiotrophoblasts. *Eur J Immunol*. 1996 Jul;26(7):1668-1671.
12. Baril L, Briles DE, Crozier P, et al. Natural materno-fetal transfer of antibodies to PspA and to PsaA. *Clin Exp Immunol*. 2004 Mar;135(3):474-477.
13. Garty BZ, Ludomirsky A, Danon YL, et al. Placental transfer of immunoglobulin G subclasses. *Clin Diagn Lab Immunol*. 1994 Nov;1(6):667-669. PMC 368387.
14. Hanson LA, Silfverdal SA, Korotkova M, et al. Immune system modulation by human milk. *Adv Exp Med Biol*. 2002;503:99-106.

15. Bednar-Tantscher E, Mudde GC, Rot A, et al. Maternal antigen stimulation downregulates via mother's milk the specific immune responses in young mice. *Int Arch Allergy Immunol.* 2001 Dec;126(4):300-308.
16. Watanaveeradej V, Endy TP, Samakoses R, et al. Transplacentally transferred maternal-infant antibodies to dengue virus. *Am J Trop Med Hyg.* 2003 Aug;69(2):123-128.
17. Thornton CA, Holloway JA, Popplewell EJ, et al. Fetal exposure to intact immunoglobulin E occurs via the gastrointestinal tract. *Clin Exp Allergy.* 2003 Mar;33(3):306-311.
18. Vassella CC, Odelram H, Kjellman NI, et al. High anti-IgE levels at birth are associated with a reduced allergy prevalence in infants at risk: A prospective study. *Clin Exp Allergy.* 1994 Aug;24(8):771-777.
19. Van de Perre P. Transfer of antibody via mother's milk. *Vaccine.* 2003 Jul 28;21(24):3374-3376.
20. de Souza Campos Fernandes RC, Quintana Flores VM, Medina-Acosta E. Prevalent transfer of human colostral IgA antibody activity for the enteropathogenic Escherichia coli bundle-forming pilus structural repeating subunit A in neonates. *Diagn Microbiol Infect Dis.* 2002 Dec;44(4):331-336.
21. Israel EJ, Taylor S, Wu Z, et al. Expression of the neonatal Fc receptor, FcRn, on human intestinal epithelial cells. *Immunology.* 1997 Sep;92(1):69-74. PMC 1363983.
22. Hanson LA, Korotkova M. The role of breastfeeding in prevention of neonatal infection. *Semin Neonatol.* 2002 Aug;7(4):275-281.
23. Pabst HF, Spady DW. Effect of breast-feeding on antibody response to conjugate vaccine. *Lancet.* 1990 Aug 4;336(8710):269-270.
24. Kelleher SL, Lonnerdal B. Immunological activities associated with milk. *Adv Nutr Res.* 2001;10:39-65.
25. Wingen AM, Dohner H, Scharer K, et al. Evidence for developmental changes of type IV collagen in glomerular basement membrane. *Nephron.* 1987;45(4):302-305.
26. Jeraj K, Fish AJ, Yoshioka K, et al. Development and heterogeneity of antigens in the immature nephron. Reactivity with human antiglomerular basement membrane autoantibodies. *Am J Pathol.* 1984 Nov;117(2):180-183. PMC 1900438.
27. Hirsch R, Anderson J, Weinberg JM, et al. Neonatal pemphigus foliaceus. *J Am Acad Dermatol.* 2003 Aug;49(2 Suppl Case Reports):S187-S189.
28. Okoko BJ, Wesumperuma HL, Fern J, et al. The transplacental transfer of IgG subclasses: Influence of prematurity and low birthweight in the Gambian population. *Ann Trop Paediatr.* 2002 Dec;22(4):325-332.
29. Lemons PK, Lemons JA. Transition to breast/bottle feedings: The premature infant. *J Am Coll Nutr.* 1996 Apr;15(2):126-135.
30. Askanase AD, Miranda-Carus ME, Tang X, et al. The presence of IgG antibodies reactive with components of the SSA/Ro-SSB/La complex in human breast milk: Implications in neonatal lupus. *Arthritis Rheum.* 2002 Jan;46(1):269-271.
31. Wright AL, Holberg CJ, Taussig LM, et al. Factors influencing the relation of infant feeding to asthma and recurrent wheeze in childhood. *Thorax.* 2001 Mar;56(3):192-197. PMC 1758780.
32. Oddy WH, Peat JK, de Klerk NH, et al. Maternal asthma, infant feeding, and the risk of asthma in childhood. *J Allergy Clin Immunol.* 2002 Jul;110(1):65-67.
33. Friedman NJ, Zeiger RS. The role of breast-feeding in the development of allergies and asthma. *J Allergy Clin Immunol.* 2005 Jun;115(6):1238-1248.
34. Rothenbacher D, Weyermann M, Beermann C, et al. Breastfeeding, soluble CD14 concentration in breast milk and risk of atopic dermatitis and asthma in early childhood: Birth cohort study. *Clin Exp Allergy.* 2005 Aug;35(8):1014-1021.
35. Leme AS, Hubeau C, Xiang Y, et al. Role of breast milk in a mouse model of maternal transmission of asthma susceptibility. *J Immunol.* 2006 Jan 15;176(2):762-769.
36. Cimaz R, Biggioggero M, Catelli L, et al. Ultraviolet light exposure is not a requirement for the development of cutaneous neonatal lupus. *Lupus.* 2002;11(4):257-260.
37. Martin DA, Elkon KB. Mechanisms of apoptosis. *Rheum Dis Clin North Am.* 2004 Aug;30(3):441-454, vii.
38. Polak M. Hyperthyroidism in early infancy: Pathogenesis, clinical features and diagnosis with a focus on neonatal hyperthyroidism. *Thyroid.* 1998 Dec;8(12):1171-1177.
39. Muller R, Svoboda V, Wenzel E, et al. IgG reactivity against non-conformational NH-terminal epitopes of the desmoglein 3 ectodomain relates to clinical activity and phenotype of pemphigus vulgaris. *Exp Dermatol.* 2006 Aug;15(8):606-614.
40. Rothenberg SP, da Costa MP, Sequeira JM, et al. Autoantibodies against folate receptors in women with a pregnancy complicated by a neural-tube defect. *N Engl J Med.* 2004 Jan 8;350(2):134-142.
41. Bar-Shany S, Herbert V. Transplacentally acquired antibody to intrinsic factor with vitamin B12 deficiency. *Blood.* 1967 Dec;30(6):777-784.
42. Chertow BS, Baranetsky NG, Sivitz WI, et al. The effects of human insulin on antibody formation in pregnant diabetics and their newborns. *Obstet Gynecol.* 1988 Nov;72(5):724-728.
43. Dotta F, Gargiulo P, Tiberti C, et al. Humoral and cellular immune abnormalities in neonates of diabetic mothers: Any pathological role? *Exp Clin Endocrinol.* 1987 Aug;89(3):333-339.
44. Setiady YY, Samy ET, Tung KS, et al. Maternal autoantibody triggers de novo T cell-mediated neonatal autoimmune disease. *J Immunol.* 2003;170(9):4656-4664.
45. Okajima S, Cho K, Chiba H, et al. Two sibling cases of hydrops fetalis due to alloimmune anti-CD36 (Nak a) antibody. *Thromb Haemost.* 2006 Feb;95(2):267-271.

46. Debiec H, Nauta J, Coulet F, et al. Role of truncating mutations in MME gene in fetomaternal alloimmunisation and antenatal glomerulopathies. *Lancet*. 2004 Oct 2-8;364(9441):1252-1259.
47. Ristic AD, Maisch B. Cardiac rhythm and conduction disturbances: What is the role of autoimmune mechanisms? *Herz*. 2000 May;25(3):181-188.
48. Camusso JJ, Borda ES, Bacman S, et al. Antibodies against beta adrenoceptors in mothers of children with congenital heart block. *Acta Physiol Pharmacol Ther Latinoam*. 1994;44(3):94-99.
49. Maisch B, Ristic AD. Immunological basis of the cardiac conduction and rhythm disorders. *Eur Heart J*. 2001 May;22(10):813-824.
50. Julkunen H, Miettinen A, Walle TK, et al. Autoimmune response in mothers of children with congenital and postnatally diagnosed isolated heart block: A population-based study. *J Rheumatol*. 2004 Jan;31(1):183-189.
51. Borrego L, Rodriguez J, Soler E, et al. Neonatal lupus erythematosus related to maternal leukocytoclastic vasculitis. *Pediatr Dermatol*. 1997 May-Jun;14(3):221-225.
52. Penate Y, Lujan D, Rodriguez J, et al. [Neonatal lupus erythematosus: 4 cases and clinical review]. *Actas Dermosifiliogr*. 2005 Dec;96(10):690-696.
53. Izmirly PM, Rivera TL, Buyon JP. Neonatal lupus syndromes. *Rheum Dis Clin North Am*. 2007 May; 33(2):267-285, vi.
54. Buyon JP, Clancy RM. Neonatal lupus syndromes. *Curr Opin Rheumatol*. 2003;15(5):535-541.
55. Martin V, Lee LA, Askanase AD, et al. Long-term followup of children with neonatal lupus and their unaffected siblings. *Arthritis Rheum*. 2002 Sep;46(9):2377-2383.
56. Burch JM, Lee LA, Weston WL, et al. Neonatal lupus erythematosus. *Dermatol Nurs*. 2002 Jun;14(3): 157-160.
57. Boh EE. Neonatal lupus erythematosus. *Clin Dermatol*. 2004 Mar-Apr;22(2):125-128.
58. Cimaz R, Spence DL, Hornberger L, et al. Incidence and spectrum of neonatal lupus erythematosus: A prospective study of infants born to mothers with anti-Ro autoantibodies. *J Pediatr*. 2003;142(6): 678-683.
59. Lee LA. Transient autoimmunity related to maternal autoantibodies: Neonatal lupus. *Autoimmun Rev*. 2005 Apr;4(4):207-213.
60. Watson RM, Scheel JN, Petri M, et al. Neonatal lupus erythematosus. Report of serological and immunogenetic studies in twins discordant for congenital heart block. *Br J Dermatol*. 1994; 130(3):342-348.
61. Batard ML, Sainte-Marie D, Clity E, et al. [Cutaneous neonatal lupus erythematosus: Discordant expression in identical twins]. *Ann Dermatol Venereol*. 2000 Oct;127(10):814-817.
62. Solomon BA, Laude TA, Shalita AR. Neonatal lupus erythematosus: Discordant disease expression of U1RNP-positive antibodies in fraternal twins—is this a subset of neonatal lupus erythematosus or a new distinct syndrome? *J Am Acad Dermatol*. 1995;32(5 Pt 2):858-862.
63. Fesslova V, Mannarino S, Salice P, et al. Neonatal lupus: Fetal myocarditis progressing to atrioventricular block in triplets. *Lupus*. 2003;12(10):775-778.
64. Siren MK, Julkunen H, Kaaja R, et al. Role of HLA in congenital heart block: Susceptibility alleles in children. *Lupus*. 1999;8(1):60-67.
65. Miyagawa S, Fukumoto T, Hashimoto K, et al. Neonatal lupus erythematosus: Haplotypic analysis of HLA class II alleles in child/mother pairs. *Arthritis Rheum*. 1997;40(5):982-983.
66. Brucato A, Ramoni V, Penco S, et al. Passively acquired anti-SSA/Ro antibodies are required for congenital heart block following ovodonation but maternal genes are not. *Arthritis Rheum*. 2010 Oct;62(10):3119-3121.
67. Selander B, Cedergren S, Domanski H, et al. A case of severe neonatal lupus erythematosus without cardiac or cutaneous involvement. *Acta Paediatr*. 1998 Jan;87(1):105-107.
68. Buyon JP, Hiebert R, Copel J, et al. Autoimmune-associated congenital heart block: Demographics, mortality, morbidity and recurrence rates obtained from a national neonatal lupus registry. *J Am Coll Cardiol*. 1998 Jun;31(7):1658-1666.
69. Scott JS, Maddison PJ, Taylor PV, et al. Connective-tissue disease, antibodies to ribonucleoprotein, and congenital heart block. *N Engl J Med*. 1983 Jul 28;309(4):209-212.
70. Buyon J, Szer I. Passively acquired autoimmunity and the maternal fetal dyad in systemic lupus erythematosus. *Springer Semin Immunopathol*. 1986;9(2-3):283-304.
71. Buyon JP, Rupel A, Clancy RM, et al. Neonatal lupus syndromes. *Lupus*. 2004;13(9):705-712.
72. Lee LA. Neonatal lupus erythematosus. *J Invest Dermatol*. 1993 Jan;100(1):9S-13S.
73. Cimaz R, Duquesne A. [Neonatal lupus syndromes.]. *Arch Pediatr*. 2006 May;13(5):473-478.
74. Brucato A, Frassi M, Franceschini F, et al. Risk of congenital complete heart block in newborns of mothers with anti-Ro/SSA antibodies detected by counterimmunoelectrophoresis: A prospective study of 100 women. *Arthritis Rheum JID—0370605*. 2001;44(8):1832-1835.
75. Raboisson MJ, Fouron JC, Sonesson SE, et al. Fetal Doppler echocardiographic diagnosis and successful steroid therapy of Luciani-Wenckebach phenomenon and endocardial fibroelastosis related to maternal anti-Ro and anti-La antibodies. *J Am Soc Echocardiogr*. 2005 Apr;18(4):375-380.
76. Costedoat-Chalumeau N, Amoura Z, Villain E, et al. Anti-SSA/Ro antibodies and the heart: More than complete congenital heart block? A review of electrocardiographic and myocardial abnormalities and of treatment options. *Arthritis Res Ther*. 2005;7(2):69-73.
77. Nield LE, Silverman ED, Taylor GP, et al. Maternal anti-Ro and anti-La antibody-associated endocardial fibroelastosis. *Circulation*. 2002 Feb 19;105(7):843-848.
78. Moak JP, Barron KS, Hougen TJ, et al. Congenital heart block: Development of late-onset cardiomyopathy, a previously underappreciated sequela. *J Am Coll Cardiol*. 2001 Jan;37(1):238-242.

10

79. Neufing PJ, Clancy RM, Jackson MW, et al. Exposure and binding of selected immunodominant La/SSB epitopes on human apoptotic cells. *Arthritis Rheum.* 2005 Dec;52(12):3934-3942.

80. Tran HB, Macardle PJ, Hiscock J, et al. Anti-La/SSB antibodies transported across the placenta bind apoptotic cells in fetal organs targeted in neonatal lupus. *Arthritis Rheum.* 2002;46(6): 1572-1579.

81. Clancy RM, Askanase AD, Kapur RP, et al. Transdifferentiation of cardiac fibroblasts, a fetal factor in anti-SSA/Ro-SSB/La antibody-mediated congenital heart block. *J Immunol.* 2002 Aug 15;169(4): 2156-2163.

82. Clancy RM, Buyon JP. Autoimmune-associated congenital heart block: Dissecting the cascade from immunologic insult to relentless fibrosis. *Anat Rec A Discov Mol Cell Evol Biol.* 2004 Oct;280(2): 1027-1035.

83. Nii M, Hamilton RM, Fenwick L, et al. Assessment of fetal atrioventricular time intervals by tissue Doppler and pulse Doppler echocardiography: Normal values and correlation with fetal electrocardiography. *Heart.* 2006 Dec;92(12):1831-1837. PMC 1861294.

84. Claus R, Hickstein H, Kulz T, et al. Identification and management of fetuses at risk for, or affected by, congenital heart block associated with autoantibodies to SSA (Ro), SSB (La), or an HsEg5-like autoantigen. *Rheumatol Int.* 2006 Jan 10:1-10.

85. Hickstein H, Kulz T, Claus R, et al. Autoimmune-associated congenital heart block: Treatment of the mother with immunoadsorption. *Ther Apher Dial.* 2005 Apr;9(2):148-153.

86. Buyon JP, Swersky SH, Fox HE, et al. Intrauterine therapy for presumptive fetal myocarditis with acquired heart block due to systemic lupus erythematosus. Experience in a mother with a predominance of SS-B (La) antibodies. *Arthritis Rheum.* 1987 Jan;30(1):44-49.

87. Jaeggi ET, Silverman ED, Yoo SJ, et al. Is immune-mediated complete fetal atrioventricular block reversible by transplacental dexamethasone therapy? *Ultrasound Obstet Gynecol.* 2004 Jun;23(6): 602-605.

88. Jaeggi ET, Fouron JC, Silverman ED, et al. Transplacental fetal treatment improves the outcome of prenatally diagnosed complete atrioventricular block without structural heart disease. *Circulation.* 2004 Sep 21;110(12):1542-1548.

89. Saleeb S, Copel J, Friedman D, et al. Comparison of treatment with fluorinated glucocorticoids to the natural history of autoantibody-associated congenital heart block: Retrospective review of the research registry for neonatal lupus. *Arthritis Rheum.* 1999 Nov;42(11): 2335-2345.

90. Buyon JP, Waltuck J, Kleinman C, et al. In utero identification and therapy of congenital heart block. *Lupus.* 1995 Apr;4(2):116-121.

91. Pisoni CN, Brucato A, Ruffatti A, et al. Failure of intravenous immunoglobulin to prevent congenital heart block: Findings of a multicenter, prospective, observational study. *Arthritis Rheum.* 2010 Apr; 62(4):1147-1152.

92. Friedman DM, Llanos C, Izmirly PM, et al. Evaluation of fetuses in a study of intravenous immunoglobulin as preventive therapy for congenital heart block: Results of a multicenter, prospective, open-label clinical trial. *Arthritis Rheum.* 2010 Apr;62(4):1138-1146.

93. Matsui S, Fu ML, Shimizu M, et al. Dilated cardiomyopathy defines serum autoantibodies against G-protein-coupled cardiovascular receptors. *Autoimmunity.* 1995;21(2):85-88.

94. Baba A, Yoshikawa T, Fukuda Y, et al. Autoantibodies against M2-muscarinic acetylcholine receptors: New upstream targets in atrial fibrillation in patients with dilated cardiomyopathy. *Eur Heart J.* 2004 Jul;25(13):1108-1115.

95. Zhang L, Hu D, Li J, et al. Autoantibodies against the myocardial beta1-adrenergic and M2-muscarinic receptors in patients with congestive heart failure. *Chin Med J (Engl).* 2002 Aug; 115(8):1127-1131.

96. Wallukat G, Nissen E, Morwinski R, et al. Autoantibodies against the beta- and muscarinic receptors in cardiomyopathy. *Herz.* 2000 May;25(3):261-266.

97. Matsui S, Fu ML. Myocardial injury due to G-protein coupled receptor-autoimmunity. *Jpn Heart J.* 1998 May;39(3):261-274.

98. Ferrari I, Levin MJ, Wallukat G, et al. Molecular mimicry between the immunodominant ribosomal protein P0 of Trypanosoma cruzi and a functional epitope on the human beta 1-adrenergic receptor. *J Exp Med.* 1995 Jul 1;182(1):59-65.

99. Elies R, Ferrari I, Wallukat G, et al. Structural and functional analysis of the B cell epitopes recognized by anti-receptor autoantibodies in patients with Chagas' disease. *J Immunol.* 1996 Nov 1; 157(9):4203-4211.

100. Bacman S, Sterin-Borda L, Camusso JJ, et al. Circulating antibodies against neurotransmitter receptor activities in children with congenital heart block and their mothers. *Faseb J.* 1994 Nov;8(14): 1170-1176.

101. Mijares A, Lebesgue D, Wallukat G, et al. From agonist to antagonist: Fab fragments of an agonist-like monoclonal anti-beta(2)-adrenoceptor antibody behave as antagonists. *Mol Pharmacol.* 2000 Aug;58(2):373-379.

102. Quan CP, Ruffet E, Arihiro K, et al. High affinity serum-derived Fab fragments as another source of antibodies in the gut lumen of both neonates and adults. *Scand J Immunol.* 1996 Aug;44(2): 108-114.

103. Wedeking-Schohl H, Maisch B, Schonian UH, et al. [Fetal arrhythmias—new immunologic studies and results]. *Z Geburtshilfe Perinatol.* 1993 May-Jun;197(3):144-147.

104. Kleinman CS, Nehgme RA. Cardiac arrhythmias in the human fetus. *Pediatr Cardiol.* 2004 May-Jun;25(3):234-251.

105. Moise KJ Jr. Management of rhesus alloimmunization in pregnancy. *Obstet Gynecol*. 2002 Sep; 100(3):600-611.

106. Lambin P, Debbia M, Puillandre P, et al. IgG1 and IgG3 anti-D in maternal serum and on the RBCs of infants suffering from HDN: Relationship with the severity of the disease. *Transfusion*. 2002 Dec;42(12):1537-1546.

107. Fung Kee Fung K, Eason E, Crane J, et al. Prevention of Rh alloimmunization. *J Obstet Gynaecol Can*. 2003 Sep;25(9):765-773.

108. Maayan-Metzger A, Schwartz T, Sulkes J, et al. Maternal anti-D prophylaxis during pregnancy does not cause neonatal haemolysis. *Arch Dis Child Fetal Neonatal Ed*. 2001 Jan;84(1):F60-F62. PMC 1721201.

109. Collinet P, Subtil D, Puech F, et al. Successful treatment of extremely severe fetal anemia due to Kell alloimmunization. *Obstet Gynecol*. 2002 Nov;100(5 Pt 2):1102-1105.

110. Denomme GA, Ryan G, Seaward PG, et al. Maternal ABO-mismatched blood for intrauterine transfusion of severe hemolytic disease of the newborn due to anti-Rh17. *Transfusion*. 2004 Sep;44(9): 1357-1360.

111. Mundy CA. Intravenous immunoglobulin in the management of hemolytic disease of the newborn. *Neonatal Netw*. 2005 Nov-Dec;24(6):17-24.

112. Miqdad AM, Abdelbasit OB, Shaheed MM, et al. Intravenous immunoglobulin G (IVIG) therapy for significant hyperbilirubinemia in ABO hemolytic disease of the newborn. *J Matern Fetal Neonatal Med*. 2004 Sep;16(3):163-166.

113. Narang A, Jain N. Haemolytic disease of newborn. *Indian J Pediatr*. 2001 Feb;68(2):167-172.

114. Sarici SU, Yurdakok M, Serdar MA, et al. An early (sixth-hour) serum bilirubin measurement is useful in predicting the development of significant hyperbilirubinemia and severe ABO hemolytic disease in a selective high-risk population of newborns with ABO incompatibility. *Pediatrics*. 2002 Apr;109(4):e53.

115. Dinesh D. Review of positive direct antiglobulin tests found on cord blood sampling. *J Paediatr Child Health*. 2005 Sep-Oct;41(9-10):504-507.

116. Dikshit SK, Gupta PK. Exchange transfusion in neonatal hyperbilirubinemia. *Indian Pediatr*. 1989 Nov;26(11):1139-1145.

117. Amato M, Blumberg A, Hermann U Jr, et al. Effectiveness of single versus double volume exchange transfusion in newborn infants with ABO hemolytic disease. *Helv Paediatr Acta*. 1988 Nov;43(3): 177-186.

118. Geifman-Holtzman O, Wojtowycz M, Kosmas E, et al. Female alloimmunization with antibodies known to cause hemolytic disease. *Obstet Gynecol*. 1997 Feb;89(2):272-275.

119. Wenk RE, Goldstein P, Felix JK, et al. Kell alloimmunization, hemolytic disease of the newborn, and perinatal management. *Obstet Gynecol*. 1985 Oct;66(4):473-476.

120. Mochizuki K, Ohto H, Hirai S, et al. Hemolytic disease of the newborn due to anti-Di: A case study and review of the literature. *Transfusion*. 2006 Mar;46(3):454-460.

121. Moise KJ. Fetal anemia due to non-Rhesus-D red-cell alloimmunization. *Semin Fetal Neonatal Med*. 2008 Aug;13(4):207-214.

122. Vaughan JI, Manning M, Warwick RM, et al. Inhibition of erythroid progenitor cells by anti-Kell antibodies in fetal alloimmune anemia. *N Engl J Med*. 1998 Mar 19;338(12):798-803.

123. Grant SR, Kilby MD, Meer L, et al. The outcome of pregnancy in Kell alloimmunisation. *BJOG*. 2000 Apr;107(4):481-485.

124. Dhodapkar KM, Blei F. Treatment of hemolytic disease of the newborn caused by anti-Kell antibody with recombinant erythropoietin. *J Pediatr Hematol Oncol*. 2001 Jan;23(1):69-70.

125. Hromadnikova I, Vechetova L, Vesela K, et al. Non-invasive fetal RHD exon 7 and exon 10 genotyping using real-time PCR testing of fetal DNA in maternal plasma. *Fetal Diagn Ther*. 2005 Jul-Aug;20(4):275-280.

126. Daniels G, Finning K, Martin P, et al. Noninvasive prenatal diagnosis of fetal blood group phenotypes: Current practice and future prospects. *Prenat Diagn*. 2009 Feb;29(2):101-107.

127. Illanes S, Soothill P. Management of red cell alloimmunisation in pregnancy: The non-invasive monitoring of the disease. *Prenat Diagn*. 2010 Jul;30(7):668-673.

128. Szczepura A, Osipenko L, Freeman K, et al. A new fetal RHD genotyping test: Costs and benefits of mass testing to target antenatal anti-D prophylaxis in England and Wales. *BMC Pregnancy Childbirth*. 2011;11:5. PMC 3034710.

129. Uhrynowska M, Maslanka K, Zupanska B, et al. Neonatal thrombocytopenia: Incidence, serological and clinical observations. *Am J Perinatol*. 1997 Aug;14(7):415-418.

130. Kaplan C, Morel-Kopp MC, Clemenceau S, et al. Fetal and neonatal alloimmune thrombocytopenia: Current trends in diagnosis and therapy. *Transfus Med*. 1992 Dec;2(4):265-271.

131. Manno CS. Management of bleeding disorders in children. *Hematology (Am Soc Hematol Educ Program)*. 2005:416-422.

132. Deaver JE, Leppert PC, Zaroulis CG, et al. Neonatal alloimmune thrombocytopenic purpura. *Am J Perinatol*. 1986 Apr;3(2):127-131.

133. Davoren A, Saving K, McFarland JG, et al. Neonatal neutropenia and bacterial sepsis associated with placental transfer of maternal neutrophil-specific autoantibodies. *Transfusion*. 2004 Jul;44(7):1041-1046.

134. Maheshwari A, Christensen RD, Calhoun DA, et al. Immune neutropenia in the neonate. *Adv Pediatr*. 2002;49:317-339.

135. Minchinton RM, McGrath KM. Alloimmune neonatal neutropenia—a neglected diagnosis? *Med J Aust*. 1987 Aug 3;147(3):139-141.

10

136. Han TH, Chey MJ, Han KS, et al. A case of neonatal alloimmune neutropenia associated with anti-human neutrophil antigen-1a (HNA-1a) antibody. *J Korean Med Sci.* 2006 Apr;21(2):351-354. PMC 2734018.

137. Curtis BR, Reno C, Aster RH, et al. Neonatal alloimmune neutropenia attributed to maternal immunoglobulin G antibodies against the neutrophil alloantigen HNA-1c (SH): A report of five cases. *Transfusion.* 2005 Aug;45(8):1308-1313.

138. Hagimoto R, Koike K, Sakashita K, et al. A possible role for maternal HLA antibody in a case of alloimmune neonatal neutropenia. *Transfusion.* 2001 May;41(5):615-620.

139. Tomicic M, Starcevic M, Bux J, et al. Severe neonatal neutropenia due to anti-human leucocyte antigen B49 alloimmunization only: a case report. *Transfus Med.* 2003 Aug;13(4):233-237.

140. Kameoka J, Funato T, Miura T, et al. Autoimmune neutropenia in pregnant women causing neonatal neutropenia. *Br J Haematol.* 2001 Jul;114(1):198-200.

141. Lee LA. Neonatal lupus: clinical features and management. *Paediatr Drugs.* 2004;6(2):71-78.

142. Kanagasegar S, Cimaz R, Kurien BT, et al. Neonatal lupus manifests as isolated neutropenia and mildly abnormal liver functions. *J Rheumatol.* 2002 Jan;29(1):187-191.

143. Fung YL, Pitcher LA, Taylor K, et al. Managing passively acquired autoimmune neonatal neutropenia: A case study. *Transfus Med.* 2005 Apr;15(2):151-155.

144. Bastian JF, Williams RA, Ornelas W, et al. Maternal isoimmunisation resulting in combined immunodeficiency and fatal graft-versus-host disease in an infant. *Lancet.* 1984;1(8392): 1435-1437.

145. Fu J, Jiang Y, Liang L, et al. Risk factors of primary thyroid dysfunction in early infants born to mothers with autoimmune thyroid disease. *Acta Paediatr.* 2005 Aug;94(8):1043-1048.

146. Vargova V, Pytliak M, Mechirova V, et al. Maternal autoimmune thyroiditis and congenital malformations of newborns in a cohort of Slovak women. *Wien Med Wochenschr.* 2010 Sep;160(17-18): 470-474.

147. Lazarus JH. Thyroid disease in pregnancy and childhood. *Minerva Endocrinol.* 2005 Jun;30(2): 71-87.

148. Svensson J, Lindberg B, Ericsson UB, et al. Thyroid autoantibodies in cord blood sera from children and adolescents with autoimmune thyroiditis. *Thyroid.* 2006 Jan;16(1):79-83.

149. Pop VJ, de Vries E, van Baar AL, et al. Maternal thyroid peroxidase antibodies during pregnancy: A marker of impaired child development? *J Clin Endocrinol Metab.* 1995 Dec;80(12):3561-3566.

150. Biro E, Szekanecz Z, Czirjak L, et al. Association of systemic and thyroid autoimmune diseases. *Clin Rheumatol.* 2006 Mar;25(2):240-245.

151. McDonagh JE, Isenberg DA. Development of additional autoimmune diseases in a population of patients with systemic lupus erythematosus. *Ann Rheum Dis.* 2000 Mar;59(3):230-232. PMC 1753089.

152. Ruggeri RM, Galletti M, Mandolfino MG, et al. Thyroid hormone autoantibodies in primary Sjogren syndrome and rheumatoid arthritis are more prevalent than in autoimmune thyroid disease, becoming progressively more frequent in these diseases. *J Endocrinol Invest.* 2002 May;25(5): 447-454.

153. Spence D, Hornberger L, Hamilton R, et al. Increased risk of complete congenital heart block in infants born to women with hypothyroidism and anti-Ro and/or anti-La antibodies. *J Rheumatol.* 2006 Jan;33(1):167-170.

154. Alexander EK, Marqusee E, Lawrence J, et al. Timing and magnitude of increases in levothyroxine requirements during pregnancy in women with hypothyroidism. *N Engl J Med.* 2004 Jul 15;351(3):241-249.

155. Kvetny J, Poulsen H. Transient hyperthyroxinemia in newborns from women with autoimmune thyroid disease and raised levels of thyroid peroxidase antibodies. *J Matern Fetal Neonatal Med.* 2006 Dec;19(12):817-822.

156. Zimmerman D. Fetal and neonatal hyperthyroidism. *Thyroid.* 1999 Jul;9(7):727-733.

157. Kung AW, Lau KS, Kohn LD, et al. Epitope mapping of tsh receptor-blocking antibodies in Graves' disease that appear during pregnancy. *J Clin Endocrinol Metab.* 2001 Aug;86(8):3647-3653.

158. Luton D, Le Gac I, Vuillard E, et al. Management of Graves' disease during pregnancy: The key role of fetal thyroid gland monitoring. *J Clin Endocrinol Metab.* 2005 Nov;90(11):6093-6098.

159. Nachum Z, Rakover Y, Weiner E, et al. Graves' disease in pregnancy: Prospective evaluation of a selective invasive treatment protocol. *Am J Obstet Gynecol.* 2003 Jul;189(1):159-165.

160. Kamishlian A, Matthews N, Gupta A, et al. Different outcomes of neonatal thyroid function after Graves' disease in pregnancy: Patient reports and literature review. *J Pediatr Endocrinol Metab.* 2005 Dec;18(12):1357-1363.

161. Naserke HE, Bonifacio E, Ziegler AG, et al. Immunoglobulin G insulin autoantibodies in BABYDIAB offspring appear postnatally: Sensitive early detection using a protein A/G-based radiobinding assay. *J Clin Endocrinol Metab.* 1999 Apr;84(4):1239-1243.

162. Di Mario U, Fallucca F, Gargiulo P, et al. Insulin-anti-insulin complexes in diabetic women and their neonates. *Diabetologia.* 1984 Jul;27(Suppl):83-86.

163. Poletaev AB, Gnedenko BB, Makarova AA, et al. Possible mechanisms of diabetic fetopathy. *Hum Antibodies.* 2000;9(4):189-197.

164. Koczwara K, Ziegler AG, Bonifacio E, et al. Maternal immunity to insulin does not affect diabetes risk in progeny of non obese diabetic mice. *Clin Exp Immunol.* 2004 Apr;136(1):56-59.

165. Greeley SA, Katsumata M, Yu L, et al. Elimination of maternally transmitted autoantibodies prevents diabetes in nonobese diabetic mice. *Nat Med.* 2002 Apr;8(4):399-402.

10

166. Melanitou E, Devendra D, Liu E, et al. Early and quantal (by litter) expression of insulin autoantibodies in the nonobese diabetic mice predict early diabetes onset. *J Immunol*. 2004 Dec 1;173(11):6603-6610.

167. Naserke HE, Bonifacio E, Ziegler AG, et al. Prevalence, characteristics and diabetes risk associated with transient maternally acquired islet antibodies and persistent islet antibodies in offspring of parents with type 1 diabetes. *J Clin Endocrinol Metab*. 2001 Oct;86(10):4826-4833.

168. Ludvigsson J, Wahlberg J. Diabetes-related autoantibodies in cord blood from children of healthy mothers have disappeared by the time the child is one year old. *Ann N Y Acad Sci*. 2002 Apr; 958:289-292.

169. Hamalainen AM, Savola K, Kulmala PK, et al. Disease-associated autoantibodies during pregnancy and at birth in families affected by type 1 diabetes. *Clin Exp Immunol*. 2001 Nov;126(2):230-235.

170. Lindsay RS, Ziegler AG, Hamilton BA, et al. Type 1 diabetes-related antibodies in the fetal circulation: Prevalence and influence on cord insulin and birth weight in offspring of mothers with type 1 diabetes. *J Clin Endocrinol Metab*. 2004 Jul;89(7):3436-3439.

171. Weiss PA, Kainer F, Purstner P, et al. Anti-insulin antibodies and birth weight in pregnancies complicated by diabetes. *Early Hum Dev*. 1998 Dec;53(2):145-154.

172. Gamlen TR, Aynsley-Green A, Irvine WJ, et al. Immunological studies in the neonate of a mother with Addison's disease and diabetes mellitus. *Clin Exp Immunol*. 1977 Apr;28(1):192-195. PMC 1540872.

173. Betterle C, Pra CD, Pedini B, et al. Assessment of adrenocortical function and autoantibodies in a baby born to a mother with autoimmune polyglandular syndrome Type 2. *J Endocrinol Invest*. 2004 Jul-Aug;27(7):618-621.

174. Evoli A. Acquired myasthenia gravis in childhood. *Curr Opin Neurol*. 2010 Oct;23(5):536-540.

175. Lefvert AK, Bergstrom K, Matell G, et al. Determination of acetylcholine receptor antibody in myasthenia gravis: Clinical usefulness and pathogenetic implications. *J Neurol Neurosurg Psychiatry*. 1978 May;41(5):394-403.

176. Sisman J, Ceri A, Nafday SM. Seronegative neonatal myasthenia gravis in one of the twins. *Indian Pediatr*. 2004 Sep;41(9):938-940.

177. Podciechowski L, Brocka-Nitecka U, Dabrowska K, Bielak A, et al. Pregnancy complicated by myasthenia gravis—twelve years experience. *Neuro Endocrinol Lett*. 2005 Oct;26(5):603-608.

178. Lefvert AK, Osterman PO. Newborn infants to myasthenic mothers: A clinical study and an investigation of acetylcholine receptor antibodies in 17 children. *Neurology*. 1983 Feb;33(2):133-138.

179. Cantagrel S, Maury L, Yamamoto AM, et al. Akinesia, arthrogryposis, craniosynostosis: A presentation of neonatal myasthenia with fetal onset. *Am J Perinatol*. 2002 Nov;19(6):297-301.

180. Riemersma S, Vincent A, Beeson D, et al. Association of arthrogryposis multiplex congenita with maternal antibodies inhibiting fetal acetylcholine receptor function. *J Clin Invest*. 1996 Nov 15; 98(10):2358-2363.

181. Hesselmans LF, Jennekens FG, Van den Oord CJ, et al. Development of innervation of skeletal muscle fibers in man: Relation to acetylcholine receptors. *Anat Rec*. 1993 Jul;236(3):553-562.

182. Gardnerova M, Eymard B, Morel E, et al. The fetal/adult acetylcholine receptor antibody ratio in mothers with myasthenia gravis as a marker for transfer of the disease to the newborn. *Neurology*. 1997 Jan;48(1):50-54.

183. Kane SV, Acquah LA. Placental transport of immunoglobulins: A clinical review for gastroenterologists who prescribe therapeutic monoclonal antibodies to women during conception and pregnancy. *Am J Gastroenterol*. 2009 Jan;104(1):228-233.

184. Eymard B, Morel E, Harpey JP, et al. [Assay of anti-acetylcholine receptor antibodies in myasthenic syndromes of newborn infants]. *Presse Med*. 1986 May 31;15(22):1019-1022.

185. Rieder AA, Conley SF, Rowe L, et al. Pediatric myasthenia gravis and velopharyngeal incompetence. *Int J Pediatr Otorhinolaryngol*. 2004 Jun;68(6):747-752.

186. Barnes PR, Kanabar DJ, Brueton L, et al. Recurrent congenital arthrogryposis leading to a diagnosis of myasthenia gravis in an initially asymptomatic mother. *Neuromuscul Disord*. 1995 Jan;5(1): 59-65.

187. Ferrero S, Pretta S, Nicoletti A, et al. Myasthenia gravis: Management issues during pregnancy. *Eur J Obstet Gynecol Reprod Biol*. 2005 Aug 1;121(2):129-138.

188. Verspyck E, Mandelbrot L, Dommergues M, et al. Myasthenia gravis with polyhydramnios in the fetus of an asymptomatic mother. *Prenat Diagn*. 1993 Jun;13(6):539-542.

189. Donat JF, Donat JR, Lennon VA, et al. Exchange transfusion in neonatal myasthenia gravis. *Neurology*. 1981 Jul;31(7):911-912.

190. Tagher RJ, Baumann R, Desai N, et al. Failure of intravenously administered immunoglobulin in the treatment of neonatal myasthenia gravis. *J Pediatr*. 1999 Feb;134(2):233-235.

191. Hamrock DJ. Adverse events associated with intravenous immunoglobulin therapy. *Int Immunopharmacol*. 2006 Apr;6(4):535-542.

192. Siegel J. Safety considerations in IGIV utilization. *Int Immunopharmacol*. 2006 Apr;6(4):523-527.

193. Schmidt-Ott R, Schmidt H, Feldmann S, et al. Improved serological diagnosis stresses the major role of Campylobacter jejuni in triggering Guillain-Barre syndrome. *Clin Vaccine Immunol*. 2006 Jul;13(7):779-783. PMC 1489570.

194. Caporale CM, Papola F, Fioroni MA, et al. Susceptibility to Guillain-Barre syndrome is associated to polymorphisms of CD1 genes. *J Neuroimmunol*. 2006 Aug;177(1-2):112-118.

195. Jackson AH, Baquis GD, Shah BL, et al. Congenital Guillain-Barre syndrome. *J Child Neurol*. 1996 Sep;11(5):407-410.

10

196. Bamford NS, Trojaborg W, Sherbany AA, et al. Congenital Guillain-Barre syndrome associated with maternal inflammatory bowel disease is responsive to intravenous immunoglobulin. *Eur J Paediatr Neurol*. 2002;6(2):115-119.

197. Buchwald B, de Baets M, Luijckx GJ, et al. Neonatal Guillain-Barre syndrome: Blocking antibodies transmitted from mother to child. *Neurology*. 1999 Oct 12;53(6):1246-1253.

198. Attarian S, Azulay JP, Chabrol B, et al. Neonatal lower motor neuron syndrome associated with maternal neuropathy with anti-GM1 IgG. *Neurology*. 2004 Jul 27;63(2):379-381.

199. Bansal PJ, Tobin MC. Neonatal microscopic polyangiitis secondary to transfer of maternal myeloperoxidase-antineutrophil cytoplasmic antibody resulting in neonatal pulmonary hemorrhage and renal involvement. *Ann Allergy Asthma Immunol*. 2004 Oct;93(4):398-401.

200. Silva F, Specks U, Sethi S, et al. Successful pregnancy and delivery of a healthy newborn despite transplacental transfer of antimyeloperoxidase antibodies from a mother with microscopic polyangiitis. *Am J Kidney Dis*. 2009 Sep;54(3):542-545.

201. Lee BH, Stoll BJ, McDonald SA, et al. Adverse neonatal outcomes associated with antenatal dexamethasone versus antenatal betamethasone. *Pediatrics*. 2006 May;117(5):1503-1510.

202. Finer NN, Powers RJ, Ou CH, et al. Prospective evaluation of postnatal steroid administration: A 1-year experience from the California Perinatal Quality Care Collaborative. *Pediatrics*. 2006 Mar;117(3):704-713.

203. Mildenhall LF, Battin MR, Morton SM, et al. Exposure to repeat doses of antenatal glucocorticoids is associated with altered cardiovascular status after birth. *Arch Dis Child Fetal Neonatal Ed*. 2006 Jan;91(1):F56-F60. PMC 2672653.

204. Bakker JM, Kavelaars A, Kamphuis PJ, et al. Neonatal dexamethasone treatment increases susceptibility to experimental autoimmune disease in adult rats. *J Immunol*. 2000 Nov 15;165(10):5932-5937.

205. Dolfin T, Pomeranz A, Korzets Z, et al. Acute renal failure in a neonate caused by the transplacental transfer of a nephrotoxic paraprotein: Successful resolution by exchange transfusion. *Am J Kidney Dis*. 1999 Dec;34(6):1129-1131.

206. Laugel V, Goetz J, Wolff S, et al. Neonatal management of symptomatic transplacental cryoglobulinaemia. *Acta Paediatr*. 2004 Apr;93(4):556-558.

207. Tissot JD, Schneider P, Hohlfeld P, et al. Monoclonal gammopathy in a 30 weeks old premature infant. *Appl Theor Electrophor*. 1992;3(2):67-68.

208. Rosenblatt DS, Cooper BA. Inherited disorders of vitamin B12 metabolism. *Blood Rev*. 1987 Sep;1(3):177-182.

209. Whittingham S, Mackay IR. Autoimmune gastritis: historical antecedents, outstanding discoveries, and unresolved problems. *Int Rev Immunol*. 2005 Jan-Apr;24(1-2):1-29.

210. Kondo H, Imamura T. Pernicious anemia (PA) subsequent to insulin-dependent diabetes mellitus and idiopathic thrombocytopenic purpura, and effects of oral cobalamin on PA. *Am J Hematol*. 1999 Sep;62(1):61-62.

211. Perros P, Singh RK, Ludlam CA, et al. Prevalence of pernicious anaemia in patients with Type 1 diabetes mellitus and autoimmune thyroid disease. *Diabet Med*. 2000 Oct;17(10):749-751.

212. Durand JM, Cretel E, Juhan V, et al. Systemic lupus erythematosus associated with pernicious anemia. *Clin Exp Rheumatol*. 1994 Mar-Apr;12(2):233.

213. Hertl M, Veldman C. Pemphigus—paradigm of autoantibody-mediated autoimmunity. *Skin Pharmacol Appl Skin Physiol*. 2001 Nov-Dec;14(6):408-418.

214. Mahoney MG, Hu Y, Brennan D, et al. Delineation of diversified desmoglein distribution in stratified squamous epithelia: Implications in diseases. *Exp Dermatol*. 2006 Feb;15(2):101-109.

215. Wu H, Wang ZH, Yan A, et al. Protection against pemphigus foliaceus by desmoglein 3 in neonates. *N Engl J Med*. 2000 Jul 6;343(1):31-35.

216. Parlowsky T, Welzel J, Amagai M, et al. Neonatal pemphigus vulgaris: IgG4 autoantibodies to desmoglein 3 induce skin blisters in newborns. *J Am Acad Dermatol*. 2003 Apr;48(4):623-625.

217. Campo-Voegeli A, Muniz F, Mascaro JM, et al. Neonatal pemphigus vulgaris with extensive mucocutaneous lesions from a mother with oral pemphigus vulgaris. *Br J Dermatol*. 2002 Oct;147(4):801-805.

218. Fenniche S, Benmously R, Marrak H, et al. Neonatal pemphigus vulgaris in an infant born to a mother with pemphigus vulgaris in remission. *Pediatr Dermatol*. 2006 Mar-Apr;23(2):124-127.

219. Diaz LA, Arteaga LA, Hilario-Vargas J, et al. Anti-desmoglein-1 antibodies in onchocerciasis, leishmaniasis and Chagas disease suggest a possible etiological link to Fogo selvagem. *J Invest Dermatol*. 2004 Dec;123(6):1045-1051.

220. Nagasaka T, Nishifuji K, Ota T, et al. Defining the pathogenic involvement of desmoglein 4 in pemphigus and staphylococcal scalded skin syndrome. *J Clin Invest*. 2004 Nov;114(10):1484-1492.

221. Chiossi MP, Costa RS, Roselino AM, et al. Dermal dendritic cell number correlates with serum autoantibody titers in Brazilian pemphigus foliaceus patients. *Braz J Med Biol Res*. 2004 Mar;37(3):337-341.

222. Shieh S, Fang YV, Becker JL, et al. Pemphigus, pregnancy, and plasmapheresis. *Cutis*. 2004 May;73(5):327-329.

223. Fainaru O, Mashiach R, Kupferminc M, et al. Pemphigus vulgaris in pregnancy: A case report and review of literature. *Hum Reprod*. 2000 May;15(5):1195-1197.

10

224. Nguyen VT, Arredondo J, Chernyavsky AI, et al. Pemphigus vulgaris IgG and methylprednisolone exhibit reciprocal effects on keratinocytes. *J Biol Chem.* 2004 Jan 16;279(3):2135-2146.

225. Ortiz-Urda S, Elbe-Burger A, Smolle J, et al. The plant lectin wheat germ agglutinin inhibits the binding of pemphigus foliaceus autoantibodies to desmoglein 1 in a majority of patients and prevents pathomechanisms of pemphigus foliaceus in vitro and in vivo. *J Immunol.* 2003 Dec 1;171(11):6244-6250.

226. Burch JM, Sokol RJ, Narkewicz MR, et al. Autoantibodies in mothers of children with neonatal liver disease. *J Pediatr Gastroenterol Nutr.* 2003 Sep;37(3):262-267.

227. Whitington PF, Kelly S, Ekong UD. Neonatal hemochromatosis: Fetal liver disease leading to liver failure in the fetus and newborn. *Pediatr Transplant.* 2005 Oct;9(5):640-645.

228. Kelly AL, Lunt PW, Rodrigues F, et al. Classification and genetic features of neonatal haemochromatosis: A study of 27 affected pedigrees and molecular analysis of genes implicated in iron metabolism. *J Med Genet.* 2001 Sep;38(9):599-610.

229. Ekong UD, Kelly S, Whitington PF, et al. Disparate clinical presentation of neonatal hemochromatosis in twins. *Pediatrics.* 2005 Dec;116(6):e880-884.

230. Whitington PF, Malladi P. Neonatal hemochromatosis: Is it an alloimmune disease? *J Pediatr Gastroenterol Nutr.* 2005 May;40(5):544-549.

231. Whitington PF, Kelly S. Outcome of pregnancies at risk for neonatal hemochromatosis is improved by treatment with high-dose intravenous immunoglobulin. *Pediatrics.* 2008 Jun;121(6):e1615-1621.

232. Whitington PF, Hibbard JU. High-dose immunoglobulin during pregnancy for recurrent neonatal haemochromatosis. *Lancet.* 2004 Nov 6-12;364(9446):1690-1698.

233. Pall H, Jonas MM. Pediatric hepatobiliary disease. *Curr Opin Gastroenterol.* 2005 May;21(3):344-347.

234. Flynn DM, Mohan N, McKiernan P, et al. Progress in treatment and outcome for children with neonatal haemochromatosis. *Arch Dis Child Fetal Neonatal Ed.* 2003 Mar;88(2):F124-F127. PMC 1721526.

235. Rand EB, Karpen SJ, Kelly S, et al. Treatment of neonatal hemochromatosis with exchange transfusion and intravenous immunoglobulin. *J Pediatr.* 2009 Oct;155(4):566-571.

236. Gleicher N. Autoantibodies and pregnancy loss. *Lancet.* 1994 Mar 26;343(8900):747-748.

237. Wallukat G, Neichel D, Nissen E, et al. Agonistic autoantibodies directed against the angiotensin II AT1 receptor in patients with preeclampsia. *Can J Physiol Pharmacol.* 2003 Feb;81(2):79-83.

238. Xia Y, Wen H, Bobst S, et al. Maternal autoantibodies from preeclamptic patients activate angiotensin receptors on human trophoblast cells. *J Soc Gynecol Investig.* 2003 Feb;10(2):82-93.

239. Bobst SM, Day MC, Gilstrap LC 3rd, et al. Maternal autoantibodies from preeclamptic patients activate angiotensin receptors on human mesangial cells and induce interleukin-6 and plasminogen activator inhibitor-1 secretion. *Am J Hypertens.* 2005 Mar;18(3):330-336.

240. Dechend R, Muller DN, Wallukat G, et al. Activating auto-antibodies against the AT1 receptor in preeclampsia. *Autoimmun Rev.* 2005 Jan;4(1):61-65.

241. Dragun D, Muller DN, Brasen JH, et al. Angiotensin II type 1-receptor activating antibodies in renal-allograft rejection. *N Engl J Med.* 2005 Feb 10;352(6):558-569.

242. Kutteh WH, Rote NS, Silver R. Antiphospholipid antibodies and reproduction: The antiphospholipid antibody syndrome. *Am J Reprod Immunol.* 1999 Feb;41(2):133-152.

243. Nishiguchi T, Kobayashi T. Antiphospholipid syndrome: Characteristics and obstetrical management. *Curr Drug Targets.* 2005 Aug;6(5):593-605.

244. Wu S, Stephenson MD. Obstetrical antiphospholipid syndrome. *Semin Reprod Med.* 2006 Feb;24(1):40-53.

245. Zurgil N, Bakimer R, Tincani A, et al. Detection of anti-phospholipid and anti-DNA antibodies and their idiotypes in newborns of mothers with anti-phospholipid syndrome and SLE. *Lupus.* 1993 Aug;2(4):233-237.

246. el-Roeiy A, Gleicher N, Isenberg D, et al. A common anti-DNA idiotype and other autoantibodies in sera of offspring of mothers with systemic lupus erythematosus. *Clin Exp Immunol.* 1987 Jun;68(3):528-534. PMC 1542743.

247. Silver RK, MacGregor SN, Pasternak JF, et al. Fetal stroke associated with elevated maternal anti-cardiolipin antibodies. *Obstet Gynecol.* 1992 Sep;80(3 Pt 2):497-499.

248. Pierangeli SS, Girardi G, Vega-Ostertag M, et al. Requirement of activation of complement C3 and C5 for antiphospholipid antibody-mediated thrombophilia. *Arthritis Rheum.* 2005 Jul;52(7):2120-2124.

249. Girardi G, Redecha P, Salmon JE, et al. Heparin prevents antiphospholipid antibody-induced fetal loss by inhibiting complement activation. *Nat Med.* 2004 Nov;10(11):1222-1226.

250. Inagaki J, Kondo A, Lopez LR, et al. Pregnancy loss and endometriosis: Pathogenic role of anti-laminin-1 autoantibodies. *Ann N Y Acad Sci.* 2005 Jun;1051:174-184.

251. Klaffky EJ, Gonzales IM, Sutherland AE, et al. Trophoblast cells exhibit differential responses to laminin isoforms. *Dev Biol.* 2006 Apr 15;292(2):277-289.

252. Matalon ST, Blank M, Matsuura E, et al. Immunization of naive mice with mouse laminin-1 affected pregnancy outcome in a mouse model. *Am J Reprod Immunol.* 2003 Aug;50(2):159-165.

253. Inagaki J, Matsuura E, Nomizu M, et al. IgG anti-laminin-1 autoantibody and recurrent miscarriages. *Am J Reprod Immunol.* 2001 Apr;45(4):232-238.

254. Ludvigsson JF, Falth-Magnusson K, Ludvigsson J, et al. Tissue transglutaminase auto-antibodies in cord blood from children to become celiacs. *Scand J Gastroenterol.* 2001 Dec;36(12):1279-1283.

10

255. Eliakim R, Sherer DM. Celiac disease: Fertility and pregnancy. *Gynecol Obstet Invest*. 2001;51(1): 3-7.
256. Hager H, Gliemann J, Hamilton-Dutoit S, et al. Developmental regulation of tissue transglutaminase during human placentation and expression in neoplastic trophoblast. *J Pathol*. 1997 Jan;181(1): 106-110.
257. Robinson NJ, Glazier JD, Greenwood SL, et al. Tissue transglutaminase expression and activity in placenta. *Placenta*. 2006 Feb-Mar;27(2-3):148-157.
258. Di Simone N, Silano M, Castellani R, et al. Anti-tissue transglutaminase antibodies from celiac patients are responsible for trophoblast damage via apoptosis in vitro. *Am J Gastroenterol*. 2010 Oct;105(10):2254-2261.
259. Hoff JM, Daltveit AK, Gilhus NE, et al. Myasthenia gravis: Consequences for pregnancy, delivery, and the newborn. *Neurology*. 2003 Nov 25;61(10):1362-1366.
260. Hoff JM, Daltveit AK, Gilhus NE, et al. Asymptomatic myasthenia gravis influences pregnancy and birth. *Eur J Neurol*. 2004 Aug;11(8):559-562.
261. Ghafoor F, Mansoor M, Malik T, et al. Role of thyroid peroxidase antibodies in the outcome of pregnancy. *J Coll Physicians Surg Pak*. 2006 Jul;16(7):468-471.
262. Mecacci F, Parretti E, Cioni R, et al. Thyroid autoimmunity and its association with non-organ-specific antibodies and subclinical alterations of thyroid function in women with a history of pregnancy loss or preeclampsia. *J Reprod Immunol*. 2000 Feb;46(1):39-50.
263. Peleg D, Cada S, Peleg A, Ben-Ami M, et al. The relationship between maternal serum thyroid-stimulating immunoglobulin and fetal and neonatal thyrotoxicosis. *Obstet Gynecol*. 2002 Jun;99(6): 1040-1043.
264. Shanske AL, Bernstein L, Herzog R, et al. Chondrodysplasia punctata and maternal autoimmune disease: A new case and review of the literature. *Pediatrics*. 2007 Aug;120(2):e436-441.
265. Schulz SW, Bober M, Johnson C, et al. Maternal mixed connective tissue disease and offspring with chondrodysplasia punctata. *Semin Arthritis Rheum*. 2010 Apr;39(5):410-416. PMC 2844477.
266. Chitayat D, Keating S, Zand DJ, et al. Chondrodysplasia punctata associated with maternal autoimmune diseases: Expanding the spectrum from systemic lupus erythematosus (SLE) to mixed connective tissue disease (MCTD) and scleroderma report of eight cases. *Am J Med Genet A*. 2008 Dec 1;146A(23):3038-3053.
267. Curry CJ. Chondrodysplasia punctata associated with maternal collagen vascular disease. A new etiology? David W Smith Workshop on Morphogenesis and Malformations; Mont Tremblant, Quebec 1993.
268. Viskari H, Ludvigsson J, Uibo R, et al. Relationship between the incidence of type 1 diabetes and maternal enterovirus antibodies: Time trends and geographical variation. *Diabetologia*. 2005 Jul;48(7):1280-1287.
269. Sadeharju K, Hamalainen AM, Knip M, et al. Enterovirus infections as a risk factor for type I diabetes: Virus analyses in a dietary intervention trial. *Clin Exp Immunol*. 2003 May;132(2): 271-277.
270. Harkonen T, Paananen A, Lankinen H, et al. Enterovirus infection may induce humoral immune response reacting with islet cell autoantigens in humans. *J Med Virol*. 2003 Mar;69(3):426-440.
271. Green I, Inkelas M, Allen LB. Hodgkin's disease: A maternal-to fetal lymphocyte chimaera? *The Lancet*. 1960;1:30-32.
272. Desai RG, Creger WP. Maternofetal passage of leukocytes and platelets in man. *Blood*. 1963;21(6):665-673.
273. Lo ES, Lo YM, Hjelm NM, et al. Transfer of nucleated maternal cells into fetal circulation during the second trimester of pregnancy [letter; comment]. *Br J Haematol*. 1998;100(3):605-606.
274. Piotrowski P, Croy BA. Maternal cells are widely distributed in murine fetuses in utero. *Biol Reprod*. 1996;54(5):1103-1110.
275. Berry SM, Hassan SS, Russell E, et al. Association of maternal histocompatibility at class II HLA loci with maternal microchimerism in the fetus. *Pediatr Res*. 2004 Jul;56(1):73-78.
276. Lambert NC, Erickson TD, Yan Z, et al. Quantification of maternal microchimerism by HLA-specific real-time polymerase chain reaction: Studies of healthy women and women with scleroderma. *Arthritis Rheum*. 2004;50(3):906-914.
277. Zarou DM, Lichtman HC, Hellman LM. The transmission of chromium-51 tagged maternal erythrocytes from mother to fetus. *Am J Obstet Gynecol*. 1964 Mar 1;88:565-571.
278. Petit T, Gluckman E, Carosella E, et al. A highly sensitive polymerase chain reaction method reveals the ubiquitous presence of maternal cells in human umbilical cord blood. *Exp Hematol*. 1995;23(14):1601-1605.
279. Socie G, Gluckman E, Carosella E, et al. Search for maternal cells in human umbilical cord blood by polymerase chain reaction amplification of two minisatellite sequences. *Blood*. 1994;83(2): 340-344.
280. Lo YM, Lo ES, Watson N, et al. Two-way cell traffic between mother and fetus: Biologic and clinical implications. *Blood*. 1996;88(11):4390-4395.
281. Lo YM. Fetal DNA in maternal plasma. *Ann N Y Acad Sci*. 2000;906:141-147.
282. Loubiere LS, Lambert NC, Flinn LJ, et al. Maternal microchimerism in healthy adults in lymphocytes, monocyte/macrophages and NK cells. *Lab Invest*. 2006 Nov;86(11):1185-1192.
283. Reed AM, McNallan K, Wettstein P, et al. Does HLA-dependent chimerism underlie the pathogenesis of juvenile dermatomyositis? *J Immunol*. 2004;172(8):5041-5046.

10

284. Artlett CM, Ramos R, Jiminez SA, et al. Chimeric cells of maternal origin in juvenile idiopathic inflammatory myopathies. Childhood Myositis Heterogeneity Collaborative Group. *Lancet*. 2000; 356(9248):2155-2156.

285. Keller MA, Rodgriguez AL, Alvarez S, et al. Transfer of tuberculin immunity from mother to infant. *Pediatr Res*. 1987 Sep;22(3):277-281.

286. Osada S, Horibe K, Oiwa K, et al. A case of infantile acute monocytic leukemia caused by vertical transmission of the mother's leukemic cells. *Cancer*. 1990;65(5):1146-1149.

287. Catlin EA, Roberts JD Jr, Erana R, et al. Transplacental transmission of natural-killer-cell lymphoma. *N Engl J Med*. 1999;341(2):85-91.

288. Tolar J, Coad JE, Neglia JP. Transplacental transfer of small-cell carcinoma of the lung. *N Engl J Med*. 2002;346(19):1501-1502.

289. Alexander A, Samlowski WE, Grossman D, et al. Metastatic melanoma in pregnancy: Risk of transplacental metastases in the infant. *J Clin Oncol*. 2003 Jun 1;21(11):2179-2186.

290. Stevens AM, Hermes HM, Rutledge JC, et al. Myocardial-tissue-specific phenotype of maternal microchimerism in neonatal lupus congenital heart block. *Lancet*. 2003 Nov 15;362(9396): 1617-1623.

291. Stevens AM, Mullarkey ME, Pang JM, et al. Differentiated maternal and fetal cells in tissues from patients with and without autoimmune disease. *Arthritis Rheumatism*. [Abstract]. 2003;48:S511.

292. Khosrotehrani K, Guegan S, Fraitag S, et al. Presence of chimeric maternally derived keratinocytes in cutaneous inflammatory diseases of children: The example of pityriasis lichenoides. *J Invest Dermatol*. 2006 Feb;126(2):345-348.

293. Sugimoto H, Mundel TM, Sund M, et al. Bone-marrow-derived stem cells repair basement membrane collagen defects and reverse genetic kidney disease. *Proc Natl Acad Sci U S A*. 2006 May 9;103(19):7321-7326.

294. Holzgreve W, Ghezzi F, Di Naro E, et al. Disturbed feto-maternal cell traffic in preeclampsia. *Obstet Gynecol*. 1998;91(5 Pt 1):669-672.

295. Smid M, Vassallo A, Lagona F, et al. Quantitative analysis of fetal DNA in maternal plasma in pathological conditions associated with placental abnormalities. *Ann NY Acad Sci*. 2001;945:132-137.

296. Zhong XY, Laivuori H, Livingston JC, et al. Elevation of both maternal and fetal extracellular circulating deoxyribonucleic acid concentrations in the plasma of pregnant women with preeclampsia. *Am J Obstet Gynecol*. 2001;184(3):414-419.

297. Bianchi DW, Farina A, Weber W, et al. Significant fetal-maternal hemorrhage after termination of pregnancy: Implications for development of fetal cell microchimerism. *Am J Obstet Gynecol*. 2001; 184(4):703-706.

298. Lo YM, Lau TK, Zhang J, et al. Increased fetal DNA concentrations in the plasma of pregnant women carrying fetuses with trisomy 21. *Clin Chem*. 1999;45(10):1747-1751.

299. Kaplan J, Land S. Influence of maternal-fetal histocompatibility and MHC zygosity on maternal microchimerism. *J Immunol*. 2005 Jun 1;174(11):7123-7128.

300. Lambert NC, Evans PC, Hashizumi TL, et al. Cutting edge: Persistent fetal microchimerism in T lymphocytes is associated with HLA-DQA1*0501: Implications in autoimmunity. *J Immunol*. 2000;164(11):5545-5548.

301. Stevens AM, Hermes H, Tylee T, et al. Maternal microchimerism in the human thymus. *Arthritis Rheumatism*. [Abstract]. 2001;44(9):S340.

302. Marrack P, Kappler J. Control of T cell viability. *Annu Rev Immunol*. 2004;22:765-787.

303. van Dijk BA, Boomsma DI, de Man AJ. Blood group chimerism in human multiple births is not rare. *AmJ Med Genet*. 1996;61(3):264-268.

304. Kuhl-Burmeister R, Simeoni E, Weber-Matthiesen K, et al. Equal distribution of congenital blood cell chimerism in dizygotic triplets after in-vitro fertilization. *Hum Reprod*. 2000 May;15(5): 1200-1204.

305. Hall JG. Twinning. *Lancet*. 2003;362(9385):735-743.

306. Stevens AM, Hermes HM, Lambert NC, et al. Maternal and sibling microchimerism in twins and triplets discordant for neonatal lupus syndrome-congenital heart block. *Rheumatology (Oxford)*. 2005 Feb;44(2):187-191.

307. Sudik R, Jakubiczka S, Nawroth F, et al. Chimerism in a fertile woman with 46,XY karyotype and female phenotype. *Hum Reprod*. 2001 Jan;16(1):56-58.

308. Bianchi DW, Zickwolf GK, Weil GJ, et al. Male fetal progenitor cells persist in maternal blood for as long as 27 years postpartum. *Proc Natl Acad Sci U S A*. 1996;93(2):705-708.

309. Lambert NC, Pang JM, Yan Z, et al. Male microchimerism in women with systemic sclerosis and healthy women who have never given birth to a son. *Ann Rheum Dis*. 2005 Jun;64(6):845-848. PMC 1755528.

310. Yan Z, Lambert NC, Guthrie KA, et al. Male microchimerism in women without sons: Quantitative assessment and correlation with pregnancy history. *Am J Med*. 2005 Aug;118(8):899-906.

311. Guettier C, Sebagh M, Buard J, et al. Male cell microchimerism in normal and diseased female livers from fetal life to adulthood. *Hepatology*. 2005 Jul;42(1):35-43.

312. Lo ES, Lo YM, Hjelm NM, et al. Transfer of nucleated maternal cells into fetal circulation during the second trimester of pregnancy. *Br J Haematol*. 1998 Mar;100(3):605-606.

313. Carrier E, Lee TH, Busch MP, et al. Induction of tolerance in nondefective mice after in utero transplantation of major histocompatibility complex-mismatched fetal hematopoietic stem cells. *Blood*. 1995 Dec 15;86(12):4681-4690.

10

10

314. Hayward A, Ambruso D, Battaglia F, et al. Microchimerism and tolerance following intrauterine transplantation and transfusion for alpha-thalassemia-1. *Fetal Diagn Ther*. 1998 Jan-Feb;13(1): 8-14.

315. Peranteau WH, Hayashi S, Hsieh M, et al. High-level allogeneic chimerism achieved by prenatal tolerance induction and postnatal nonmyeloablative bone marrow transplantation. *Blood*. 2002 Sep 15;100(6):2225-2234.

316. Vietor HE, Hallensleben E, van Bree SP, et al. Survival of donor cells 25 years after intrauterine transfusion. *Blood*. 2000 Apr 15;95(8):2709-2714.

317. Kim HB, Shaaban AF, Milner R, et al. In utero bone marrow transplantation induces donor-specific tolerance by a combination of clonal deletion and clonal anergy. *J Pediatr Surg*. 1999 May;34(5):726-729; discussion 729-730.

318. Carrier E, Gilpin E, Lee TH, et al. Microchimerism does not induce tolerance after in utero transplantation and may lead to the development of alloreactivity. *J Lab Clin Med*. 2000; 136(3):224-235.

319. van der Veen FM, Rolink AG, Gleichmann E, et al. Autoimmune disease strongly resembling systemic lupus erythematosus (SLE) in F1 mice undergoing graft-versus-host reaction (GVHR). *Adv ExpMedBiol*. 1982;149:669-677.

320. Parkman R, Mosier D, Umansky I, et al. Graft-versus-host disease after intrauterine and exchange transfusions for hemolytic disease of the newborn. *N Engl J Med*. 1974 Feb 14;290(7):359-363.

321. Donahue J, Gilpin E, Lee TH, et al. Microchimerism does not induce tolerance and sustains immunity after in utero transplantation. *Transplantation*. 2001 Feb 15;71(3):359-368.

322. Moustafa ME, Srivastava AS, Nedelcu E, et al. Chimerism and tolerance post-in utero transplantation with embryonic stem cells. *Transplantation*. 2004 Nov 15;78(9):1274-1282.

323. Andrassy J, Kusaka S, Jankowska-Gan E, et al. Tolerance to noninherited maternal MHC antigens in mice. *J Immunol*. 2003;171(10):5554-5561.

324. Molitor ML, Haynes LD, Jankowska-Gan E, et al. HLA class I noninherited maternal antigens in cord blood and breast milk. *Hum Immunol*. 2004;65(3):231-239.

325. Davis MK. Breastfeeding and chronic disease in childhood and adolescence. *Pediatr Clin North Am*. 2001 Feb;48(1):125-141, ix.

326. Bertotto A, Castellucci G, Fabietti G, et al. Lymphocytes bearing the T cell receptor gamma delta in human breast milk. *Arch Dis Child*. 1990 Nov;65(11):1274-1275. PMC 1792611.

327. Bertotto A, Gerli R, Fabietti G, et al. Human breast milk T lymphocytes display the phenotype and functional characteristics of memory T cells. *Eur J Immunol*. 1990 Aug;20(8):1877-1880.

328. Wirt DP, Adkins LT, Palkowetz KH, et al. Activated and memory T lymphocytes in human milk. *Cytometry*. 1992;13(3):282-290.

329. Goldman AS. The immune system of human milk: Antimicrobial, antiinflammatory and immunomodulating properties. *Pediatr Infect Dis J*. 1993 Aug;12(8):664-671.

330. Losonsky GA, Ogra PL. Maternal-neonatal interactions and human breast milk. *Prog Clin Biol Res*. 1981;70:171-182.

331. Shimamura M, Huang YY, Goji H, et al. Antibody production in early life supported by maternal lymphocyte factors. *Biochim Biophys Acta*. 2003 Jan 20;1637(1):55-58.

332. Vernochet C, Caucheteux SM, Gendron MC, et al. Affinity-dependent alterations of mouse B cell development by noninherited maternal antigen. *Biol Reprod*. 2005 Feb;72(2):460-469.

333. Reber AJ, Hippen AR, Hurley DJ, et al. Effects of the ingestion of whole colostrum or cell-free colostrum on the capacity of leukocytes in newborn calves to stimulate or respond in one-way mixed leukocyte cultures. *Am J Vet Res*. 2005 Nov;66(11):1854-1860.

334. Reber AJ, Lockwood A, Hippen AR, et al. Colostrum induced phenotypic and trafficking changes in maternal mononuclear cells in a peripheral blood leukocyte model for study of leukocyte transfer to the neonatal calf. *Vet Immunol Immunopathol*. 2006 Jan 15;109(1-2):139-150.

335. Tuboly S, Bernath S. Intestinal absorption of colostral lymphoid cells in newborn animals. *Adv Exp Med Biol*. 2002;503:107-114.

336. Pollack MS, Kirkpatrick D, Kapoor N, et al. Identification by HLA typing of intrauterine-derived maternal T cells in four patients with severe combined immunodeficiency. *N Engl J Med*. 1982; 307(11):662-666.

337. Pollack MS, Kapoor N, Sorell M, et al. DR-positive maternal engrafted T cells in a severe combined immunodeficiency patient without graft-versus-host disease. *Transplantation*. 1980;30(5):331-334.

338. Thompson LF, O'Connor RD, Bastian JF, et al. Phenotype and function of engrafted maternal T cells in patients with severe combined immunodeficiency. *J Immunol*. 1984 Nov;133(5):2513-2517.

339. Knobloch C, Goldmann SF, Friedrich W, et al. Limited T cell receptor diversity of transplacentally acquired maternal T cells in severe combined immunodeficiency. *J Immunol*. 1991;146(12): 4157-4164.

340. Muller SM, Ege M, Pottharst A, et al. Transplacentally acquired maternal T lymphocytes in severe combined immunodeficiency: A study of 121 patients. *Blood*. 2001 Sep 15;98(6):1847-1851.

341. Wahn V, Yokota S, Meyer KL, et al. Expansion of a maternally derived monoclonal T cell population with CD3+/CD8+/T cell receptor-gamma/delta+ phenotype in a child with severe combined immunodeficiency. *J Immunol*. 1991 Nov 1;147(9):2934-2941.

342. Zhou M, Mellor AL. Expanded cohorts of maternal CD8+ T-cells specific for paternal MHC class I accumulate during pregnancy. *J Reprod Immunol*. 1998 Oct;40(1):47-62.

343. Lambert N, Erickson T. Fetal and maternal microchimerism are simultaneously present in multiple organs in systemic sclerosis: A quantitative study. *Arthritis Rheum*. 2003;46(9S).

344. Morse JH, Barst RJ, Whitman HH, 3rd, Fotino M, Jacobs JC, et al. Isolated pulmonary hypertension in the grandchild of a kindred with scleroderma (systemic sclerosis): "Neonatal scleroderma"? *J Rheumatol.* 1989 Dec;16(12):1536-1541.

345. Barba A, Rosina P, Chieregato C, et al. Morphoea in a newborn boy. *Br J Dermatol.* 1999 Feb;140(2):365-366.

346. Ohtaki N, Miyamoto C, Orita M, et al. Concurrent multiple morphea and neonatal lupus erythematosus in an infant boy born to a mother with SLE. *Br J Dermatol.* 1986 Jul;115(1):85-90.

347. Sato S, Ishida W, Takehara K, et al. A case of juvenile systemic sclerosis with disease onset at six months old. *Clin Rheumatol.* 2003 May;22(2):162-163.

348. Brucato A, Doria A, Frassi M, et al. Pregnancy outcome in 100 women with autoimmune diseases and anti-Ro/SSA antibodies: A prospective controlled study. *Lupus.* 2002;11(11):716-721.

349. Reed A, Picinorell YJ, Harwood A, et al. Chimerism in children with juvenile dermatomyositis. *Lancet.* 2000;356:2156-2157.

350. Harney S, Newton J, Milicic A, et al. Non-inherited maternal HLA alleles are associated with rheumatoid arthritis. *Rheumatology (Oxford).* 2003;42(1):171-174.

351. Kowalzick L, Artlett CM, Thoss K, et al. Chronic graft-versus-host-disease-like dermopathy in a child with CD4+ cell microchimerism. *Dermatology.* 2005;210(1):68-71.

352. Vajsar J, Jay V, Babyn P. Infantile myositis presenting in the neonatal period. *Brain Dev.* 1996 Sep-Oct;18(5):415-419.

353. McNeil SM, Woulfe J, Ross C, et al. Congenital inflammatory myopathy: A demonstrative case and proposed diagnostic classification. *Muscle Nerve.* 2002 Feb;25(2):259-264.

354. Morrow J, Nelson J, Watts R, et al. The Immune System-Order and Disorder, In: Morrow J, editor. *Autoimmune Rheumatic Disease.* New York: Oxford University Press; 1999.

355. Stevens AM, Tsao BP, Hahn BH, et al. Maternal HLA class II compatibility in men with systemic lupus erythematosus. *Arthritis Rheum.* 2005 Sep;52(9):2768-2773.

356. Barrera P, Balsa A, Alves H, et al. Noninherited maternal antigens do not increase the susceptibility for familial rheumatoid arthritis. European Consortium on Rheumatoid Arthritis Families (ECRAF). *J Rheumatol.* 2001 May;28(5):968-974.

357. van Rood JJ, Claas F. Noninherited maternal HLA antigens: A proposal to elucidate their role in the immune response. *Hum Immunol.* 2000 Dec;61(12):1390-1394.

358. Barrera P, Balsa A, Alves H, et al. Noninherited maternal antigens do not play a role in rheumatoid arthritis susceptibility in Europe. European Consortium on Rheumatoid Arthritis Families. *Arthritis Rheum.* 2000 Apr;43(4):758-764.

359. van der Horst-Bruinsma IE, Hazes JM, Schreuder GM, et al. Influence of non-inherited maternal HLA-DR antigens on susceptibility to rheumatoid arthritis. *Ann Rheum Dis.* 1998 Nov;57(11): 672-675.

360. Guthrie KA, Tishkevich NR, Nelson JL, et al. Non-inherited maternal human leukocyte antigen alleles in susceptibility to familial rheumatoid arthritis. *Ann Rheum Dis.* 2009 Jan;68(1):107-109. PMC 2760537.

361. Lee LA, Bias WB, Arnett FC Jr, et al. Immunogenetics of the neonatal lupus syndrome. *Ann Intern Med.* 1983;99(5):592-596.

362. Watson RM, Lane AT, Barnett NK, et al. Neonatal lupus erythematosus. A clinical, serological and immunogenetic study with review of the literature. *Medicine (Baltimore).* 1984;63(6):362-378.

363. Brucato A, Franceschini F, Gasparini M, et al. Isolated congenital complete heart block: Longterm outcome of mothers, maternal antibody specificity and immunogenetic background. *J Rheumatol.* 1995;22(3):533-540.

364. Siren MK, Julkunen H, Kaaja R, et al. Role of HLA in congenital heart block: Susceptibility alleles in mothers. *Lupus.* 1999;8(1):52-59.

365. Colombo G, Brucato A, Coluccio E, et al. DNA typing of maternal HLA in congenital complete heart block: Comparison with systemic lupus erythematosus and primary Sjogren's syndrome. *Arthritis Rheum.* 1999;42(8):1757-1764.

366. Matsuoka K, Ichinohe T, Hashimoto D, et al. Fetal tolerance to maternal antigens improves the outcome of allogeneic bone marrow transplantation by a CD4+ CD25+ T-cell-dependent mechanism. *Blood.* 2006 Jan 1;107(1):404-409.

367. Owen RD, Wood HR, Foord AG, et al. Evidence for actively acquired tolerance to Rh antigens. *Proc Natl Acad Sci U S A.* 1954 Jun;40(6):420-424. PMC 534062.

368. Claas FH, Gijbels Y, Munck VDV-D, et al. Induction of B cell unresponsiveness to noninherited maternal HLA antigens during fetal life. *Science.* 1988;241(4874):1815-1817.

369. van den Boogaardt DE, van Rood JJ, Roelen DL, et al. The influence of inherited and noninherited parental antigens on outcome after transplantation. *Transpl Int.* 2006 May;19(5):360-371.

370. Opelz G. Analysis of the "NIMA effect" in renal transplantation. Collaborative Transplant Study. *Clin Transpl.* 1990:63-67.

371. Sakaguchi S. Naturally arising Foxp3-expressing CD25+CD4+ regulatory T cells in immunological tolerance to self and non-self. *Nat Immunol.* 2005 Apr;6(4):345-352.

372. Maggi E, Cosmi L, Liotta F, et al. Thymic regulatory T cells. *Autoimmun Rev.* 2005 Nov;4(8): 579-586.

373. Chatila TA. Role of regulatory T cells in human diseases. *J Allergy Clin Immunol.* 2005 Nov;116(5):949-959; quiz 960.

374. Cupedo T, Nagasawa M, Weijer K, et al. Development and activation of regulatory T cells in the human fetus. *Eur J Immunol.* 2005 Feb;35(2):383-390.

10

375. Piccirillo CA, Letterio JJ, Thornton AM, et al. CD4(+)CD25(+) regulatory T cells can mediate suppressor function in the absence of transforming growth factor beta1 production and responsiveness. *J Exp Med.* 2002 Jul 15;196(2):237-246. PMC 2193919.

376. Schaub B, Campo M, He H, et al. Neonatal immune responses to TLR2 stimulation: Influence of maternal atopy on Foxp3 and IL-10 expression. *Respir Res.* 2006;7:40. PMC 1435749.

377. Somerset DA, Zheng Y, Kilby MD, et al. Normal human pregnancy is associated with an elevation in the immune suppressive CD25+ CD4+ regulatory T-cell subset. *Immunology.* 2004 May;112(1):38-43. PMC 1782465.

378. Godfrey WR, Spoden DJ, Ge YG, et al. Cord blood CD4(+)CD25(+)-derived T regulatory cell lines express FoxP3 protein and manifest potent suppressor function. *Blood.* 2005 Jan 15;105(2):750-758.

379. Wing K, Larsson P, Sandstrom K, et al. CD4+ CD25+ FOXP3+ regulatory T cells from human thymus and cord blood suppress antigen-specific T cell responses. *Immunology.* 2005 Aug;115(4):516-525. PMC 1782183.

10

CHAPTER 11

CMV: Diagnosis, Treatment, and Considerations on Vaccine-Mediated Prevention

Shannon A. Ross, MD, MSPH, and Suresh B. Boppana, MD

- **The Virus**
- **Epidemiology**
- **Transmission of CMV**
- **Pathogenesis**
- **Immune Response to Infection**
- **Pathogenesis of Congenital Infection**
- **Pathology**
- **Clinical Manifestations**
- **Laboratory Diagnosis**
- **Diagnosis During Pregnancy**
- **Treatment**
- **Prognosis**
- **Prevention**

The Virus

CMV (human herpesvirus 5) is the largest and most complex member of the family of herpesviruses. The virion consists of three regions: the capsid containing the double-stranded DNA viral genome, the tegument, and the envelope. The viral genome consists of more than 235 kilobase pairs, which contain more than 252 open reading frames.[1] The complexity of the genetic makeup of CMV confers extensive genetic variability among strains. Restriction fragment length polymorphism analysis, as well as DNA sequence analysis, has demonstrated that no two clinical isolates are alike.[2] The viral tegument contains viral proteins that function to maintain the structural integrity of the virion, are important for assembly of an infectious particle, and are involved in regulatory activities in the replicative cycle of the virus. The viral envelope contains eight glycoproteins that have been described, as well as an unknown number of additional proteins. The most abundant envelope glycoproteins are the gM/gN, gB, and gH/gL/gO complexes, all of which are important for virus infectivity. In addition, gB, gH, and gM/gN have been shown to induce an antibody response in the infected host and are major components of the protective response of the infected host to the virus.[3,4]

Epidemiology

Cytomegalovirus infections have been recognized in all human populations. CMV is acquired early in life in most populations, with the exception of people in the economically well developed countries of northern Europe and North America.

Patterns of CMV acquisition vary greatly on the basis of geographic and socio-economic backgrounds, and seroprevalence generally increases with age. Studies have shown that most preschool children (>90%) in South America, Sub-Saharan Africa, East Asia, and India are CMV antibody positive.[5] In contrast, seroepidemiologic surveys in Great Britain and in the United States have found that less than 20% of children of similar age are seropositive.[5] A recent study of CMV seroprevalence that utilized samples from the National Health and Examination Survey (NHANES) 1988–2004 showed that overall age-adjusted CMV seroprevalence in the United States was 50.4%.[6] That study also showed that CMV seroprevalence was higher among non-Hispanic black children and Mexican-American children compared with non-Hispanic white children.[6]

Transmission of CMV

Although the exact mode of CMV acquisition is unknown, it is assumed to be acquired through direct contact with body fluids from an infected person. Breast-feeding, group care of children, crowded living conditions, and sexual activity have all been associated with high rates of CMV infection. Sources of the virus include oropharyngeal secretions, urine, cervical and vaginal secretions, semen, breast milk, blood products, and allografts (Table 11-1). Presumably, exposure to saliva and other body fluids containing infectious virus is a primary mode of spread because infected infants typically excrete significant amounts of CMV for months to years following infection. Even older children and adults shed virus for prolonged periods (>6 months) following primary CMV infection. In addition, a significant proportion of seropositive individuals continue to shed virus intermittently. An important determinant of the frequency of congenital and perinatal CMV infection is the seroprevalence rate in women of child-bearing age. Studies from the United States and Europe have shown that the seropositivity rates in young women range from less than 50% to 85%.[5,6] In contrast, most women of child-bearing age in less developed regions are CMV antibody positive.[7,8]

Vertical Transmission

CMV can be transmitted from mother to child transplacentally, during birth, and in the postpartum period via breast milk. Congenital CMV infection rates are directly related to maternal seroprevalence rates (Table 11-2). Rates of congenital CMV infection are higher in developing countries and among low-income groups in developed

Table 11-1 SOURCES AND ROUTES OF TRANSMISSION OF CMV INFECTION

Mode of Exposure and Transmission	
Community Acquired	
Age Perinatal	Intrauterine fetal infection (congenital); intrapartum exposure to virus; breast milk acquired; mother-to-infant transmission
Infancy and childhood	Exposure to saliva and other body fluids; child-to-child transmission
Adolescence and adulthood	Exposure to young children; sexual transmission; possible occupational exposures
Hospital Acquired	
Source Blood products	Blood products from seropositive donors; multiple transfusions; white blood cell containing blood products
Allograft recipients	Allograft from seropositive donors

Reproduced with permission from Boppana SB, Fowler KB. Persistence in the population: Epidemiology and transmission. In: Arvin A, Campadelli-Fiume G, Mocarski E, et al, eds. *Human Herpesviruses*. Cambridge: Cambridge University Press; 2007.

Table 11-2 RATES OF MATERNAL CMV SEROPREVALENCE AND CONGENITAL CMV INFECTION IN DIFFERENT POPULATIONS

Location	Maternal CMV Seroprevalence, %	Congenital CMV Infection, %
Aarhus-Viborg, Denmark	52	0.4
Abidjan, Ivory Coast	100	1.4
Birmingham, United States		
Low income	77	1.25
Middle income	36	0.53
Hamilton, Ontario, Canada	44	0.42
London, United Kingdom	56	0.3
Seoul, South Korea	96	1.2
New Delhi, India	99	2.1
Ribeirão Preto, Brazil	96	1.1
Sukuta, The Gambia	96	5.4

countries.[7-9] Although the reasons for this increased rate of congenital CMV in populations with high seroprevalence rates are not clear, recent demonstration that infection with new or different virus strains occurs commonly in previously seropositive individuals in a variety of settings suggests that frequent exposure to CMV could be an important determinant of maternal reinfection and subsequent intrauterine transmission.[10-12] Studies of risk factors for congenital CMV infection showed that young maternal age, nonwhite race, single marital status, and history of sexually transmitted disease (STD) have been associated with increased rates of congenital CMV infection.[13]

Preexisting Maternal Immunity and Intrauterine Transmission

The factors responsible for transmission and severity of congenital CMV infection are not well understood. Unlike rubella and toxoplasmosis, for which intrauterine transmission occurs only as a result of primary infection acquired during pregnancy, congenital CMV infection has been shown to occur in children born to mothers who have had CMV infection before pregnancy (nonprimary infection).[7,8,14] Preexisting maternal CMV seroimmunity provides significant protection against intrauterine transmission; however, this protection is incomplete. Birth prevalence of congenital CMV infection is directly related to maternal seroprevalence rates such that higher rates are seen in populations with higher CMV seroprevalence in women of childbearing age.[15] As depicted in Figure 11-1, the rate of transplacental transmission of CMV decreases from 25% to 40% in mothers with primary infection during pregnancy to less than 2% in women with preexisting seroimmunity. Although the reasons for failure of maternal immunity to provide complete protection against intrauterine transmission are not well defined, recent studies examining strain-specific antibody responses have suggested that reinfection with a different strain of CMV can lead to intrauterine transmission and symptomatic congenital infection.[10,11] It was previously thought that maternal immunity also provides protection against symptomatic CMV infection and long-term sequelae in congenitally infected infants.[16] However, recent accumulation data, especially from studies in highly seropositive populations, suggest that once intrauterine transmission occurs, preexisting maternal immunity may not modify the severity of fetal infection and the frequency of long-term sequelae.[7,8,14,17,18]

Intrapartum Transmission

Transmission of CMV during delivery occurs in approximately 50% of infants born to mothers shedding CMV from the cervix or vagina at the time of delivery.[19] Genital

11

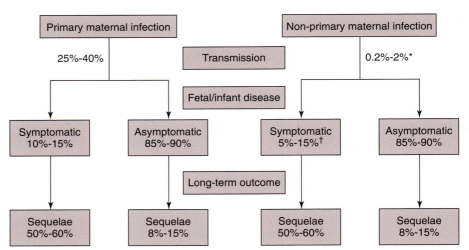

Figure 11-1   Schematic representation of consequences of cytomegalovirus (CMV) infection during pregnancy. *The transmission rate varies depending on the population. Transmission rates are as high as 2% in women of lower income groups, whereas women from middle and upper income groups have rates less than 0.2%. †The exact prevalence of symptomatic infection following nonprimary maternal infection is not well defined. However, studies of newborn CMV screening in populations with high maternal seroprevalence demonstrate that the rates of symptomatic infection are similar to those observed following primary maternal CMV infection.

tract shedding of CMV has been associated with younger age, other STDs, and a greater number of sexual partners.[20]

Postnatal Transmission

Breast-feeding practices have a major influence on the epidemiology of postnatal CMV infection.[21] CMV has been detected in breast milk in 13% to 50% of lactating women tested with conventional virus isolation techniques.[22] Recent studies utilizing the more sensitive polymerase chain reaction (PCR) technology have demonstrated the presence of CMV DNA in breast milk from more than 90% of seropositive women.[23] The early appearance of viral DNA in milk whey, the presence of infectious virus in milk whey, and a higher viral load in breast milk have been shown to be risk factors for transmission of CMV infection.[23] Treating maternal milk by freeze-storing or pasteurization has been shown to reduce the viral load; however, transmission of CMV to infants that have received treated milk has been documented.[24]

Nosocomial Transmission

Blood products and transplanted organs are the most important vehicles of transmission of CMV in the hospital setting; the latter are unlikely to be of concern during pregnancy. Transmission of CMV through packed red blood cell, leukocyte, and platelet transfusions poses a risk of severe disease for seronegative small premature infants and immunocompromised patients. Prevention of blood product transmission of CMV can be achieved by using seronegative donors or special filters that remove white blood cells. Person-to-person transmission of CMV requires contact with infected body fluids and therefore should be prevented by routine hospital infection control precautions. Studies in health care settings found no evidence of increased risk of CMV infection in settings in which patients shedding CMV are encountered.[25]

Pathogenesis

The pathogenesis of CMV infection in the naïve host has been characterized in human and animal models.[26,27] After entry into a naïve host, cytomegalovirus infection induces a primary viremia, with initial viral replication occurring in reticuloendothelial organs (liver and spleen). Secondary viremia subsequently ensues with viral dissemination to end organs. In healthy humans, both primary and secondary viremia may be asymptomatic, or secondary viremia may be associated with mononucleosis-like symptoms such as fever, transaminase elevation, and atypical lymphocytosis.

After immune-mediated clearance of acute viremia, the immunocompetent host may remain asymptomatic for life. Reservoirs of latent infection are not clearly defined but are thought to include monocytes and marrow progenitors of myeloid lineage, as well as possibly endothelium and secretory glandular epithelium such as salivary, breast, prostate, and renal epithelium.[28] Control of latency and reactivation is not well understood and has been intensively studied both in vitro and in animal models. It is believed that viral reactivation occurs intermittently in the immuno-competent host but fails to induce clinical disease secondary to intact immune control mechanisms. Up to 10% of the memory T lymphocyte repertoire may be directed against CMV in the healthy host, and immune senescence ("T cell exhaustion") may contribute to susceptibility to reactivation and reduced immunity to other infections among the elderly.[29,30]

Immune Response to Infection

The innate immune system, particularly natural killer (NK) cells, is responsible for initial control of viremia in the normal host. Animal models demonstrate that activation of NK cells by virus-infected host cells contributes to viral clearance.[31] Consistent with this, patients with NK cell deficiencies may develop life-threatening CMV disease, as well as disease from other herpesviruses.[32] Long-term control of CMV is maintained by adaptive immunity. Serum antibodies against CMV gB, gM/gN, and gH neutralize infection in vitro.[3,4,33] IgM and IgG titers are used to determine clinical immunity and history of past infection. IgM is an indicator of recent infection, although IgM may persist for many months after primary infection. In addition, IgM antibodies can appear during reactivation of CMV infection. However, hypogam-maglobulinemia does not appear to be a risk factor for severe CMV disease, except in conjunction with other forms of immunosuppression (e.g., transplant recipients). CMV-specific T lymphocytes are critical for long-term control of chronic infection.

Pathogenesis of Congenital Infection

The pathogenesis of central nervous system (CNS) disease and sequelae, including hearing loss, in congenital CMV infection is not well understood. Few autopsy specimens are available for study, and because of the species specificity of the virus, human congenital CMV infection lacks a well-developed animal model that truly emulates human disease. Imaging studies of infants and children with congenital CMV infection reveal a variety of CNS abnormalities including periventricular cal-cifications, ventriculomegaly, and loss of white-gray matter demarcations.[34] Histo-logic examination from CMV-infected fetuses has demonstrated evidence of virus by immunohistochemical staining for CMV proteins in a variety of brain tissues, includ-ing cortex, white matter, germinal matrix, neurons of the basal ganglia and thalamus, ependyma, endothelium, and leptomeningeal epithelial cells. In most cases, virus was accompanied by an inflammatory response, sometimes severe and associated with necrosis.[35] These findings together suggest that lytic infection, as well as inflam-mation in response to infection, contributes to the pathology in CNS infection. The neurologic manifestations are unique in congenital CMV infection, leading to the hypothesis that the immature brain is more susceptible to infection. Animal models have supported this theory, wherein infection of the developing CNS leads to wide-spread lytic virus replication in neuronal progenitor cells of the subventricular gray area and endothelium.[36,37]

A few temporal bones from congenitally infected children have been studied and described in the literature. Specimens displayed evidence of endolabyrinthitis, and virus has been isolated from the endolymph and the perilymph. Cochlear and vestibular findings were variable, ranging from an occasional inclusion-bearing cell within or adjacent to sensory epithelium of the cochlea or vestibular system to more extensive involvement of the nonsensory epithelium. It is interesting to note that inflammatory cell infiltrates were minimal and were reported in only three cases.[38] In contrast to the findings in infants, a study of the temporal bones from a 14-year-old with severe congenital CMV infection revealed extensive cellular degeneration, fibrosis, and calcifications in the cochlea and the vestibular system.[39] Studies in the guinea pig model of congenital CMV infection have shed some additional information on the possible mechanisms of CMV-related hearing loss and have demonstrated not only that viral gene expression was a prerequisite for damage to the inner ear and auditory abnormalities, but that an intact host immune response was required.[40]

From these studies in animal models and from limited studies of human temporal bones, two mechanisms of hearing loss in congenital CMV infection are suggested. The presence of viral antigens or inclusions in the cochlea and/or the vestibular apparatus of human temporal bones suggests that CMV can readily infect both the epithelium and neural cells in the inner ear, and that hearing loss can occur as a result of direct virus-mediated damage to neural tissue. Alternatively, the host-derived inflammatory responses secondary to viral infection in the inner ear could be responsible for damage leading to sensorineural hearing loss (SNHL).

Because of the great variability of CMV clinical strains, diversity within a host could play a role in outcome in congenital CMV infection. A recent study in 28 children with congenital CMV demonstrated that approximately 1/3 of the infants harbored multiple CMV strains in the saliva, urine, and blood within the first few weeks of life. Interestingly, four infants demonstrated distinct CMV strains in different compartments of shedding.[41] The relationship of specific genotypes and the implications of infection with multiple viral strains in the pathogenesis of CMV sequelae is currently under investigation.

Pathology

Cytomegalovirus was originally named for the cytomegalic changes and intracellular inclusions observed within infected cells during histologic analysis of infected tissues. The classic histologic finding in CMV pathology is the "owl's eye" nucleus, which is a large intranuclear basophilic viral inclusion spanning half the nuclear diameter, surrounded by a clear intranuclear halo beneath the nuclear membrane. Smaller cytoplasmic basophilic inclusions may also be seen in infected cells. Infected cell types include epithelial and endothelial cells, neurons, and macrophages, and can be found in biopsies of numerous tissues, including brain, lung, liver, salivary glands, and kidneys. CMV-infected tissues may show minimal inflammation or may demonstrate an interstitial mononuclear infiltrate with focal necrosis. In the intestine, CMV may induce ulceration and pseudomembrane formation. In congenital infection, chorioretinitis may be found in the eye, and pathologic findings in the central nervous system include microcephaly, focal calcifications, ventricular dilatation, cysts, and lenticulostriate vasculopathy.

Clinical Manifestations

Pregnancy

Most CMV infections in healthy pregnant women are asymptomatic. A small proportion of patients may have symptoms, which can include a mononucleosis-like syndrome with fever, malaise, myalgia, sore throat, lymphocytosis, lymphadenopathy, pharyngeal erythema, and hepatic dysfunction.[19]

Congenital Infection

Of the 20,000 to 40,000 children born with congenital CMV infection each year, most (approximately 85% to 90%) exhibit no clinical abnormalities at birth (asymptomatic congenital CMV infection). The remaining 10% to 15% are born with clinical abnormalities and thus are classified as having clinically apparent or symptomatic congenital infection. The infection involves multiple organ systems with a particular predilection for the reticuloendothelial and central nervous systems (Table 11-3).

Table 11-3   CLINICAL FINDINGS IN 106 INFANTS WITH SYMPTOMATIC CONGENITAL CMV INFECTION IN THE NEWBORN PERIOD

Abnormality	Positive/Total Examined, %
Prematurity[a]	36/106 (34)
Small for gestational age[b]	56/106 (50)
Petechiae	80/106 (76)
Jaundice	69/103 (67)
Hepatosplenomegaly	63/105 (60)
Purpura	14/105 (13)
Microcephaly[c]	54/102 (53)
Lethargy/hypotonia	25/104 (27)
Poor suck	20/103 (19)
Seizures	7/105 (7)

Adapted from Boppana SB, Pass RF, Britt WJ, et al. Symptomatic congenital cytomegalovirus infection: Neonatal morbidity and mortality. *Pediatr Infect Dis J.* 1992;11:93-99, with permission.
[a]Gestational age less than 38 weeks.
[b]Weight less than 10th percentile for gestational age.
[c]Head circumference less than 10th percentile.

The most commonly observed physical signs are petechiae, jaundice, and hepato-splenomegaly; neurologic abnormalities such as microcephaly and lethargy affect a significant proportion of symptomatic children. Ophthalmologic examination is abnormal in approximately 10%, with chorioretinitis and/or optic atrophy most commonly observed.[42,43]

Approximately half of symptomatic children are small for gestational age, and one third are born before 38 weeks' gestation. It has been thought that symptomatic congenital CMV infection occurs exclusively in infants born to women with primary CMV infection during pregnancy. However, data accumulated over the past 10 years demonstrate that symptomatic congenital CMV infection can occur at a similar frequency in infants born following primary maternal infection and in those born to women with preexisting immunity (see Fig. 11-1).[7,14,17]

Laboratory findings in children with symptomatic infection reflect involvement of the hepatobiliary and reticuloendothelial systems and include conjugated hyper-bilirubinemia, thrombocytopenia, and elevation of hepatic transaminases in more than half of symptomatic newborns. Transaminases and bilirubin levels typically peak within the first 2 weeks of life and can remain elevated for several weeks thereafter, but thrombocytopenia reaches its nadir by the second week of life and normalizes within 3 to 4 weeks of age.[42,43] Radiographic imaging of the head is abnormal in approximately 50% to 70% of children with symptomatic infection at birth. The most common finding is intracranial calcifications, with ventricular dilatation, cysts, and lenticulostriate vasculopathy also observed.[34,44]

Perinatal Infection

As discussed in previous sections, perinatal CMV infection can be acquired through exposure to CMV in the maternal genital tract at delivery, through blood transfusions, or, most commonly, from breast milk. CMV infection acquired perinatally in a healthy, full-term infant is typically asymptomatic and without sequelae.[22] In contrast, very low birth weight (VLBW) preterm infants who acquire CMV postnatally may be completely asymptomatic or can have a sepsis-like syndrome with abdominal distention, apnea, hepatomegaly, bradycardia, poor perfusion, and respiratory distress.[23,45,46] Some of the earlier prospective studies on CMV transmission to preterm infants by breast milk were conducted by investigators in Germany. They reported that approximately 50% of infants who acquired CMV postnatally had clinical or laboratory abnormalities, the most common being neutropenia and thrombocytopenia. All symptoms resolved without antiviral therapy, and low birth weight and early postnatal virus transmission were risk factors for symptomatic infection.[23] Subsequent studies from many different countries have reported lower rates of CMV transmission (6% to 29%), but symptomatic infection was noted in all studies.[46]

Laboratory Diagnosis

Serology

Serologic tests are useful for determining whether an individual has had CMV infection in the past, determined by the presence or absence of CMV IgG antibodies. The detection of IgM antibodies has been used as an indicator of acute or recent infection. However, assays for IgM antibody lack specificity for primary infection because IgM can persist for months after primary infection, and because IgM can be positive in reactivated CMV infection, leading to false-positive results.[47] Because of the limitations of IgM assays, IgG avidity assays are utilized in some populations to help distinguish primary from nonprimary CMV infection. These assays are based on the observation that IgG antibodies of low avidity are present during the first few months after onset of infection, and avidity increases over time, reflecting maturation of the immune response. Thus, the presence of high-avidity anti-CMV IgG is considered evidence of long-standing infection in an individual.[47]

Viral Culture

The traditional method for detecting CMV is conventional cell culture. Clinical specimens are inoculated onto human fibroblast cells and incubated and observed for the appearance of characteristic cytopathic effect (CPE) for a period ranging from 2 to 21 days. The shell vial assay is a viral culture modified by a centrifugation-amplification technique designed to decrease the length of time needed for virus detection. Centrifugation of the specimen onto the cell monolayer assists adsorption of virus, effectively increasing infectivity of the viral inoculum.[48] Viral antigens may then be detected by monoclonal antibody directed at a CMV immediate-early (IE) antigen by indirect immunofluorescence after 16 hours of incubation. This method was adapted to be performed in 96-well microtiter plates, allowing the screening of larger numbers of samples.[49]

Antigen Detection Assays

The antigenemia assay has been commonly used for longer than a decade for CMV virus quantification in blood specimens. Antigenemia is measured by the quantitation of positive leukocyte nuclei in an immunofluorescence assay for the CMV matrix phosphoprotein pp65 in a cytospin preparation of 2×10^5 peripheral blood leukocytes (PBL).[50] The disadvantages of the antigenemia assay are that it is labor-intensive with low throughput and is not amenable to automation. It may also be affected by subjective bias. The samples have to be processed immediately (within 6 hours) because delay greatly reduces the sensitivity of the assay. The utility of this assay in diagnosing CMV infection in neonates has not been examined.

Polymerase Chain Reaction

Polymerase chain reaction (PCR) is a widely available rapid and sensitive method of CMV detection based on amplification of nucleic acids. The techniques usually target highly conserved regions of major IE and late antigen genes,[51] but several other genes have also been used as targets for detection of CMV DNA. DNA can be extracted from whole blood, leukocytes, plasma, or any other tissue (biopsy samples) or fluid (urine, cerebrospinal fluid [CSF], bronchoalveolar lavage [BAL] fluid). PCR for CMV DNA can be qualitative or quantitative, in which the amount of viral DNA in the sample is measured. Qualitative PCR has been largely replaced by quantitative assays owing to increased sensitivity for detecting CMV, and because quantitative PCR (real-time PCR) allows continuous monitoring of immunocompromised individuals to identify patients at risk for CMV disease for preemptive therapy and to determine response to treatment. This method generally is more expensive than the antigenemia assay, but it is rapid and can be automated. Results usually are reported as number of copies per milliliter of blood or plasma.

Immunohistochemistry

Immunohistochemistry is performed primarily on tissue or body fluid samples. Slides are made from frozen or paraffin-embedded sections of biopsy tissue samples (e.g., liver, lung) or by centrifuging cells onto a slide. Monoclonal or polyclonal antibodies against early CMV antigens are applied to the slides and are visualized by fluorescently labeled antibodies or enzyme-labeled secondary antibodies, which are detected by the change in color of the substrate. The stained slides are examined by fluorescent or light microscopy.

Diagnosis During Pregnancy

Maternal Infection

The diagnosis of primary CMV infection is accomplished by documenting seroconversion through the de novo appearance of virus-specific IgG antibodies in the serum of a pregnant woman known previously to be seronegative. The presence of IgG antibodies indicates past infection ranging from 2 weeks' to many years' duration. Detection of IgM in the serum of a pregnant woman may indicate a primary infection. However, IgM can be produced in pregnant women with nonprimary CMV infection, and false-positive results are common in patients with other viral infections.[52] In addition, anti-CMV IgM can persist for 6 to 9 months following primary CMV infection.[47,53] Because of the limitations of IgM assays, IgG avidity assays are utilized to help distinguish primary from nonprimary CMV infection. When IgM testing in addition to IgG avidity is performed at 20 to 23 weeks' gestation, the sensitivity of detecting a mother who transmits CMV to her offspring is around 8%. Based on these data, some investigators propose screening pregnant women with serum IgG and IgM. If IgM is positive, then serum IgG avidity could be performed to help determine recent or past infection. Using this algorithm, some argue that the sensitivity is similar to documenting de novo seroconversion.[53,54] Identification of primary maternal infection is important because of the high rate of intrauterine transmission—25% to 40%—in this setting. However, in populations with high CMV seroprevalence, it is estimated that most infants with congenital CMV infection are born to women with preexisting seroimmunity.[15]

Fetal Infection

Detection of CMV in the amniotic fluid has been the standard for the diagnosis of infection of the fetus. Viral isolation in tissue culture was first utilized; however, the sensitivity was found to be moderate (70% to 80%) and the rate of false-negative results high. With the advent of PCR, detection of CMV DNA in amniotic fluid has been shown to improve prenatal diagnosis of congenital CMV infection.[55] The highest sensitivity of this assay (90% to 100%) has been shown when amniotic fluid samples are obtained after the 21st week of gestation, and at least 6 weeks after the first positive maternal serologic assay. This allows adequate time for maternal transmission of the virus to the fetus and shedding of the virus by the fetal kidney. However, even when PCR on amniotic fluid is performed at the optimal time, false-negative results may be obtained. A recent study showed that among 194 women who underwent prenatal diagnosis of congenital CMV infection, 8 mothers with negative amniotic fluid PCR results for CMV delivered infants who were confirmed to be CMV-infected.[56]

Recently, CMV DNA quantification in amniotic fluid samples has been proposed as a means of evaluating the risk that a fetus can develop infection or disease. Several groups of investigators have shown that higher CMV DNA viral load in the amniotic fluid ($\geq 10^5$ genome equivalents [GE]/mL) was associated with symptomatic infection in the newborn or fetus.[57,58] However, other studies have failed to confirm a correlation between CMV DNA levels and clinical status at birth.[59] Rather, CMV viral load in the amniotic fluid correlated with the time during pregnancy when amniocentesis was performed, and higher CMV viral loads were observed later in gestation.[57,59]

11

However, as with qualitative PCR on amniotic fluid, even when sampling was done at the appropriate time, very low or undetectable CMV DNA by quantitative PCR was found in some infants infected with CMV.[58,59]

Fetal blood sampling has been evaluated to determine the prognostic value of virologic assays in the diagnosis of congenital infection and in the determination of severity of CMV disease. The utility of CMV viremia, antigenemia, DNAemia, and IgM antibody assays on fetal blood was examined for the diagnosis of congenital infection. Although these assays were highly specific, the sensitivity was shown to be poor (41.1% to 84.8%) for identifying fetuses infected with CMV.[47] More recently, fetal thrombocytopenia has been shown to be associated with more severe disease in the fetus/newborn. However, investigators have documented fetal loss after funipuncture. Thus, it is important to balance the value of cordocentesis against that known risk of miscarriage.[60]

Fetal imaging by ultrasound can reveal structural and/or growth abnormalities and thus can help the clinician identify fetuses with congenital CMV infection that will be symptomatic at birth. The more common abnormalities on ultrasound include ascites, fetal growth restriction, microcephaly, and structural abnormalities of the brain.[55] However, most infected fetuses will not have abnormalities on ultrasound examination.[61] In a recent retrospective study of 650 mothers with primary CMV infection, among 131 infected fetuses/neonates with normal sonographic findings in utero, 52% were symptomatic at birth. Furthermore, when fetal infection status was unknown, ultrasound abnormalities predicted symptomatic congenital infection in only one third of infected infants.[62]

Fetal magnetic resonance imaging (MRI) has been evaluated in a few small, retrospective studies to assess its utility in detecting fetal abnormalities in utero. MRI appears to add to the diagnostic value of ultrasound with increased sensitivity and positive predictive value (PPV) of both studies versus ultrasound or MRI alone.[63,64] However, more studies are needed to determine the true diagnostic and prognostic value of MRI in CMV-infected fetuses.

Congenital Infection

The diagnosis of congenital CMV infection is typically made by demonstration of the virus, viral antigens, or viral genome in newborn urine or saliva (Table 11-4). Detection of virus in urine or saliva within the first 2 weeks of life is considered the gold standard for the diagnosis of congenital CMV infection. Because detection of the virus or viral genome in samples obtained from infants after the first 2 to 3 weeks of life may represent natal or postnatal acquisition of CMV, it is not possible to confirm congenital CMV infection in infants older than 3 weeks. Serologic methods are unreliable for the diagnosis of congenital infection. Detection of CMV IgG antibody is complicated by transplacental transfer of maternal antibodies; currently available CMV IgM antibody assays do not have the high level of sensitivity and specificity of virus culture or PCR.

Traditional tissue culture techniques and shell vial assay for the detection of CMV in saliva or urine are considered standard methods for the diagnosis of congenital CMV infection (see Table 11-4).[65] Rapid culture methods have comparable sensitivity and specificity to standard cell culture assays, and the results are available within 24 to 36 hours. A rapid method using a 96-well microtiter plate and a monoclonal antibody to the CMV IE antigen was shown to be 94.5% sensitive and

Table 11-4   LABORATORY DIAGNOSIS OF CYTOMEGALOVIRUS INFECTION BY PATIENT POPULATION

Congenital infection	Detection of virus or viral antigens in saliva or urine using standard or rapid culture methods; CMV PCR of blood is highly specific but insufficiently sensitive; PCR assays of saliva and urine are promising
Perinatal infection	Viral culture or PCR of urine or saliva; proof of absence of CMV shedding in the first 2 weeks of life

CMV, Cytomegalovirus; *PCR,* polymerase chain reaction.

100% specific for detecting CMV in the urine of congenitally infected infants.[49] This microtiter plate assay has been adapted for use with saliva specimens with comparable sensitivity and specificity.[66] The utility of antigenemia assay in the diagnosis of congenital CMV infection has not been established.

Although PCR amplification of virus DNA is a very sensitive method for the detection of CMV in a variety of clinical specimens, the utility of PCR or other nucleic acid amplification assays for the diagnosis of congenital CMV infection has not been defined. Several studies have shown that PCR of saliva and urine specimens could be useful for the identification of infants with congenital CMV infection.[67,68] Because dried blood spots (DBS) are collected for routine metabolic screening from all infants born in the United States, interest has been increasing in utilizing PCR-based assays for the detection of CMV in newborn DBS samples. Most early reports have studied selected infant populations and did not include a direct comparison of PCR versus a standard (i.e., tissue culture) method for identifying CMV infection.[69-72] The sensitivity of DBS PCR in the diagnosis of congenital CMV infection may vary with the amount of blood collected on the filter card, the method used for DNA extraction, and the PCR protocol.

Early studies examined the utility of PCR on DBS obtained from infants in the nursery to diagnose congenital CMV infection retrospectively at the time of detection of SNHL.[70] A number of studies from a group of investigators in Italy examined DBS from newborns and reported a sensitivity of the DBS PCR assay approaching 100% with a specificity of 99%.[69] However, in a large multicenter study of more than 20,000 newborns, a DBS real-time PCR assay was compared with saliva rapid culture for identification of infants with congenital CMV infection; it was demonstrated that DBS PCR could detect less than 40% of congenitally infected infants.[73] The sensitivity and specificity of the DBS PCR assay when compared with the saliva rapid culture were 34.4% (95% confidence interval [CI], 18.6% to 53.2%) and 99.9% (95% CI, 99.9% to 100%), respectively. These results indicate that such methods as currently performed will not be suitable for the mass screening of newborns for congenital CMV infection. The high specificity of the DBS PCR assay suggests that a positive DBS PCR result will identify infants with congenital CMV infection. However, the negative DBS PCR assay result does not exclude congenital CMV infection. These findings underscore the need for further evaluation of high-throughput methods performed on saliva or other samples that can be adapted to large-scale newborn CMV screening.

Several previous studies examined the utility of testing saliva samples with PCR-based methods and demonstrated the feasibility and high sensitivity of these methods.[8,68] However, none of these studies included screening of unselected newborns or direct comparison of a saliva PCR assay versus the standard rapid culture method on saliva or urine. Although a more recent study from Brazil in which more than 8000 newborns were screened for congenital CMV infection demonstrated the utility of a saliva PCR assay to screen newborns for CMV, the PCR assay was not directly compared with the standard culture-based assay.[7] The utility of real-time PCR of saliva samples in identifying infants with congenital CMV infection was evaluated in a multicenter newborn screening study of approximately 35,000 infants who were screened for CMV using rapid culture and PCR of saliva specimens.[74] Findings of this study showed that PCR testing of both liquid and dried saliva specimens has excellent sensitivity (>97%) and specificity (99.9%).

Interest is growing in examining the feasibility of a newborn CMV screening program combined with universal newborn hearing screening. Although DBS PCR assays have been shown to have insufficient sensitivity for the identification of most infants with congenital CMV infection, saliva PCR assays have the potential to adapt these methods in a high-throughput approach to screen large number of newborns for congenital CMV infection.

Perinatal Infection

For definitive diagnosis of perinatal CMV infection, it is important to demonstrate no viral shedding in the first 2 weeks of life to rule out congenital infection because

11

CMV excretion does not begin until 3 to 12 weeks after exposure (see Table 11-4).[5] There is no agreed-upon standard method for diagnosis of perinatal CMV infection, however. Viral culture and CMV DNA detection by PCR using urine or saliva are the preferred diagnostic methods.

Treatment

Pregnancy

Antivirals have not been used extensively in pregnancy to treat fetal CMV infection. Ganciclovir (GCV) is a nucleoside analogue of guanosine that inhibits the CMV DNA polymerase. Ganciclovir has teratogenic and hematopoietic adverse effects; this contraindicates its use in pregnant women. Acyclovir, which also inhibits viral DNA polymerase, has less activity against CMV but is safe for use in pregnancy. A pilot study utilizing the oral pro-drug of acyclovir, valacyclovir, in 21 women with confirmed fetal CMV infection demonstrated placental transfer of acyclovir to the fetus and a decrease in fetal CMV viral load. This study was not designed to evaluate efficacy for preventing sequelae in the fetuses. However, three infants had sequelae on follow-up, and six cases required termination of pregnancy for in utero progression of disease.[75] These results led to a randomized, placebo-controlled trial that is currently being conducted to assess the safety and efficacy of valacyclovir in pregnancy with documented fetal disease (http://clinicaltrials.gov/ct2/results?term=NCT01037712).

Passive immunization with intravenous CMV hyperimmune globulin (HIG) for prevention and treatment of fetal infection and disease was studied in Italy, and results were reported in 2005. The study identified women with primary CMV infection through serologic screening during pregnancy. Women were offered therapy, and those who accepted were compared with women who declined therapy with hyperimmune globulin. Passive transfer of antibodies reduced the frequency of transmission of virus to the fetus and reduced the incidence of disease in infected infants. However, the study was uncontrolled, with women receiving anywhere from one to six doses of hyperimmune globulin; thus, skepticism regarding the validity of the findings has been raised by some investigators.[76] Evaluation of placentas among women who received HIG and a control group of CMV-seropositive pregnant women demonstrated reduced placental size in the treated group, suggesting that the benefits of HIG could be related to anti-inflammatory effects on the placenta.[77] To properly study the effects of hyperimmune globulin on viral transmission and outcome in congenital infection, a randomized, double-blind, placebo-controlled multicenter trial of hyperimmune globulin in pregnancy is currently recruiting participants (http://clinicaltrials.gov/ct2/results?term=NCT00881517).

Congenital Infection

Antiviral therapy for congenital CMV infection is limited. Only one randomized controlled trial has been performed to assess the effects of 6 weeks of intravenous ganciclovir therapy on hearing outcomes in infants with symptomatic congenital infection with involvement of the central nervous system.[78] Although this study suffered from patient attrition, treatment suggested a possible benefit, with hearing thresholds declining in 20% of ganciclovir recipients at 1 year of age or older compared with worsening of hearing in 70% of subjects who did not receive treatment. Time to resolution of clinical symptoms, including splenomegaly, hepatomegaly, and retinitis, was not different between control and treatment groups. Treatment was associated with significant neutropenia in 63% of ganciclovir recipients. The American Academy of Pediatrics Committee on Infectious Diseases thus states, "therapy is not recommended routinely in this population of infected infants because of possible toxicities and adverse events associated with prolonged intravenous therapy…"[79] Because congenital CMV infection is a chronic infection, few data are available to suggest the best time to begin therapy and the ideal length of therapy. Currently, the National Institute of Allergy and Infectious Diseases Collaborative Antiviral Study Group is conducting a randomized placebo-controlled study to compare a 6-week versus 6-month course of oral valganciclovir in babies born with symptomatic

CMV infection to assess safety and efficacy with regard to hearing and development outcomes (http://clinicaltrials.gov/ct2/show/NCT00466817?term=congenital+cmv+ infection&rank=3). No studies have been conducted in children with asymptomatic infection at birth; antiviral therapy generally is not recommended in these patients because the risks of treatment far outweigh the potential benefit.

Perinatal Infection

Antiviral therapy has not been studied in preterm infants with symptomatic, perinatally acquired CMV infection. Some experts recommend parenteral ganciclovir for 2 weeks if evidence of end-organ disease (pneumonitis, hepatitis, thrombocytopenia) is found, and continuation of therapy for an additional 1 to 2 weeks if symptoms and signs of infection have not resolved.[79]

Some investigators have suggested that intravenous immunoglobulin (IVIG) might be useful in preventing or treating CMV infection in preterm neonates. Mosca and colleagues noted that rates of CMV were low in their population of preterm infants, despite a high rate of CMV exposure, and hypothesized that routine use of IVIG in their neonatal intensive care unit (NICU) might be protective.[80] However, no randomized, controlled trials have been performed to assess the efficacy of IVIG or CMV-specific IVIG for prevention or treatment of neonatal CMV disease.

Prognosis

Congenital Infection

Early studies of outcome in symptomatic congenital CMV infection demonstrated that approximately 10% of symptomatic infants will die in the newborn period. However, more recent data suggest that the mortality rate is probably less than 5%.[14,42] However, a majority of symptomatic children will suffer sequelae ranging from mild to severe psychomotor and perceptual handicaps. Multiple prospective studies have shown that approximately half of the children born with symptomatic infection will develop SNHL, mental retardation with IQ less than 70, and microcephaly.[43,81] Predictors of adverse neurologic outcome in children with symptomatic congenital CMV infection include microcephaly, chorioretinitis, the presence of other neurologic abnormalities at birth or in early infancy, and cranial imaging abnormalities detected within the first month of life.[34,44,82] In one study, Rivera and associates analyzed newborn findings and hearing outcome data on 190 children with symptomatic infection to identify clinical predictors of hearing loss. Univariate analysis revealed that intrauterine growth retardation, petechiae, hepatosplenomegaly, hepatitis, thrombocytopenia, and intracerebral calcifications were associated with the development of hearing loss. Logistic regression analysis showed that petechiae and intrauterine growth retardation were the only factors that were independently predictive of hearing loss.[83]

In general, asymptomatic children have a better long-term prognosis than children with symptomatic congenital infection. However, approximately 10% of asymptomatic children will develop SNHL (Table 11-5). Many prospective studies of children with asymptomatic CMV infection have been performed to define the natural history of hearing loss in this group. These studies show that approximately one half of children with asymptomatic infection who develop hearing loss will have bilateral deficits, which can vary from mild high-frequency loss to profound impairment.[14,84-87] Additionally, hearing loss in these children is often progressive and/or of delayed onset, requiring ongoing audiologic evaluation.[84,85,87] Other neurologic complications can occur in asymptomatic congenital CMV infection but at a much lower frequency than in symptomatic infection.[88]

Predictors of outcome, particularly hearing loss, in children with asymptomatic congenital CMV infection have not been identified. It was thought that children born to mothers with primary CMV infection during pregnancy are at higher risk for adverse sequelae. However, recent data argue against this notion (see Fig. 11-1).[7,14,18] Several studies have examined the relationship between peripheral blood viral load and outcome in congenital CMV. Children with symptomatic infection at birth

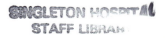

Table 11-5 AUDIOLOGIC RESULTS FOR CHILDREN WITH CONGENITAL CYTOMEGALOVIRUS INFECTION

	Symptomatic	Asymptomatic
Children with SNHL, %	40.7	7.4
Bilateral loss, %	67.1	47.9
High-frequency loss only (4000–8000 Hz)	12.9	37.5
Delayed-onset loss, %	27.1	37.5
Median age (range) of delayed onset	33 mo (6–197 mo)	44 mo (24–182 mo)
Progressive loss, %	54.1	54.2
Fluctuating loss, %	29.4	54.1
Improvement of loss, %	21.1	47.9

Adapted from Dahle AJ, Fowler KB, Wright JD, et al. Longitudinal investigations of hearing disorders in children with congenital cytomegalovirus. *J Am Acad Audiol.* 2000;11:283-290, with permission.

SNHL, Sensorineural hearing loss.

appear to have higher viral load compared with children with asymptomatic infection.[89,90] However, the most recent study, which utilized peripheral blood samples from 135 children with congenital infection, demonstrated no difference in CMV viral load levels in the first months of life and beyond, among children with and without SNHL.[90] Because the frequency and natural history of SNHL in children with symptomatic and asymptomatic infection differ, data from the two groups of children were analyzed independently (Fig. 11-2). These data indicate that in individual children with congenital CMV infection, an elevated viral load measurement may not be useful in identifying a child at risk for CMV-related hearing loss.

Perinatal Infection

Asymptomatic perinatal CMV infection in full-term healthy infants does not have adverse effects on neurodevelopmental or hearing outcome. In VLBW preterm infants, studies have failed to show an association between perinatal CMV infection and sensorineural hearing loss or delay in neuromotor development.[91,92] Vollmer and associates performed a matched pair outcome analysis in 44 children followed for 4.5 years and found no difference in neurodevelopment or hearing sequelae between CMV-infected infants and infants without preterm perinatal CMV infection.[92] A

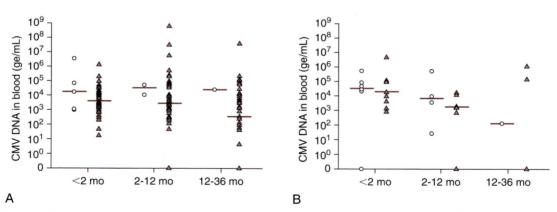

Figure 11-2 Results of tests measuring levels of cytomegalovirus (CMV) DNA in peripheral blood (PB) at three different age ranges from children with congenital CMV infection with **(A)** asymptomatic and **(B)** symptomatic infection at birth who had hearing loss (o) and normal hearing (▲). Results are expressed as genomic equivalents per mL of blood (GE/mL). The horizontal bars represent median values. (Adapted from Ross SA, Novak Z, Fowler KB, Arora N, Britt WJ, Boppana SB. Cytomegalovirus blood viral load and hearing loss in young children with congenital infection. *Pediatr Infect Dis J.* 2009;28:588-592, with permission.)

similar study in Israel with 24 months of follow-up showed no adverse outcomes among infants with perinatal CMV.[91]

Prevention

Hand washing is considered an effective means of limiting the spread of CMV in the community among immunocompetent hosts, as well as nosocomial spread. Disinfectants such as chlorine, alcohol, and detergents (soap) destroy the viral envelope and render the virus noninfectious. It has been suggested that all women of child-bearing age should know their CMV serostatus; however, this is controversial. Evidence suggests that hygiene counseling and change in behavior can decrease the rate of primary CMV infection in seronegative women during pregnancy.[93,94] For immunocompromised hosts, contact precautions including gown and gloves with hand washing/disinfection may prevent transmission in the hospital setting but are not feasible in the community.

Vaccine prevention of congenital CMV infection has been considered since the 1970s and has been directed toward prevention of primary CMV infection during pregnancy.[95] A 2000 report by the Institute of Medicine listed CMV vaccine development as a high priority because of the public health impact of congenital CMV infection as a leading cause of hearing loss (www.niaid.gov/newsroom/IOM.htm). Several vaccine candidates have been studied, including an attenuated, replication-competent virus and an adjuvanted glycoprotein subunit vaccine. Both appear to induce an immune response, and both produce at least some level of cellular immunity.[96-99] In a phase II trial that included 464 CMV-seronegative women of child-bearing age, an MF59-adjuvanted CMV glycoprotein B subunit vaccine had 50% efficacy (95% CI, 7% to 73%) in preventing CMV infection. Overall benefits were modest, and the study was not powered to assess efficacy in preventing maternal–fetal transmission.[100] In addition, the strategy of preventing primary maternal infection does not address CMV-associated hearing loss and other neurologic sequelae noted in congenitally infected children born to women with pre-existing CMV immunity.[7,10,18] Additional candidate vaccines that are in clinical trials include alphavirus replicon particle vaccines, DNA vaccines, and live attenuated vaccines.

References

1. Murphy E, Yu D, Grimwood J, et al. Coding potential of laboratory and clinical strains of human cytomegalovirus. *Proc Natl Acad Sci U S A*. 2003;100:14976-14981.
2. Rasmussen L, Geissler A, Winters M. Inter- and intragenic variations complicate the molecular epidemiology of human cytomegalovirus. *J Infect Dis*. 2003;187:809-819.
3. Klein M, Schoppel K, Amvrossiadis N, Mach M. Strain-specific neutralization of human cytomegalovirus isolates by human sera. *J Virol*. 1999;73:878-886.
4. Shimamura M, Mach M, Britt WJ. Human cytomegalovirus infection elicits a glycoprotein M (gM)/gN-specific virus-neutralizing antibody response. *J Virol*. 2006;80:4591-4600.
5. Stagno S, Britt WJ. Cytomegalovirus. In: Remington JS, Klein JO, WIlson CB, Baker CJ, eds. *Infectious Diseases of the Fetus and Newborn Infant*. 6th ed. Philadelphia: Elsevier Saunders; 2006:740-781.
6. Bate SL, Dollard SC, Cannon MJ. Cytomegalovirus seroprevalence in the United States: The National Health and Nutrition Examination Surveys, 1988-2004. *Clin Infect Dis*. 2010;50:1439-1447.
7. Mussi-Pinhata MM, Yamamoto AY, Moura Brito RM, et al. Birth prevalence and natural history of congenital cytomegalovirus infection in a highly seroimmune population. *Clin Infect Dis*. 2009;49: 522-528.
8. Dar L, Pati SK, Patro AR, et al. Congenital cytomegalovirus infection in a highly seropositive semi-urban population in India. *Pediatr Infect Dis J*. 2008;27:841-843.
9. van der Sande MAB, Kaye S, Miles DJC, et al. Risk factors for and clinical outcome of congenital cytomegalovirus infection in a peri-urban West-African birth cohort. *PLos One*. 2007;2:e492.
10. Boppana SB, Rivera LB, Fowler KB, Mach M, Britt WJ. Intrauterine transmission of cytomegalovirus to infants of women with preconceptional immunity. *N Engl J Med*. 2001;344:1366-1371.
11. Yamamoto AY, Mussi-Pinhata MM, Boppana SB, et al. Human cytomegalovirus reinfection is associated with intrauterine transmission in a highly cytomegalovirus-immune maternal population. *Am J Obstet Gynecol*. 2010;202:297.e291-297.e298.
12. Ross SA, Arora N, Novak Z, Fowler KB, Britt WJ, Boppana SB. Cytomegalovirus reinfections in healthy seroimmune women. *J Infect Dis*. 2010;201:386-389.

11

13. Fowler KB, Stagno S, Pass RF. Maternal age and congenital cytomegalovirus infection: Screening of two diverse newborn populations, 1980-1990. *J Infect Dis*. 1993;168:552-556.

14. Ahlfors K, Ivarsson SA, Harris S. Report on a long-term study of maternal and congenital cytomegalovirus infection in Sweden. Review of prospective studies available in the literature. *Scand J Infect Dis*. 1999;31:443-457.

15. Kenneson A, Cannon MJ. Review and meta-analysis of the epidemiology of congenital cytomegalovirus (CMV) infection. *Rev Med Virol*. 2007;17:253-276.

16. Fowler KB, Stagno S, Pass RF, Britt WJ, Boll TJ, Alford CA. The outcome of congenital cytomegalovirus infection in relation to maternal antibody status. *N Engl J Med*. 1992;326:663-667.

17. Boppana SB, Fowler KB, Britt WJ, Stagno S, Pass RF. Symptomatic congenital cytomegalovirus infection in infants born to mothers with preexisting immunity to cytomegalovirus. *Pediatrics*. 1999;104:55-60.

18. Ross SA, Fowler KB, Ashrith G, et al. Hearing loss in children with congenital cytomegalovirus infection born to mothers with preexisting immunity. *J Pediatr*. 2006;148:332-336.

19. Preece PM, Tookey P, Ades A, Peckham CS. Congenital cytomegalovirus infection: Predisposing maternal factors. *J Epidemiol Community Health*. 1986;40:205-209.

20. Stagno S, Reynolds DW, Tsiantos A, et al. Cervical cytomegalovirus excretion in pregnant and nonpregnant women: Suppression in early gestation. *J Infect Dis*. 1975;131:522-527.

21. Stagno S, Cloud G. Working parents: The impact of day care and breast-feeding on cytomegalovirus infections in offspring. *Proc Natl Acad Sci U S A*. 1994;91:2384-2389.

22. Dworsky M, Yow M, Stagno S, Pass RF, Alford CA. Cytomegalovirus infection of breast milk and transmission in infancy. *Pediatrics*. 1983;72:295-299.

23. Hamprecht K, Maschmann J, Vochem M, Dietz K, Speer CP, Jahn G. Epidemiology of transmission of cytomegalovirus from mother to preterm infants by breastfeeding. *Lancet*. 2001;357:513-518.

24. Doctor S, Friedman S, Dunn MS, et al. Cytomegalovirus transmission to extremely low-birthweight infants through breast milk. *Acta Paediatr*. 2005;94:53-58.

25. Balcarek KB, Bagley R, Cloud GA, Pass RF. Cytomegalovirus infection among employees of a children's hospital: No evidence for increased risk associated with patient care. *JAMA*. 1990;263:840-844.

26. Klemola E, Robert von E, Henle G, Henle W. Infectious-mononucleosis-like disease with negative heterophil agglutination test. Clinical features in relation to Epstein-Barr virus and cytomegalovirus antibodies. *J Infect Dis*. 1970;121:608-614.

27. Collins TM, Quirk MR, Jordan MC. Biphasic viremia and viral gene expression in leukocytes during acute cytomegalovirus infection of mice. *J Virol*. 1994;68:6305-6311.

28. Hendrix RM, Wagenaar M, Slobbe RL, Bruggeman CA. Widespread presence of cytomegalovirus DNA in tissues of healthy trauma victims. *J Clin Pathol*. 1997;50:59-63.

29. Fletcher JM, Vukmanovic-Stejic M, Dunne PJ, et al. Cytomegalovirus-specific CD4+ T cells in healthy carriers are continuously driven to replicative exhaustion. *J Immunol*. 2005;175:8218-8225.

30. Sylvester AW, Mitchell BL, Edgar JB, et al. Broadly targeted human cytomegalovirus-specific CD4+ and CD8+ T cells dominate the memory compartments of exposed subjects. *J Exp Med*. 2005;202:673-685.

31. Bubic I, Wagner M, Krmpotic A, et al. Gain of virulence caused by loss of a gene in murine cytomegalovirus. *J Virol*. 2004;78:7536-7544.

32. Bernard F, Picard C, Cormier-Daire V, et al. A novel developmental and immunodeficiency syndrome associated with intrauterine growth retardation and a lack of natural killer cells. *Pediatrics*. 2004;113:136-141.

33. Rasmussen L, Matkin C, Spaete R, Pachl C, Merigan TC. Antibody response to human cytomegalovirus glycoproteins gB and gH after natural infection in humans. *J Infect Dis*. 1991;164:835-842.

34. Boppana SB, Fowler KB, Vaid Y, et al. Neuroradiographic findings in the newborn period and long-term outcome in children with symptomatic congenital cytomegalovirus infection. *Pediatrics*. 1997;99:409-414.

35. Gabrielli L, Bonasoni MP, Lazzarotto T, et al. Histological findings in foetuses congenitally infected by cytomegalovirus. *J Clin Virol*. 2009;46(Suppl 4):S16-S21.

36. van den Pol AN, Reuter JD, Santarelli JG. Enhanced cytomegalovirus infection of developing brain independent of the adaptive immune system. *J Virol*. 2002;76:8842-8854.

37. Koontz T, Bralic M, Tomac J; et al. Altered development of the brain after focal herpesvirus infection of the central nervous system. *J Exp Med*. 2008;205:423-435.

38. Strauss M. Human cytomegalovirus labyrinthitis. *Am J Otolaryngol*. 1990;11:292-298.

39. Rarey KE, Davis LE. Temporal bone histopathology 14 years after cytomegalic inclusion disease: A case study. *Laryngoscope*. 1993;103:904-909.

40. Harris JP, Fan JT, Keithley EM. Immunologic responses in experimental cytomegalovirus labyrinthitis. *Am J Otolaryngol*. 1990;11:304-308.

41. Ross SA, Novak Z, Pati S, et al. Mixed infection and strain diversity in congenital cytomegalovirus infection. *J Infect Dis*. 2011;204:1003-1007.

42. Boppana SB, Pass RF, Britt WJ, Stagno S, Alford CA. Symptomatic congenital cytomegalovirus infection: Neonatal morbidity and mortality. *Pediatr Infect Dis J*. 1992;11:93-99.

43. Conboy TJ, Pass RF, Stagno S, et al. Early clinical manifestations and intellectual outcome in children with symptomatic congenital cytomegalovirus infection. *J Pediatr*. 1987;111:343-348.

44. Ancora G, Lanari M, Lazzarotto T, et al. Cranial ultrasound scanning and prediction of outcome in newborns with congenital cytomegalovirus infection. *J Pediatr*. 2007;150:157-161.
45. Lawrence RM. Cytomegalovirus in human breast milk: Risk to the premature infant. *Breastfeed Med*. 2006;1:99-107.
46. Hamprecht K, Maschmann J, Jahn G, Poets CF, Goelz R. Cytomegalovirus transmission to preterm infants during lactation. *J Clin Virol*. 2008;41:198-205.
47. Revello MG, Gerna G. Diagnosis and management of human cytomegalovirus infection in the mother, fetus, and newborn infant. *Clin Microbiol Rev*. 2002;15:680-715.
48. Chou SW, Scott KM. Rapid quantitation of cytomegalovirus and assay of neutralizing antibody by using monoclonal antibody to the major immediate-early viral protein. *J Clin Microbiol*. 1988;26:504-507.
49. Boppana SB, Smith R, Stagno S, Britt WJ. Evaluation of a microtiter plate fluorescent antibody assay for rapid detection of human cytomegalovirus infections. *J Clin Microbiol*. 1992;30:721-723.
50. van der Bij W, Schirm J, Torensma R, van Son WJ, Tegzess AM, The TH. Comparison between viremia and antigenemia for detection of cytomegalovirus in blood. *J Clin Microbiol*. 1988;26:2531-2535.
51. Rasmussen L, Geissler A, Cowan C, Chase A, Winters M. The genes encoding the gCIII complex of human cytomegalovirus exist in highly diverse combinations in clinical isolates. *J Virol*. 2002;76:10841-10848.
52. Lazzarotto T, Gabrielli L, Lanari M, et al. Congenital cytomegalovirus infection: Recent advances in the diagnosis of maternal infection. *Hum Immunol*. 2004;65:410-415.
53. Mace M, Sissoeff L, Rudent A, Grangeot-Keros L. A serological testing algorithm for the diagnosis of primary CMV infection in pregnant women. *Prenat Diagn*. 2004;24:861-863.
54. Lazzarotto T, Guerra B, Lanari M, Gabrielli L, Landini MP. New advances in the diagnosis of congenital cytomegalovirus infection. *J Clin Virol*. 2008;41:192-197.
55. Enders G, Bader U, Lindemann L, Schalasta G, Daiminger A. Prenatal diagnosis of congenital cytomegalovirus infection in 189 pregnancies with known outcome. *Prenat Diagn*. 2001;21:362-377.
56. Revello MG, Furione M, Zavattoni M, et al. Human cytomegalovirus (HCMV) DNAemia in the mother at amniocentesis as a risk factor for iatrogenic HCMV infection of the fetus. *J Infect Dis*. 2008;197:593-596.
57. Gouarin S, Gault E, Vabret A, et al. Real-time PCR quantification of human cytomegalovirus DNA in amniotic fluid samples from mothers with primary infection. *J Clin Microbiol*. 2002;40:1767-1772.
58. Guerra B, Lazzarotto T, Quarta S, et al. Prenatal diagnosis of symptomatic congenital cytomegalovirus infection. *Am J Obstet Gynecol*. 2000;183:476-482.
59. Goegebuer T, Van Meensel B, Beuselinck K, et al. Clinical predictive value of real-time PCR quantification of human cytomegalovirus DNA in amniotic fluid samples. *J Clin Microbiol*. 2009;47:660-665.
60. Benoist G, Salomon LJ, Jacquemard F, Daffos F, Ville Y. The prognostic value of ultrasound abnormalities and biological parameters in blood of fetuses infected with cytomegalovirus. *BJOG*. 2008;115:823-829.
61. Coll O, Benoist G, Ville Y, et al. Guidelines on CMV congenital infection. *J Perinat Med*. 2009;37:433-445.
62. Guerra B, Simonazzi G, Puccetti C, et al. Ultrasound prediction of symptomatic congenital cytomegalovirus infection. *Am J Obstet Gynecol*. 2008;198:380 e381-387.
63. Benoist G, Salomon LJ, Mohlo M, Suarez B, Jacquemard F, Ville Y. Cytomegalovirus-related fetal brain lesions: Comparison between targeted ultrasound examination and magnetic resonance imaging. *Ultrasound Obstet Gynecol*. 2008;32:900-905.
64. Picone O, Simon I, Benachi A, Brunelle F, Sonigo P. Comparison between ultrasound and magnetic resonance imaging in assessment of fetal cytomegalovirus infection. *Prenat Diagn*. 2008;28:753-758.
65. Pass RF, Britt WJ, Stagno S. Cytomegalovirus. In: Lennette EH, Lennette DA, Lennette ET, eds. *Diagnostic Procedures for Viral, Rickettsial, and Chlamydial Infections*. 5th ed. Washington D.C.: American Public Health Association; 1995:253-271.
66. Balcarek KB, Warren W, Smith RJ, Lyon MD, Pass RF. Neonatal screening for congenital cytomegalovirus infection by detection of virus in saliva. *J Infect Dis*. 1993;30:1433-1436.
67. Warren WP, Balcarek KB, Smith R, Pass RF. Comparison of rapid methods of detection of cytomegalovirus in saliva with virus isolation in tissue culture. *J Clin Microbiol*. 1992;30:786-789.
68. Yamamoto AY, Mussi-Pinhata MM, Marin LJ, Brito RM, Oliveira PF, Coelho TB. Is saliva as reliable as urine for detection of cytomegalovirus DNA for neonatal screening of congenital CMV infection? *J Clin Virol*. 2006;36:228-230.
69. Barbi M, Binda S, Primache V, et al. Cytomegalovirus DNA detection in Guthrie cards: A powerful tool for diagnosing congenital infection. *J Clin Virol*. 2000;17:159-165.
70. Johansson PJH, Jonsson M, Ahlfors K, Ivarsson SA, Svanberg L, Guthenberg C. Retrospective diagnosis of congenital cytomegalovirus infection performed by polymerase chain reaction in blood stored on filter paper. *Scand J Infect Dis*. 1997;29:465-468.
71. Scanga L, Chaing S, Powell C, et al. Diagnosis of human congenital cytomegalovirus infection by amplification of viral DNA from dried blood spots on perinatal cards. *J Mol Diagn*. 2006;8:240-245.

11

72. Yamagishi Y, Miyagawa H, Wada K, et al. CMV DNA detection in dried blood spots for diagnosing congenital CMV infection in Japan. *J Med Virol*. 2006;78:923-925.
73. Boppana SB, Ross SA, Novak Z, et al. Dried blood spot real-time polymerase chain reaction assays to screen newborns for congenital cytomegalovirus infection. *JAMA*. 2010;303:1375-1382.
74. Boppana SB, Ross SA, Shimamura M, et al. Saliva polymerase chain reaction assays for cytomegalovirus screening in newborns. *N Engl J Med*. 2011;364:2011-2018.
75. Jacquemard F, Yamamoto M, Costa JM, et al. Maternal administration of valaciclovir in symptomatic intrauterine cytomegalovirus infection. *BJOG*. 2007;114:1113-1121.
76. Nigro G, Adler SP, La Torre R, Best AM. Passive immunization during pregnancy for congenital cytomegalovirus infection. *N Engl J Med*. 2005;353:1350-1362.
77. La Torre R, Nigro G, Mazzocco M, Best AM, Adler SP. Placental enlargement in women with primary maternal cytomegalovirus infection is associated with fetal and neonatal disease. *Clin Infect Dis*. 2006;43:994-1000.
78. Kimberlin DW, Lin CY, Sanchez PJ, et al. Effect of ganciclovir therapy on hearing in symptomatic congenital cytomegalovirus disease involving the central nervous system: A randomized, controlled trial. *J Pediatr*. 2003;143:16-25.
79. Cytomegalovirus. In: Pickering LK, Baker CJ, Kimberlin DW, Long SS, eds. *Red Book: 2009 Report of the Committee of Infectious Diseases*. 29th ed. Elk Grove Village: American Academy of Pediatrics; 2009:275-280.
80. Mosca F, Pugni L, Barbi M, Binda S. Transmission of cytomegalovirus. *Lancet*. 2001;357:1800.
81. Williamson WD, Desmond MM, LaFevers N, Taber LH, Catlin FI, Weaver TG. Symptomatic congenital cytomegalovirus. Disorders of language, learning and hearing. *Am J Dis Child*. 1982;136:902-905.
82. Noyola DE, Demmler GJ, Nelson CT, et al. Early predictors of neurodevelopmental outcome in symptomatic congenital cytomegalovirus infection. *J Pediatr*. 2001;138:325-331.
83. Rivera LB, Boppana SB, Fowler KB, Britt WJ, Stagno S, Pass RF. Predictors of hearing loss in children with symptomatic congenital cytomegalovirus infection. *Pediatrics*. 2002;110:762-767.
84. Dahle AJ, Fowler KB, Wright JD, Boppana SB, Britt WJ, Pass RF. Longitudinal investigations of hearing disorders in children with congenital cytomegalovirus. *J Am Acad Audiol*. 2000;11:283-290.
85. Fowler KB, McCollister FP, Dahle AJ, Boppana SB, Britt WJ, Pass RF. Progressive and fluctuating sensorineural hearing loss in children with asymptomatic congenital cytomegalovirus infection. *J Pediatr*. 1997;130:624-630.
86. Harris S, Ahlfors K, Ivarsson SA, Lernmark B, Svanberg L. Congenital cytomegalovirus infection and sensorineural hearing loss. *Ear Hear*. 1984;5:352-355.
87. Williamson WD, Demmler GJ, Percy AK, Catlin FI. Progressive hearing loss in infants with asymptomatic congenital cytomegalovirus infection. *Pediatrics*. 1992;90:862-866.
88. Williamson WD, Percy AK, Yow MD, et al. Asymptomatic congenital cytomegalovirus infection: Audiologic, neuroradiologic, and neurodevelopmental abnormalities during the first year. *Am J Dis Child*. 1990;144:1365-1368.
89. Lanari M, Lazzarotto T, Venturi V, et al. Neonatal cytomegalovirus blood load and risk of sequelae in symptomatic and asymptomatic congenitally infected newborns. *Pediatrics*. 2006;117:e76-e83.
90. Ross SA, Novak Z, Fowler KB, Arora N, Britt WJ, Boppana SB. Cytomegalovirus blood viral load and hearing loss in young children with congenital infection. *Pediatr Infect Dis J*. 2009;28:588-592.
91. Miron D, Brosilow S, Felszer K, et al. Incidence and clinical manifestations of breast milk-acquired cytomegalovirus infection in low birth weight infants. *J Perinatol*. 2005;25:299-303.
92. Vollmer B, Seibold-Weiger K, Schmitz-Salue C, et al. Postnatally acquired cytomegalovirus infection via breast milk: Effects on hearing and development in preterm infants. *Pediatr Infect Dis J*. 2004;23:322-327.
93. Adler SP, Finney JW, Manganello AM, Best AM. Prevention of child-to-mother transmission of cytomegalovirus among pregnant women. *J Pediatr*. 2004;145:485-491.
94. Picone O, Vauloup-Fellous C, Cordier AG, et al. A 2-year study on cytomegalovirus infection during pregnancy in a French hospital. *BJOG*. 2009;116:818-823.
95. Stern H. Live cytomegalovirus vaccination of healthy volunteers: Eight-year follow-up studies. *Birth Defects Orig Artic Ser*. 1984;20:263-269.
96. Adler SP, Plotkin SA, Gonczol E, et al. A canarypox vector expressing cytomegalovirus (CMV) glycoprotein B primes for antibody responses to a live attenuated CMV vaccine (Towne). *J Infect Dis*. 1999;180:843-846.
97. Gonczol E, Ianacone J, Ho WZ, Starr S, Meignier B, Plotkin S. Isolated gA/gB glycoprotein complex of human cytomegalovirus envelope induces humoral and cellular immune-responses in human volunteers. *Vaccine*. 1990;8:130-136.
98. Pass RF, Zhang C, Evans A, et al. Vaccine prevention of maternal cytomegalovirus infection. *N Engl J Med*. 2009;360:1191-1199.
99. Plotkin SA. Cytomegalovirus vaccine. *Am Heart J*. 1999;138:S484-S487.
100. Dekker CL, Arvin AM. One step closer to a CMV vaccine. *N Engl J Med*. 2009;360:1250-1252.

Neonatal T Cell Immunity and Its Regulation by Innate Immunity and Dendritic Cells

David B. Lewis, MD

12

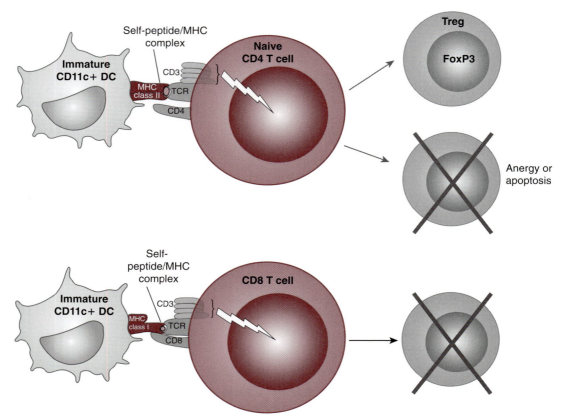

Figure 12-1   Immature dendritic cells (DCs) play an important role in T cell tolerance. The CD11c⁺ DC subset presents self-peptides associated with major histocompatibility complex (MHC) molecules to naïve CD4 or CD8 T cells without costimulation. In the case of CD4 T cells, which are recognized by their T cell receptor (TCR) peptides associated with MHC class II molecules, this may lead to differentiation of self-reactive CD4 T cells into regulatory T cells (Tregs), which express the FoxP3 transcription factor, or to the induction of CD4 T cell anergy or apoptosis. In the case of self-reactive CD8 T cells, which recognize peptides associated with MHC class I molecules, this may lead to anergy or apoptosis.

Dendritic cells (DCs), which have been aptly referred to as the sentinels of the immune system, are bone marrow–derived myeloid cells that integrate signals from receptors that recognize pathogen products and signs of inflammation, damage, or cellular stress that often occur in the setting of infection.[1,2] In the absence of these warning signs of infection, the default program of DCs is to maintain tolerance by presenting peptides derived from self-proteins to T cells (Fig. 12-1). The presentation by DCs of self-peptides bound to major histocompatibility complex (MHC) molecules without concurrent co-stimulatory signals leads T cells to undergo clonal deletion, anergy, or differentiation into suppressive regulatory T cells (Tregs).[3] Alternatively, if DCs are activated by the engagement of receptors indicating infection or a potential infection-related stress, they increase their internalization of extracellular fluid and particulate debris from perturbed tissues and process internalized proteins into peptides, which are loaded onto MHC molecules (Fig. 12-2). If these peptides are derived from foreign pathogens and are recognized by the αβ–T cell receptor (TCR) on the T cell surface, the T cell undergoes activation, proliferation, and differentiation into effector cells that carry out adaptive immune responses. In general, cluster of differentiation (CD)4 T cells are programmed during their development in the thymus to recognize peptides bound to MHC class II molecules, whereas CD8 T cells recognize peptides bound to MHC class I molecules. Full T cell activation of naïve CD4 or CD8 T cells requires that the DCs also express co-stimulatory ligands, such as CD80 and CD86, for molecules on the T cell, such as CD28. Because

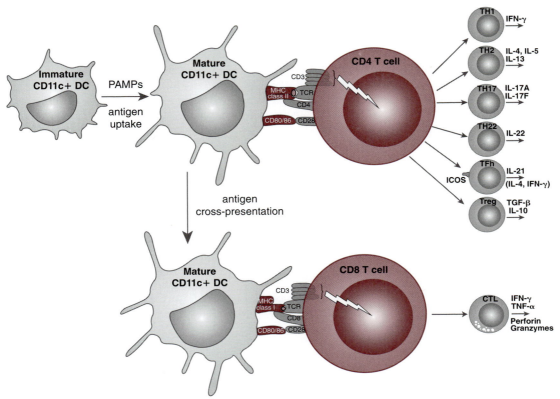

Figure 12-2   Recognition by immature dendritic cells (DCs) of pathogen-associated molecular patterns (PAMPs) by innate immune receptors results in DC maturation and enhanced capacity to activate CD4 and CD8 T cells, owing in part to increased expression of CD80/86 costimulatory molecules. CD4 T cell activation involves presentation of antigenic peptides bound to major histocompatibility complex (MHC) class II molecules. Activated CD4 T cells may differentiate into at least five different types of effector populations, characterized by specialized cytokine secretion patterns, which are indicated in parentheses, including T helper (Th)-1 (interferon [IFN]-γ), Th-2 (interleukin [IL]-4, IL-5, and IL-13), Th-17 (IL-17A and IL-17F), Th-22 (IL-22), and T follicular helper (TFh) cells (IL-21, variably IL-4, IFN-γ), or into regulatory T cells (Tregs) (transforming growth factor [TGF]-β, IL-10), which suppress the function of effector T cells. CD11c⁺ DCs activated by PAMPs are also efficient in cross-presentation of antigens taken up by endocytosis or pinocytosis by MHC class I molecules; this activates CD8 T cells, leading to their differentiation into effector cells that secrete cytokines, such as IFN-γ and tumor necrosis factor (TNF)-α, and cytotoxins, such as perforin and granzymes.

activated DCs display very high levels of peptide/MHC complexes and co-stimulatory ligands, they are the most efficient antigen-presenting cells (APCs) for initiating the T cell immune response to new antigens that have not been previously encountered, also referred to as *neoantigens*. However, DCs are also important for maximizing the memory T cell response to bacterial and viral pathogens.[4]

In the case of DCs located in nonlymphoid tissue, such as the skin or gut, activation results in their migration from infected/perturbed tissue to peripheral lymphoid organs via afferent lymphatics. Once reaching the peripheral lymphoid organ (e.g., a locally draining lymph node), the migratory DC, or a lymphoid tissue resident DC to which the migratory DC transfers, presents antigen to T cells.[5] DC-derived signals have an important influence on the type of effector responses that are elicited from naïve T cells. For example, naïve CD4 T cells may become T helper (Th)-1, Th-2, Th-9, Th-17, Th-22, or T follicular helper (TFh) effector cells, each with a distinct cytokine secretion profile and role in host defense[6-8] (see Fig. 12-2). Given that the role of DCs in regulating T cell immunity is highly nuanced and potentially involves the recognition of diverse types of pathogens in different tissues, it is perhaps not surprising that DCs are heterogeneous in their ontogeny, location, migration, phenotype, and function.

12

Because substantial evidence suggests that neonatal and infant T cell function, particularly that mediated by CD4 T cells, is reduced compared with that of the adult in response to infection,[9] it is plausible that immaturity and/or altered DC function could contribute to this age-related limitation in adaptive immunity. This chapter will provide a brief summary of the major phenotypes and functions of the major subsets of human DCs and their usage of innate immune receptors for pathogen recognition; will summarize clinical and immunologic studies indicating decreased T cell immune function in the neonate; and will provide evidence that functional immaturity of DCs may contribute to limitations of T cell immunity in early postnatal life.

Dendritic Cells and Their Development

DCs, which derive their name from the characteristic cytoplasmic protrusions or "dendrites" found on their mature form, are found in all tissues. DCs also circulate in the blood, where they represent approximately 0.5% to 1% of peripheral blood mononuclear cells (PBMCs). Human DCs express high levels of the CD11c/CD18 β2 integrin protein, with the exception of the plasmacytoid DC (pDC) subset, which is CD11c⁻. Hereafter, we collectively refer to these "conventional" nonplasmacytoid DC populations as CD11c⁺ DCs. The DC cell surface lacks molecules that characterize other bone marrow–derived cell lineages—a feature that is termed lineage (Lin)⁻, including molecules that are typically expressed on T cells (e.g., CD3-ε), monocytes or neutrophils (e.g., CD14), B cells (e.g., CD19, CD20), and natural killer (NK) cells (e.g., CD16, CD56). Resting DCs express MHC class II, and, upon activation/maturation, express greater amounts than any other cell type in the body. Relatively high levels of MHC class I are also expressed.

DCs in the circulation and tissues are heterogeneous based on their surface phenotype and functional attributes. A population of CD11c⁺ lymphoid tissue (LT) DCs resides in the thymus and peripheral lymphoid tissues, such as lymph nodes and spleen. In the absence of infection-related signals or inflammation, LT DCs, which are referred as being "immature," are highly effective in the uptake of self-antigens in soluble or particulate form and present self-antigens for the maintenance of T cell tolerance. CD11c⁺ migratory DCs with a similar immature phenotype and function as LT DCs are found in the interstitial areas of all nonlymphoid tissues. Based on murine studies, a small number of these immature migratory DCs move via the lymphatics to draining lymphoid tissue, where they present self-peptides to maintain T cell tolerance. Also based on murine studies, a small number of bone marrow–derived pre-DCs enter into the blood and then exit into the lymphoid and nonlymphoid tissues for their final stages of differentiation into immature LT and migratory DCs, respectively. In humans, the extent to which immature CD11c⁺ LT and migratory DCs recirculate (re-enter the bloodstream) is unclear, as are the surface phenotype and frequency of circulating pre-DCs.

Most populations of human DCs are capable of internally transferring proteins taken up from the external environment, which would normally be destined for MHC class II antigen presentation to CD4 T cells. Instead, these external environmental proteins are loaded onto the MHC class I antigen presentation pathway for CD8 T cells through a process known as cross-presentation. Although the mechanisms by which cross-presentation occurs in DCs remains poorly understood, this process is important not only for activation of CD8 T cells to pathogen-derived antigens but also for maintenance of CD8 T cell tolerance by immature DCs.

When the results of gene expression profiling are combined with phenotype, function, tissue location, and ontogeny, human DCs can be divided into three major subgroups: (1) resident CD11c⁺ LT DCs and CD11c- plasmacytoid DCs (pDCs); (2) migratory CD11c⁺ DCs of nonlymphoid tissues (e.g., dermal DCs); and (3) inflammatory DCs that are derived from mature mononuclear phagocytes.[10] Murine studies[1] suggest that the DC and monocyte lineages are derived from a common bone marrow cell precursor—the monocyte and DC progenitor—which can differentiate into monocytes or committed DC progenitors (CDPs). The CDP gives rise to CD11c⁺

pre-DCs, which enter the blood and then are presumed to rapidly enter into lymphoid or nonlymphoid organs, where they respectively differentiate in situ into immature LT DCs or migratory DCs. In the mouse this final differentiation step includes the acquisition of their final DC subset surface phenotype, characteristic cytoplasmic protrusions, and probing behavior.[11] In contrast to CD11c[+] DCs, pDCs leaving the bone marrow appear to be immature functionally but otherwise fully differentiated. Unlike CD11c[+] DCs, pDCs acquire cytoplasmic protrusions and high levels of MHC class II only after they undergo terminal maturation through exposure to pathogen-derived products or viral infection. Finally, inflammatory DCs are generated from mononuclear phagocytes that enter through the endothelium of inflamed tissues sites.[12]

PAMP Receptors Used by Dendritic Cells

DCs use four major families of innate immune receptors to detect pathogen-associated molecular patterns (PAMPs): Toll-like receptors (TLRs), nucleotide-binding domain (NOD)- and leucine-rich repeat (LRR)-containing receptors (NLRs), C-type lectin receptors (CLRs), and retinoic acid inducible gene (RIG)-I–like receptors (RLRs).[13,14] Although each of these families has distinct ligand-binding specificity, their engagement ultimately generates pro-inflammatory signals by canonical pathways, such as those involving nuclear factor kappa light chain enhancer of activated B cells (NFκB) and activator protein-1 (AP-1).[13] Also, depending on the local tissue context, these innate immune receptors may be involved in DCs, inducing tolerance rather than promoting T cell activation.[3] Appropriate regulation of innate immune receptor activity in leukocytes is important to prevent autoinflammatory or autoimmune disease and involves receptor proteins containing cytoplasmic immunoreceptor tyrosine-based inhibitory motifs, such as those of the Siglec (sialic acid–binding immunoglobulin-like lectin) family.[15] These negative regulatory pathways have been extensively exploited by microbes to evade initiation of the innate immune response.[16]

TOLL-Like Receptors

The TLR family of transmembrane proteins recognizes microbial structures, particularly those that are highly evolutionarily conserved and typically essential for the function of the microbe. These microbial structures are relatively invariant and are not present in normal mammalian cells. For this reason, recognition of these pathogen-associated molecular patterns by TLRs provides infallible evidence for microbial invasion, alerting the innate immune system to respond appropriately. TLRs are a family of structurally related pattern recognition receptors for pathogen-derived molecules. Ten different TLRs are expressed in humans with distinct ligand specificities.[14] TLR-1, -2, -4, -5, -6, and -10 are expressed on the cell surface and are involved in the recognition of pathogen-derived non–nucleic acid products found in the extracellular environment, whereas TLR-3, -7, -8, and -9 are found in endosomal compartments and recognize nucleic acids.[17] Some of the better characterized surface TLRs in terms of their ligand specificity[14] include the following: TLR-2, which heterodimerizes with TLR-1 or TLR-6 and recognizes bacterial lipopeptides, lipoteichoic acid, and peptidoglycans of Gram-positive bacteria and fungi, such as *Candida* species; TLR-4, which recognizes lipopolysaccharide (LPS) on Gram-negative bacteria and respiratory syncytial virus (RSV) fusion protein; and TLR-5, which recognizes bacterial flagellin protein. TLRs with nucleic acid ligand specificity[17] include the following: TLR-3, which recognizes double-stranded RNA; TLR-7 and -8, which recognize single-stranded RNA; and TLR-9, which recognizes unmethylated CpG (a TLR-9 ligand)–containing DNA. The nucleic acid–binding TLRs appear to play a role mainly in antiviral recognition and defense. This is supported by the finding that individuals lacking TLR-3, tumor necrosis factor (TNF) receptor–associated factor-3 (TRAF3) (which is required for TLR-3 signaling), or uncoordinated-93B (UNC-93B, which is required for proper localization of TLR-3,

12

TLR-7, TLR-8, and TLR-9 to endosomes), are highly susceptible to developing encephalitis following primary infection with herpes simplex virus (HSV).[18,19]

The efficient presentation by DCs of peptide antigens to T cells requires that the foreign proteins internalized by DCs should be contained in phagosomes that also have TLR ligands.[20] Signals derived from interaction of these TLR ligands with TLRs induce maturation of migratory and LT DCs. Most cytokine production by CD11c$^+$ DCs in response to TLR engagement requires the adaptor molecule myeloid differentiation factor 88 (MyD88) and the interferon response factor (IRF)-5 transcription factor.[21] The production of type I interferons (IFNs) by pDCs through engagement of TLR-7, -8, and -9 is dependent on MyD88 and the IRF-7 transcription factor.[22]

In mice, DCs can upregulate their surface expression of MHC class II and T cell costimulatory molecules, such as CD80 and CD86, by exposure to inflammatory mediators. However, these CD11c$^+$ DCs are not able to produce interleukin (IL)-12p70 (a heterodimer consisting of the IL-12/23 p40 subunit and the IL-12 p35 subunit) and effectively drive naïve CD4 T cell differentiation toward Th-1 cells unless they also receive a second signal by concurrent engagement of their TLRs.[23] This "two-signal" requirement, which is reminiscent of T cell activation needing both peptide/MHC and a separate costimulatory signal, may be important in preventing inappropriate T cell activation by CD11c$^+$ DCs.

NOD- and LRR-Containing Receptors

NLRs are encoded by 22 genes in humans.[24] NLRs have a characteristic three-domain structure consisting of a C-terminal LRR domain that is involved in ligand recognition and modulates their activity, a central NOD domain involved in nucleotide oligomerization and binding, and an N-terminal effector domain that is linked to intracellular signaling molecules.[25-28] NOD1 and NOD2 are NLRs that sense intracellular products of the synthesis, degradation, and remodeling of the peptidoglycan component of bacterial cell walls (e.g., γ-D-glutamyl-meso-diaminopimelic acid and muramyl dipeptide) and activate the NFκB and AP-1 pro-inflammatory pathways, often in synergy with TLRs. This synergy may account for the more efficient production of interleukin (IL)-23 by peptidoglycan, a TLR-2 ligand, than bacterial lipopeptides, which activate TLR-2 but not NODs.[29] NOD2 is also activated by viral infection,[30] leading to its association with components of the RIG-I complex, which is discussed later.[31] Several NLRs, including NLRP3 (also known as NALP3 or cryopyrin), are part of the multiprotein complex called the *inflammasome,* in which ligand recognition results in the activation of caspase 1. Activated caspase 1 cleaves pro–IL-1-β and –IL-18, resulting in secretion of the mature forms of these cytokines.[28] Caspase 1 is activated by the NLRP3 inflammasome in response to non–nucleic acid components of bacteria (e.g., LPS, muramyl dipeptide), including toxins,[32] *Candida albicans,*[33] bacterial RNA and DNA, viral RNA, products of injured host cells (e.g., uric acid), danger signals (e.g., low intracellular potassium concentrations that are triggered by extracellular adenosine triphosphate [ATP] binding to purinergic receptors that mediate potassium efflux), and foreign substances, including asbestos.[25,28,30] Studies of gain-of-function mutations of NLRP3 in humans and mice also demonstrate that the NLRP3 inflammasome promotes Th-17 cell development.[34] The activated in melanoma 2 (AIM2) inflammasome is activated by cytosolic DNA that occurs during viral or bacterial infection.[30]

C-Type Lectin Receptors

CLRs are a heterogeneous and large group of transmembrane proteins that have C-type lectin-like domains and that mediate diverse infections, including cell adhesion, tissue remodeling, endocytosis, phagocytosis, and innate immune recognition.[35] CLRs include dendritic cell–specific intercellular adhesion molecule-3-grabbing non-integrin (DC-SIGN, also known as CD209), a receptor on DCs that is involved in their interaction with human immunodeficiency virus (HIV), langerin (CD207; a protein that is expressed at particularly high levels by Langerhans DCs), and DC-associated C-type lectin (DECTIN)-1 (also known as CLEC7A) and DECTIN-2 (also known as CLEC6A).[36] DEs are expressed by DCs and macrophages, with DECTIN-1 recognizing β-1,3-linked glucans and DECTIN-2 recognizing high mannose α-mannans; these sugar residues are found in fungi and mycobacteria but not in mammalian cells.[35] DECTIN-1 and DECTIN-2 synergize with TLR-2 ligands present on fungi to stimulate production of tumor necrosis factor (TNF)-α, IL-6, IL-10, IL-12, and IL-23.

RIG-I–Like Receptors

Three members of the RLR family have been identified: retinoic acid inducible gene-I (RIG-I), melanoma differentiation associated gene 5 (MDA-5), and laboratory of genetics and physiology 2 (LGP-2).[14,37,38] RIG-I and MDA-5 have a helicase domain that binds viral RNA, a regulatory domain, and an N-terminal caspase recruitment domain (CARD) that links these receptors to signaling pathways. These pathways include those involved in the production of type I IFNs (IRF-3 and IRF-7) and NFκB, as well as inflammasome activation.[39] LGP-2 has a helicase and regulatory domain but lacks a CARD domain, and appears to positively regulate responses by RIG-I and MDA-5.[14] RLRs are expressed in the cytoplasm of nearly all mammalian cells, which provides a ubiquitous, cell-intrinsic, and rapid viral surveillance system for double-stranded RNAs found in healthy mammalian cells. RIG-I mainly recognizes parainfluenza and other paramyxoviruses, influenza, and flaviviruses, such as hepatitis C, whereas MDA-5 is important for resistance to picornaviruses, such as enteroviruses. RIG-I and MDA-5 interact with a common signaling adaptor interferon-β promoter stimulator-1 (IPS-1), which, like the TRIF signal adapter molecule in the TLR-3/4 pathway, induces the phosphorylation of IRF-3/IRF-7 to stimulate type I IFN production.[14] RIG-I and MDA-5 are able to trigger the production of type I IFN.[40] These RNA helicases are able to detect viral RNA found in the cytoplasm; in contrast, recognition of viral nucleic acids by TLR-3, and TLR-7, -8, and -9 can occur only in the lumen of endosomes.

CD11c⁺ Lymphoid Tissue Dendritic Cells

Human CD11c⁺ LT DCs are found in the thymus, spleen, peripheral lymph nodes, and other secondary lymphoid tissues, and in small numbers in the blood. They can be divided into two major subsets: blood DC antigen (BDCA)-1⁺ and BDCA-3⁺ CD11c⁺ DCs. These and other CD11c⁺ DC populations that are not pDCs are often referred to in the older literature as *conventional DCs.* The term *myeloid DCs,* which has also been used, is obsolete and should be avoided, because all DC populations are myeloid derived. CD11c⁺ LT DC development in the bone marrow requires expression by DC precursors of Flt3, a cytokine receptor, and its binding of FMS-related tyrosine kinase 3 (Flt3)-ligand, which is produced by nonhematopoietic stromal cells.[41]

The subset of circulating CD11c⁺ DCs, which are likely the human equivalent of the murine CD11b⁺ subset of LT and migratory DCs, basally express high levels of MHC class II and other proteins involved in MHC class II antigen. As activated/mature DCs, they appear to be specialized for initiating immune responses by naïve CD4 T cells or, as immature DCs, for their tolerance induction. BDCA-1⁺ CD11c⁺ DCs express a number of receptors for PAMPs, which include TLRs, NLRs, CLRs, and RLRs (see later). PAMP receptor engagement results in their switching from a tolerance program to an activation program that initiates the T cell immune response. The BDCA-1 molecule (CD1c) is involved in nonclassic antigen presentation of mycobacterial products (mycoketides and lipopeptides) to T cells,[42] but it is unclear whether CD1c has additional roles in CD11c⁺ DC function.

BDCA-3⁺ CD11c⁺ DCs are likely the human equivalent of the murine CD8α⁺ subset of LT and migratory DCs in that they share a number of characteristic features.[43] These include expression of the basic leucine zipper transcription factor, ATF-like 3 (BATF3), and IRF-8 transcription factors; the C-type LECtin domain family 9 member A (CLEC9A) of the CLR family; langerin; nectin-like 2; the XCR1 chemokine receptor (for lymphotactin);[44-46] and expression of TLR-3 but not TLR-7.[47] BDCA3+ CD11c+ DCs are a discrete LT DC population of the human spleen[47] and tonsils,[48] and are also present at a low frequency in the circulation (1 in 10^4 of PBMCs). Similar to murine CD8α+ DCs, BDCA-3+ CD11c+ DCs are capable of efficiently phagocytosing dead cells and cross-presenting cell-associated and soluble antigens to CD8 T cells,[47] and the CLEC9A protein may facilitate their recognition and uptake of necrotic cellular material.[49] Most other human CD11c+ DCs populations besides BDCA-3+ DCs also have the capacity to cross-present, whereas murine CD8α+ DCs are highly specialized for this purpose.[43] Engagement of TLR-3 (e.g., using polyinosinic:polycytidylic acid [poly I:C], a mimic of double-stranded RNA) induces high levels of IFN-λ (IL-28/29) production by human BDCA-3+ CD11c+ and murine CD8α+ DCs.[50] BDCA-3+ CD11c+ DCs of the spleen produce IL-12p70 in response to a mixture of TLR agonists, antigen-specific CD8 T cell clones, and antigenic peptide;[47] BDCA-3+ CD11c+-like DCs, generated from cord blood hematopoietic stem cell and progenitor cells using a cocktail of cytokines, produce IL-6 in response to agonists for TLR-8 but not for TLR-7, which suggests that they express TLR-8.[47] BDCA-3, also known as CD141 or thrombomodulin, binds to thrombin, but its role in human DC function remains unclear.

CD11c+ Migratory Dendritic Cells and Langerhans Cells

The migratory DCs of nonlymphoid tissues, as in the dermis of the skin, appear to be derived from a common circulating pre-DC pool that also can give rise to LT DCs. Dermal DCs have been among the best studied and will be used as an example here. Similar to LT DCs, migratory DCs appear to be derived from the sequential differentiation of a common progenitor into committed DC progenitors in an Flt3-ligand–dependent manner. Migratory DCs in noninflamed nonlymphoid tissues are mainly immature, and express low to moderate quantities of MHC class I and class II molecules on their surface. These dermal CD11c+ populations include both BDCA-1+ and BDCA-3+ subsets,[51] analogous to those found in the blood and lymphoid tissues. Small numbers of pDCs are also found in normal dermis.[52]

Based largely on murine data, in the steady-state conditions that prevail in uninfected individuals, a constant low-level turnover of migratory DCs occurs; these cells enter into tissues from the blood and migrate via lymphatics to secondary lymphoid tissues, where they play a central role in maintaining a state of tolerance to self-antigens. This tolerance appears to be the result of migratory DCs presenting self-antigens to T cells in the absence of costimulatory signals required for T cell activation. Support for this idea comes from a recent study of lymph nodes that drain uninfected and noninflamed skin, which revealed small numbers of skin-derived dermal DCs and Langerhans cells (described in detail later) that were relatively ineffective in stimulating T cells in vitro compared with LT resident DCs.[53]

In response to infection of the tissue, the immature migratory DC undergoes maturation, which includes increased surface expression of the CC-chemokine receptor 7 (CCR7), and loss of chemokine receptors that help retain the DC within the tissues. This change in chemokine receptor expression enhances CD11c+ DC migration via lymphatics to T cell–rich areas of the draining lymph nodes. Migratory DC maturation and entry into the draining lymphatics can be triggered by a variety of stimuli, including pathogen-derived products that are recognized directly by innate immune receptors; by cytokines, including IL-1β, TNF-α, and type I IFNs; and by engagement of CD40 on the DC surface by CD40 ligand (CD154) on the surface of activated CD4 T cells. Migratory DCs also express multiple TLRs, NLRs, CLRs, and RLRs (see later) that when engaged also promote maturation and migration to draining lymph nodes via the afferent lymphatics.

Langerhans cells are a unique type of DC found only in the epidermis, where they can be differentiated from dermal CD11c+ DCs by their expression of CD1a and Birbeck granules and lack of expression of the factor XIIIa coagulation factor.[54] Langerhans cells are distinct from other DC populations in their ability to undergo local self-renewal in the epidermis and their dependence on macrophage colony-stimulating factor (M-CSF) for their development, rather than Flt3-ligand or granulocyte-monocyte colony-stimulating factor (GM-CSF). Expression of langerin is not specific for Langerhans cells, and recent cell lineage tracing studies suggest that Langerhans cells may play a relatively minor role compared with migratory dermal DCs in the activation of T cells in draining lymph nodes, at least in certain contexts.[55] Nevertheless, they appear to be able to cross-present protein antigens as efficiently as CD11c+ DCs.[56]

Plasmacytoid Dendritic Cells

Human plasmacytoid dendritic cells (pDCs), which are BDCA-2+ CD11c−, were formerly considered to represent a distinct lymphoid DC population. However, currently, pDCs are included with the CD11c+ LT DC subgroup based on gene expression profiling[10] and the fact that murine studies have shown that pDCs, similar to CD11c+ DCs, are derived from a bone marrow CDP population. The differentiation of pDCs from CDPs appears to require high levels of expression of the E protein 2-2 (E2-2) transcription factor.[10,57] Human pDC-lineage cells have a characteristic surface phenotype of high expression of the IL-3 receptor α chain (CD123), low but detectable expression of CD4, and lack of immunoglobulin-like transcript 1 (ILT1). BDCA-2, also known as CD303 or CLEC4C, is a C-type lectin that appears to be involved in the negative regulation of intracellular pDC signaling. pDCs appear to complete their differentiation in the bone marrow and enter into the lymphoid tissues and the liver from the circulation. pDCs are found in the blood, secondary lymphoid organs, and particularly inflamed lymph nodes.[57,58] The difference in the pDC pattern of localization from that of most immature DCs of the tissues is attributable to their expression of adhesion molecules, such as L-selectin (CD62-L), which promotes entry into peripheral lymphoid tissue via high endothelial venules.[57] In contrast to immature/unactivated CD11c+ DCs of the lymphoid and nonlymphoid tissues, immature/unactivated pDCs have a limited capacity for antigen uptake and presentation. Although with maturation signals, pDCs acquire a substantial ability to present and cross-present antigen to CD4 and CD8 T cells, respectively,[57] their predominant function appears not to be antigen presentation but, rather, the production of large numbers of type I IFNs. Secretion of type I IFNs results in systemic antiviral protection and helps promote CD8 T cell and Th-1 CD4 T cell responses that contribute to antiviral protection. Consistent with this function, and discussed later, pDCs do not appear to employ NLRs, CLRs, or RLRs to recognize and respond to microbes. Rather, recognition and type I IFN response are triggered through the three TLRs they express in abundance: TLR-7, -8, and -9. TLR-7 and TLR-8 are activated by binding ssRNA from RNA viruses such as influenza, and TLR-9 is activated by binding to DNA from viruses such as HSV, or from bacteria.[14]

Inflammatory and Monocyte-Derived Dendritic Cells

Murine studies have demonstrated that monocytes can differentiate into DC populations at sites of marked inflammation, as occurs in infection with *Listeria*, *Leishmania*, or influenza virus. In murine infection models, these inflammatory DCs characteristically secrete high levels of TNF-α and produce inducible nitric oxide synthase, which contributes to pathogen clearance.[59] The extent to which inflammatory DC generation occurs in vivo in humans is unclear, but one of the best described examples is found in the skin of certain patients with severe leprosy.[60,61] The phenotype of these DCs (CD1b+DC-SIGN−) suggests that they may differentiate from monocytes that are activated by TLR engagement, and that they differentiate by a GM-CSF/GM-CSF receptor pathway.[61] Thus, unlike the differentiation of LT DCs and migratory DCs, in vivo generation of inflammatory DCs is GM-CSF rather than Flt3-ligand dependent. Culturing of monocytes with GM-CSF plus IL-4 to produce monocyte-derived DCs (MDDCs) probably more closely mimics the generation of inflammatory DCs than of migratory or LT DCs; this is supported by comparative gene expression studies.[10]

12

Combinatorial PAMP Receptor Recognition by Dendritic Cells

The innate immune system of DCs identifies the nature of the microbial threat based on the combination of innate immune receptors that are engaged, and then tailors the early innate response and the subsequent antigen-specific T cell response to combat that specific type of infection. For example, extracellular bacteria characteristically engage TLR-2, -4, and/or -5 on the cell surface; they also activate NLRs. This leads to the production of pro-inflammatory cytokines and IL-23, which recruits neutrophils and favors the development of a Th-17 CD4 T cell response. Fungal products engage TLR-2 and DECTIN-1 and -2, and activate the NLRP3 RLR, which leads to a similar neutrophil/Th-17–predominant response.[29,62] Viruses activate TLR-3, -7, -8, and -9, RLRs, and cytoplasmic receptors for DNA, such as DNA-dependent activator of IFN-regulatory factors (DAI) and others yet to be characterized, resulting in the robust induction of type I IFNs and IFN-induced chemokines; this promotes the differentiation and recruitment of CD8 T cells and Th-1 CD4 T cells. Nonviral intracellular bacterial pathogens, such as *Mycobacteria, Salmonella,* and *Listeria,* also induce type I IFNs, which collaborate with signals from cell surface TLRs and NLRs to induce the production of IL-12-p70, resulting in Th-1–type responses. The importance of these innate sensing mechanisms is indicated by the frequency with which pathogenic microbes and viruses have evolved strategies to evade them and their downstream mediators.[16,63]

T Cell Activation by Dendritic Cells

DC maturation and, in the case of nonlymphoid tissue CD11c[+] DCs, migration can be triggered by a variety of stimuli. These include pathogen-derived products that are recognized through innate immune receptors of the TLR, NLR, RLR, and CLR families and cytokines (e.g., IL-1β, TNF-α, and GM-CSF), and by engagement of CD40 on the CD11c[+] DC surface by CD154 expressed on activated CD4 T cells. Thus, the function and localization of DCs can be rapidly modulated by direct recognition of microbes or their products, by cytokines produced by neighboring DCs[64] or other cells of the innate system,[65] or by products of T cells to which they present antigens (e.g., CD154). Exposure of immature CD11c[+] DCs to inflammatory stimuli prevents further antigen uptake and, instead, leads to increased surface expression of MHC class II and class I molecules displaying antigenic peptides derived from previously internalized particles.[66] Concurrently, in the case of migratory DCs of nonlymphoid tissues, this maturation results in their migration to the T cell–dependent areas of secondary lymphoid organs by afferent lymphatics. This migration is orchestrated, in part, by an increase in CD11c[+] DC surface expression of the CCR7 chemokine receptor and a decrease in expression of most other chemokine receptors. This favors migration to T cell–rich areas of secondary lymphoid organs that express the CCR7 ligands, CCL19 and CCL21. Once migratory DCs home to these T cell–rich areas, they can present foreign peptide–MHC complexes to antigenically naïve T cells bearing cognate αβ-TCR for these peptides. Studies of HSV antigen presentation to CD8 T cells after skin infection in mice suggest that migratory DCs that reach the draining lymph nodes may not all directly present to T cells; instead, some may transfer their antigen to LT DCs that reside in the lymph nodes and that carry out such antigen presentation.[67] Such a transfer between migratory DCs to LT DCs may also occur in the mediastinal draining lymph nodes during influenza A infection of the respiratory epithelium.[68] In cases of skin immunization of mice, both Langerhans cell and dermal CD11c[+] DCs are induced to migrate to draining lymph nodes. However, dermal CD11c[+] DCs arrive in the lymph nodes first, at approximately 2 days post immunization. In contrast, Langerhans cells, which probably are delayed because they must first detach from adjacent keratinocytes, arrive in the lymph nodes at approximately 4 days post immunization.[69]

Activated CD11c[+] DCs not only play a critical role in T cell activation, but through the production of cytokines, they influence the quality of the T cell response that ensues.[70] For example, IL-12, IL-27, and type I IFNs produced by activated DCs instruct naïve CD4 T cells to produce IFN-γ and to differentiate into Th-1 cells (IFN-γ secretors), which help to protect against intracellular bacteria and viruses. IL-6, transforming growth factor (TGF)-β, and IL-23 induce naïve T cells to become Th-17 cells (secretors of IL-17A and IL-17F), which help to protect against extracellular bacteria and fungi by promoting neutrophil influx and activation. Th-2 cells (secretors of IL-4, IL-5, and IL-13) develop in the absence of exposures to Th-1–promoting cytokines and in the presence of thymic stromal lymphopoietin, IL-25, and IL-33 produced by epithelial cells, as well as IL-4 produced by basophils and innate lymphoid cells such as nuocytes.[71] Th-2 responses, which promote effector functions by mast cells, basophils, and eosinophils, are important in protection against large extracellular parasites and are characteristic of classic immunoglobulin (Ig)E-mediated allergic disease. CD11c$^+$ DCs also appear to be important for TFh differentiation from naïve CD4 T cells; for human TFh differentiation, IL-12p70, possibly from a DC source, plays an important role.[72] TFh cells provide help to follicular B cells for antibody responses and secrete IL-10, IL-21, and other cytokines that regulate immunoglobulin production.[73] CD11c$^+$ DCs, particularly those of the gut, may also promote the differentiation of naïve CD4 T cells into adaptive Tregs, which help limit the development of immune response to antigens from commensal intestinal flora.[70] Thus, the function and localization of CD11c$^+$ DCs are highly plastic and rapidly modulated in response to infection and inflammation; this in turn allows them to induce and instruct the nature of the T cell response. The role of DCs in instructing naïve CD4 T cells to become Th22 cells (IL-22 and TNF-α secretors) remains unclear. Th-22 cells appear to be particularly important for cutaneous immunity to fungal and bacteria pathogens.[7]

CD11c$^+$ DCs are also essential for activating CD8 T cells and have the unique ability among APCs to internally transfer proteins taken up from the external environment from a MHC class II antigen presentation pathway to the MHC class I pathway—a process called *cross-presentation*. How cross-presentation occurs in CD11c$^+$ DCs remains poorly understood, but genetic studies indicate that a protein called uncoordinated-93B (UNC-93B) that is mainly found in the endoplasmic reticulum is required for appropriate trafficking of intracellular TLRs to the endosome and cross-presentation.[74] UNC-93B is also required for intact signaling by TLR-3, -7, and -9. A recent and unexpected finding is that cross-presentation may also be facilitated by the NADPH oxidase complex, which is critical for the oxidative mechanism of killing bacteria and fungi internalized into neutrophils.[75] Naïve CD8 T cells that are effectively activated by CD11c$^+$ DCs expressing peptide/MHC class I complexes differentiate into effector cells, expressing cytotoxins that are important for killing virally infected cells. CD8 T cells are also rich sources of cytokines such as IFN-γ and TNF-α, which have antiviral activity and may help overcome viral-mediated immunosubversive effects, such as inhibition of antigen presentation.

Upon maturation, mature CD11c$^+$ DCs express high levels of peptide-MHC complexes and molecules that act as costimulatory signals for T cell activation, such as CD80 (B7-1) and CD86 (B7-2), and consequently are highly efficient for presenting antigen in a manner that effectively activates naïve CD4 and CD8 T cells for clonal expansion. In the case of naïve CD4 T cell activation and differentiation into effector cells in vivo, TLR-induced cytokine production as well as TLR ligand maturation of CD11c$^+$ DCs is required. TLR signals act on CD11c$^+$ DCs to promote effector CD4 T cell differentiation by enhancing effective antigen presentation and activation of naïve CD4, but also by limiting the inhibitory effects of Tregs.[76]

Clinical Evidence for Deficiencies of T Cell–Mediated Immunity in the Neonate and Young Infant

Term newborns are highly vulnerable to severe infection with HSV-1 and -2, and neonatal infection frequently results in death or severe neurologic damage, despite administration of high doses of antiviral agents, such as acyclovir, to which HSV is susceptible.[77,78] Death from disseminated primary HSV infection is distinctly unusual

12

after the neonatal period, except in cases of genetic T cell immunodeficiency, or among recipients of T cell ablative chemotherapy or immunosuppression. Neonates with primary HSV infection have delayed and diminished appearance of HSV-specific Th-1 responses (i.e., CD4 T cell proliferation, secretion of IFN-γ and TNF-α, and production of HSV-specific T cell–dependent antibody) compared with adults with primary infection.[79] These decreased responses ex vivo suggest that poor adaptive immune responses in vivo may allow HSV to disseminate, causing profound organ destruction for days to weeks after infection. This impairment of Th-1 immunity is potentially important given a recent study of intravaginally inoculated HSV in mice, which found that Th-1 immunity protected against infection by a noncytolytic mechanism, and that Th-1 cytokine secretion also required local antigen presentation by DCs and B cells.[80] A recent study also found that pDCs are closely associated with activated T cells at sites of recurrent HSV infection and have the capacity to enhance the proliferation of HSV-specific T cells.[81] Thus, it is plausible that limitations in pDC function in the neonate could impair the control of local viral replication. Whether the postinfection appearance of HSV-specific CD8 T cell immunity is also delayed in the neonate is unknown. It is also unclear by what age after birth the capacity to generate an HSV-specific CD4 T cell immune response to primary infection becomes similar to that of adults.

The delayed Th-1 immunity observed in neonatal HSV infection may also apply to other herpes viruses acquired during infancy. For example, we compared cytomegalovirus (CMV)-specific CD4 and CD8 T cell immune responses in infants and young children versus those in adults following primary CMV infection, and found that infants and young children had persistently reduced Th-1 immune responses.[82] In contrast, CD8 T cell responses, including the expression of cytotoxin molecules, were similar.[82,83] Decreased CMV-specific CD4 T cell responses were associated with persistent viral shedding in the urine,[82] suggesting that CD4 T cell immunity may be particularly important for the local control of viral replication in the mucosa. It is likely that this selective decrease in CD4 T cell immunity to CMV also applies to infection acquired perinatally and in the neonatal period, which is characterized by persistent viral shedding. Congenital CMV infection can result in a robust CMV-specific CD8 T cell response in the fetus, suggesting possible major differences in the capacity for generation of CD4 versus CD8 T cell responses to CMV very early in ontogeny.[84]

The otherwise healthy term newborn is also susceptible to severe infection from enteroviruses,[85,86] which have a relatively small RNA genome, indicating that limitations in antiviral immunity are not unique to herpes viruses, which have a large DNA genome. The most severe form of infection (i.e., hepatic necrosis with disseminated intravascular coagulation and liver failure) is highly unusual outside the neonatal period, except in cases of severe T cell immunodeficiency, such as early after hematopoietic cell transplantation before T cell reconstitution, or in cases of severe combined immunodeficiency. This complication is particularly common in neonates with overt infection during the first week after birth,[85] in contrast to HSV, which can present with severe disseminated infection up to several weeks of age.[77] It is not known whether the vulnerability of the neonate to severe enteroviral infection is paralleled by delayed or diminished T cell responses compared with older children upon their first infection with this class of viruses.

The severity or persistence of nonviral infections in which T cells also play a critical role in control also suggests a general limitation in T cell–mediated immunity to pathogens in early human development. Examples include congenital infections, such as toxoplasmosis,[87] which frequently disseminates to the retina, even when acquired during the last trimester of gestation. Mucocutaneous candidiasis, particularly thrush, is common during the first year of life.[88,89] The high prevalence of thrush in early infancy may reflect, at least in part, decreased fungus-specific CD4 T cell immunity by Th-17 cells, because thrush is also characteristic of adults with acquired defects in Th-17 immunity, such as human immunodeficiency virus (HIV)-1 infection[90] or autoimmune regulator (AIRE) deficiency, in which autoantibodies to IL-17A and IL-17F are frequent.[36]

In the case of *Mycobacterium tuberculosis* infection, the tendency for the neonate and the young infant to develop miliary disease and tuberculous meningitis is paralleled by decreased cell-mediated immunity compared with older children and young adults, as assessed by delayed-type sensitivity skin tests.[91] The young infant is able to mount substantial levels of IFN-γ production by CD4 T cells following neonatal vaccination with bacillus Calmette-Guérin (BCG), a live attenuated strain of *Mycobacterium bovis*.[92,93] The BCG response of these young infants includes CD8 T cells, which suggests that the newborn immune system has the ability to effectively cross-present BCG antigens to CD8 T cells.[94] However, these robust BCG responses do not rule out a reduced or delayed T cell response to virulent *M. tuberculosis* or *bovis* in infants compared with adults.

Major Phenotypes and Levels of Circulating Neonatal Dendritic Cells

Although most DCs are found in the tissues, small numbers, consisting of immature CD11c$^+$ DCs and pDCs, and representing approximately 0.5% of circulating blood mononuclear cells, are found in the circulation. Several studies found that DCs with an immature pDC surface phenotype (Lin$^-$HLA-DR^{mid}CD11c$^-$CD33$^-$CD123^{hi}) predominated in cord blood and early infancy, constituting about 75% of the total Lin$^-$HLA-DR$^+$ DCs[72] and about 0.75% of total blood mononuclear cells.[95,96] The remaining 25% of cells had an HLA-DR^{high}CD11c$^+$CD33$^+$CD123^{low} surface phenotype consistent with conventional CD11c$^+$ DCs found in adults, except that CD83 expression was absent.[97] The "cocktail" of Lin monoclonal antibodies (mAbs) used to enrich for DCs by negative selection included those for CD3 (T cells), CD14 (monocytes), CD16 (natural killer [NK] cells), CD19 (B cells), CD34 (hematopoietic precursor cells), CD56 (NK cells), CD66b (granulocytes), and glycophorin A (erythroid cells).

More recent work has shown that circulating CD11c$^+$ DCs can be divided into four nonoverlapping subsets that express CD16, CD34, BDCA-1, or BDCA-3.[98,99] Moreover, a portion of the CD16$^+$ and BDCA-1$^+$ DC subsets may also express low levels of CD14.[98,99] Thus, the inclusion of mAbs for CD16, CD34, and, perhaps, CD14 in lineage cocktails used for depletion will substantially reduce the final yield of CD11c$^+$ DCs. On the other hand, genomic profiling suggests that the CD11c$^+$CD16$^+$Lin$^-$ subset is likely an NK cell population rather than a bona fide DC subset,[100] so that CD16 depletion may be sufficient for CD11c$^+$ DC purification. In addition, both CD11c$^+$ DCs and pDCs may be lost by forming complexes with T cells during the purification of mononuclear cells by density gradient centrifugation (e.g., with Ficoll-Hypaque).[101]

More accurate determination of the circulating levels of DCs can be achieved by staining whole blood with mAbs, followed by red cell lysis and flow cytometry. Using this whole-blood approach for the identification of CD11c$^+$ DCs indicates that adult peripheral blood and cord blood have similar concentrations of CD11c$^+$ DCs that are Lin$^-$CD16$^-$HLA-DR^{high} ($\approx$70 to 76 cells/μL). In contrast, the concentration of Lin$^-$CD123^{high} pDCs in cord blood was significantly higher than in adult peripheral blood ($\approx$17.5 vs. 10.5 cells/μL, respectively[101]). Other workers, using the whole-blood method and a Lin cocktail that removes both CD16$^+$ and CD34$^+$ cells, have found that the levels of cord blood CD11c$^+$ DCs and pDCs are higher than those in adult peripheral blood.[102] After the neonatal period, the number of pDC lineage cells declines with increasing postnatal age, whereas the number of CD11c$^+$ DCs does not.[103] The biological significance of the predominance of pDCs in the neonatal circulation is uncertain but may reflect their relatively high rate of colonization of lymphoid tissue, which is undergoing rapid expansion at this age. The pDC concentration in the cord blood of prematurely born infants appears to be modestly but significantly lower than that of infants born at term.[104]

One study,[105] using the whole-blood analytic technique, found that cord blood may have an increased proportion of immature DCs with a distinct Lin$^-$HLA-DR$^+$CD11c$^-$CD34$^-$CD123^{mid} phenotype. These less differentiated DCs[105] may represent a precursor of more mature pDCs, because they have been reported to stain with monoclonal antibody against BDCA-4, which is a marker of the pDC lineage.[99]

In cord blood, the concentrations of less differentiated DCs and CD123[high] pDCs are similar. The concentration of less differentiated DCs declines with age, so that they are essentially absent by early adulthood. Confirmation of these results using additional markers that distinguish pDCs and CD11c[+] DCs and compares their function is required.

Circulating Neonatal Cd11c[+] Dendritic Cells: Activation by PAMP Receptors

Basal expression of MHC class II (HLA-DR) on cord blood and adult peripheral blood CD11c[+] DCs is similar,[106,107] although the level of the CD86 costimulatory molecule on both CD11c[+]CD16[-] DCs is lower in cord blood.[108] Stimulation with LPS (a TLR-4 ligand) and poly (I:C) (a TLR-3 ligand and activator of RLRs) increased expression of HLA-DR and CD86 on CD11c[+] DCs to a similar extent by neonatal compared with adult CD11c[+] DCs. However, compared with adult peripheral blood CD11c[+] DCs, CD11c[+] DCs from cord blood decreased upregulation of CD40 after incubation with ligands for TLR-2/6 (*Mycoplasma fermetans*), TLR-3 or RLR (poly [I:C]), TLR-4 (LPS), or TLR-7 (imiquimod),[107] and decreased upregulation of CD80 by TLR-3 and TLR-4 ligands.[106,107] A recent flow cytometric study has revealed that cord blood CD11c[+] DCs of prematurely born infants (compared with those born at term) have significantly reduced IL-6 expression in response to TLR-2 agonists (PAM3CSK4 or FSL-1).[104]

Neonatal blood cells produce less IFN-α than is produced by adult blood cells in response to poly (I:C);[107] this most likely reflects decreased production by neonatal CD11c[+] DCs, which express TLR-3, rather than by pDCs, which do not. LPS-induced expression of TNF-α by cord blood CD11c[+] DCs was also reduced compared with adult CD11c[+] DCs, in terms of the percentage of cells that expressed this cytokine and the amount of cytokine produced among cytokine-positive cells;[109] in contrast, LPS-induced expression of IL-1α by cord blood and adult CD11c[+] DCs was similar. TLR-4 surface expression was similar on cord blood and adult CD11c[+] DCs, consistent with the selective nature of diminished responses to LPS by cord blood DCs.[109]

The production of bioactive IL-12p70 by cord blood mononuclear cells also appears to be reduced in response to LPS alone or in combination with IFN-γ or pertussis toxin, which also activates CD11c[+] DCs via TLR-4,[110] compared with older children or adults.[111,112] The cellular source of IL-12p70 in these in vitro cultures is probably CD11c[+] DCs.[111,112] Based on murine studies, pertussis toxin may also activate RLRs associated with the inflammasome,[32] which could contribute to IL-12 production under these conditions. Moreover, decreased IL-12 production by cord blood CD11c[+] DCs may not apply to all stimuli. For example, neonatal and adult blood mononuclear cells stimulated with *Staphylococcus aureus*, other Gram-positive and Gram-negative bacterial cells, or meningococcal outer membrane proteins have been reported to produce equivalent amounts of IL-12.[113-116]

TLR-8 ligands, such as single-stranded RNA enriched in GU sequences, are particularly potent activators of both cord blood and adult CD11c[+] DCs (e.g., for increased expression of CD40); these cell types also have similar levels of intracellular TLR-8 expression.[117] This raises the possibility that TLR-8 ligands might be particularly effective in enhancing CD11c[+] DC function in neonates compared with other TLR ligands, although it remains to be shown that TLR-8 engagement is also effective in inducing neonatal CD11c[+] DCs to produce pro-inflammatory cytokines and to allostimulate T cells for Th-1 differentiation.

Circulating Neonatal Plasmacytoid Dendritic Cells: Activation by PAMP Receptors

Similar to pDCs from the tonsils of older children,[118,119] cord blood pDCs are ineffective in uptake of protein or peptide antigens.[120] It is unclear whether maturation of pDCs in the neonate (e.g., by exposure to viruses) results in a similar increase in capacity for antigen presentation as is observed with adult pDCs. Stimulation with unmethylated CpG DNA (a TLR-9 ligand) increased expression of HLA-DR on cord blood and adult pDCs to a similar extent[121] and, in combination with IL-3–containing medium, induced higher levels of CD80 and CD86 on cord blood pDCs than on adult pDCs.[122] The levels of CD80 and CD86 on cord blood pDCs after incubation with IL-3–containing medium alone for 20 hours were markedly lower than on adult pDCs,[122] suggesting that these differences are likely to apply to circulating pDCs in vivo.

Type I IFN production and the frequency of IFN-α–producing cells in response to HSV were diminished in cord blood mononuclear cells, particularly from prematurely born infants, compared with adult PBMCs.[123] Similar results were obtained with whole-blood preparations stimulated with unmethylated CpG DNA.[106] Decreased production of type I IFN by neonatal PBMCs or whole-blood cells (persisting until at least 4 days of age) in response to viruses or unmethylated CpG DNA likely reflected decreased production by pDC lineage cells signaling through TLR-9,[106] as reduced production of type I IFN was also shown using purified cord blood pDCs in response to CpG, a TLR-7 agonist (R-848), or CMV or HSV exposure, compared with adult pDCs.[124] Single-cell flow cytometric analysis has extended these findings by showing that the production of type I IFN and TNF-α by cord blood pDCs is lower compared with that of adult pDCs after stimulation with CpG or TLR-7 agonists,[125] and that these responses by pDCs from prematurely born neonates are significantly less than those from neonates born at term.[104] This decreased production of type I IFN is not attributable to diminished TLR-9 expression by cord blood pDCs,[122] but rather appears to be due to reduced nuclear translocation of IRF-7, a transcription factor that is essential for the induction of type I IFN.[124] Cord blood pDCs also have reduced induction of surface expression of CD40, CD80, and CCR7, and reduced production of TNF-α, after TLR-7 agonist treatment compared with adult pDCs.[124,126] Taken together, these findings suggest that NFκB-mediated gene transcription may also be reduced in neonatal pDCs.[124] The extent to which decreased cord blood pDC responses are due to the presence in cord blood of pDCs with CD123^{dim} staining (the ldDCs described earlier)[108] is unclear, but it is plausible that these phenotypically immature pDCs might also have reduced function compared with CD123^{high} pDCs.

Allostimulation of T Cells by Circulating Neonatal Dendritic Cells

The first study to directly test the ability of cord blood DCs to activate T cells was done before markers became available that allow them to be isolated relatively rapidly and in high purity. In these studies, cells cultured overnight in vitro were substantially less effective than adult cells in activating allogeneic T cell proliferation.[127,128] This decreased activity was associated with reduced levels of expression of HLA-DR and the adhesion molecule ICAM-1.[127] In more recent studies cited earlier,[106,107] in which expression of HLA-DR was evaluated on uncultured DCs, HLA-DR expression on neonatal and adult CD11c$^+$ DCs and pDCs did not differ significantly. The lower level of HLA-DR expression by neonatal DC in studies by Hunt and colleagues[127] probably reflects the overnight culture or the predominance of pDCs among DCs isolated from neonatal blood obtained using certain enrichment strategies. These pDCs express lower levels of HLA-DR than CD11c$^+$ DCs,[97] and pDC lineage cells are highly prone to die during culture in vitro. Therefore, the use of an overnight protocol for cell isolation may adversely affect cord blood DCs, in which pDCs are predominant.

Several studies found that circulating DCs from cord blood can allogeneically stimulate cord blood T cells in vitro;[97,120,129] however, their efficiency was not compared with that of adult DCs. Virtually all of the allostimulatory activity of partially purified cord blood DCs is mediated by the CD11c$^+$ DC subset rather than by the pre-pDC subset.[97] It should also be noted that activation of allogeneic T cells does not require uptake, processing, and presentation of exogenous antigens, and thus is not as stringent a test of APC function as is activation of foreign antigen-specific T cells.

As was discussed previously, DCs have a major influence on whether naïve CD4 T cells differentiate into producers of Th-1 cytokines, Th-2 cytokines, Th-17 cytokines (i.e., IL-17), TFh cells, or adaptive Tregs, or into less committed "nonpolarized" effector cells that lack the capacity to produce any of these cytokines.[70,130] For example, antigen presentation by pDCs favors the differentiation of naïve T cells into Th-2 cells, unless these cells have been activated by viruses or unmethylated CpG DNA, which causes them to release IFN-α or IL-12 and, in turn, to drive potent Th-1 polarization.[131] Thus it is plausible that limitations in the production of IL-12 by neonatal CD11c$^+$ DCs and of type I IFN by pDCs (via engagement of TLR-7 and TLR-9) and CD11c$^+$ DCs (via engagement of TLR-3) in the fetus and neonate may account for the tendency to have Th-2 skewing of immune responses to environmental allergens, limited responses to intracellular pathogens, maintenance of fetal-maternal tolerance during pregnancy, and lower risk of graft-versus-host disease following cord blood transplantation.

Adenosine and Neonatal Dendritic Cell Function

Adenosine is a purine metabolite induced by hypoxia and other stresses that has a variety of effects on innate and adaptive immune function. Adenosine levels are elevated in cord blood plasma, likely in association with perinatal hypoxic stress, and are thought to rapidly decline after birth to normal homeostatic levels. In studies comparing neonatal versus adult monocyte cytokine production, Levy and colleagues[132,133] found decreased production of TNF-α and greater or equal production of IL-6 in response to LPS and TLR-2 agonists; these events were accounted for by elevated adenosine levels in cord blood plasma. This selective impact on TNF-α but not IL-6 production also appeared to be due, in part, to heightened sensitivity of adenosine A3 receptors on cord blood monocytes compared with those of the adult, which resulted in higher intracellular levels of cyclic adenosine monophosphate (cAMP).[132] These effects of adenosine may apply to pDC-derived cytokine production, because elevated IL-6/TNF-α ratios were obtained by comparison of cord blood versus adult blood after incubation with an agonist for TLR-9,[133] which is expressed only by human pDCs. Whether these effects of adenosine also apply to cord blood CD11c$^+$ DCs is unclear. Recent murine studies have found that adenosine treatment of CD11c$^+$ DCs and inflammatory-type DCs acting through the A2B adenosine receptor skews naïve CD4 T cell differentiation toward a Th-17 outcome.[134] If applicable to human DCs, this effect of adenosine might contribute to Th-17 skewing of CD4 T cell responses in the newborn.

Neonatal Monocyte-Derived Dendritic Cells (MDDCs)

Cells phenotypically similar to CD11c$^+$ DCs can be generated in vitro from a variety of precursor cells, including blood monocytes, immature pDCs, CD34$^+$ cells, and even granulocytes, depending on the cytokines and culture conditions employed.[135,136] The generation of MDDCs by culture of freshly isolated blood monocytes with GM-CSF and IL-4 has been a particularly useful experimental system for evaluating human DCs, because a relatively large number of cells can be generated in vitro within a short period.[137] These MDDCs have features of immature CD11c$^+$ DCs and with further stimulation (e.g., incubation with LPS or TNF-α) acquire phenotypic and functional features characteristic of mature CD11c$^+$ DCs (e.g., increased expression of HLA-DR and costimulatory molecules). Expression of various DC markers (e.g., CD1a) and the functional capacity of MDDCs to produce cytokines in vitro (e.g., IL-12p40) and to allostimulate T cells are substantially influenced by the serum concentrations of the growth media.[138]

Adult peripheral and cord blood MDDCs generated by GM-CSF and IL-4 incubation give rise to immature DCs, similar to the CD11c$^+$ DC lineage. However, immature MDDCs from cord blood express less HLA-DR, fewer costimulatory molecules (CD40 and CD80), and less CD1a than are seen with adult MDDCs;[139,140] the expression of CD11c, CD86, CCR5, and mannose receptor by cord blood MDDCs appears to be similar or only moderately less than by adult MDDCs.[139,141] The internalization of fluorescein isothiocyanate (FITC)-dextran by cord blood MDDCs is substantially less compared with adult peripheral blood MDDCs.[141] LPS stimulation is also significantly less effective in increasing HLA-DR and CD86 expression by cord blood–derived MDDCs than by those generated from adult peripheral blood.[141]

Consistent with these reductions in HLA-DR and costimulatory molecules, MDDCs from cord blood matured by LPS stimulation have decreased allostimulatory activity for the production of IFN-γ by T cells compared with adult MDDCs.[139,141] The ability of neonatal MDDCs to allogeneically induce T cell proliferation has been reported as reduced in one study[140] but not in two others.[111,139] Reduced IFN-γ production[141] during allostimulation of T cells is likely due to a markedly reduced capacity of immature neonatal MDDCs to produce IL-12p70. IL-12p70 production by isolated cord blood MDDCs was reduced compared with that by adult MDDCs after LPS stimulation (a TLR-4 ligand) in some studies[139,141] but not all;[111] the reasons for these discrepant results are not clear. Decreased IL-12p70 production by cord blood MDDCs was also observed after engagement of CD40 (which is the likely physiologic stimulus for IL-12 production during allostimulation) or incubation with double-stranded RNA (poly [I:C]), a TLR-3 or RLR ligand,[139,141] or CMV.[142] The decreased IL-12 production by cord blood MDDCs is accounted for by a selective decrease in mRNA expression of the IL-12 p35 chain component,[139] a decrease that can be overcome by incubating these cells with the combination of LPS and IFN-γ. Decreased IL-12 p35 expression appears to be due to a chromatin configuration of the IL-12 p35 genetic locus in neonatal MDDCs that limits access to transcriptional activator proteins such as IRF3.[143,144] In contrast to the results obtained for IL-12p70, adult and cord blood MDDCs produce similar levels of TNF-α, IL-6, IL-8, and IL-10 after stimulation.[139,140,145]

Cord blood MDDCs produce significantly higher levels of IL-23 than adult MDDCs after stimulation by LPS or the TLR-8 ligand resiquimod (R-848).[146] These two cell populations also produce similar amounts of IL-23 after incubation with (S-[2,3-bis{palmitoyloxy}-{2-RS}-propyl]-N-palmitoyl-[R]-Cys-[S]-Ser-Lys4-OH trihydrochloride) (PAM3CSK4), a TLR-2 ligand, and poly (I:C),[146] indicating that signaling via TLR-2 and TLR-3 for IL-23 production is intact in cord blood MDDCs. Moreover, culture supernatants from LPS-stimulated cord blood or adult MDDCs are effective in inducing IL-17 production by neonatal T cells, especially those of the CD8 subset. This preferential induction of IL-17 by cord blood CD8 T cells rather than CD4 T cells is also observed after polyclonal activation and incubation with recombinant IL-23. These findings raise the possibility that the Th-17 pathway of immunity might be intact in neonates. Results obtained for poly (I:C)-induced IL-23 production are surprising given the report by Porras and associates,[147] which demonstrates that basal and poly (I:C)–induced TLR-3 expression is markedly lower in cord blood MDDCs than in adult MDDCs. One potential explanation for this discrepancy is that IL-23 production might be the result of poly (I:C)–activating RLRs rather than TLR-3.[14]

These findings using MDDCs provide an explanation for limitations in Th-1 immunity, such as delayed-type hypersensitivity skin reactions and antigen-specific CD4 T cell IFN-γ production, which are discussed later. The relevance of these findings obtained with MDDCs is supported by observations in mice suggesting that inflammatory DCs can directly differentiate from monocytes in vivo (e.g., in response to *Listeria* or *Leishmania* infection). However, it remains unclear to what extent inflammatory DCs occur in human infection in vivo or in response to other pro-inflammatory stimuli, including those found in the neonate.

Fetal Tissue Dendritic Cells

Immature CD11c$^+$ DC lineage cells of the migratory (nonlymphoid tissue) subtype have been identified in the interstitium of solid organs, including the kidney,

12

heart, pancreas, and lung, but not the brain, by 12 weeks' gestation.[148] The numbers of these cells in tissues other than the brain progressively increase by 21 weeks' gestation. Epidermal HLA-DR[+] DC-like cells are found in the skin even earlier (7 weeks' gestation)[149] and appear to be derived from CD45[+] HLA-DR[+] cells that enter the epidermis, extensively proliferate, and then acquire CD1c, langerin, and CD1a in a stepwise manner.[150] These HLA-DR[+] DC epidermal populations between 9 and 14 weeks' gestation upregulate costimulatory molecules (CD80 and CD86) during in vitro culture, and the CD1c[+] fraction efficiently induces the proliferation of allogeneic T cells.[150] In contrast to postnatal skin, these fetal Langerhans-lineage DCs are mainly CD1a[−] until 12 to 13 weeks' gestation,[149] and CD1a[+] Langerhans cells do not predominate before about 27 weeks' gestation.[151] These findings indicate that colonization and differentiation of Langerhans cells in the fetal skin are developmentally regulated independent of exposure to inflammatory mediators.

Cells with features of DCs, possibly of the pDC lineage, are found in fetal lymph nodes between 19 and 21 weeks' gestation;[118] they have an immature phenotype and are not recent emigrants from inflamed tissues. An early study found S100[+] T zone histiocyte cells, which had the histologic appearance of pDCs, in the fetal liver between 2 and 3 months' gestation—a time when the liver is a major hematopoietic organ;[152] this was followed by the appearance of these cells in the thymic medulla at 4 months, and in the spleen, lymph nodes, tonsils, and Peyer's patches by 4 to 5 months' gestation. These findings require confirmation using better-characterized and more definitive histologic markers.

Postnatal Ontogeny of Human Dendritic Cell Phenotype and Function

The recent application of multiparameter flow cytometry using fluorochrome-conjugated monoclonal antibodies (e.g., 6 to 10 parameters/cell) in conjunction with whole-blood stimulation with TLR ligands has allowed a better definition of the postnatal ontogeny of the phenotype and function of circulating DCs. This approach confirmed earlier studies that basal HLA-DR expression and CD80 expression induced by LPS on cord blood CD11c[+] DCs were significantly lower than in adult peripheral blood. By 3 months of age, HLA-BR and CD80 expression reached the levels of adult CD11c[+] DCs.[153] Corbett and colleagues[154] longitudinally studied a cohort of Gambian infants at birth and 1 year and 2 years of age by analyzing single-cell cytokine production (TNF-α, IL-6, and IL-12/23 p40 subunit) through multiparameter flow cytometry after whole-blood stimulation with TLR agonists. Investigators found that, at 1 year of age, cytokine responses by CD11[+] DCs in response to LPS (TLR-4) were significantly greater than those at birth or compared with those of adults; all three time points in neonates/infants had high levels of cytokine production in response to PAM (a TLR-2 agonist) or 3M-003 (a TLR-7/8 agonist).

In contrast, for pDCs, adult levels of HLA-DR and CD80 expression induced by CpG (a TLR-9 ligand) were not achieved until 6 to 9 months of age. Consistent with this finding, which suggested maturation of pDC function by 9 months of age, Corbett and coworkers[154] found that pDC production of TNF-α and IL-6, in response to TLR-7/8 or TLR-9 agonists at 1 year of age, was similar to that of adult pDCs.

Given that pDCs are the main sources of cytokines in response to CpG stimulation, pDC-derived chemokine production (interferon-gamma induced protein 10 (IP-10), also known as CXCL10, and monokine induced by gamma interferon (MIG), also known as CXCL10) was less during the first year of life compared with that in the adult. pDC-derived IL-6, IL-8, IL-10, and IL-1β were significantly higher than values from 3 months of age onward, suggesting that neonatal pDCs have a unique cytokine profile that may inhibit Th-1 responses (i.e., IL-10) and may promote Th-17 responses (IL-6 and IL-1β). In future studies, the application of single-cell mass cytometry,[155] in which 35 parameters per cell can be analyzed, should allow an even more comprehensive assessment of the postnatal ontogeny of DC function and phenotype.

Postnatal Studies of Tissue-Associated Dendritic Cells in Children

A study of nasal wash samples obtained from children with acute viral respiratory infection demonstrated that CD11c[+] DCs and pDCs can be identified as part of these secretions by multiparameter flow cytometry.[156,157] Increased numbers of both DC populations were observed after acute infection with RSV or with other respiratory viral pathogens (parainfluenza and influenza). In the case of RSV infection, the number of these cells was correlated positively with the viral load and persisted in the nasal mucosa for 2 to 8 weeks after acute infection. No CD83 expression by these DCs was detected, consistent with their being more tissue-associated DCs. Infection with RSV, not influenza or parainfluenza, led to decreased circulating levels of CD11c[+] DCs and pDCs.[156] It will be of interest to determine whether these DC populations accumulate to a similar degree in neonates and young infants, and to assess the ability of these cells to function ex vivo.

Postnatal Ontogeny of Murine Dendritic Cell Function

It is technically more difficult, particularly in humans, to assess the capabilities of DCs that are resident in peripheral tissues. To address this issue, we examined the impact of TLR-4 signaling on CD11c[+] DCs in young mice.[158] CD11c[+] DCs from the spleens of 6- to 12-week-old TLR-4–deficient (C3He/J) mice were similar to those of wild-type mice in terms of the proportion of cells that were immature (MHC class II[low]) compared with mature (MHC class II[high]) (Fig. 12-3). However, mature splenic CD11c[+] DCs from TLR-4–deficient mice had reduced expression of costimulatory proteins (e.g., CD86) in response to incubation with GM-CSF alone or together with CD40 engagement (Fig. 12-4). Moreover, myeloid CD11c[+] DCs from TLR-4–deficient mice also had significantly reduced capacity to produce IL-12 in response to CD40 engagement compared with those from wild-type mice (Fig. 12-5), a feature that would probably limit Th-1 differentiation.

It is interesting to speculate that CD11c[+] DCs from neonates born from a sterile uterine environment are functionally immature until exposures to bacterial products

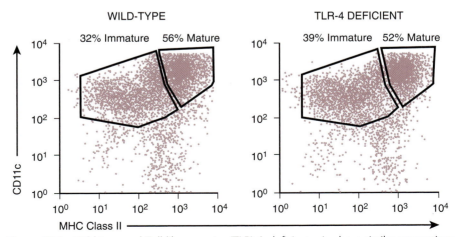

Figure 12-3 Wild-type and Toll-like receptor (TLR)-4–deficient mice have similar proportions of splenic CD11c[+] dendritic cells that are mature and immature as assessed by the level of major histocompatibility complex (MHC) class II surface expression. CD11c and MHC class II surface expression was determined by flow cytometry, with the cell numbers shown expressed as the percentage of total CD11c[+] cells.

12

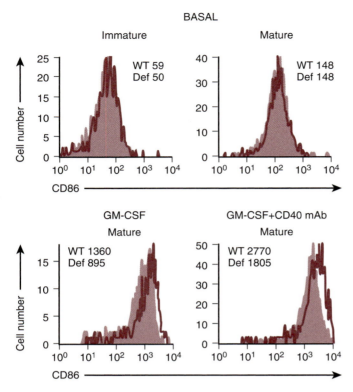

Figure 12-4 Toll-like receptor (TLR)-4–deficient CD11c⁺ dendritic cells express substantially less surface CD86 (B72) co-stimulatory molecule after activation with granulocyte-monocyte colony-stimulating factor (GM-CSF) alone or in combination with CD40 engagement. CD86 expression was determined on immature (major histocompatibility complex [MHC] class II^{low}) and mature (MHC class II^{high}) splenic dendritic cell populations immediately following purification (basal), with the use of gating for the mature (MHC class II^{high}) cell population, 24 hours after incubation with GM-CSF ± anti-CD40 monoclonal antibody (mAb). The mean fluorescence index of positive cells is shown in the inserts for dendritic cells from wild-type (WT; *clear histogram*) and TLR-4–defective (Def; *filled histogram*) mice.

in the extrauterine environment have occurred. Consistent with this idea is the capacity of purified murine splenic CD11c⁺ DCs, particularly those of the CD8α⁺ subset, to produce IL-12p70 increases between 1 to 2 weeks and 6 weeks of age in response to CpG (TLR-9 is expressed by CD11c⁺ DCs in mice) and a combination of cytokines.[159] Also supportive of this model is the fact that expression of a number of surface markers on CD11c⁺ DCs (e.g., CD8α, CD11b, F4/80) gradually increases after birth, achieving adult levels at approximately 4 weeks of age.[160] Early postnatal exposure of mice to certain microbial stimuli (e.g., heat-killed *Chlamydia muridarum*) appears to result in an "immune-educating effect," whereby an alteration occurs in the phenotype and function of DCs from these animals as young adults (i.e., 6 to 8 weeks of age).[161] Whether this is truly a persistent DC "reprogramming" for the life of the animal remains unclear.

IFN-α production by purified murine splenic pDCs at 1 to 2 weeks of age was similar to or higher than that seen in these cells at 6 weeks of age,[159] indicating that developmental limitations in DC function may be limited to CD11c⁺ DCs rather than occurring in pDCs as well. This is consistent with the robust induction of T cell immunity in the neonatal mouse with the addition of unmethylated CpG DNA to protein vaccines.[162] Moreover, in contrast to human neonatal CD11c⁺ DCs, those of

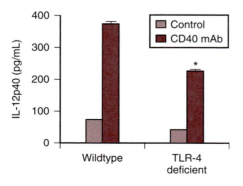

Figure 12-5 Splenic conventional dendritic cells from Toll-like receptor (TLR)-4–deficient mice produce less interleukin (IL)-12 compared with wild-type dendritic cells. Levels of IL-12p40 in supernatants of splenic conventional dendritic cells activated with anti-CD40 monoclonal antibody (mAb) for 48 hours are shown. Data represent means ± standard error of the mean (SEM) and are representative of three experiments. *P < 0.05 versus the wild-type CD40 mAb-treated group with the two-tailed unpaired Student's t-test.

the neonatal mouse respond robustly to LPS and are able to effectively activate naïve T cells for differentiation into effector cells.[163] Although it remains to be determined whether circulating CD11c+ DCs in neonatal mice have reduced function compared with those in older mice, available in vivo data strongly suggest that neonatal mice may not accurately model the apparently more prolonged and intrinsic limitations in CD11c+ DC function noted in early postnatal life in humans.

Commensal bacterially derived products, such as gut flora DNA, act as natural adjuvants in promoting the development of effector CD4 T cell responses, such as Th-17 cytokine secretion, rather than Treg development. Skewing toward Treg development in mice lacking TLR-9 was shown to impair the immune response to oral infection or vaccination.[164] Similar mechanisms could be operative in humans, such that delayed gut colonization could have similar effects in limiting the development of immunity by CD4 T cells of the gastrointestinal tract.

12

Neonatal CD4 T Cells Have Intrinsic Limitations in Th-1 Differentiation

Numerous studies have demonstrated decreased Th-1 function in human neonatal CD4 T cells.[9] These findings can be accounted for by the increased numbers of differentiated memory T cells of the Th-1 subset observed in adult blood compared with neonatal blood.[165,166] Naïve (CD45RA^{high}CD45RO^{low}) cells account for approximately 60% of the CD4 T cells in most adults, but they represent more than 90% of cells in infants.[9] Thus any direct comparison of cord blood T cells versus unfractionated adult cells involves comparing a relatively pure population of naïve cells with a mixed population containing both naïve and memory cells. However, even when purified naïve adult CD4+ T cells are used for comparison, major functional differences are apparent. For example, we recently investigated the capacity of neonatal T cells to mount Th-1 responses.[167] To avoid questions of inadequate antigen presentation by neonatal DCs, a pool of allogeneic adult dendritic cells (MDDCs) were used as stimulators. Compared with purified adult naïve CD4 T cells, neonatal naïve CD4 T cells from cord blood secreted much less IL-2 and IFN-γ and expressed less CD154 on their cell surface.[168] A decrease in IL-12p70 was detected in culture supernatants, indicating decreased induction of DC-dependent IL-12p70 secretion by neonatal CD4 T cells. The capacity for neonatal CD4 T cells to induce IL-12p70 expression by neonatal DCs in vivo is unknown. However, it is plausible that the combination of decreased neonatal CD154 expression and intrinsic functional limitations of neonatal DCs could result in markedly impaired IL-12p70 secretion. Neonatal CD4 T cells were impaired in their differentiation into Th-1 cells because they expressed less signal transduction and activator of transcription (STAT)-4 and had lower levels of STAT-4 tyrosine phosphorylation,[168] which are required for signaling by the IL-12 receptor. Such decreases in STAT-4 signaling would be expected to impair Th-1 differentiation.[70]

No evidence of increased skewing toward Th2 cells was noted, based on the low level of IL-4 produced in both neonatal and adult CD4 T cell cultures with allogeneic dendritic cells. Also, no evidence suggested increased levels of immunosuppressive cytokines, such as IL-10, to account for reduced neonatal CD4 T cell differentiation. We also found that neonatal naïve CD4 T cells in these experiments had relatively reduced numbers of regulatory CD25^{high} CD4 T cells (Tregs), based on their intracellular expression of the Forkhead Box P3 Foxp3 transcription factor.[168] This strongly argues that the reduced ability of neonatal naïve CD4 T cells to differentiate into Th-1 cells in response to a potent allogeneic stimulus is not accounted for by an increased number of Tregs, a cell population that is able to inhibit CD4 T cell activation.[137]

Epigenetic mechanisms may also regulate IFN-γ gene expression in neonatal T cells. Studies using methylation-sensitive restriction mapping demonstrated a hypermethylated CpG site in the IFN-γ promoter of neonatal and adult naive (CD45RA^{high}) CD4 T cells compared with memory/effector (CD45RO^{high}) CD4+ T cells.[169] This finding correlated with decreased IFN-γ expression in cells with hypermethylation

12

of the IFN-γ promoter. A more sensitive bisulfite sequencing technique was used by Holt and colleagues[170] to show that the IFN-γ promoter is hypermethylated at various sites in neonatal CD4 T cells compared with naïve adult CD4 T cells. The IFN-γ promoter in neonatal CD8[+] T cells did not show the same degree of hypermethylation; indeed, stimulated neonatal CD8 T cells were capable of making significant amounts of IFN-γ, albeit not as much as is made by adult CD8 T cells. These differences in methylation of the IFN-γ gene in neonatal versus adult T cells are specific in that they are not associated with the general decrease in the overall level of methylation in T cells noted with aging.[171]

Neonatal CD4 T Cells Have Features of CD4⁺CD8⁻ Thymocytes and Recent Thymic Emigrants

Mature CD4[hi]CD8[−] and CD4[−]CD8[hi] single-positive thymocytes enter into the circulation as recent thymic emigrants (RTEs), joining the antigenically naïve CD4 and CD8 αβ T cell compartments, respectively. In humans, RTEs of CD4 T cell lineage are identified by their expression of protein tyrosine kinase 7 (PTK7), a member of the receptor tyrosine kinase family.[172] The function of PTK7 in immune function is unclear, although studies in acute myelogenous leukemia cells suggest that it may act to inhibit apoptosis.[173] PTK7 has no known ligands and appears to be a catalytically inactive kinase, because it lacks a functional ATP-binding cassette in its cytoplasmic domain.[174] Approximately 5% of circulating naïve CD4 T cells from healthy young adults are PTK7[+]; these cells are highly enriched in their signal joint T cell receptor excision circle content compared with PTK7-naïve CD4 T cells, consistent with their recent emigration from the thymus. Otherwise, PTK7[+] CD4 T cells in the adult circulation have a similar surface phenotype for αβ-TCR/CD3, CD4, CD5, CD28, CD31, CD38, CD45RA, L-selectin (CD62L), and CD127 (the IL-7 receptor α chain) surface expression as PTK7-naïve CD4 T cells.[172] As expected for an RTE cell population, PTK7[+]-naïve CD4 T cells have a highly diverse αβ-TCR repertoire, similar to that of the overall naïve CD4 T cell population, and rapidly decline in the circulation following complete thymectomy (performed for the treatment of myasthenia gravis).[172] As described later, PTK7[+]-naïve CD4 T cells (hereafter referred to as PTK7[+] CD4 RTEs) from healthy adults have reduced activation-dependent function compared with PTK7[−]-naïve CD4 T cells.

Virtually all CD4 T cells and most CD8 T cells of the neonate express high levels of surface protein and mRNA transcripts for PTK7, which is a marker for CD4 RTEs in older children and adults[172] (D.B. Lewis, unpublished observations, 2009). Lower levels of PTK7 on neonatal CD8 T cells compared with CD4 T cells reflect differences manifest in the thymus, because CD3[high] (mature) CD4[−]CD8[+] single-positive thymocytes also have reduced expression of PTK7 compared with CD4[+]CD8[−] thymocytes.[172] Although this high level of PTK7 expression by neonatal naïve CD4 T cells may be explained, in part, by their being highly enriched in RTEs, it is likely that PTK7 expression is regulated differently in neonatal CD4 T cells compared with adult naïve CD4 T cells based on two observations. First, a higher level of expression of PTK7 occurs per neonatal naïve CD4 T cell compared with adult PTK7 CD4 RTEs.[172] Second, few if any PTK7[−] cells are found among circulating neonatal naïve CD4 T cells, even though studies of older children undergoing complete thymectomy suggest that most PTK7[+] CD4 RTEs are converted to PTK7-naïve CD4 T cells over a 3-month period,[172] and at least some neonatal T cells are likely to have emigrated from the thymus more than 6 months previously.

Fetal T cell development begins at the end of the first trimester, with rapid expansion of cell numbers through early childhood. This expansion involves de novo production by the thymus of transitional T cells, which are also referred to as *recent thymic emigrants (RTEs)*. Our recent studies of human CD4 RTEs, which are identified by their surface expression of PTK7,[172] indicate that in adults and older children, RTEs become fully mature naïve CD4 T cells and lose PTK7 in about 2 months. This maturation is accompanied by an increased capacity for naïve CD4 T cells to be activated and become Th-1 effector cells.[172] Whether PTK7 expression itself contributes to the decreased capacity for CD4 T lineage cells to become Th-1 effectors remains unclear and is under investigation. Regardless, neonatal naïve CD4 T cells have features suggestive of RTEs, including uniformly high levels of surface expression of PTK7.[172] It is plausible that the predominance of RTEs in the peripheral neonatal CD4 T cell compartment may contribute to limitations in the capacity of the neonate to mount a Th-1 type of immune response. Other findings suggest that maturational arrest (i.e., retention of thymocyte-type phenotype and function) by neonatal CD4 T cells also contributes to their reduced capacity to carry out effector mechanisms. For example, neonatal CD4 T cells and their immediate intrathymic precursors, CD4$^+$CD8$^-$ thymocytes, express high levels of CD38[9] and have a markedly reduced capacity to produce CD154[9] (see later), whereas adult naïve CD4 T cells, including the PTK7$^+$ subset, lack CD38 expression and have a greater capacity to produce CD154.[172]

Reduced CD154 Expression

Interactions between CD154, which is expressed at high levels by activated CD4 T cells, and CD40, which is expressed by B cells, dendritic cells, and mononuclear phagocytes, are critical for induction of immunoglobulin class switching and memory formation by B cells, dendritic cell maturation, and cytokine secretion (e.g., IL-12 secretion), and increased microbicidal activity by mononuclear phagocytes for pathogens, such as *Pneumocystis*. Patients with genetic deficiency of CD154 also lack vaccine-specific T cells that proliferate and produce IFN-γ, indicating the importance of the CD154-CD40 interaction in the accumulation of functional memory T cells, including those of the Th-1 subset.[175,176] Part of the defect in Th-1 differentiation probably lies in the inability of neonatal CD4 T cells to upregulate CD154, which in turn results in decreased IL-12 production from dendritic cells. We and others have shown that stimulated neonatal T cells fail to upregulate CD154, in spite of upregulation of other activation markers such as CD69.[9,177,178] Decreased expression of CD154 was due to decreased transcription after engagement of the αβ-TCR–CD3 complex.[177] However, even when the TCR was pharmacologically bypassed using ionomycin and phorbol myristate acetate, transcription of CD154 remained low.[9,178] As mentioned previously, decreased CD154 expression was also observed when neonatal naïve CD4 T cells were stimulated by fully mature allogeneic dendritic cells.[168] This indicates that the defect in CD154 expression is intrinsic to the neonatal T cell and is likely to apply to activation in vivo in response to foreign antigens. As noted earlier, adult PTK7$^+$ CD4 RTEs have a capacity for CD154 expression that is similar to that of adult mature naïve CD4 T cells, indicating that reduced CD154 expression by neonatal CD4 T cells is not accounted for by their being enriched in RTEs.

Conclusion

Immaturity of dendritic cells and the innate immune mechanisms that activate them, including Toll-like receptors and other innate immune receptor molecules, probably contributes to decreased T cell immunity after birth, particularly in the immediate postnatal period. Although the circulating concentrations of CD11c$^+$ and plasmacytoid dendritic cells are similar in the neonate and the adult, some functions of both of these cell types may be selectively reduced in the neonate, as in response to certain Toll-like receptor ligands. A particularly consistent finding has been the reduced secretion of type I interferons by neonatal plasmacytoid dendritic cells. This finding, taken with those indicating that plasmacytoid dendritic cells may play a role in the activation of herpes simplex virus–specific T cells in nonlymphoid tissues, suggests that reduced plasmacytoid dendritic cell function could contribute to the vulnerability of the newborn to herpes simplex virus infection. The function of dendritic cells derived from neonatal monocytes in vitro is also reduced, particularly for the secretion of IL-12p70. However, it is unclear to what extent these in vitro decreases in dendritic cell function apply to cells found in the tissues where most dendritic cell

12

interaction takes place with T cells. In particular, these studies with monocyte-derived dendritic cells are most relevant to in vivo immune responses by inflammatory dendritic cells, a cell type that may be involved only when marked inflammation of the tissues occurs. Studies of the phenotype and function of tissue-associated dendritic cells in the newborn have been limited for practical and ethical reasons, but in the future, it should be possible to continue to evaluate myeloid and plasmacytoid dendritic cells that are found in respiratory secretions during viral infections. Murine studies also indicate that postnatal exposure to commensal bacteria may play a role in conventional dendritic cell maturation, suggesting that early postnatal limitations in dendritic cells may be, in part, a normal physiologic consequence of a sterile intrauterine environment. Mouse models also raise the possibility of persistent "programming" of dendritic cell function by infections in early life, and it will be interesting to determine whether such mechanisms apply to humans. In addition to potential limitations in dendritic cell function, intrinsic limitations in T cell activation and Th-1 differentiation (including the production of CD154, CD154-mediated expression of interleukin-12p70 by DCs, expression of the interferon-γ gene, and interleukin-12p70–induced tyrosine phosphorylation of STAT-4) may contribute to an impaired ability of T cells in the neonate to respond to antigenic challenges. These limitations are likely to be important in explaining the increased vulnerability of the neonate to intracellular pathogens, the relatively low incidence of acute graft-versus-host disease when cord blood mononuclear cells are used for hematopoietic stem cell transplantation, and the inability of the neonate to reject allogeneic skin grafts.

References

1. Liu K, Nussenzweig MC. Origin and development of dendritic cells. *Immunol Rev*. 2010;234: 45-54.
2. Steinman RM, Idoyaga J. Features of the dendritic cell lineage. *Immunol Rev*. 2010;234:5-17.
3. Manicassamy S, Pulendran B. Dendritic cell control of tolerogenic responses. *Immunol Rev*. 2011; 241:206-227.
4. Zammit DJ, Cauley LS, Pham QM, et al. Dendritic cells maximize the memory CD8 T cell response to infection. *Immunity*. 2005;22:561-570.
5. Villadangos JA, Schnorrer P. Intrinsic and cooperative antigen-presenting functions of dendritic-cell subsets in vivo. *Nat Rev Immunol*. 2007;7:543-555.
6. Zhu J, Yamane H, Paul WE. Differentiation of effector CD4 T cell populations. *Ann Rev Immunol*. 2010;28:445-489.
7. Eyerich S, Wagener J, Wenzel V, et al. IL-22 and TNF-alpha represent a key cytokine combination for epidermal integrity during infection with *Candida albicans*. *Eur J Immunol*. 2011;41:1894-1901.
8. Qiao D, Yang BY, Li L, et al. ESAT-6- and CFP-10-specific Th1, Th22 and Th17 cells in tuberculous pleurisy may contribute to the local immune response against Mycobacterium tuberculosis infection. *Scand J Immunol*. 2011;73:330-337.
9. Lewis DB, Wilson CB. Developmental immunology and role of host defenses in the fetal and neonatal susceptibility to infection. In: Remington JS, Klein JO, Wilson CB, Nizet V, Maldonado YA, eds. *Infectious Diseases of the Fetus and Newborn Infant*. Philadelphia: Elsevier; 2010:80-191.
10. Crozat K, Guiton R, Guilliams M, et al. Comparative genomics as a tool to reveal functional equivalences between human and mouse dendritic cell subsets. *Immunol Rev*. 2010;234:177-198.
11. Cahalan MD, Parker I. Choreography of cell motility and interaction dynamics imaged by two-photon microscopy in lymphoid organs. *Annu Rev Immunol*. 2008;26:585-626.
12. Randolph GJ, Ochando J, Partida-Sanchez S. Migration of dendritic cell subsets and their precursors. *Ann Rev Immunol*. 2008;26:293-316.
13. Takeuchi O, Akira S. Pattern recognition receptors and inflammation. *Cell*. 2010;140:805-820.
14. Kumar H, Kawai T, Akira S. Pathogen recognition by the innate immune system. *Int Rev Immunol*. 2011;30:16-34.
15. O'Reilly MK, Paulson JC. Multivalent ligands for siglecs. *Methods Enzymology*. 2010;478:343-363.
16. Hajishengallis G, Lambris JD. Microbial manipulation of receptor crosstalk in innate immunity. *Nat Rev Immunol*. 2011;11:187-200.
17. Blasius AL, Beutler B. Intracellular toll-like receptors. *Immunity*. 2010;32:305-315.
18. Zhang SY, Jouanguy E, Ugolini S, et al. TLR3 deficiency in patients with herpes simplex encephalitis. *Science*. 2007;317:1522-1527.
19. Perez de Diego R, Sancho-Shimizu V, Lorenzo L, et al. Human TRAF3 adaptor molecule deficiency leads to impaired Toll-like receptor 3 response and susceptibility to herpes simplex encephalitis. *Immunity*. 2010;33:400-411.
20. Blander JM, Medzhitov R. Toll-dependent selection of microbial antigens for presentation by dendritic cells. *Nature*. 2006;440:808-812.
21. Takaoka A, Yanai H, Kondo S, et al. Integral role of IRF-5 in the gene induction programme activated by Toll-like receptors. *Nature*. 2005;434:243-249.

22. Kawai T, Akira S. Toll-like receptors and their crosstalk with other innate immune receptors in infection and immunity. *Immunity*. 2011; 34:637-650.

23. Sporri R, Reis E, Sousa C. Inflammatory mediators are insufficient for full dendritic cell activation and promote expansion of CD4+ T cell populations lacking helper function. *Nat Immunol*. 2005;6: 163-170.

24. Ting JP, Lovering RC, Alnemri ES, et al. The NLR gene family: A standard nomenclature. *Immunity*. 2008;28:285-287.

25. Jha S, Ting JP. Inflammasome-associated nucleotide-binding domain, leucine-rich repeat proteins and inflammatory diseases. *J Immunol*. 2009;183:7623-7629.

26. Franchi L, Eigenbrod T, Munoz-Planillo R, Nunez G. The inflammasome: A caspase-1-activation platform that regulates immune responses and disease pathogenesis. *Nat Immunol*. 2009;10: 241-247.

27. Dunne A. Inflammasome activation: From inflammatory disease to infection. *Biochem Soc Trans*. 2011;39:669-673.

28. Davis BK, Wen H, Ting JP. The inflammasome NLRs in immunity, inflammation, and associated diseases. *Ann Rev Immunol*. 2011;29:707-735.

29. Goriely S, Neurath MF, Goldman M. How microorganisms tip the balance between interleukin-12 family members. *Nat Rev Immunol*. 2008;8:81-86.

30. Kanneganti TD. Central roles of NLRs and inflammasomes in viral infection. *Nat Rev Immunol*. 2010;10:688-698.

31. Ting JP, Duncan JA, Lei Y. How the noninflammasome NLRs function in the innate immune system. *Science*. 2010;327:286-290.

32. Dunne A, Ross PJ, Pospisilova E, et al. Inflammasome activation by adenylate cyclase toxin directs Th17 responses and protection against Bordetella pertussis. *J Immunol*. 2010;185:1711-1719.

33. Gross O, Poeck H, Bscheider M, et al. Syk kinase signalling couples to the Nlrp3 inflammasome for anti-fungal host defence. *Nature*. 2009;459:433-436.

34. Meng G, Zhang F, Fuss I, et al. A mutation in the Nlrp3 gene causing inflammasome hyperactivation potentiates Th17 cell-dominant immune responses. *Immunity*. 2009;30:860-874.

35. Osorio F, Reis E, Sousa C. Myeloid C-type lectin receptors in pathogen recognition and host defense. *Immunity*. 2011;34:651-664.

36. Vautier S, Sousa Mda G, Brown GD. C-type lectins, fungi and Th17 responses. *Cytokine Growth Factor Rev*. 2010;21:405-412.

37. Takeuchi O, Akira S. MDA5/RIG-I and virus recognition. *Curr Opin Immunol*. 2008;20:17-22.

38. Onoguchi K, Yoneyama M, Fujita T. Retinoic acid-inducible gene-I-like receptors. *J Interferon Cytokine Res*. 2011;31:27-31.

39. Poeck H, Bscheider M, Gross O, et al. Recognition of RNA virus by RIG-I results in activation of CARD9 and inflammasome signaling for interleukin 1 beta production. *Nat Immunol*. 2010;11: 63-69.

40. Kawai T, Akira S. Innate immune recognition of viral infection. *Nat Immunol*. 2006;7:131-137.

41. Lisovsky M, Braun SE, Ge Y, et al. Flt3-ligand production by human bone marrow stromal cells. *Leukemia*. 1996;10:1012-1018.

42. Kasmar A, Van Rhijn I, Moody DB. The evolved functions of CD1 during infection. *Curr Opin Immunol*. 2009;21:397-403.

43. Villadangos JA, Shortman K. Found in translation: The human equivalent of mouse CD8+ dendritic cells. *J Exp Med*. 2010;207:1131-1134.

44. Bachem A, Guttler S, Hartung E, et al. Superior antigen cross-presentation and XCR1 expression define human CD11c+CD141+ cells as homologues of mouse CD8+ dendritic cells. *J Exp Med*. 2010;207:1273-1281.

45. Crozat K, Guiton R, Contreras V, et al. The XC chemokine receptor 1 is a conserved selective marker of mammalian cells homologous to mouse CD8alpha+ dendritic cells. *J Exp Med*. 2010;207:1283-1292.

46. Yamazaki C, Miyamoto R, Hoshino K, et al. Conservation of a chemokine system, XCR1 and its ligand, XCL1, between human and mice. *Biochem Biophys Res Commun*. 2010;397:756-761.

47. Poulin LF, Salio M, Griessinger E, et al. Characterization of human DNGR-1+ BDCA3+ leukocytes as putative equivalents of mouse CD8alpha+ dendritic cells. *J Exp Med*. 2010;207:1261-1271.

48. Jongbloed SL, Kassianos AJ, McDonald KJ, et al. Human CD141+ (BDCA-3)+ dendritic cells (DCs) represent a unique myeloid DC subset that cross-presents necrotic cell antigens. *J Exp Med*. 2010; 207:1247-1260.

49. Sancho D, Joffre OP, Keller AM, et al. Identification of a dendritic cell receptor that couples sensing of necrosis to immunity. *Nature*. 2009;458:899-903.

50. Lauterbach H, Bathke B, Gilles S, et al. Mouse CD8alpha+ DCs and human BDCA3+ DCs are major producers of IFN-lambda in response to poly IC. *J Exp Med*. 2010;207:2703-2717.

51. Zaba LC, Krueger JG, Lowes MA. Resident and "inflammatory" dendritic cells in human skin. *J Invest Derm*. 2009;129:302-308.

52. Zaba LC, Fuentes-Duculan J, Steinman RM, et al. Normal human dermis contains distinct populations of CD11c+BDCA-1+ dendritic cells and CD163+FXIIIA+ macrophages. *J Clin Invest*. 2007; 117:2517-2525.

53. van de Ven R, van den Hout MF, Lindenberg JJ, et al. Characterization of four conventional dendritic cell subsets in human skin-draining lymph nodes in relation to T-cell activation. *Blood*. 2011;118: 2502-2510.

54. Banchereau J, Briere F, Caux C, et al. Immunobiology of dendritic cells. *Annu Rev Immunol*. 2000;18: 767-811.

55. Kissenpfennig A, Malissen B. Langerhans cells—revisiting the paradigm using genetically engineered mice. *Trends Immunol*. 2006;27:132-139.

56. Cao T, Ueno H, Glaser C, et al. Both Langerhans cells and interstitial DC cross-present melanoma antigens and efficiently activate antigen-specific CTL. *Eur J Immunol*. 2007;37:2657-2667.

57. Reizis B, Bunin A, Ghosh HS, et al. Plasmacytoid dendritic cells: Recent progress and open questions. *Ann Rev Immunol*. 2011;29:163-183.

58. Cella M, Jarrossay D, Facchetti F, et al. Plasmacytoid monocytes migrate to inflamed lymph nodes and produce large amounts of type I interferon. *Nat Med*. 1999;5:919-923.

59. Serbina NV, Salazar-Mather TP, Biron CA, et al. TNF/iNOS-producing dendritic cells mediate innate immune defense against bacterial infection. *Immunity*. 2003;19:59-70.

60. Poulter LW, Janossy G. The involvement of dendritic cells in chronic inflammatory disease. *Scand J Immunol*. 1985;21:401-407.

61. Krutzik SR, Tan B, Li H, et al. TLR activation triggers the rapid differentiation of monocytes into macrophages and dendritic cells. *Nat Med*. 2005;11:653-660.

62. Hise AG, Tomalka J, Ganesan S, et al. An essential role for the NLRP3 inflammasome in host defense against the human fungal pathogen *Candida albicans*. *Cell Host Microbe*. 2009;5:487-497.

63. Cunningham AL, Donaghy H, Harman AN, et al. Manipulation of dendritic cell function by viruses. *Curr Opin Microbiol*. 2010;13:524-529.

64. Kuwajima S, Sato T, Ishida K, et al. Interleukin 15-dependent crosstalk between conventional and plasmacytoid dendritic cells is essential for CpG-induced immune activation. *Nat Immunol*. 2006;7:740-746.

65. Munz C, Steinman RM, Fujii S. Dendritic cell maturation by innate lymphocytes: Coordinated stimulation of innate and adaptive immunity. *J Exp Med*. 2005;202:203-207.

66. Guermonprez P, Valladeau J, Zitvogel L, et al. Antigen presentation and T cell stimulation by dendritic cells. *Annu Rev Immunol*. 2002;20:621-667.

67. Allan RS, Waithman J, Bedoui S, et al. Migratory dendritic cells transfer antigen to a lymph node-resident dendritic cell population for efficient CTL priming. *Immunity*. 2006;25:153-162.

68. Smith CM, Wilson NS, Waithman J, et al. Cognate CD4(+) T cell licensing of dendritic cells in CD8(+) T cell immunity. *Nat Immunol*. 2004;5:1143-1148.

69. Kissenpfennig A, Henri S, Dubois B, et al. Dynamics and function of Langerhans cells in vivo: dermal dendritic cells colonize lymph node areas distinct from slower migrating Langerhans cells. *Immunity*. 2005;22:643-654.

70. Zhu J, Paul WE. Peripheral CD4+ T-cell differentiation regulated by networks of cytokines and transcription factors. *Immunol Rev*. 2010;238:247-262.

71. Barlow JL, McKenzie AN. Nuocytes: Expanding the innate cell repertoire in type-2 immunity. *J Leukoc Biol*. 2011. 2011 Jun 28. [Epub ahead of print].

72. Ma CS, Suryani S, Avery DT, et al. Early commitment of naive human CD4(+) T cells to the T follicular helper (T(FH)) cell lineage is induced by IL-12. *Immunol Cell Biol*. 2009;87:590-600.

73. Chevalier N, Jarrossay D, Ho E, et al. CXCR5 expressing human central memory CD4 T cells and their relevance for humoral immune responses. *J Immunol*. 2011;186:5556-5568.

74. Tabeta K, Hoebe K, Janssen EM, et al. The Unc93b1 mutation 3d disrupts exogenous antigen presentation and signaling via Toll-like receptors 3, 7 and 9. *Nat Immunol*. 2006;7:156-164.

75. Savina A, Jancic C, Hugues S, et al. NOX2 controls phagosomal pH to regulate antigen processing during crosspresentation by dendritic cells. *Cell*. 2006;126:205-218.

76. Pasare C, Medzhitov R. Toll-dependent control mechanisms of CD4 T cell activation. *Immunity*. 2004;21:733-741.

77. Kimberlin DW. Herpes simplex virus infections of the newborn. *Semin Perinatol*. 2007;31:19-25.

78. Muller WJ, Jones CA, Koelle DM. Immunobiology of herpes simplex virus and cytomegalovirus infections of the fetus and newborn. *Curr Immunol Rev*. 2010;6:38-55.

79. Sullender WM, Miller JL, Yasukawa LL, et al. Humoral and cell-mediated immunity in neonates with herpes simplex virus infection. *J Infect Dis*. 1987;155:28-37.

80. Iijima N, Linehan MM, Zamora M, et al. Dendritic cells and B cells maximize mucosal Th1 memory response to herpes simplex virus. *J Exp Med*. 2008;205:3041-3052.

81. Donaghy H, Bosnjak L, Harman AN, et al. Role for plasmacytoid dendritic cells in the immune control of recurrent human herpes simplex virus infection. *J Virol*. 2009;83:1952-1961.

82. Tu W, Chen S, Sharp M, et al. Persistent and selective deficiency of CD4+ T cell immunity to cytomegalovirus in immunocompetent young children. *J Immunol*. 2004;172:3260-3267.

83. Chen SF, Tu WW, Sharp MA, et al. Antiviral CD8 T cells in the control of primary human cytomegalovirus infection in early childhood. *J Infect Dis*. 2004;189:1619-1627.

84. Marchant A, Appay V, Van Der Sande M, et al. Mature CD8(+) T lymphocyte response to viral infection during fetal life. *J Clin Invest*. 2003;111:1747-1755.

85. Lin TY, Kao HT, Hsieh SH, et al. Neonatal enterovirus infections: Emphasis on risk factors of severe and fatal infections. *Pediatr Infect Dis J*. 2003;22:889-894.

86. Ventura KC, Hawkins H, Smith MB, et al. Fatal neonatal echovirus 6 infection: Autopsy case report and review of the literature. *Mod Pathol*. 2001;14:85-90.

87. Rorman E, Zamir CS, Rilkis I, et al. Congenital toxoplasmosis—prenatal aspects of *Toxoplasma gondii* infection. *Reprod Toxicol*. 2006;21:458-472.

88. Marodi L. Neonatal innate immunity to infectious agents. *Infect Immun*. 2006;74:1999-2006.

89. Marodi L, Johnston Jr RB. Invasive *Candida* species disease in infants and children: Occurrence, risk factors, management, and innate host defense mechanisms. *Curr Opin Pediatr*. 2007;19:693-697.

90. Klatt NR, Brenchley JM. Th17 cell dynamics in HIV infection. *Curr Opin HIV AIDS*. 2010;5:135-140.

91. Smith S, Jacobs RF, Wilson CB. Immunobiology of childhood tuberculosis: A window on the ontogeny of cellular immunity. *J Pediatr.* 1997;131:16-26.
92. Marchant A, Goetghebuer T, Ota MO, et al. Newborns develop a Th1-type immune response to *Mycobacterium bovis* bacillus Calmette-Guerin vaccination. *J Immunol.* 1999;163:2249-2255.
93. Vekemans J, Amedei A, Ota MO, et al. Neonatal bacillus Calmette-Guerin vaccination induces adult-like IFN-gamma production by CD4+ T lymphocytes. *Eur J Immunol.* 2001;31:1531-1535.
94. Murray RA, Mansoor N, Harbacheuski R, et al. Bacillus Calmette Guerin vaccination of human newborns induces a specific, functional CD8+ T cell response. *J Immunol.* 2006;177:5647-5651.
95. De Wit D, Olislagers V, Goriely S, et al. Blood plasmacytoid dendritic cell responses to CpG oligo-deoxynucleotides are impaired in human newborns. *Blood.* 2004;103:1030-1032.
96. Teig N, Moses D, Gieseler S, et al. Age-related changes in human blood dendritic cell subpopulations. *Scand J Immunol.* 2002;55:453-457.
97. Borras FE, Matthews NC, Lowdell MW, et al. Identification of both myeloid CD11c+ and lymphoid CD11c– dendritic cell subsets in cord blood. *Br J Haematol.* 2001;113:925-931.
98. MacDonald KP, Munster DJ, Clark GJ, et al. Characterization of human blood dendritic cell subsets. *Blood.* 2002;100:4512-4520.
99. Dzionek A, Fuchs A, Schmidt P, et al. BDCA-2, BDCA-3, and BDCA-4: Three markers for distinct subsets of dendritic cells in human peripheral blood. *J Immunol.* 2000;165:6037-6046.
100. Robbins SH, Walzer T, Dembele D, et al. Novel insights into the relationships between dendritic cell subsets in human and mouse revealed by genome-wide expression profiling. *Genome Biology.* 2008;9:R17.
101. Vuckovic S, Gardiner D, Field K, et al. Monitoring dendritic cells in clinical practice using a new whole blood single-platform TruCOUNT assay. *J Immunol Methods.* 2004;284:73-87.
102. Szabolcs P, Park KD, Reese M, et al. Absolute values of dendritic cell subsets in bone marrow, cord blood, and peripheral blood enumerated by a novel method. *Stem Cells.* 2003;21:296-303.
103. Vakkila J, Thomson AW, Vettenranta K, et al. Dendritic cell subsets in childhood and in children with cancer: Relation to age and disease prognosis. *Clin Exp Immunol.* 2004;135:455-461.
104. Lavoie PM, Huang Q, Jolette E, et al. Profound lack of interleukin (IL)-12/IL-23p40 in neonates born early in gestation is associated with an increased risk of sepsis. *J Infect Dis.* 2010;202:1754-1763.
105. Hagendorens MM, Ebo DG, Schuerwegh AJ, et al. Differences in circulating dendritic cell subtypes in cord blood and peripheral blood of healthy and allergic children. *Clin Exp Allergy.* 2003;33:633-639.
106. De Wit D, Olislagers V, Goriely S, et al. Blood plasmacytoid dendritic cell responses to CpG oligo-deoxynucleotides are impaired in human newborns. *Blood.* 2004;103:1030-1032.
107. De Wit D, Tonon S, Olislagers V, et al. Impaired responses to toll-like receptor 4 and toll-like receptor 3 ligands in human cord blood. *J Autoimmun.* 2003;21:277-281.
108. Crespo I, Paiva A, Couceiro A, et al. Immunophenotypic and functional characterization of cord blood dendritic cells. *Stem Cells Dev.* 2004;13:63-70.
109. Drohan L, Harding JJ, Holm B, et al. Selective developmental defects of cord blood antigen-presenting cell subsets. *Hum Immunol.* 2004;65:1356-1369.
110. Kerfoot SM, Long EM, Hickey MJ, et al. TLR4 contributes to disease-inducing mechanisms resulting in central nervous system autoimmune disease. *J Immunol.* 2004;173:7070-7077.
111. Upham JW, Lee PT, Holt BJ, et al. Development of interleukin-12-producing capacity throughout childhood. *Infect Immun.* 2002;70:6583-6588.
112. Tonon S, Goriely S, Aksoy E, et al. Bordetella pertussis toxin induces the release of inflammatory cytokines and dendritic cell activation in whole blood: Impaired responses in human newborns. *Eur J Immunol.* 2002;32:3118-3125.
113. Lee SM, Suen Y, Chang L, et al. Decreased interleukin-12 (IL-12) from activated cord versus adult peripheral blood mononuclear cells and upregulation of interferon-gamma, natural killer, and lymphokine-activated killer activity by IL-12 in cord blood mononuclear cells. *Blood.* 1996;88:1945-1954.
114. Lee SM, Suen Y, Chang L, et al. Decreased interleukin-12 (IL-12) from activated cord versus adult peripheral blood mononuclear cells and upregulation of interferon-gamma, natural killer, and lymphokine-activated killer activity by IL-12 in cord blood mononuclear cells. *Blood.* 1996;88:945-954.
115. Perez-Melgosa M, Ochs HD, Linsley PS, et al. Carrier-mediated enhancement of cognate T cell help: The basis for enhanced immunogenicity of meningococcal outer membrane protein polysaccharide conjugate vaccine. *Eur J Immunol.* 2001;31:2373-2381.
116. Karlsson H, Hessle C, Rudin A. Innate immune responses of human neonatal cells to bacteria from the normal gastrointestinal flora. *Infect Immun.* 2002;70:6688-6696.
117. Levy O, Suter EE, Miller RL, et al. Unique efficacy of Toll-like receptor 8 agonists in activating human neonatal antigen-presenting cells. *Blood.* 2006;108:1284-1290.
118. Olweus J, BitMansour A, Warnke R, et al. Dendritic cell ontogeny: A human dendritic cell lineage of myeloid origin. *Proc Natl Acad Sci U S A.* 1997;94:12551-12556.
119. Grouard G, Rissoan MC, Filgueira L, et al. The enigmatic plasmacytoid T cells develop into dendritic cells with interleukin (IL)-3 and CD40-ligand. *J Exp Med.* 1997;185:1101-1111.
120. Sorg RV, Kogler G, Wernet P. Identification of cord blood dendritic cells as an immature CD11c– population. *Blood.* 1999;93:2302-2307.
121 Prescott SL, Irwin S, Taylor A, et al. Cytosine-phosphate-guanine motifs fail to promote T-helper type 1-polarized responses in human neonatal mononuclear cells. *Clin Exp Allergy.* 2005;35:358-366.

12

12

122. Gold MC, Donnelly E, Cook MS, et al. Purified neonatal plasmacytoid dendritic cells overcome intrinsic maturation defect with TLR agonist stimulation. *Pediatr Res.* 2006;60:34-37.
123. Cederblad B, Riesenfeld T, Alm GV. Deficient herpes simplex virus-induced interferon-alpha production by blood leukocytes of preterm and term newborn infants. *Pediatr Res.* 1990;27:7-10.
124. Danis B, George TC, Goriely S, et al. Interferon regulatory factor 7-mediated responses are defective in cord blood plasmacytoid dendritic cells. *Eur J Immunol.* 2008;38:507-517.
125. Wilson CB, Kollmann TR. Induction of antigen-specific immunity in human neonates and infants. *Nestle Nutr Workshop Ser Pediatr Program.* 2008;61:183-195.
126. Kollmann TR, Crabtree J, Rein-Weston A, et al. Neonatal innate TLR-mediated responses are distinct from those of adults. *J Immunol.* 2009;183:7150-7160.
127. Hunt DW, Huppertz HI, Jiang HJ, et al. Studies of human cord blood dendritic cells: Evidence for functional immaturity. *Blood.* 1994;84:4333-4343.
128. Petty RE, Hunt DW. Neonatal dendritic cells. *Vaccine.* 1998;16:1378-1382.
129. Sorg RV, Kogler G, Wernet P. Functional competence of dendritic cells in human umbilical cord blood. *Bone Marrow Transplant.* 1998;22(Suppl 1):S52–S54.
130. Lozza L, Rivino L, Guarda G, et al. The strength of T cell stimulation determines IL-7 responsiveness, secondary expansion, and lineage commitment of primed human CD4+IL-7Rhi T cells. *Eur J Immunol.* 2008;38:30-39.
131. Cella M, Facchetti F, Lanzavecchia A, et al. Plasmacytoid dendritic cells activated by influenza virus and CD40L drive a potent TH1 polarization. *Nat Immunol.* 2000;1:305-310.
132. Levy O, Zarember KA, Roy RM, et al. Selective impairment of TLR-mediated innate immunity in human newborns: Neonatal blood plasma reduces monocyte TNF-alpha induction by bacterial lipopeptides, lipopolysaccharide, and imiquimod, but preserves the response to R-848. *J Immunol.* 2004;173:4627-4634.
133. Angelone DF, Wessels MR, Coughlin M, et al. Innate immunity of the human newborn is polarized toward a high ratio of IL-6/TNF-alpha production in vitro and in vivo. *Pediatr Res.* 2006;60:205-209.
134. Wilson JM, Kurtz CC, Black SG, et al. The A2B adenosine receptor promotes Th17 differentiation via stimulation of dendritic cell IL-6. *J Immunol.* 2011;186:6746-6752.
135. Borras FE, Matthews NC, Patel R, et al. Dendritic cells can be successfully generated from CD34+ cord blood cells in the presence of autologous cord blood plasma. *Bone Marrow Transplant.* 2000;26:371-376.
136. Canque B, Camus S, Dalloul A, et al. Characterization of dendritic cell differentiation pathways from cord blood CD34(+)CD7(+)CD45RA(+) hematopoietic progenitor cells. *Blood.* 2000;96:3748-3756.
137. Sallusto F, Lanzavecchia A. Efficient presentation of soluble antigen by cultured human dendritic cells is maintained by granulocyte/macrophage colony-stimulating factor plus interleukin 4 and downregulated by tumor necrosis factor alpha. *J Exp Med.* 1994;179:1109-1118.
138. Jakobsen MA, Moller BK, Lillevang ST. Serum concentration of the growth medium markedly affects monocyte-derived dendritic cells' phenotype, cytokine production profile and capacities to stimulate in MLR. *Scand J Immunol.* 2004;60:584-591.
139. Goriely S, Vincart B, Stordeur P, et al. Deficient IL-12(p35) gene expression by dendritic cells derived from neonatal monocytes. *J Immunol.* 2001;166:2141-2146.
140. Liu E, Tu W, Law HK, et al. Decreased yield, phenotypic expression and function of immature monocyte-derived dendritic cells in cord blood. *Br J Haematol.* 2001;113:240-246.
141. Langrish CL, Buddle JC, Thrasher AJ, et al. Neonatal dendritic cells are intrinsically biased against Th-1 immune responses. *Clin Exp Immunol.* 2002;128:118-123.
142. Renneson J, Dutta B, Goriely S, et al. IL-12 and type I IFN response of neonatal myeloid DC to human CMV infection. *Eur J Immunol.* 2009;39:2789-2799.
143. Goriely S, Lint Van C, Dadkhah R, et al. A defect in nucleosome remodeling prevents IL-12(p35) gene transcription in neonatal dendritic cells. *J Exp Med.* 2004;199:1011-1016.
144. Goriely S, Molle C, Nguyen M, et al. Interferon regulatory factor 3 is involved in Toll-like receptor 4 (TLR4)- and TLR3-induced IL-12p35 gene activation. *Blood.* 2006;107:1078-1084.
145. Zheng Z, Takahashi M, Narita M, et al. Generation of dendritic cells from adherent cells of cord blood by culture with granulocyte-macrophage colony-stimulating factor, interleukin-4, and tumor necrosis factor-alpha. *J Hematother Stem Cell Res.* 2000;9:453-464.
146. Vanden Eijnden S, Goriely S, De Wit D, et al. Preferential production of the IL-12(p40)/IL-23(p19) heterodimer by dendritic cells from human newborns. *Eur J Immunol.* 2006;36:21-26.
147. Porras A, Kozar S, Russanova V, et al. Developmental and epigenetic regulation of the human TLR3 gene. *Mol Immunol.* 2008;46:27-36.
148. Hofman FM, Danilovs JA, Taylor CR. HLA-DR (Ia)-positive dendritic-like cells in human fetal nonlymphoid tissues. *Transplantation.* 1984;37:590-594.
149. Foster CA, Holbrook KA. Ontogeny of Langerhans cells in human embryonic and fetal skin: Cell densities and phenotypic expression relative to epidermal growth. *Am J Anat.* 1989;184:157-164.
150. Schuster C, Vaculik C, Fiala C, et al. HLA-DR+ leukocytes acquire CD1 antigens in embryonic and fetal human skin and contain functional antigen-presenting cells. *J Exp Med.* 2009;206:169-181.
151. Drijkoningen M, De Wolf-Peeters C, Van der Steen K, et al. Epidermal Langerhans' cells and dermal dendritic cells in human fetal and neonatal skin: An immunohistochemical study. *Pediatr Dermatol.* 1987;4:11-17.
152. Watanabe S, Nakajima T, Shimosato Y, et al. T-zone histiocytes with S100 protein. Development and distribution in human fetuses. *Acta Pathol Jpn.* 1983;33:15-22.

153. Nguyen M, Leuridan E, Zhang T, et al. Acquisition of adult-like TLR4 and TLR9 responses during the first year of life. *PLoS One*. 2010;5:e10407.
154. Corbett NP, Blimkie D, Ho KC, et al. Ontogeny of Toll-like receptor mediated cytokine responses of human blood mononuclear cells. *PLoS One*. 2010;5:e15041.
155. Bendall SC, Simonds EF, Qiu P, et al. Single-cell mass cytometry of differential immune and drug responses across a human hematopoietic continuum. *Science*. 2011;332:687-696.
156. Gill MA, Palucka AK, Barton T, et al. Mobilization of plasmacytoid and myeloid dendritic cells to mucosal sites in children with respiratory syncytial virus and other viral respiratory infections. *J Infect Dis*. 2005;191:1105-1115.
157. Gill MA, Long K, Kwon T, et al. Differential recruitment of dendritic cells and monocytes to respiratory mucosal sites in children with influenza virus or respiratory syncytial virus infection. *J Infect Dis*. 2008;198:1667-1676.
158. Dabbagh K, Dahl ME, Stepick-Biek P, et al. Toll-like receptor 4 is required for optimal development of Th2 immune responses: role of dendritic cells. *J Immunol*. 2002;168:4524-4530.
159. Dakic A, Shao QX, D'Amico A, et al. Development of the dendritic cell system during mouse ontogeny. *J Immunol*. 2004;172:1018-1027.
160. Muthukkumar S, Goldstein J, Stein KE. The ability of B cells and dendritic cells to present antigen increases during ontogeny. *J Immunol*. 2000;165:4803-4813.
161. Jiao L, Han X, Wang S, et al. Imprinted DC mediate the immune-educating effect of early-life microbial exposure. *Eur J Immunol*. 2009;39:469-480.
162. Wood N, Siegrist CA. Neonatal immunization: Where do we stand? *Curr Opin Infect Dis*. 2011;24:190-195.
163. Dadaglio G, Sun CM, Lo-Man R, et al. Efficient in vivo priming of specific cytotoxic T cell responses by neonatal dendritic cells. *J Immunol*. 2002;168:2219-2224.
164. Hall JA, Bouladoux N, Sun CM, et al. Commensal DNA limits regulatory T cell conversion and is a natural adjuvant of intestinal immune responses. *Immunity*. 2008;29:637-649.
165. Ehlers S, Smith KA. Differentiation of T cell lymphokine gene expression: the in vitro acquisition of T cell memory. *J Exp Med*. 1991;173:25-36.
166. Lewis DB, Prickett KS, Larsen A, et al. Restricted production of interleukin 4 by activated human T cells. *Proc Natl Acad Sci U S A*. 1988;85:9743-9747.
167. Lewis DB, Yu CC, Meyer J, English BK, et al. Cellular and molecular mechanisms for reduced interleukin 4 and interferon-gamma production by neonatal T cells. *J Clin Invest*. 1991;87:194-202.
168. Chen L, Cohen AC, Lewis DB. Impaired allogeneic activation and T-helper 1 differentiation of human cord blood naive CD4 T cells. *Biol Blood Marrow Transplant*. 2006;12:160-171.
169. Melvin AJ, McGurn ME, Bort SJ, et al. Hypomethylation of the interferon-gamma gene correlates with its expression by primary T-lineage cells. *Eur J Immunol*. 1995;25:426-430.
170. White GP, Watt PM, Holt BJ, et al. Differential patterns of methylation of the IFN-gamma promoter at CpG and non-CpG sites underlie differences in IFN-gamma gene expression between human neonatal and adult CD45RO- T cells. *J Immunol*. 2002;168:2820-2827.
171. Tra J, Kondo T, Lu Q, et al. Infrequent occurrence of age-dependent changes in CpG island methylation as detected by restriction landmark genome scanning. *Mech Ageing Dev*. 2002;123:1487-1503.
172. Haines CJ, Giffon TD, Lu LS, et al. Human CD4+ T cell recent thymic emigrants are identified by protein tyrosine kinase 7 and have reduced immune function. *J Exp Med*. 2009;206:275-285.
173. Prebet T, Lhoumeau AC, Arnoulet C, et al. The cell polarity PTK7 receptor acts as a modulator of the chemotherapeutic response in acute myeloid leukemia and impairs clinical outcome. *Blood*. 2010;2010:2315-2323.
174. Blume-Jensen P, Hunter T. Oncogenic kinase signalling. *Nature*. 2001;411:355-365.
175. Ameratunga R, Lederman HM, Sullivan KE, et al. Defective antigen-induced lymphocyte proliferation in the X-linked hyper-IgM syndrome. *J Pediatr*. 1997;131:147-150.
176. Jain A, Atkinson TP, Lipsky PE, et al. Defects of T-cell effector function and post-thymic maturation in X-linked hyper-IgM syndrome. *J Clin Invest*. 1999;103:1151-1158.
177. Jullien P, Cron RQ, Dabbagh K, et al. Decreased CD154 expression by neonatal CD4+ T cells is due to limitations in both proximal and distal events of T cell activation. *Int Immunol*. 2003;15:1461-1472.
178. Nonoyama S, Penix LA, Edwards CP, et al. Diminished expression of CD40 ligand by activated neonatal T cells. *J Clin Invest*. 1995;95:66-75.

12

CHAPTER 13

Breast Milk and Viral Infection

Marianne Forsgren, MD, PhD; Björn Fischler, MD, PhD; and Lars Navér, MD, PhD

- HIV and Breast-feeding
- HTLV-I and Breast-feeding
- Hepatitis B Infection and Breast-feeding
- Hepatitis C Infection and Breast-feeding
- Cytomegalovirus and Breast-feeding

Breast milk is the most important nutrient for all newborn babies—preterm and full-term. Breast milk supplies the infant not only with essential nutrition but also with factors for its immune defense.[1]

The immune system of a full-term newborn infant is still undergoing structural and functional maturation at the time of birth. During this period of ongoing immunologic development, passive transfer of maternal immune factors across the placenta and in breast milk protects the young infant. Active transport of maternal immunoglobulin (Ig)G via an Fcγ receptor in placental cells starts slowly in the second trimester.[2] At the time of delivery, the full-term neonate has about 90% of the maternal total IgG level for its defense, and certain antibodies such as those against rubella may reach higher levels in the newborn than in the mother. The more preterm a child is born, the lower are the levels of maternal antibodies and passive protection. Gradual decay of maternal antibodies occurs after birth with a half-life of 25 to 30 days,[2] although protective effects may last for the first 6 to 12 months until the infant's own IgG antibodies are produced. IgG synthesis starts during infancy at about 3 to 4 months of age.

Breast milk–borne immune factors include humoral components such as secretory IgA, which compensates for the inability of the fetus to produce IgA, cellular components such as lymphocytes, and a number of inhibitory substances. The protective role of these components may vary with specific insults and the age of the infant. Whereas lactoferrin when tested in vitro is reported to inhibit many enveloped and naked viruses such as human immunodeficiency virus (HIV), herpes simplex, hepatitis C, influenza, rotavirus, and adenoviruses,[3] it actually may stimulate the growth of human T cell lymphotropic virus type I (HTLV-I).[4,5]

Passively transferred maternal immune factors may protect an infant from many but not all microbial threats. In some instances, maternal breast milk may be a source of infection, as during the acute phase of a primary generalized viral infection such as varicella, parvovirus, hepatitis A, or rubella. At this early stage of infection, these mothers have no protection to transfer to the infant, and the breast milk frequently contains the virus. Transfer by breast milk is probably of minor importance in most instances because the child may already have been exposed to the virus by other routes, and continuation of breast-feeding is probably in the best interests of both the infant and the mother. Some exceptions may be noted, as exemplified by a case report that indicates that transmission of West Nile virus from an infected mother to her infant by breast milk may have resulted in neurologic disease.[6] However, in other reports, transmission of the virus did not always cause symptomatic infection in the neonate.[7,8]

Breast milk can also carry low titers of live vaccine viruses to a child, such as after administration of the rubella vaccine in the postpartum period.[9] Early neonatal exposure to rubella vaccine virus does not cause clinical symptoms or enhance or suppress responses to rubella vaccination in early childhood.[10] On the other hand, varicella vaccine virus is not detected in breast milk and virus is not transferred to the breast-fed infant.[11] One report describes a case of neurologic disease in an infant after transmission of yellow fever vaccine 17D virus from the vaccinated mother to her breast-fed child.[12] The child recovered with no observed sequelae at follow-up at 6 months of age. The risk for 17D vaccine–associated neurologic disease is known to be increased in infants, and 17D vaccine is not recommended in children younger than 6 months. Although the actual risk of transmission from breast milk based on this case report—and on one other suspected case[13]—is not known, current Centers for Disease Control and Prevention (CDC) recommendations are not to vaccinate breast-feeding mothers except when traveling to high-risk yellow fever–endemic areas.[14]

Viruses that can evade immune defenses and establish chronic infection with free and/or cellular viremia can infect cells or whey in breast milk. Chronic infection in these mothers as a rule is not disclosed by clinical signs. Identification of infected individuals may be possible through large-scale testing now enabled by recent advances in microbiological technology. Because currently no clinically useful tissue culture or animal model system is easily available for use in measuring the degree of infectivity of the mother (except CMV), qualitative and quantitative detection methods of viral nucleic acid are frequently used as surrogate markers. See Table 13-1.

HIV and Breast-feeding

HIV is transmitted through infected blood and body fluids. Routes of transmission include sexual intercourse, blood products, needle sharing during intravenous drug use, unsterile health care procedures, and mother-to-child transmission. Once infection is established, proviral DNA is integrated in the human genome. Antiviral drugs targeting different steps in viral replication may suppress viral replication. Two types of HIV can be distinguished—HIV-1 and HIV-2—of which HIV-1 is by far the most important. The risk of mother-to-child transmission is lower for HIV-2 than for HIV-1, probably because most HIV-2–infected mothers have low plasma viral load even without antiretroviral treatment.[15-17] This chapter will address only aspects of breast-feeding and HIV-1 (referred to as HIV).

One of the most tragic aspects of the global HIV epidemic is the vertical transmission of the virus to the next generation. UNAIDS estimated 1.6 million deaths of acquired immunodeficiency syndrome (AIDS) in 2009, of which 260,000 were children younger than 15 years. Approximately 15.7 million women were infected worldwide, most of them young and poor—a population for whom breast-feeding is critical for the survival of their infants.

Table 13-1   PATHOGENS

The most important pathogen transmitted by breast milk is HIV, human immunodeficiency virus, the causative agent of acquired immunodeficiency syndrome (AIDS)—a huge problem of global dimensions.

A second retrovirus, human T cell lymphotropic virus type I (HTLV-I), strongly associated with long-term risk of a special form of leukemia and demyelinating disease, is transmitted from mother to child mainly by breast-feeding; this is an important problem in endemic areas.

Hepatitis B and C viruses are globally spread chronic infections of the liver. The role of transmission by breast-feeding seems low as compared with highly effective transmission of hepatitis B through contact with infectious maternal blood at delivery.

Cytomegalovirus (CMV) is the pathogen most commonly transmitted by breast milk. CMV seems to have a potential pathogenic role as a cofactor aggravating the clinical course of a preexisting pulmonary, hematologic, or hepatic condition. CMV disease and symptoms are infrequent in the normal child—full-term or preterm.

Diagnosis of HIV Infection

Detection of viral antibodies is the cornerstone in individuals older than 18 months and as a screening test that is widely adapted to field conditions. Confirmatory tests and a set-up of analyses for proviral DNA and virus RNA for direct diagnosis of infant infection and determination of viral load, subtyping of virus, and resistance against antiviral drugs are available in the specialized laboratory, and the full potential of molecular microbiology is applied to HIV research.

Mother-to-Child Transmission

Transmission of HIV from an infected mother to her child can occur before, during, or after birth. Before the era of antiretroviral prophylaxis, HIV was vertically transmitted in 15% to 25% of all infected mothers in the industrialized countries, provided the mother did not breast-feed.[17,18] Studies from breast-feeding settings in Africa showed transmission rates as high as 30% to 42%.[19]

Among children of non–breast-feeding women, approximately 60% to 70% become infected during delivery, and the remaining 30% to 40% are thought to be infected in utero.[20,21] A vast majority of the children infected in utero are infected during the last months of pregnancy.[22,23] Transmission during the first trimester appears to be rare,[24] whereas the infection rate during the second trimester may be around 2% to 5%.[25,26]

Breast Milk: Transmission

HIV transmission through breast-feeding has been demonstrated in several clinical trials of formula feeding versus breast-feeding,[27,28] although only one of these study groups was properly randomized. In the randomized study from Kenya,[27] the cumulative probability of HIV infection by 24 months was 20.5% among children who were bottle-fed and 36.7% among those who were breast-fed. The estimated risk of HIV transmission through breast-feeding was 16.2% by the age of 24 months.[28] In a meta-analysis,[29] the additional risk of mother-to-child transmission of HIV through breast-feeding was found to be 16%, and the contribution of breast-feeding to overall mother-to-child transmission of HIV was estimated to be 47%.[29]

HIV in Breast Milk

HIV is present in breast milk as both free[30-32] and cell-associated virus.[32-34] Cell-free virus was detected in 34% to 63% of breast milk samples from HIV-infected women at different time points after delivery. Median virus load in colostrum/early milk was significantly higher than that in more mature breast milk collected 14 days after delivery.[31] The prevalence and mean cell-free viral load in breast milk collected longer than 1 week after delivery were not affected by postnatal age.[31,35] Cell-free viral load in breast milk correlates positively with viral load in plasma,[30] even though the plasma load is generally higher,[31] and negatively with maternal CD4+ cell count.[30,35] The relative contribution of the cell-free and cell-associated virus in breast-feeding–related mother-to-child transmission remains unclear.

The prevalence of cell-associated virus in breast milk ranges from 21% to 70% in different studies.[33,34] The number of infected breast milk cells per million cells was associated with the level of cell-free HIV RNA in breast milk,[34] and the concentration of infected cells was higher in colostrum and early milk than in more mature milk.[34] Although the origin of HIV in breast milk is not well defined, resting HIV-infected CD4+ T lymphocytes have been identified with a capacity to produce viral particles after activation.[36,37] Cells, including macrophages and lymphocytes, and cell-free virus may migrate from the systemic compartment to breast milk. HIV can infect and reproduce in mammary epithelial cells in vitro,[38] but it is not known whether the ductal or alveolar cells contribute to local viral replication in vivo. In paired samples, the HIV populations in blood and breast milk have been found to be similar. No unique variants existed in either compartment, suggesting that viruses in blood plasma and breast milk are well equilibrated.[39]

HIV Transmission: Mechanisms

The mechanism for mother-to-child transmission via breast-feeding is not well described, and it is unclear whether infection occurs through cell-free virus or through infected cells. The infant gut mucosal surface is the most likely site at which transmission occurs. Cell-free or cellular virus may penetrate to the submucosa in the setting of mucosal breaches or lesions, via transcytosis.[40,41] Oral transmission has been demonstrated in a macaque simian immunodeficiency model, and this pathway probably exists in humans as well.[42] In vitro models suggest that secretory IgA and IgM may inhibit transcytosis of HIV across enterocytes,[40,41] but HIV-specific secretory IgA in breast milk does not appear to be a protective factor against HIV transmission among breast-fed infants.[43]

A higher cell-free viral load in breast milk,[30,44] as well as a higher viral load in plasma,[45,46] is associated with a higher risk of mother-to-child transmission. Infants who acquired the infection after birth ingested significantly more cell-free virus particles from breast milk than did uninfected infants.[47] The presence of HIV-infected cells in milk 15 days postpartum was strongly predictive of HIV infection in the child,[33] and a higher cell-associated viral load in breast milk was associated with an increase in postnatal HIV transmission.[32] Primary HIV infection is associated with high levels of virus in plasma and probably also in breast milk, and a high risk of postnatal transmission.[28] Another study demonstrated a sixfold risk increase if the mother seroconverted while breast-feeding.[48] A reduction in both cell-associated and cell-free virus in breast milk might significantly reduce HIV transmission by breast-feeding.[32]

Timing of Transmission

The risk of HIV transmission through breast milk seems to be higher in young infants than in older children.[27,49] In the Kenyan randomized study of breast-feeding versus formula feeding, major breast milk–related transmission occurred early, with 75% of the risk difference between the two arms noted by 6 months, although transmission continued throughout the entire period of exposure.[27] Possible risk factors for increased transmission early in life include an immature immune system and increased permeability of the gut in combination with higher virus content in early breast milk.[33] The increase in risk of virus transmission with even a few weeks of breast-feeding in the early postnatal period supports the importance of early risk factors.[28,50] As was previously mentioned, both the cell-free viral load[45] and the concentration of infected cells[34] are higher in colostrum and early milk. However, a study from Brazil did not show that intake of colostrum affected the transmission rate.[50] The risk of HIV transmission correlates with the duration of breast-feeding.[45,51-53] In a meta-analysis, the risk for breast milk transmission was 21% among women who breast-fed for 3 months or longer compared with 13% among those who breast-fed for less than 2 months.[29] In a meta-analysis of late postnatal transmission in breast-fed children uninfected by 4 weeks of age, the transmission rate through breast milk was 1.6% at 3 months and increased gradually to 9.3% at 18 months.[54] The analysis demonstrated that the risk of late postnatal transmission was cumulative and fairly constant throughout breast-feeding. The overall risk of late postnatal transmission was 8.9 transmissions/100 child-years of breast-feeding, which represents approximately 0.8% risk for each additional month throughout the breast-feeding period. The overall probability of breast milk transmission of HIV has been estimated to be approximately 1 infected child/1500 L breast milk. The average breast-feeding infant in the studied cohort consumed 150 L of breast milk during the course of breast-feeding.[55]

Exclusive versus Mixed Breast-feeding

The only way to eliminate breast-feeding–associated HIV transmission is to completely avoid breast-feeding, but this is not an option in most areas where HIV is endemic. Exclusive breast-feeding during the first 6 months of life is associated with less morbidity and mortality from other infectious diseases than from HIV.[56-58] In a study from Botswana, breast-feeding with zidovudine prophylaxis was not as effective as formula feeding in preventing postnatal HIV transmission, but cumulative all-cause infant mortality at 7 months was significantly higher in formula-fed infants than in those assigned to breast-feeding and zidovudine.[59] Exclusive breast-feeding is advantageous over mixed feeding (breast milk and formula, cow's milk, tea, juice, or water) also with regard to mother-to-child transmission of HIV. In a randomized, controlled study from Durban, South Africa, which investigated the effect of vitamin A on the risk of mother-to-child transmission, women chose to breast-feed or formula-feed after they had been counseled. The mode of feeding was not randomized, and the study was retrospectively reanalyzed to evaluate the effect of feeding pattern on mother-to-child transmission of HIV. The cumulative probability of mother-to-child transmission at 6 months of age in never breast-fed and exclusively breast-fed infants was similar—19.4% and 19.4%, respectively. Transmission in the mixed breast-fed group was 26.1%.[60] It is noteworthy that at 3 months, the transmission rate in those exclusively breast-fed was lower (14.6%) than in those never breast-fed (18.8%), which could indicate a selection bias.

Another trial of a vitamin A intervention showed that HIV postnatal transmission risk and mortality were higher in mixed breast-fed infants than in those who were exclusively breast-fed. Compared with exclusive breast-feeding, early mixed feeding was associated with 4.03, 3.79, and 2.6 greater risk of postnatal transmission at 6, 12, and 18 months, respectively.[61] In a nonrandomized cohort study, breast-fed infants who received solid foods in addition to breast milk had an 11-fold increased risk of acquiring HIV compared with those exclusively breast-fed, and infants who received both breast milk and formula doubled their risk of HIV acquisition. Mortality in the first 3 months of life was roughly doubled in the group receiving replacement feeding compared with the exclusively breast-feeding group (15% vs. 6%).[62] Although observational, this was the first study in which measurement of transmission by feeding method was the primary aim.

Mixed feedings (breast milk and solids, formula, cow's milk, tea, juice, or water) have been hypothesized to enhance the rate of mother-to-child transmission owing to the introduction of contaminated fluids that predispose to gastrointestinal infection, inflammation, and increased gut permeability.[63] Breast milk viral load has been shown to be substantially higher after rapid weaning—a fact that may explain the increased risk of transmission when breast-feeding is resumed after a period of cessation.[64]

Antiretroviral Therapy and Transmission

The antiretroviral drugs nevirapine, lamivudine, and zidovudine administered during the last trimester of pregnancy and after delivery reached concentrations in breast milk similar to or higher than in plasma and significantly reduced HIV RNA levels in breast milk.[65] Passage of didanosine, stavudine, abacavir, delavirdine, indinavir, ritonavir, saquinavir, and amprenavir can be detected in the breast milk of lactating rats.[66] Combination antiretroviral therapy given to the mother during lactation or to the infant during breast-feeding has been shown to reduce the risk of transmission with similar efficacy. When provided as chemoprophylaxis to the infant during breast-feeding, combination therapy reduced postnatal transmission at 9 months to around 5%.[67,68] In breast-feeding mothers, combination antiretroviral therapy reduced transmission rates at 12 months postpartum to 5%.[69,70] It is not clear whether infants of women on combination antiretroviral therapy with undetectable viral load are at risk for transmission of HIV through breast milk.

Antiretroviral drug resistance has been observed in infants infected through breast milk during both infant and maternal antiretroviral prophylaxis interventions during breast-feeding.[71,72] Resistant virus may emerge in the infant as a consequence of suboptimal infant drug levels.

The 2010 World Health Organization infant feeding recommendations for HIV-infected mothers in settings where replacement feeding is neither safe nor affordable are to breast-feed the infant for the first year, with antiretroviral treatment and/or prophylaxis provided for mothers or their infants.[73]

Table 13-2   HIV: RECOMMENDATIONS

- HIV screening of pregnant women is crucial for effective MTCT prevention programs, including counseling about feeding practices.
- Appropriate strategies need to be developed to increase the number of pregnant women who are tested for HIV and who are able to accept available interventions.
- If possible, HIV-infected women are strongly recommended to avoid breast-feeding completely. This is of interest only if alternatives to breast-feeding are feasible, affordable, safe, and available.
- If complete avoidance is not possible, the current WHO recommendation for mothers known to be HIV-infected is to exclusively breast-feed their infants for the first 6 months of life, introducing appropriate complementary foods thereafter, and to continue breast-feeding for the first 12 months of life with antiretroviral treatment and/or prophylaxis provided for mothers or their infants.
- Treatment of breast milk with heat or chemical agents is an option, but these methods would be difficult to utilize in many affected settings.

HIV, Human immunodeficiency virus; *MTCT,* mother-to-child transmission; *WHO,* World Health Organization.

Additional Risk Factors

The risk of mother-to-child transmission is increased in the presence of maternal breast pathologies such as mastitis, breast abscess, and nipple lesions[45,48,74] or oral candidiasis in the infant.[48]

Inactivation of HIV

HIV is heat sensitive and is inactivated by boiling[75] and pasteurization at temperatures between 56° C and 62.5° C.[76,77] HIV-infected milk was pasteurized at 62.5° C for 30 minutes[76] by a simplified technique developed for low-income settings—Pretoria pasteurization.[77] No infective virus was recovered after processing. On the other hand, HIV RNA levels were remarkably stable in whole milk after three freeze-thaw cycles[53] and 6 to 30 hours at room temperature was inadequate to destroy HIV.[75,78] The conclusion in a review by Rollins and colleagues was that correctly applied heat treatment of expressed breast milk reliably inactivated HIV within the milk.[79] However, freezing and inherited lipolytic activity of breast milk are inadequate for destruction of HIV.[75,78] The use of alkyl sulfate microbicides to treat HIV-infected breast milk may be an alternative for preventing/reducing transmission through breast-feeding.[80] See Tables 13-2 and 13-3.

HTLV-I and Breast-feeding

Infection with the retrovirus HTLV-I is followed by a latent period, and after 30 to 60 years, 3% to 5% of carriers develop adult T cell leukemia or HTLV-associated progressive and spastic paresis in lower limbs caused by demyelinating myelopathy.[6,81,82] HTLV-I enters the body inside infected CD4+ lymphocytes in breast milk, blood, or semen and is transmitted by breast-feeding, sexual intercourse, blood transfusion, and sharing of contaminated needles and syringes. No curative therapy or vaccine is available. More than a million people (even up to 15 to 20 million) are estimated to be infected,[81] particularly in countries in the Caribbean,[83] southern Japan,[84] equatorial Africa,[81] Papua New Guinea,[85] and parts of South America,[81] where a combination of vertical and horizontal transmission can maintain 5% to 30% levels of infection from generation to generation. Highest figures are reported from areas of southwestern Japan, with up to 10% of pregnant women being seropositive.[86]

Table 13-3   HIV: RESEARCH DIRECTIONS

Several urgent research directions in the field of HIV and breast-feeding include study of the following:
- The effects and safety of antiretroviral therapy given to the mother and/or child during breast-feeding, especially in women on combination antiretroviral therapy with undetectable viral load
- The effects of early cessation of breast-feeding on HIV transmission, morbidity, and mortality
- Mechanisms by which HIV is transmitted through breast milk

HIV, Human immunodeficiency syndrome.

In the United States and Europe, adult T cell leukemia and HTLV-associated myelopathy are found in immigrants from endemic areas. The rate is very low among blood donors, and spread among drug users is limited, although these conditions were reported in New York and Brazil in the early 1990s.[81,87,88] A closely related virus, HTLV-II, which is transmitted similarly, is linked to HTLV-associated myelopathy[89] but not to lymphoproliferative disease.[90] Infection is more prevalent than HTLV-I among intravenous drug users in the United States and Europe and has been introduced at a low rate in the general population and among blood donors.

Diagnosis of Infection

Antibody tests used for screen testing for HTLV cross-react between HTLV types I and II. Confirmatory tests and demonstration of type-specific HTLV proviral DNA are required to confirm true infection and the HTLV type.

Mother-to-Child Transmission

Virus transmission in utero seems to be of minor importance. The major transmission route is through breast milk.[86,91-93]

Breast Milk: Transmission

About 1 out of 5 children breast-fed by HTLV-I mothers become infected.[86,91,92] Long-term breast-feeding (>6 months), high provirus load in milk, and high antibody level in maternal blood are risk factors that predict infection.[94,95] Studies in Japan demonstrate that bottle-feeding reduces the infection rate in the child to a few percent (2.5%; 5.6%).[86,91,93] The transmission risk after short-term breast-feeding (<6 months) is of the same magnitude (3.9%; 3.8%), but it is high after long-term breast-feeding (14.5% to 20.3%).

The virus is cell associated because it is present in CD4+ lymphocytes and macrophages.[96] Procedures that inactivate cells in breast milk—heating, freeze-thawing—eliminate the infectivity and viral transmission. Feeding the infant with mother's milk after freeze-thawing may thus be an alternative to bottle-feeding.[97] See Table 13-4.

Hepatitis B Infection and Breast-feeding

Chronic hepatitis B virus (HBV) infection is estimated to occur in 350 million people globally.[98] HBV is transmitted via contaminated blood or blood products, but also through sexual contacts. Currently, no clinically useful tissue culture or animal model system is available to test infectivity of the virus.

Diagnosis of HBV Infection

Detection of the viral antigens HBsAg (surface antigen of HBV) and HBeAg (the hepatitis "e" antigen) and their corresponding antibodies is the cornerstone of diagnostic management of HBV infection. Thus, the presence of HBsAg in serum for

Table 13-4   HTLV: RECOMMENDATIONS

- Prenatal screening of pregnant women from endemic areas and counseling of seropositive mothers regarding risk of transmission through breast-feeding have substantially reduced the transmission and infection rates.[76]
- In other areas, prenatal screening should be recommended for immigrants from endemic areas and should be encouraged in pregnant women from risk populations in which HTLV-I has emerged.
- If possible, HTLV-I–infected women are strongly recommended to avoid breast-feeding completely. This is of interest only if alternatives to breast-feeding are feasible, affordable, safe, and available.
- If complete avoidance is not possible, early weaning from breast milk (e.g., at 3 to 6 months of age), if feasible, would limit exposure to HTLV-I–infected breast milk.
- Feeding the infant with the mother's milk after freeze-thawing may be an alternative to bottle-feeding.
- The prospective risk with maternal HTLV-II is not known. However, authorities recommend that HTLV-II–infected mothers refrain from breast-feeding when and where safe nutritional alternatives exist.

HTLV, Human T cell lymphotropic virus.

6 months or longer is defined as a chronic infection. Furthermore, concomitant detection of HBeAg denotes a high level of viremia, indicating infectivity. On the other hand, if HBeAg is not detected, but rather its antibody anti-HBe is found, a lower grade of viremia and infectivity has been assumed. In the 1990s, with the availability of new diagnostic tools of molecular virology, such as polymerase chain reaction (PCR), the latter assumption was proved right in most but not all such situations. The exception, that is, when high levels of viremia and infectivity occur despite the presence of anti-HBe and the absence of HBeAg, is associated with the presence of mutated HBV virus. Certain mutated viral strains do not produce HBeAg and therefore can avoid the immune system and replicate in high numbers despite the presence of anti-HBe. In such cases, HBV DNA quantification by PCR methods is very useful for determining the level of viremia.

Mother-to-Child Transmission

Pregnant women who are HBV infected run a high risk of passing the virus on to their offspring. The most efficient route of infection seems to be the perinatal one. Prenatal infection may also occur, although in a much lower proportion of cases. It is also well established that HBV infection acquired early in life will become chronic in most cases. In contrast, if the virus is acquired in adulthood, development of chronic infection is uncommon. The introduction of HBV immunization, in combination with the administration of HBV-specific immune globulins, has greatly decreased the risk of mother-to-infant transmission.[99]

Breast Milk: Transmission Mechanisms

Most available studies suggest that the virus can be found in breast milk from infected mothers. Thus, both HBsAg and HBeAg have been detected in the breast milk of a large proportion of infected mothers, and later PCR studies have confirmed the presence of HBV-DNA as well.[100-103] The virus has been detected in both the cellular and whey fractions of centrifuged colostrum. The levels of viral antigens in breast milk are lower than in serum.[102] The highest levels in breast milk were found in mothers with the highest levels of antigenemia.[102] The failure of other investigators to detect viral antigens in breast milk may be due to differences in the sensitivity of methods used or to differences in the levels of antigens present in breast milk.[104]

It is still unclear whether the presence of viral antigen in breast milk will influence the risk of the infant's becoming infected. In a study from Taiwan, 147 infants of HBsAg-positive mothers were studied. The study was performed before any preventive measures were available, and the HBeAg status of the mothers was not reported. The rate of infection was high but not different in breast-fed (49% infected) versus bottle-fed (53% infected) children, all of whom were followed for a mean of 11 months.[104]

In studies performed in Italian infants of infected mothers, the effect of feeding habits on the vaccination effect was investigated. No differences were detected in the risk of developing hepatitis B when breast-fed and bottle-fed infants were compared.[105] The vaccine effect was similar in the two groups with regard to the rate of seroconversion. It is interesting to note that bottle-fed infants had transient but significantly higher antibody levels to HBs. In general, no or very few data are available on the possible HBV immune-modulating effect of breast milk.

In practice, for HBV-vaccinated babies of infected mothers, breast-feeding is not looked upon as an additional risk factor. The rate of successful vaccinations is high (90% to 95%), and in those few unfortunate cases where a chronic infection still develops, it is thought to be associated with prenatal transmission. It is still unclear whether nonvaccinated babies of infected mothers could be breast-fed. Indeed, some authors argue against such a practice, although we have no data supporting the possible risk of such feeding.[102] Caution may also be suggested in the case of bleeding nipple lesions, if the mother has high levels of viremia.

Very few data are available on the risk of transferring the infection via banked breast milk. Given the findings of the virus in colostrum, as discussed previously, compulsory HBV testing of breast milk donors seems appropriate.[106] In particular,

Table 13-5   HEPATITIS B: RECOMMENDATIONS

- In practice, for HBV-vaccinated babies of infected mothers, breast-feeding is not looked upon as an additional risk factor. The rate of successful vaccinations is high (90% to 95%), and in those few unfortunate cases where a chronic infection still develops, it is thought to be associated with prenatal transmission.
- It is still unclear whether nonvaccinated babies of infected mothers should be breast-fed. Indeed, some authors argue against such a practice, although we have no data supporting the possible risk of such feeding.[84] Caution may be suggested in the case of bleeding nipple lesions, if the mother has high levels of viremia.
- Few data are available on the risk of transferring infection via banked breast milk. Given the findings of the virus in colostrum, both before and after Holder pasteurization (62.5° C for 30 minutes), compulsory HBV testing of breast milk donors seems appropriate. In particular, it should be considered in areas of the world where universal HBV vaccination is not yet established.

HBV, Hepatitis B virus.

it should be considered in areas of the world where universal HBV vaccination is not yet established.

In most centers, pasteurization of banked breast milk is mandatory. However, in one study from Brazil,[107] HBsAg and HBV DNA were detected in breast milk from infected mothers both before and after pasteurization by the Holder method (62.5° C for 30 minutes). Although the biologic importance of this finding is unclear, it suggests that serologic screening should be universal before milk is donated. If such screening is not feasible, early routine HBV vaccination of newborns would be of importance to protect recipients of donated milk. See Table 13-5.

Hepatitis C Infection and Breast-Feeding

Chronic hepatitis C virus (HCV) infection, which is transmitted mainly via the blood-borne route, occurs in approximately 170 million people around the world.[98] Most infected individuals develop chronic infection.

Diagnosis of HCV Infection

The clinical diagnosis relies on the detection of antibodies to the virus (anti-HCV) in serum. Additionally, for information on the infectivity of the individual, a PCR test is needed to detect HCV-RNA, that is, the viral genome, in serum. PCR methods are also routinely used for HCV-RNA quantification before and during antiviral therapy, and to determine the genotype of the virus.

Mother-to-Child Transmission

The transmission rate from an HCV-infected mother to her infant is approximately 5%.[108-110] To date, no preventive measures that could lower this figure have been defined. Thus, no vaccine or immune globulin is available, and routine use of cesarean section does not seem to improve the situation.[111,112] The timing of viral transmission seems to be prenatal in one third of infected cases, and perinatal transmission accounts for most of the remaining cases.[113] The maternal level of HCV viremia has been suggested as a risk factor for transmission to the infant. However, no clear cutoff level has been defined for viremia between mothers transmitting and not transmitting the virus. Theoretically, antiviral treatment during the latter parts of pregnancy and at the time of birth to selected mothers with high levels of viremia could be of value. However, the positive effects in a rather low number of infants might not balance the possibly negative effects of such drugs given to a large number of fetuses/infants.

Breast Milk: Transmission

Several studies have addressed the question of infection via breast milk. Data concerning viral content in breast milk are contradictory. Some authors report exclusively negative findings regarding HCV-RNA in breast milk, and others report positive findings in each studied sample.[114-116] The reasons for this discrepancy may include differences in viremia levels among study subjects, differences in sensitivity in PCR methods used, or the fact that different portions of breast milk were studied. In a Taiwanese study, all 15 mothers had HCV-RNA detected in the colostrum, at consistently lower levels than in the corresponding serum sample. It is interesting to note that none of the children was infected on follow-up.[115] On the other hand, Kumar and coworkers, who studied 65 infected mothers, all of whom had HCV-RNA in their breast milk, diagnosed HCV infection in three of the children. The authors noted that all three seemed to have been infected postnatally and had mothers with clinical signs of advanced HCV infection.[114]

When larger cohorts of HCV-infected mothers and their exposed children are used, the rate of infection can be compared between breast-fed and bottle-fed children. In a retrospective study of HCV-infected mothers performed by the European Paediatric Hepatitis C Network (EPHN), no differences were seen in transmission rates between these two groups of infants.[98] Increased risk of HCV transmission has been reported among infants of mothers with HIV-HCV coinfection. When children whose mothers had such coinfection were analyzed separately, an increase in the risk of HCV transmission was seen among breast-fed subjects.[117] However, in a more recent, prospective study from EPHN, no such difference was seen, most probably owing to the secondary effects of modern HIV therapy on the HCV viremia.[118] Current recommendations from EPHN and other authors conclude that breast-feeding need not be avoided in the case of maternal HCV. However, if the mother has HCV-HIV coinfection, breast-feeding should be discouraged.[119]

Data concerning HCV and banked breast milk are sparse, suggesting that caution as described in the same setting for hepatitis B earlier (i.e., donor testing and pasteurization procedures) is recommended.[120] The latter seems efficient in reducing the risk of transmitting HCV via plasma-derived products.[121] Donated breast milk is often used for premature babies, who may be more prone to acquiring viral infection than term infants owing to immaturity of the immune system. See Table 13-6.

Cytomegalovirus and Breast-Feeding

Cytomegalovirus (CMV) infections are ubiquitous and are rarely symptomatic in the immuno-competent individual. Primary infection is followed by lifelong latency of virus with intermittent activation and excretion of virus. Virus is spread vertically from mother to child and horizontally by close contact with body secretions from children—later by kissing, sexual intercourse, and blood or organ transfusion. The epidemiology varies greatly in different populations, and susceptibility among women of fertile age varies from none in close-living societies to about half of women living in highly hygienic surroundings. CMV infection may cause serious disease in the immuno-incompetent patient and in the fetus.[122] A vaccine approach so far has been used with limited success. Antiviral agents may suppress viral replication, but toxicity restricts their use in pregnant women and infants.[123]

Diagnosis of Infection

The presence of CMV-specific IgG in maternal serum denotes past or present infection. If simultaneously, CMV IgM is demonstrable and CMV IgG is of low avidity,

Table 13-6   HEPATITIS C: RECOMMENDATIONS

- Current recommendations from the European Paediatric Hepatitis C Network and other authors are that breast-feeding need not be avoided in the case of maternal HCV. However, if the mother has HCV-HIV coinfection, breast-feeding should be discouraged.[100]
- Data concerning HCV and banked breast milk are sparse, suggesting that caution as described in the same setting for hepatitis B (i.e., donor testing and pasteurization procedures) is recommended.[101] The latter seems efficient in reducing the risk of transmitting HCV via plasma-derived products.[88]

HCV, Hepatitis C virus; *HIV,* human immunodeficiency virus.

the mother has an ongoing primary infection. If this is not the case, she has previous experience of CMV and her latent virus infection may be reactivated. If neither CMV IgG nor IgM is found, the mother has no latent CMV infection, and virus cannot be reactivated. Viral DNA is used to demonstrate the presence of CMV virus in, for example, breast milk or the infant's throat or urine and may be quantitated to measure viral load. Ongoing replication of virus is indicated by the presence of viral RNA and infectious virus by culture isolation.

Mother-to-Child Transmission

CMV is a very common viral pathogen that may be transmitted in utero, at delivery by exposure to CMV in the birth canal, or—in most cases—through breast-feeding by mothers reactivating CMV in the mammary gland. Congenital infection has been reported in 0.2% to 2% of all children. Neonatal disease is seen in 10% to 15%, and about 18% of all children with congenital CMV will have long-term sequelae such as neurodevelopmental handicaps, including sensorineural hearing impairment and mental retardation. Severe handicap may result from infection in any period of fetal life, although the highest risk is believed to occur in the early phase.

Breast Milk: Transmission

Although the child may be infected by CMV in the birth canal, the major source of postnatal CMV infection is viral excretion in maternal breast milk.[122,124] With sensitive analysis, CMV reactivation may be seen in breast milk from most CMV-seropositive individuals and is found in milk whey and cells.[125,126] Excretion time varies between individuals but seems low in the first week postpartum, reaches a maximum at about 4 to 8 weeks after delivery, and ends at about 9 to 12 weeks.[125,126] The presence of virus is not equal to transmission. The risk of transmission is correlated with viral load in the milk whey, and transmission occurs close to maximal excretion in the milk. Virus in breast milk is readily inactivated by pasteurization at 65° C or 62.5° C for 30 minutes—a procedure that destroys not only infectivity, but also beneficial factors in the milk. More of these factors are preserved after freeze-thawing—a procedure previously reported to lower or abolish CMV infectivity.[124] New data indicate that although the virus load may be reduced, transmission may still occur.[124,127]

An important question is whether breast milk–transmitted CMV from a mother to her own child may cause disease in the infant. Among term infants, subclinical infections are very common; morbidity from postnatal CMV is held to be very low and transitory, although a potential role (e.g., in the development of neonatal cholestatic disease) has been suggested.[128,129] Protection of the infant from disease has been attributed to passively transferred maternal CMV IgG, as well as to nutritional and immunologic factors in the breast milk.[130] However, a very premature infant with an immature immune system who was born before the major transfer of immunoglobulin (at 28 weeks and later) may be more vulnerable. Significant disease, even with fatal outcome, was observed in preterm infants with CMV infection acquired by transfusion of blood from CMV-seropositive donors.[131] This problem is largely eliminated by the use of CMV-free blood products from CMV-negative donors and/or leukocyte-depleted blood. Disease related to breast milk–transmitted CMV with risk of long-term neurologic but not auditory sequelae was reported in the 1980s.[132,133]

This question was then re-addressed in several studies.[124] The transmission rate was, with one exception, higher when the infant was fed fresh breast milk (25% to 55%) than when frozen milk was given (10% to 15%). Reported rates of symptoms interpreted as CMV related were divergent, but severe sepsis-like illness at the time of onset of viral excretion was reported after feeding fresh milk, and in some cases also when frozen milk was fed. Risk factors for proposed CMV disease include preterm infant weighing less than 1000 g and gestational age less than 30 weeks. No cases were lethal, and in available follow-up studies at 2 to 4 years and at 6 months, respectively, no increased risk of delay in neuromotor development or sensorineural hearing loss was found.[134-136] Although studies seem to indicate that severe CMV disease may occur, episodes of sepsis-like illness are not uncommon in

Table 13-7   CMV: CONCLUSIONS

- Breast milk from a CMV-seronegative donor mother does not transmit CMV.
- Breast milk from a CMV-seropositive mother transmits CMV at a high rate to her child, but symptoms appear only infrequently in a full-term healthy child.
- In very preterm children (<1000 g and gestational age <30 weeks), serious disease has previously been attributed to breast milk–acquired CMV.[114]
- Accumulated data seem to indicate that CMV transmitted from the seropositive mother to her very preterm child:
  - Generally induces mild transient symptoms, may sporadically cause serious disease
  - Does not seem to influence long-term outcome in the "normal" preterm child
  - Has not led to auditory or mental retardation attributable to CMV infection at follow-up
  - May be a cofactor, aggravating the course of some preexisting pulmonary, hematologic, or hepatic conditions
    - CMV may be inactivated through procedures that may be beneficial for selected patient groups
    - Freezing of milk can reduce the risk of transmission, but risk is not eliminated
    - Short-term pasteurization can be used to abolish infectivity
- Donated breast milk should be fully pasteurized according to present recommendations.
- CMV-seronegative donors may offer an alternative if available, and if other serious potential pathogens in the breast milk are excluded.

CMV, Cytomegalovirus.

preterm infants in the absence of CMV, and it might be difficult to specifically link these episodes to CMV. In the absence of carefully chosen controls, interpretation of these data has provoked debate. In subsequently published studies from other centers, serious CMV-like disease was observed only sporadically.[127,131,136-141] A case-control study has been published by the original reporting group,[142] wherein most neonatal symptoms attributable to postnatal CMV seemed to be mild and transient, with no major effects on the neonatal outcome of most preterm infants. From these studies and other reports,[134,142,143] it is clear that CMV transmission through breast milk may be a factor that aggravates the clinical course of some underlying preexisting pulmonary, hematologic, or hepatic conditions, and mild pasteurization-inactivating CMV infectivity[144] of a CMV-seropositive mother's milk might be of value for selected patients. A final conclusion still awaits case-control multicenter studies with well-defined criteria for CMV disease, weighing benefit versus risk; guidelines differ greatly among different countries and among different centers within the country.[141]

Donor milk from a seropositive mother should not be given without previous pasteurization to a vulnerable preterm or full-term child born of a seronegative mother.

See Table 13-7 for a summary.

References

1. Hanson LA, Korotkova M, Lundin S, et al. The transfer of immunity from mother to child. *Ann N Y Acad Sci.* 2003;987:199-206.
2. Simister NE. Placental transport of immunoglobulin G. *Vaccine.* 2003;21:3365-3369.
3. Jenssen H, Hancock REW. Antimicrobial properties of lactoferrin. Review. *Biochimie.* 2009;91: 19-29.
4. Moriuchi M, Moriuchi H. A milk protein lactoferrin enhances human T cell leukemia virus type I and suppresses HIV-1 infection. *J Immunol.* 2001;166:4231-4236.
5. Moriuchi M, Moriuchi H. Induction of lactoferrin gene expression in myeloid or mammary gland cells by human T-cell leukemia virus type 1 (HTLV-1) tax: Implications for milk-borne transmission of HTLV-1. *J Virol.* 2006;80:7118-7126.
6. Centers for Disease Control and Prevention. Possible West Nile virus transmission to an infant through breast-feeding: Michigan, 2002. *MMWR Morb Mortal Wkly Rep.* 2002;51:877-878.
7. O'Leary DR, Kuhn S, Kniss KL, et al. Birth outcomes following West Nile Virus infection of pregnant women in the United States: 2003-2004. *Pediatrics.* 2006;117:e537-e545. Comment in Pediatrics. 2006;117:936-939.
8. Hinckley AF, O'Leary DR, Hayes EB. Transmission of West Nile virus through human breast milk seems to be rare. *Pediatrics* 2007;119:e666-e671.

9. Losonsky GA, Fishaut JM, Strussenberg J, et al. Effect of immunization against rubella on lactation products. II. Maternal-neonatal interactions. *J Infect Dis.* 1982;145:661-666.

10. Krogh V, Duffy LC, Wong D, et al. Postpartum immunization with rubella virus vaccine and antibody response in breast-feeding infants. *J Lab Clin Med.* 1989;113:695-699.

11. Bohlke K, Galil K, Jackson LA, et al. Postpartum varicella vaccination: Is the vaccine virus excreted in breast milk? *Obstet Gynecol.* 2003;102:970-977.

12. Mallmann CA, Ribeiro SM, Schermann MT, et al. Transmission of yellow fever vaccine virus through breast-feeding—Brazil, 2009. *Morb & Mortal Weekly Rep.* 2010;59:30.

13. Kuhn S, Twele-Montecinos L, Macdonald J, et al. Case report: Probable transmission of vaccine strain of yellow fever virus to an infant via breast milk. *CMAJ* 2011;183:E243-E245.

14. CDC. Yellow fever vaccine; recommendations of the Advisory Committee on Immunization Practices (ACIP). *MMWR Morb Mortal Wkly Rep.* 2002;51:(No. RR-17). See also CDC Travelers' Health—Yellow Book Yellow fever: http://wwwnc.cdc.gov/travel/yellowbook/2010/chapter-2/yellow-fever.aspx

15. Andreasson PA, Dias F, Naucler A, et al. A prospective study of vertical transmission of HIV-2 in Bissau, Guinea-Bissau. *AIDS.* 1993;7:989-993.

16. European Collaborative Study. Risk factors for mother-to-child transmission of HIV-1. *Lancet.* 1992;339:1007-1012.

17. O'Donovan D, Ariyoshi K, Milligan P, et al. Maternal plasma viral RNA levels determine marked differences in mother-to-child transmission rates of HIV-1 and HIV-2 in The Gambia. MRC/Gambia Government/University College London Medical School working group on mother-child transmission of HIV. *Aids.* 2000;14:441-448.

18. The Working Group on Mother-To-Child Transmission of HIV. Rates of mother-to-child transmission of HIV-1 in Africa, America, and Europe: results from 13 perinatal studies. *J Acquir Immune Defic Syndr Hum Retrovirol.* 1995;8:506-510.

19. Read J. Prevention of mother-to-child transmission. In: Zeichner S, Read J, eds. *Textbook of pediatric HIV care.* New York: Cambridge University Press; 2005:111-133.

20. Dunn DT, Brandt CD, Krivine A, et al. The sensitivity of HIV-1 DNA polymerase chain reaction in the neonatal period and the relative contributions of intra-uterine and intra-partum transmission. *AIDS.* 1995;9:F7-F11.

21. Kuhn L, Steketee RW, Weedon J, et al. Distinct risk factors for intrauterine and intrapartum human immunodeficiency virus transmission and consequences for disease progression in infected children. Perinatal AIDS Collaborative Transmission Study. *J Infect Dis.* 1999;179:52-58.

22. Ehrnst A, Lindgren S, Dictor M, et al. HIV in pregnant women and their offspring: Evidence for late transmission. *Lancet.* 1991;338:203-207.

23. Lallemant M, Jourdain G, Le Coeur S, et al. A trial of shortened zidovudine regimens to prevent mother-to-child transmission of human immunodeficiency virus type 1. Perinatal HIV Prevention Trial (Thailand) Investigators. *N Engl J Med.* 2000;343:982-991.

24. Sprecher S, Soumenkoff G, Puissant F, Degueldre M. Vertical transmission of HIV in 15-week fetus. *Lancet.* 1986;2:288-289.

25. Brossard Y, Aubin JT, Mandelbrot L, et al. Frequency of early in utero HIV-1 infection: A blind DNA polymerase chain reaction study on 100 fetal thymuses. *AIDS.* 1995;9:359-366.

26. Phuapradit W, Panburana P, Jaovisidha A, et al. Maternal viral load and vertical transmission of HIV-1 in mid-trimester gestation. *AIDS.* 1999;13:1927-1931.

27. Nduati R, John G, Mbori-Ngacha D, et al. Effect of breastfeeding and formula feeding on transmission of HIV-1: A randomized clinical trial. *JAMA.* 2000;283:1167-1174.

28. Dunn DT, Newell ML, Ades AE, et al. Risk of human immunodeficiency virus type 1 transmission through breastfeeding. *Lancet.* 1992;340:585-588.

29. John GC, Richardson BA, Nduati RW, et al. Timing of breast milk HIV-1 transmission: A meta-analysis. *East Afr Med J.* 2001;78:75-79.

30. Pillay K, Coutsoudis A, York D, et al. Cell-free virus in breast milk of HIV-1-seropositive women. *J Acquir Immune Defic Syndr.* 2000;24:330-336.

31. Rousseau CM, Nduati RW, Richardson BA, et al. Longitudinal analysis of human immunodeficiency virus type 1 RNA in breast milk and of its relationship to infant infection and maternal disease. *J Infect Dis.* 2003;187:741-747.

32. Koulinska IN, Villamor E, Chaplin B, et al. Transmission of cell-free and cell associated HIV-1 through breast-feeding. *J Acquir Immune Defic Syndr.* 2006;41:93-99. Erratum in: *J Acquir Immune Defic Syndr.* 2006;42:650.

33. Van de Perre P, Simonon A, Hitimana DG, et al. Infective and anti-infective properties of breastmilk from HIV-1-infected women. *Lancet.* 1993;341:914-918.

34. Rousseau CM, Nduati RW, Richardson BA, et al. Association of levels of HIV-1-infected breast milk cells and risk of mother-to-child transmission. *J Infect Dis.* 2004;190:1880-1888.

35. Willumsen JF, Filteau SM, Coutsoudis A, et al. Breastmilk RNA viral load in HIV-infected South African women: Effects of subclinical mastitis and infant feeding. *AIDS.* 2003;17:407-414.

36. Becquart P, Petitjean G, Tabaa YA, et al. Detection of a large T-cell reservoir able to replicate HIV-1 actively in breast milk. *AIDS.* 2006;20:1453-1455.

37. Petitjean G, Becquart P, Tuaillon E, et al. Isolation and characterization of HIV-1- infected resting CD4+ T lymphocytes in breast milk. *J Clin Virol* 2007;39:1-8.

38. Toniolo A, Serra C, Conaldi PG, et al. Productive HIV-1 infection of normal human mammary epithelial cells. *AIDS.* 1995;9:859-866.

39. Henderson GJ, Hoffman NG, Ping LH, et al. HIV-1 populations in blood and breast milk are similar. *Virology.* 2004;330:295-303.

13

40. Bomsel M. Transcytosis of infectious human immunodeficiency virus across a tight human epithelial cell line barrier. *Nat Med*. 1997;3:42-47.

41. Bomsel M, Heyman M, Hocini H, et al. Intracellular neutralization of HIV transcytosis across tight epithelial barriers by anti-HIV envelope protein dIgA or IgM. *Immunity*. 1998;9:277-287.

42. Stahl-Hennig C, Steinman RM, Tenner-Racz K, et al. Rapid infection of oral mucosal-associated lymphoid tissue with simian immunodeficiency virus. *Science*. 1999;285:1261-1265.

43. Kuhn L, Trabattoni D, Kankasa C, et al. HIV-specific secretory IgA in breast milk of HIV-positive mothers is not associated with protection against HIV transmission among breast-fed infants. *J Pediatr*. 2006;149:611-616.

44. Semba RD, Kumwenda N, Hoover DR, et al. Human immunodeficiency virus load in breast milk, mastitis, and mother-to-child transmission of human immunodeficiency virus type 1. *J Infect Dis*. 1999;180:93-98.

45. John GC, Nduati RW, Mbori-Ngacha DA, et al. Correlates of mother-to-child human immunodeficiency virus type 1 (HIV-1) transmission: Association with maternal plasma HIV-1 RNA load, genital HIV-1 DNA shedding, and breast infections. *J Infect Dis*. 2001;183:206-212.

46. Fawzi W, Msamanga G, Spiegelman D, et al. Transmission of HIV-1 through breastfeeding among women in Dar es Salaam, Tanzania. *J Acquir Immune Defic Syndr*. 2002;31:331-338.

47. Neveu D, Viljoen J, Bland RM, et al. Cumulative exposure to cell-free HIV in breast milk, rather than feeding pattern per se, identifies postnatally infected infants. *Clin Infect Dis* 2011;52: 819-825.

48. Embree JE, Njenga S, Datta P, et al. Risk factors for postnatal mother-child transmission of HIV-1. *AIDS*. 2000;14:2535-2541.

49. Miotti PG, Taha TE, Kumwenda NI, et al. HIV transmission through breastfeeding: A study in Malawi. *JAMA*. 1999;282:744-749.

50. Tess BH, Rodrigues LC, Newell ML, et al. Infant feeding and risk of mother-to-child transmission of HIV-1 in Sao Paulo State, Brazil. Sao Paulo Collaborative Study for Vertical Transmission of HIV-1. *J Acquir Immune Defic Syndr Hum Retrovirol*. 1998;19:189-194.

51. de Martino M, Tovo PA, Tozzi AE, et al. HIV-1 transmission through breast-milk: Appraisal of risk according to duration of feeding. *AIDS*. 1992;6:991-997.

52. Bobat R, Moodley D, Coutsoudis A, et al. Breastfeeding by HIV-1-infected women and outcome in their infants: A cohort study from Durban, South Africa. *AIDS*. 1997;11:1627-1633.

53. Datta P, Embree JE, Kreiss JK, et al. Mother-to-child transmission of human immunodeficiency virus type 1: Report from the Nairobi Study. *J Infect Dis*. 1994;170:1134-1140.

54. The Breastfeeding and HIV International Transmission Study Group. Late postnatal transmission of HIV-1 in breast-fed children: An individual patient data meta-analysis. *J Infect Dis*. 2004;189: 2154-2166.

55. Richardson BA, John-Stewart GC, Hughes JP, et al. Breast-milk infectivity in human immunodeficiency virus type 1-infected mothers. *J Infect Dis*. 2003;187:736-740.

56. Brown KH, Black RE, Lopez de Romana G, et al. Infant-feeding practices and their relationship with diarrheal and other diseases in Huascar (Lima), Peru. *Pediatrics*. 1989;83:31-40.

57. Victora CG, Smith PG, Vaughan JP, et al. Evidence for protection by breast-feeding against infant deaths from infectious diseases in Brazil. *Lancet*. 1987;2:319-322.

58. Bahl R, Frost C, Kirkwood BR, et al. Infant feeding patterns and risks of death and hospitalization in the first half of infancy: Multicentre cohort study. *Bull World Health Organ*. 2005;83:418-426.

59. Thior I, Lockman S, Smeaton LM, et al. Breastfeeding plus infant zidovudine prophylaxis for 6 months vs formula feeding plus infant zidovudine for 1 month to reduce mother-to-child HIV transmission in Botswana: A randomized trial: The Mashi Study. *JAMA*. 2006;296:794-805.

60. Coutsoudis A, Pillay K, Kuhn L, et al. Method of feeding and transmission of HIV-1 from mothers to children by 15 months of age: Prospective cohort study from Durban, South Africa. *AIDS*. 2001;15:379-387.

61. Iliff PJ, Piwoz EG, Tavengwa NV, et al. Early exclusive breastfeeding reduces the risk of postnatal HIV-1 transmission and increases HIV-free survival. *AIDS*. 2005;19:699-708.

62. Coovadia HM, Rollins NC, Bland RM, et al. Mother-to-child transmission of HIV-1 infection during exclusive breastfeeding in the first 6 months of life: An intervention cohort study. *Lancet*. 2007;369: 1107-1116.

63. Rollins NC, Filteau SM, Coutsoudis A, et al. Feeding mode, intestinal permeability, and neopterin excretion: A longitudinal study in infants of HIV-infected South African women. *J Acquir Immune Defic Syndr*. 2001;28:132-139.

64. Thea DM, Aldrovandi G, Kankasa C, et al. Post-weaning breast milk HIV-1 viral load, blood prolactin levels and breast milk volume. *AIDS*. 2006;20:1539-1547.

65. Giuliano M, Guidotti G, Andreotti M, et al. Triple antiretroviral prophylaxis administered during pregnancy and after delivery significantly reduces breast milk viral load: A study within the Drug Resource Enhancement Against AIDS and Malnutrition Program. *J Acquir Immune Defic Syndr*. 2007;44:286-291.

66. AIDSInfo. Recommendations for use of antiretroviral drugs in pregnant HIV-1-infected women for maternal health and interventions to reduce perinatal HIV-transmission in the United States. http://aidsinfo.nih.gov/

67. Bedri A, Gudetta B, Isehak A, et al. Extended-dose nevirapine to 6 weeks of age for infants to prevent HIV transmission via breastfeeding in Ethiopia, India, and Uganda: An analysis of three randomised controlled trials. *Lancet*. 2008;372:300-313.

13

68. Kumwenda NI, Hoover DR, Mofenson LM, et al. Extended antiretroviral prophylaxis to reduce breast-milk HIV-1 transmission. *N Engl J Med.* 2008;359:119-129.

69. Tonwe-Gold B, Ekouevi DK, Viho I, et al. Antiretroviral treatment and prevention of peripartum and postnatal HIV transmission in West Africa: Evaluation of a two-tiered approach. *PLoS Med.* 2007;4:e257.

70. The Kesho Bora Study Group. Triple antiretroviral compared with zidovudine and single-dose nevirapine prophylaxis during pregnancy and breastfeeding for prevention of mother-to-child transmission of HIV-1 (Kesho Bora study): A randomised controlled trial. *Lancet Infect Dis.* 2011;11:171-180. See also WHO at http://www.who.int/reproductivehealth/publications/rtis/keshobora/en/index.html

71. Moorthy A, Gupta A, Bhosale R, et al. Nevirapine resistance and breast-milk HIV transmission: Effects of single and extended-dose nevirapine prophylaxis in subtype C HIV-infected infants. *PLoS One.* 2009;4:e4096.

72. Lidstrom J, Li Q, Hoover DR, et al. Addition of extended zidovudine to extended nevirapine prophylaxis reduces nevirapine resistance in infants who were HIV-infected in utero. *AIDS.* 2010;24: 381-386.

73 WHO, UNAIDS, UNFPA, UNICEF Guidelines on HIV and infant feeding 2010. Principles and recommendations for infant feeding in the context of HIV and a summary of evidence. ISBN 9789241599953 159955 http://www.who.int/child_adolescent_health/documents/9789241599535/en/index.html

74. Kantarci S, Koulinska IN, Aboud S, et al. Subclinical mastitis, cell-associated HIV-1 shedding in breast milk, and breast-feeding transmission of hIV-1. *J Acquir Immune Defic Syndr.* 2007;46: 651-654.

75. Chantry CJ, Morrison P, Panchula J, et al. Effects of lipolysis or heat treatment on HIV-1 provirus in breast milk. *J Acquir Immune Defic Syndr.* 2000;24:325-329.

76. Orloff SL, Wallingford JC, McDougal JS. Inactivation of human immunodeficiency virus type I in human milk: Effects of intrinsic factors in human milk and of pasteurization. *J Hum Lact.* 1993; 9:13-17.

77. Jeffery BS, Webber L, Mokhondo KR, et al. Determination of the effectiveness of inactivation of human immunodeficiency virus by Pretoria pasteurization. *J Trop Pediatr.* 2001;47:345-349.

78. Ghosh MK, Kuhn L, West J, et al. Quantitation of human immunodeficiency virus type 1 in breast milk. *J Clin Microbiol.* 2003;41:2465-2470.

79. Rollins N, Meda N, Becquet R, et al. Preventing postnatal transmission of HIV-1 through breast-feeding: Modifying infant feeding practices. *J Acquir Immune Defic Syndr.* 2004;35:188-195.

80. Urdaneta S, Wigdahl B, Neely EB, et al. Inactivation of HIV-1 in breast milk by treatment with the alkyl sulfate microbicide sodium dodecyl sulfate (SDS). *Retrovirology.* 2005;2:28.

81. Proietti FA, Carneiro-Proietti AB, Catalan-Soares BC, et al. Global epidemiology of HTLV-I infection and associated diseases. *Oncogene.* 2005;24:6058-6068.

82. Yamaguchi K, Watanabe T. Human T lymphotropic virus type-I and adult T-cell leukemia in Japan. *Int J Hematol.* 2002;76(Suppl 2):240-245.

83. Mortreux F, Gabet A-S, Wattel E. Molecular and cellular aspects of HTLV-1 associated leukemogenesis in vivo. *Leukemia.* 2003;17:26-38.

84. Hanchard B: Adult T-cell leukemia/lymphoma in Jamaica: 1986–1995. *J Acquir Immune Defic Syndr Hum Retrovirol Suppl.* 1996;1:S20-S25.

85. Yanagihara R: Human T-cell lymphotropic virus type I infection and disease in the Pacific basin. *Hum Biol.* 1992;64:843-854.

86. Takezaki T, Tajima K, Ito M, et al. Short-term breast-feeding may reduce the risk of vertical transmission of HTLV-I. The Tsushima ATL Study Group. *Leukemia.* 1997;11(Suppl. 3):60-62.

87. Trachtenberg AI, Gaudino JA, Hanson CV: Human T-cell lymphotrophic virus in California's injection drug users. *J Psychoactive Drugs.* 1991;23:225-232.

88. de Araujo AC, Casseb JS, Neitzert E, et al. HTLV-I and HTLV-II infections among HIV-1 seropositive patients in Sao Paulo, Brazil. *Eur J Epidemiol.* 1994;10:165-171.

89. Black FL, Biggar RJ, Lal RB, et al. Twenty-five years of HTLV type II follow-up with a possible case of tropical spastic paraparesis in the Kayapo, a Brazilian Indian tribe. *AIDS Res Hum Retroviruses.* 1996;12:1623-1627.

90. Roucoux DF, Murphy EL. The epidemiology and disease outcomes of human T-lymphotropic virus type II. *AIDS Rev.* 2004;6:144-154.

91. Oki T, Yoshinaga M, Otsuka H, et al. A sero-epidemiological study on mother-to-child transmission of HTLV-I in southern Kyushu, Japan. *Asia Oceania J Obstet Gynaecol.* 1992;18:371-377.

92. Ando Y, Matsumoto Y, Nakano S, et al. Long-term follow-up study of HTLV-I infection in bottle-fed children born to seropositive mothers. *J Infect.* 2003;46:9-11.

93. Hino S, Katamine S, Miyata H, et al. Primary prevention of HTLV-I in Japan. *J Acquir Immune Defic Syndr Hum Retrovirol.* 1996;13(Supp. 1):S199-S203.

94. Li HC, Biggar RJ, Miley WJ, et al. Provirus load in breast milk and risk of mother-to-child transmission of human T lymphotropic virus type I. *J Infect Dis.* 2004;190:1275-1278. Comment in: J Infect Dis. 191:1780, 2005; author reply 1781.

95. Yoshinaga M, Yashiki S, Oki T, et al. A maternal risk factor for mother-to-child HTLV-I transmission: Viral antigen-producing capacities in culture of peripheral blood and breast milk cells. *Jpn J Cancer Res.* 1995;86:649-654.

96. Rakeuchi H, Takahashi M, Norose Y, et al. Transformation of breast milk macrophages by HTLV-I: Implications for HTLV-I transmission via breastfeeding. *Biomed Res* 2010;31:53-61.

13

97. Ando Y, Ekuni Y, Matsumoto Y, et al. Long-term serological outcome of infants who received frozen-thawed milk from human T-lymphotropic virus type-I positive mothers. *J Obstet Gynaecol Res.* 2004;30:436-438.

98. Slowik MK, Jhaveri R. Hepatitis B and C viruses in infants and young children. *Semin Pediatr Infect Dis.* 2005;16:296-305.

99. Chang MH, Chen CJ, Lai MS, et al. Universal hepatitis B vaccination in Taiwan and the incidence of hepatocellular carcinoma in children. Taiwan Childhood Hepatoma Study Group. *N Engl J Med.* 1997;336(26):1855-1859.

100. Boxall EH, Flewett TH, Dane DS, et al. Letter: Hepatitis-B surface antigen in breast milk. *Lancet.* 1974;2:1007-1008.

101. Linnemann CC, Goldberg S. Letter: HBAg in breast milk. *Lancet.* 1974;2:155.

102. Lin HH, Hsu HY, et al. Hepatitis B virus in the colostra of HBeAg-positive carrier mothers. *J Pediatr Gastroenterol Nutr.* 1993;17:207-210.

103. Mitsuda T, Yokota S, Mori T, et al. Demonstration of mother-to-infant transmission of hepatitis B virus by means of polymerase chain reaction. *Lancet.* 1989;2:886-888.

104. Beasley RP, Stevens CE, Shiao IS, et al. Evidence against breast-feeding as a mechanism for vertical transmission of hepatitis B. *Lancet.* 1975;2:740-741.

105. de Martino M, Appendino C, Resti M, et al. Should hepatitis B surface antigen positive mothers breast feed? *Arch Dis Child.* 1985;60:972-974.

106. Cohen RS, Xiong SC, Sakamoto P, et al. Retrospective review of serological testing of potential human milk donors. *Arch Dis Child Fetal Neonatal Ed.* 2010;95:F118-F120.

107. Oliveira P, Yamamoto A, de Souza C, et al. Hepatitis B viral markers in banked human milk before and after Holder pasteurization. *J Clin Virol.* 2009;45:281-284.

108. Fischler B, Lindh G, Lindgren S, et al. Vertical transmission of hepatitis C virus infection. *Scand J Infect Dis.* 1996;28:353-356.

109. Kelly D, Skidmore S. Hepatitis C-Z: Recent advances. *Arch Dis Child.* 2002;86:339-343.

110. Thomas SL, Newell ML, Peckham CS, et al. A review of hepatitis C virus (HCV) vertical transmission: Risks of transmission to infants born to mothers with and without HCV viraemia or human immunodeficiency virus infection. *Int J Epidemiol.* 1998;27:108-117.

111. Pembreya L, Newella ML, Tovo PA. The management of HCV infected pregnant women and their children European paediatric HCV network. *J Hepatol.* 2005;43:515-525.

112. England K, Pembrey L, Tovo PA, et al. Excluding hepatitis C virus (HCV) infection by serology in young infants of HCV-infected mothers. *Acta Paediatr.* 2005;94:444-450.

113. Mok J, Pembrey L, Tovo PA, et al. When does mother to child transmission of hepatitis C virus occur? *Arch Dis Child Fetal Neonatal Ed.* 2005;90:F156-F160.

114. Kumar RM, Shahul S. Role of breast-feeding in transmission of hepatitis C virus to infants of HCV-infected mothers. *J Hepatol.* 1998;29:191-197.

115. Lin HH, Kao JH, Hsu HY, et al. Absence of infection in breast-fed infants born to hepatitis C virus-infected mothers. *J Pediatr.* 1995;126:589-591.

116. Polywka S, Schroter M, Feucht HH, et al. Low risk of vertical transmission of hepatitis C virus by breast milk. *Clin Infect Dis.* 1999;29:1327-1329.

117. European Paediatric Hepatitis C Virus Network. Effects of mode of delivery and infant feeding on the risk of mother to child transmission of hepatitis C virus. *Brit J Obstetr Gynaecol.* 2001;78:371-377.

118. European Paediatric Hepatitis C Virus Network. A significant sex—but not elective Cesarean section—effect on mother-to-child transmission of hepatitis C infection. *J Infect Dis.* 2005;192:1872-1879.

119. Pembrey L, Newell ML, Tovo PA, et al. The management of HCV infected pregnant women and their children. European paediatric HCV network. *J Hepatol.* 2005;43:515-525.

120. Lindemann PC, Foshaugen I, Lindemann R. Characteristics of breast milk and serology of women donating breast milk to a milk bank. *Arch Dis Child Fetal Neonatal Ed.* 2004;89:F440-F441.

121. Hilfenhaus J, Groner A, Nowak T, et al. Analysis of human plasma products: Polymerase chain reaction does not discriminate between live and inactivated viruses. *Transfusion.* 1997;37:935-940.

122. Stagno S, Britt W. Cytomegalovirus. In: Remington JS, Klein JO, Wilson CB, Baker C, eds. *Infectious diseases of the fetus and newborn infant.* 6th ed. Philadelphia: WB Saunders; 2006:739-781.

123. Sharland M, Luck S, Griffiths P, et al. Antiviral therapy of CMV disease in children. *Adv Exp Med Biol.* 2011;697:243-260. Review.

124. Hamprecht K, Goelz R, Maschmann J. Breast milk and cytomegalovirus infection in preterm infants. *Early Hum Dev.* 2005;81:989-996.

125. Yasuda A, Kimura H, Hayakawa M, et al. Evaluation of cytomegalovirus infections transmitted via breast milk in preterm infants with a real-time polymerase chain reaction assay. *Pediatrics.* 2003;111:1333-1336.

126. Hamprecht K, Witzel S, Maschman J, et al. Rapid detection and quantification of cell free cytomegalovirus by a high-speed centrifugation-based microculture assay: Comparison to longitudinally analyzed viral DNA load and pp67 late transcript during lactation. *J Clin Virol.* 2003;28:303-316.

127. Curtis N, Chau L, Garland S, et al. Cytomegalovirus remains viable in naturally infected breast milk despite being frozen for 10 days. *Arch Dis Child Fetal Neonatal Ed.* 2005;90:F529-F530.

128. Tarr PI, Haas JE, Christie DL. Biliary atresia, cytomegalovirus, and age at referral. *Pediatrics.* 1996;97:828-831.

13

129. Fischler B, Ehrnst A, Forsgren M, et al. The viral association of neonatal cholestasis in Sweden, a possible link between cytomegalovirus infection and extrahepatic biliary atresia. *J Pediatr Gastroenterol Nutr*. 1998;27:57-64.

130. Mussi-Pinhata MM, Pinto PC, Yamamoto AY, et al. Placental transfer of naturally acquired, maternal cytomegalovirus antibodies in term and preterm neonates. *J Med Virol*. 2003;69:232-239.

131. Forsgren M. Cytomegalovirus in breast milk: reassessment of pasteurization and freeze-thawing. *Pediatr Res*. 2004;56:526-528.

132. Paryani SG, Yeager AS, Hosford-Dunn H, et al. Sequelae of acquired cytomegalovirus infection in premature and sick term infants. *J Pediatr*. 1985;107:451-456.

133. Johnson SJ, Hosford-Dunn H, Paryani S, et al. Prevalence of sensorineural hearing loss in premature and sick term infants with perinatally acquired cytomegalovirus infection. *Ear Hear*. 1986;7: 325-327.

134. Vollmer B, Seibold-Weiger K, Schmitz-Salue C, et al. Postnatally acquired cytomegalovirus infection via breast milk: Effects on hearing and development in preterm infants. *Pediatr Infect Dis J*. 2004;23:322-327.

135. Jim WT, Shu CH, Chiu NC, et al. Transmission of cytomegalovirus from mothers to preterm infants by breast milk. *Pediatr Infect Dis J*. 2004;23:848-851.

136. Miron D, Brosilow S, Felszer K, et al. Incidence and clinical manifestations of breast milk-acquired Cytomegalovirus infection in low birth weight infants. *J Perinatol*. 2005;25:299-303.

137. Bryant P, Morley C, Garland S, et al. Cytomegalovirus transmission from breast milk in premature babies: Does it matter? *Arch Dis Child Fetal Neonatal Ed*. 2002;87:F75-F77.

138. Willeitner A. Transmission of cytomegalovirus (CMV) through human milk: Are new breastfeeding policies required for preterm infants? *Adv Exp Med Biol*. 2004;554:489-494.

139. Schanler RJ. CMV acquisition in premature infants fed human milk: Reason to worry? *J Perinatol*. 2005;25:297-298.

140. Capretti MG, Lanari M, Lazzarotto T, et al. Very low birth weight infants born to cytomegalovirus-seropositive mothers fed with their mother's milk: A prospective study. *J Pediatr*. 2009;154: 842-848.

141. Kurath S, Halwachs-Baumann G, Müller W, et al. Transmission of cytomegalovirus via breast milk to the prematurely born infant: A systematic review. *Clin Microbiol Infect*. 2010;16:1172-1178.

142. Neuberger P, Hamprecht K, Vochem M, et al. Case-control study of symptoms and neonatal outcome of human milk-transmitted cytomegalovirus infection in premature infants. *J Pediatr*. 2006;148: 326-331.

143. Omarsdottir S, Casper C, Zweygberg Wirgart B, et al. Transmission of cytomegalovirus to extremely preterm infants through breast milk. *Acta Paediatr*. 2007;96:492-494.

144. Hamprecht K, Maschmann J, Muller D, et al. Cytomegalovirus (CMV) inactivation in breast milk: Reassessment of pasteurization and freeze-thawing. *Pediatr Res*. 2004;56:529-535.

13

CHAPTER 14

Probiotics for the Prevention of Necrotizing Enterocolitis in Preterm Neonates

Simon Pirie, MBBS, MRCPCH, and
Sanjay Patole, MD, DCH, FRACP, MSc, DrPH

14

- **Pathogenesis and Prevention of NEC**
- **What Are Probiotics?**

Necrotizing enterocolitis (NEC) is the most common gastrointestinal emergency for preterm neonates. About 90% to 95% of cases occur in neonates who have been fed with milk, indicating the role of enteral substrate in the pathogenesis of the illness.[1,2] The incidence of Bell's stage II or greater NEC in very low birth weight (VLBW) neonates is 4% to 6%, and overall mortality is 20% to 25%.[1,2] The illness progresses to a stage requiring surgery for gastrointestinal gangrene and/or perforation in 30% of cases. Postoperative complications include late development of intestinal strictures, recurrent episodes of sepsis, dependence on total parenteral nutrition, hepatic failure, and survival with short bowel syndrome and its consequences.[3,4] The incidence (10% to 12%), mortality (40% to 45%), and morbidity of definite NEC are significantly higher in extremely preterm neonates with gestation less than 28 weeks.[5-9] Mortality reaches close to 100% in those with widespread full-thickness necrosis of the gut.[10,11] Neurodevelopmental impairment (NDI) is a serious concern in extremely preterm survivors of surgical NEC.[12,13]

Schulzke and associates systematically reviewed the observational studies reporting long-term neurodevelopmental outcomes in VLBW neonates surviving after stage II or greater NEC.[13] Eleven nonrandomized studies, including five with matched controls, were included in the analyses. The risk of long-term NDI was significantly higher in the presence of at least stage II NEC versus no NEC (odds ratio [OR], 1.82; 95% confidence interval [CI], 1.46 to 2.27). Those with NEC requiring surgery were at higher risk for NDI than those managed medically (OR, 1.99; 95% CI, 1.26 to 3.14). Risks of cerebral palsy and cognitive and severe visual impairment were significantly higher among neonates with NEC.[13] The economic burden of NEC is significant, given the range of complications and the prolonged hospital stay.[14-18] Bisquera and colleagues evaluated the impact of NEC on length of stay and hospital charges in a case-control study.[18] Neonates with surgical NEC had lengths of stay exceeding those of controls by 60 days, whereas lengths of stay among those with medical NEC exceeded those of controls by 22 days. Based on length of stay, the estimated total hospital charges for neonates with surgical NEC averaged $186,200 in excess of those for controls, and $73,700 more for those with medical NEC. The yearly additional hospital charges for NEC were $6.5 million, or $216,666 per survivor.[18] On the basis of these data, the projected economic burden of NEC has been reported to be as high as $1 billion per year in the United States, without accounting for the long-term care of impaired survivors and the number of deaths per year.[19]

Pathogenesis and Prevention of NEC

Despite decades of research, the pathogenesis of NEC continues to be poorly understood. An interplay of various risk factors (e.g., hypoxia, gut colonization with pathogens, formula feeding, sepsis, intestinal ischemia-reperfusion injury) against the background of an immature gut and an inappropriate gastrointestinal and systemic inflammatory response is currently thought to contribute to the development of NEC.[20] About 20% to 30% of cases of NEC are associated with sepsis. However, it is not clear whether the sepsis in such cases is a cause (causing initial gut injury) or a consequence (translocation across a compromised gut epithelial barrier) of NEC. Proinflammatory mediators such as tumor necrosis factor, platelet-activating factor, interleukin (IL)-1, IL-8, and IL-18 play a key role in initiating the inflammatory cascade that leads to intestinal necrosis.[21-26] These inflammatory cytokines disrupt the gut epithelial barrier, allowing the gut bacteria to translocate.[27] Bacterial translocation across the gut is normally prevented by an intact gut epithelial barrier with its tight junctions.[28]

Apart from an intact gut epithelial barrier, mature immunologic and nonimmunologic components of the intestinal defense system are essential for preventing/minimizing the initial gut injury and its propagation to gut necrosis.[29,30] The mucous layer, mucins, the trefoil factor, and maturation of mucus with increasing postnatal age in response to colonization of the gut with commensal organisms are important parts of the gut defense system.[31-33] Investigators have hypothesized that defects in the production and/or composition of mucus or its properties allow bacteria to invade the gut and contribute to the pathogenesis of NEC.[31-33] Toll-like receptors (TLRs) recognize specific molecular patterns, and different TLR members are expressed in a variety of cells, including macrophages and enterocytes.[34] TLRs play an important role in the pathogenesis of NEC because differences in their expression may alter a host's response to commensals or pathogens. TLR ligands are expressed by commensal organisms; they appear important for intestinal maturation and epithelial homeostasis.

Researchers have proposed that in response to significant endotoxemic/hypoxic stress, TLR4 expression and signaling are increased in the neonatal enterocyte monolayer and/or immune cells that migrate into the inflamed tissue, rendering the intestine increasingly susceptible to endotoxin following colonization by Gram-negative flora. Resultant activation of TLR4 tips the balance from intestinal homeostasis toward apoptotic injury, and impairs repair mechanisms through effects on proliferation and migration. The net effect is the development of intestinal inflammatory changes that characterize NEC.[34] Dysmotility of the gut in preterm neonates may cause stasis of luminal contents, and the bacterial overgrowth that results, particularly in the absence of human milk feeding, may promote the inflammatory cascade observed in NEC.[35]

Prevention of NEC is a difficult task given the complex interactions between a range of risk factors for this poorly understood illness. Difficulties in preventing preterm birth—the single most important risk factor for the illness—mean that cases of NEC will continue to occur despite the best efforts to prevent it. Antenatal glucocorticoids, early preferential feeding with breast milk, prevention and management of sepsis, and a cautious approach to enteral feeds are the only strategies available so far for the primary prevention of NEC.[36]

The Role of Gut Microflora

The sterile gut of a neonate is usually colonized within 12 to 24 hours. Intestinal microbes from the mother are the first source of bacteria, and colonization by anaerobes commences in the following 2 to 3 days. Breast milk lactobacilli and bifidobacteria colonize the gut subsequently.[37-40] Factors such as mode of birth, environment, and diet also influence colonization in a neonate.[41-44] The gut flora of preterm neonates differs from that of normal-term neonates because they acquire microbial flora mainly from the intensive care environment rather than from their mother.[38,45] Also, they are often exposed to antibiotics in early postnatal life and are intolerant of even small volumes of milk feeds. The appearance of *Bifidobacterium* species in VLBW neonates is delayed until the third week of life, even in those receiving only breast milk.[40] Stools of breast-fed neonates have a predominance of *Bifidobacterium* and *Lactobacillus* species, which compete with pathogens such as *Bacteroides* and *Clostridium*.[45,46]

Colonization with pathogens can alter the permeability of intestines in preterm neonates and can promote the inflammatory cascade, which facilitates NEC.[46,47] In light of the role of microorganisms in the development and modulation of many risk factors within the intestinal epithelium, and the altered gut flora noted in preterm neonates, probiotic supplementation has been proposed as a promising new intervention for the prevention of NEC.[46,47]

What Are Probiotics?

Probiotics are live microorganisms that have a positive effect on the host organism. The World Health Organization (WHO) defines them as "live microorganisms which when administered in adequate amounts confer a health benefit on the host."[48] The most common types are lactic acid bacteria and bifidobacteria. Lactic acid bacteria are so named because they produce lactic acid as the result of carbohydrate fermentation—a fact that was documented first by Louis Pasteur.[49] Bifidobacteria are anaerobic, Gram-positive, branched, rod-shaped bacteria. Microorganisms have been a part of certain diets for thousands of years and are even referred to in the Bible.[50] Fermented milk products were used in the treatment of gastroenteritis as far back as Roman times.[51] The earliest referenced scientific observations on the beneficial effects of probiotics were made by Elie Metchnikoff, who documented that Bulgarian peasants who regularly consumed lactic acid bacteria in fermented dairy products appeared to have longevity and improved health[52] (Table 14-1). In 1856 Louis Pasteur discovered lactic acid bacteria while investigating the cause of souring in a distillery.[53] In 1873, Joseph Lister isolated lactic acid bacteria from fermented milk while trying to show that a pure culture of *Bacterium lactis,* normally present in milk, uniquely caused the lactic acid fermentation of milk.[54] Henry Tissier noted that *Bifidobacteria* were the predominant bacteria in the stools of breast-fed infants.[55] These discoveries demonstrated that living organisms could be isolated from the gut, and that they produced changes in certain food products that might have a positive impact on the consumer.

Following Tissier's isolation of *Bifidobacterium, Lactobacillus acidophilus* was discovered in the early 20th century. In 1930, Minoru Shirota, a scientist at Kyoto University, discovered *Lactobacillus casei* strain *Shirota.* This organism was isolated from the human intestine and was therefore resistant to gastric acid and bile acid, so it could safely reach the lower intestine after ingestion.[56] The actual term *probiotics* was first used by Lilly and Stillwell in 1965 to represent "substances secreted by one organism which stimulate the growth of another."[57] Nine years later, Parker described probiotics as "organisms and substances which contribute to intestinal microbial balance."[58] Fuller proposed that probiotics were "live microbial supplements which beneficially affect the host animal by improving its microbial balance."[59] Later, Salminen defined probiotics as "foods containing live bacteria which are beneficial

Table 14-1 HISTORY OF PROBIOTICS

Year	Event
1856	Louis Pasteur discovers lactic acid bacteria.
1873	Joseph Lister isolates lactic acid bacteria from fermented milk.
1900	Henry Tissier reports findings of *Bifidobacterium* in the stools of breast-fed infants.
1908	Elie Metchnikoff reports his observation on the beneficial effects of probiotic ingestion.
1930	Minoru Shirota discovers *Lactobacillus casei* strain *Shirota.*
1965	Lilly and Stillwell use the term *probiotics.*
2001	Report of the Joint Food and Agriculture Organization (FAO)/World Health Organization (WHO) Expert Consultation on Probiotics is issued.

Table 14-2 MECHANISMS OF ACTION OF PROBIOTICS

Mechanism of Action	Reference
Gut flora: Reduce intraluminal pH	Servin, 2004[62]
Produce bacteriocins	Lawton et al, 2007[63]
Improved gut motility	Indrio et al, 2008[95] and 2009[96]
Barrier function: Increased mucus production	Deplancke et al, 2001[69]
Tight junction function	Martin et al, 2008[47]
Mucin and IgA production	Boivirant et al, 2007[79]
Immunologic: Inhibition of NF-κB	Claud, 2009[81]
TLR interaction to promote protective cytokines	Boivirant et al, 2007[79] Rakoff-Nahoum et al, 2004[83]
Promote Th 1 cytokines (anti-inflammatory)	Veckham et al, 2004[85]
Upregulate TGF-β_1 (anti-inflammatory)	Lavasani et al, 2010[86]
Antioxidant defense system enhancement	Spyropoulos et al, 2011[94]

IgA, Immunoglobulin A; *NF,* nuclear factor; *TGF,* transforming growth factor; *TLR,* toll-like receptor.

to health."[60] In 2002, a report published by the United Nations Food and Agriculture Organization and the WHO set out the results of an expert panel evaluation of available scientific evidence on the properties, functionality, benefits, safety, and nutritional features of probiotic foods.[48] In 2004, two of the main companies involved in probiotic production established The Global Probiotics Council "to promote and/or advance probiotics in the world."[61]

Mechanisms of Action of Probiotics in the Prevention of NEC

The beneficial effects of probiotics in the prevention of NEC (Table 14-2) are thought to be mediated via various pathways. Some of these are discussed in the following paragraphs.

1. **Gut flora:** Promoting colonization by commensals and inhibition of pathogens is essential for the gut to maintain its absorptive and barrier functions. Gastric acidity and digestive enzymes destroy ingested pathogens and associated antigens. Probiotics assist in this part of defense by reducing the intraluminal pH and producing bacteriocins, which are proteinaceous toxins that inhibit growth of other bacteria.[62,63] Strains of lactobacilli produce lactic acid, acetic acid, and propionic acid, all of which decrease the pH. An acidic pH inhibits the growth of potentially harmful Gram-negative pathogens.[64-66] One noted example of these effects is the action of *Lactobacillus* and *Bifidobacterium* strains on *Helicobacter pylori.*[67]

2. **Pathogen defense:** Mucus production protects against bacterial adherence to the gut wall.[68] Probiotics increase the production of mucus[69] and modulate mucosal permeability and intestinal tight junction function, which are an integral part of the gut's defense.[70-73] These actions prevent the diffusion and translocation of potentially damaging factors into the tissue and later into the systemic circulation. Permeability to pathogens and allergens plays a significant part in the development and exacerbation of a number of gastrointestinal diseases, including inflammatory bowel disease and celiac disease. Other barrier functions of probiotics include decreasing adhesion of pathogens and their toxins by producing a biofilm or producing receptor analogues and competing with pathogens for binding sites.[74-76] Probiotics have also been shown to displace pathogens that are already attached to the intestinal surface.[74,75]

3. **Gut barrier function:** Breakdown of the gut barrier plays an important role in the pathogenesis of NEC. Gut epithelial cells are linked by tight junctions and are covered by a glycocalyx. Probiotics have been shown to optimize

the function of these tight junctions and to inhibit bacterial translocation.[77] When challenged by a pathogen, chemokines are secreted; neutrophils approach the area and are transported into the gut to engage the pathogen.[78] Paneth cells, goblet cells, and enterocytes are also involved in this barrier function, producing bacteriocins, mucins, and immunoglobulin (Ig)A, all of which contribute to the inhibitory effect on potential pathogens.[79]

4. **Immunologic effects:** A significant part of gut defense is immunologically mediated, and the gut has certain receptors that trigger various responses. TLRs and nucleotide-binding oligomerization domain receptors (NODs) recognize specific pathogen regions, or pathogen-associated molecular patterns (PAMPs).[80] Binding of PAMPs to their corresponding recognition receptor (TLR or NOD) results in stimulation of the inflammatory cascade via nuclear factor (NF)-κB and mitogen-activated protein kinase (MAPK).[80] NF-κB translocates into the cell's nucleus and upregulates gene expression of inflammatory mediators. Commensal bacteria and probiotics are thought to exert beneficial effects by inhibiting the activation of NF-κB. IκB is a protein that, when bound to NF-κB, inhibits its translocation into cells.[47] IκB is developmentally regulated, and its expression is relatively reduced in immature fetal intestinal cells.[81] Immature intestinal cells therefore show excessive inflammation when the TLR pathway is activated; this effect is thought to be linked to the development of NEC. Recent studies have supported the hypothesis that probiotic immunomodulatory effects may be stimulatory rather than inhibitory.[82] Probiotics act via TLRs such as TLR-2 and TLR-4 to produce protective cytokines (e.g., IL-6), which mediate cell regeneration and inhibit cell apoptosis.[79,83] Different probiotics appear to affect TLR expression in different ways.[84] Probiotics manipulate immune function to improve anti-pathogen activity, but they also mediate inflammatory responses to pathogens by increasing Th1 cytokine profiles, resulting in increased anti-inflammatory cytokines and decreased inflammatory cytokines.[85] Probiotics can upregulate transforming growth factor (TGF)-β_1 signaling; this has potent anti-inflammatory effects.[86]

5. **Other areas of benefit:** Free radical injury plays a role in the pathogenesis of NEC.[87-89] Preterm neonates are known to have a limited antioxidant defense that increases with rising gestation.[90,91] Reactive oxygen species disrupt tight junctions in the gut epithelium and affect the barrier function.[92] Studies have demonstrated that probiotics can protect against this.[93] Cord serum antioxidant capacity correlates with gestational age but does not predict the risk of oxygen radical–related diseases such as NEC.[90] Research in radiation-induced enteritis and colitis indicates that probiotics play a key role in enhancement of the host's intestinal antioxidant defense systems.[94] Indrio and associates reported that probiotics promote feeding tolerance, improve bowel habits, and facilitate gastrointestinal motility in preterm neonates.[95,96] Because gut immaturity and dysmotility are important pathophysiologic variables in NEC, these positive effects of probiotics are expected to be beneficial in the prevention of NEC.

Clinical Data on Probiotics for Prevention of NEC in Preterm Neonates

Hoyos and colleagues (1999) were the first to report benefits of probiotic supplementation in reducing the incidence of NEC in neonates.[97] Daily doses of 250 million live *L. acidophilus* and 250 million *Bifidobacterium infantis* were given to all 1237 neonates admitted to the unit during 1 year, until they were discharged from the hospital; 1282 neonates hospitalized during the previous year were used as controls. Demographic and clinical characteristics were comparable between groups. The historic control group included 85 NEC cases compared with 34 cases in the probiotic prophylaxis group (P <0.0002). NEC-related mortality was significantly less in the study group versus the control group (14/34 vs. 35/85; P <0.005). No complications were attributed to daily probiotic administration.[97]

Table 14-3 CLINICAL TRIALS OF PROBIOTICS IN PRETERM NEONATES

Study	Probiotic Agents	Dose and Duration	Type of Milk	Primary Outcome
1997 Kitajima	BB	0.5×10^9 organisms once daily from first feed for 28 days	MM or FM	Gut colonization by BB
2002 Dani	LB-GG (Dicloflor)	6×10^9 CFU once daily from first feed until discharge	MM or DM or FM	UTI, sepsis, NEC
2003 Costalos	SB	10^9/kg twice daily from first feed for 30 days	FM	Gut function and stool colonization
2005 Bin Nun	BI, ST, BBB	BI: 0.35×10^9 CFU, ST: 0.35×10^9 CFU, and BBB: 0.35×10^9 CFU once daily from first feed to 36 weeks corrected age	MM or FM	NEC
2005 Lin	LB-A, BI	LB-A: 1004356, and BI: 1015697 organisms twice daily from day 7 until discharge	MM or DM	NEC or death
2006 Manzoni	LB-C (Dicloflor)	6×10^9 CFU once daily from 3rd day of life to 6 weeks or discharge from NICU	MM or DM	Gut colonization by *Candida* species
2006 Mohan*	BB-L	1.6×10^9 CFU once daily from day 1 to day 3 4.8×10^9 CFU once daily from day 4 to day 21	FM	Gut colonization by BB-L and enteric pathogens
2007 Stratki*	BB-L	Preterm formula 1×10^7 CFU/g started within 48 hours to 30 days	FM	Intestinal permeability
2008 Lin	BBB, LB-A	2×10^9 CFU daily for 6 weeks	MM or FM	NEC or death
2009 Samanta	BBB, BB-L, BI, LB-A	2.5×10^9 CFU daily until discharge	MM or FM	NEC, time to full feed, sepsis, death, and hospital stay
2009 Rouge	BB-LG, LB GG	1×10^8 CFU daily until discharge	MM or DM or FM	Enteral feed intake at day 14
2010 Mihatsch	BB-L	$6 \times 2.0 \times 10^9$ CFU/kg/day for first 6 weeks of life	MM or FM	Incidence of nosocomial infection
2010 Braga	BB, LB-C	3.5×10^7 to 3.5×10^9 CFU daily day 2 until day 30	MM or DM	NEC

*Data for <34 weeks and <1500 g obtained by contacting the authors.
BB, Bifidobacterium breve; BBB, Bifidobacterium bifidus; BB-L, Bifidobacterium lactis; BB-LG, Bifidobacterium longum; BI, Bifidobacterium infantis; CFU, colony-forming units; DM, donor milk; FM, formula milk; LB-A, Lactobacillus acidophilus; LB-C, Lactobacillus casei; LB GG, Lactobacillus GG; MM, mother's milk; SB, Saccharomyces boulardii; ST, Streptococcus thermophilus.

On the basis of these encouraging results, many randomized controlled trials (RCTs) were undertaken subsequently[98-110] (Table 14-3). Deshpande and coworkers (2007) provided the first systematic review and meta-analysis of RCTs conducted to evaluate the efficacy and safety of any probiotic supplementation (started within first 10 days, duration ≥7 days) in preventing stage II or greater NEC in preterm VLBW (birth weight <1500 g; gestation <33 weeks) neonates.[111] A total of 7 of 12 retrieved RCTs ($N = 1393$) were eligible for inclusion in the analysis. Meta-analysis using a fixed effects model (7 trials; $N = 1393$) estimated a lower risk of stage II or greater NEC (relative risk, 0.36; 95% CI, 0.20 to 0.65) in the probiotic group. The number needed to treat (NNT) with probiotics to prevent one case of NEC was 25 (95% CI, 17 to 50). The risk of death (5 trials; $N = 1268$) was reduced significantly in the probiotic versus the control group (RR, 0.47; 95% CI, 0.30 to 0.73); the NNT to prevent one death by supplementation with probiotics was 20 (95% CI, 12 to 50). Mortality due to NEC or sepsis did not differ significantly. The time to full enteral feeds (TFEF, 3 trials; $N = 316$) was significantly shorter in the probiotic group (weighted mean difference [WMD], −2.74 days; 95% CI, −4.98 to −0.51). The risk of blood culture–positive sepsis (6 trials; N = 1355) did not differ significantly between groups (RR, 0.94; 95% CI, 0.74 to 1.20).

Overall results indicate that, in general, probiotics may significantly reduce the risk of all-cause mortality and stage II or greater NEC in preterm neonates at less than 33 weeks' gestation, while significantly shortening the TFEF.[111] These results were confirmed in the Cochrane systematic review, which concluded that except for those weighing less than 1000 grams (because of lack of specific data in this high-risk population), a change in practice was supported by the data.[112] However, the systematic review by Barclay and colleagues did not include a meta-analysis on the basis that effects of probiotics are very much strain specific, and pooling data from different strains is not appropriate.[113]

Deshpande and coworkers (2010) have reported their updated meta-analysis of RCTs (11 trials; N = 2176) that investigated probiotics in preterm neonates.[114] Their results confirm the previously reported benefits of probiotics with further precision and certainty. Meta-analysis using a fixed effects model estimated a significantly lower risk of stage II or greater NEC and all-cause mortality, and a shorter TFEF, in the probiotic versus control group (NEC [11 trials, N = 2176]: RR, 0.35 [95% CI, 0.23 to 0.55), P <0.00001, NNT, 25 [95% CI, 17 to 34]; mortality (9 trials; N = 2051): RR, 0.42 [95% CI, 0.29 to 0.62], P <0.00001, NNT, 20 [95% CI, 14 to 34]; TFEF (5 trials; N = 936): WMD, −5.03 days [95% CI, −5.62 to −4.44], P <0.0001). The risk of blood culture–positive sepsis (10 trials; N = 2138) did not differ significantly between groups (RR, 0.98 [95% CI, 0.81 to 1.18]). Additionally, trial sequential analysis (TSA) indicated that probiotics reduced the incidence of NEC by at least 30%.[114]

Despite these very encouraging results, problems involving pooling data in the presence of clinical heterogeneity, heterogeneity of probiotic strains, the role of breast milk, reproducibility of results in different set-ups, pitfalls of TSA, lack of availability of safe and effective products, cross-contamination, and adverse effects such as probiotic sepsis, development of antibiotic resistance, and altered immunologic responses in the long run have been cited as the reasons for not introducing routine use of probiotics at this stage in preterm neonates.[115-119] However, considering the health burden of NEC and the fact that many level III neonatal nurseries in Japan, Italy, Finland, and Colombia have been using probiotics routinely for over a decade and have not reported any significant adverse effects, many feel that probiotics may be offered routinely if safe and clinically effective products are available.[120-127] Although it has not happened in proper sequence, it is important to note that probiotics as an intervention have completed a full circle, from basic science[128] and cohort studies[97] to conclusive meta-analysis,[114] routine use,[123-125] and long-term follow-up.[121,122]

The future of probiotics for prevention of NEC in preterm neonates depends on resolution of the current debate either by consensus or by additional large and definitive placebo-controlled trials designed to detect the smallest clinically significant effect size in extremely preterm neonates, who are at highest risk for NEC and death. Potentially preventable cases of NEC and all-cause death during the conduct of such trials will be a matter of debate. Offering probiotics routinely but still within a framework of research will help in dealing with yet unanswered questions in this high-risk but highly deserving population.

Unaddressed Issues

Optimal strains, doses, and durations of probiotic organisms are not clear. It also is not clear whether a combination of probiotics is more effective than a single probiotic. Individual strains are known to have variable rates of colonization in different populations.[98,129,130] Maturity of the host is another important factor in colonization by probiotic organisms.[98] Human breast milk contains the synergistic combination of probiotics and prebiotics.[129,131,132] However, preferential use of human breast milk alone has not eliminated NEC. Current data do not provide details on the types

14

of feeds (exclusive/predominant breast milk and formula feeds) and on antibiotic exposure for sepsis—a factor known to have a significant adverse impact on the gut flora.

Prebiotics have been shown to enhance the survival of probiotic organisms.[133,134] Whether the clinical benefits of probiotics can be improved significantly by using a combination of probiotics and prebiotics (synbiotics) remains to be determined.[135]

Evaluation of the effects of live and dead probiotics is an important issue.[136,137] Live probiotics influence the gut flora and the immune response; dead cell components exert an anti-inflammatory response. Variable quantities of dead cells may thus explain the variation in response to live probiotics.[138] Products with dead probiotics may offer several advantages, including safety and a long shelf life. Awad and associates reported the results of their randomized, controlled trial comparing the role of killed probiotics (KPs) *L. acidophilus* versus living probiotics (LPs) in reducing the incidence of sepsis and NEC in preterm neonates.[139] Sixty neonates received oral LP, 60 received KP, and 30 received placebo on day 1. LPs and KPs were preventive factors for NEC with absolute risk reductions of 16% and 15%, respectively, and 18% for sepsis compared with placebo. The incidence of NEC and sepsis did not differ significantly between neonates supplemented with LP and those with KP. Neonates supplemented with KP showed a significantly lower incidence of NEC compared with placebo, and the incidence of sepsis showed no significant differences between groups. A significant reduction in sepsis and NEC was noted among neonates with gut colonization with *Lactobacillus* compared with those without colonization at day 7 (27.9% vs. 85.9%, 0% vs. 7.8%) and day 14 (sepsis, 48.7% vs. 91.7%; NEC, 0% vs. 20.8%). Overall, these results indicate that early gut colonization with probiotic bacteria lowers the incidence of NEC and sepsis, and that the benefits of killed probiotic bacteria are similar to those of live bacteria.[139]

A few important clinical issues need to be appreciated. Benefits as significant as those reported in the meta-analysis of probiotic supplementation may not occur in populations with a low baseline rate of NEC. Tolerance of probiotic supplements with regard to volume, osmolality, and presence of dairy products such as lactose is an important issue for extremely low birth weight (ELBW) neonates.[140] It is important to note that most of the unaddressed issues can be dealt with by clinical trials not involving a placebo. Cohort studies are an attractive option for studying many of these issues.

Adverse Effects

Probiotic sepsis, development and transfer of antibiotic resistance, altered immune responses, and allergic sensitization in the long run are some of the significant potential adverse effects of probiotic supplementation in preterm neonates. Given that the effects of probiotics are strain specific, different strains are expected to have different profiles of adverse effects. Case reports of neonatal probiotic sepsis indicate the importance of this issue.[141-144] However, data from clinical trials and follow-up studies in neonates, from neonatal units using routine probiotic supplementation for over a decade, and from countries using routine probiotic supplementation at the population level are reassuring. The true safety profile of probiotics will be known only when they are introduced as routine in neonatal intensive care. Standardized high-level surveillance and reporting (postmarketing surveillance) are necessary to evaluate the safety of probiotics in preterm, especially extremely preterm (gestation <28 weeks) neonates—a population that is most deserving but also is at highest risk of short- and long-term adverse effects. Most of the reports of probiotic sepsis involve strains of the species *Lactobacillus,* and it is possible that *Bifidobacterium* strains may be safer. However, the rarity of bifidobacterial sepsis in the literature may reflect failure in isolating these strains by routine culture methods.

Development and transfer of antibiotic resistance is a significant issue with probiotic strains.[145,146] Liu and associates studied the antimicrobial resistance of commercial lactic acid bacteria by analyzing their isolated strains used for fermentation and probiotics.[147] Antimicrobial susceptibility of 41 screened isolates was tested with disk diffusion and E-test methods after species-level identification.

Resistant strains were selected and examined for the presence of resistance genes by polymerase chain reaction (PCR). All isolates were susceptible to chloramphenicol, tetracycline, ampicillin, amoxicillin/clavulanic acid, cephalothin, and imipenem. The incidence of resistance to vancomycin, rifampicin, streptomycin, bacitracin, and erythromycin was relatively low. In contrast, most strains were resistant to ciprofloxacin, amikacin, trimethoprim/sulfamethoxazole, and gentamicin. The genes *msrC, vanX,* and *dfrA* were detected in strains of *Enterococcus faecium, Lactobacillus plantarum, Streptococcus thermophilus,* and *Lactococcus lactis.*[147] Experimental studies have also shown that lactic acid bacteria (LAB) can act as a source of mobile genetic elements encoding antibiotic resistance that can spread to other LAB.[148] Knowledge of antibiotic resistance patterns among selected probiotic strains and ongoing surveillance are thus critical for optimal use of this intervention in preterm neonates.[149,150] Advances in technology have allowed removal of antibiotic-resistant gene-carrying plasmids from probiotic strains such as *Lactobacillus reuteri* ATCC 55730, resulting in daughter strains (*L. reuteri* DSM 17938), which still retain the probiotic properties.[151] Current research indicates resistance to lysozyme as a promising criterion for the selection of new probiotic bifidobacterial strains.[152]

Cross-contamination of nonrecipients is a practical issue during probiotic supplementation in a high-risk cohort. Kitajima and associates reported a 12% and a 44% contamination rate in control group neonates at 6 and 12 weeks of probiotic supplementation, whereas Costeloe and colleagues reported a rate of 35% among control group neonates in their pilot study.[98,153] Thus, a significant number of control group neonates may be exposed to the benefits, as well as the adverse effects, of probiotics.

Allergic sensitization in the long run is a concern with probiotic supplementation in the perinatal period. In a double-blind, placebo-controlled RCT, 105 pregnant women from families with at least one member (mother, father, or child) with an atopic disease were randomly assigned to receive the probiotic *Lactobacillus* GG or placebo.[154] The supplementation period started 4 to 6 weeks before expected delivery and was followed by a postnatal period of 6 months. The primary outcome was the occurrence of atopic dermatitis at the age of 2 years. Secondary outcomes included severity of atopic dermatitis, recurrent episodes of wheezing bronchitis, and allergic sensitization at the age of 2 years. Ninety-four families (89.5%) completed the trial. Atopic dermatitis was diagnosed in 14 of 50 (28%) in the *Lactobacillus* GG group and in 12 of 44 (27.3%) in the placebo group. The risk of atopic dermatitis in children on probiotics relative to placebo was 0.96 (95% CI, 0.38 to 2.33). The severity of atopic dermatitis was comparable between the two groups. Children with recurrent (≥5) episodes of wheezing bronchitis were more frequent in the *Lactobacillus* GG group (26%; $n = 13$) than in the placebo group (9.1%; $n = 4$).[154]

Similar concerns were reported by Taylor and coworkers (2007).[155] In their placebo-controlled trial, early probiotic supplementation with *Lactobacillus acidophilus* did not reduce the risk of atopic dermatitis in high-risk infants and was associated with increased allergen sensitization in infants receiving supplements. The presence of culturable *Lactobacillus* or *Bifidobacterium* in stools in the first month of life was not associated with risk of subsequent sensitization or disease; however, the presence of *Lactobacillus* at 6 months of age was associated with increased risk of subsequent cow's milk sensitization ($P = 0.012$).[155] The long-term significance of the increased rate of sensitization following probiotic supplementation needs to be investigated in further studies. Taylor and associates (2006) also studied whether probiotic supplementation in the first 6 months of life could modify allergen- and vaccine-specific immune responses.[156] Pregnant women ($n = 231$) with a history of allergic disease and positive allergen skin prick tests were recruited into an RCT. Their infants received a probiotic (3×10^9 *L. acidophilus*) or placebo daily for the first 6 months of life, given independent of feeding methods; 178 children completed the study. Those who received the probiotic showed reduced production of IL-5 and TGF-β in response to polyclonal stimulation ($P = 0.044$ and 0.015, respectively), and a significantly lower IL-10 response to tetanus toxoid (TT) vaccine antigen compared with the placebo group ($P = 0.03$); this was not due to any differences in vaccination. No significant effects of probiotics on type 1 (Th1) or type 2 (Th2) T helper cell responses to allergens or other stimuli were noted. Overall, although there was no consistent effect on allergen-specific responses, results suggest that probiotics may have immunomodulatory effects on vaccine responses.[156]

Practical Issues

Dealing with the difficulties associated with accessing a probiotic product suitable for preterm neonates, which is approved by the regulatory agencies, and ensuring its quality is an important practical issue. Probiotics are registered in many countries as food supplements that are generally considered as safe. Regulatory hurdles in accessing probiotics will be very significant in countries where probiotics ("intended to use to diagnose, cure, mitigate, treat, or prevent disease and affecting structure or function of the body") are registered as drugs rather than food supplements.[157,158] Substantial delay in access to probiotics is inevitable in such countries if phase I, II, and III studies are to be conducted before probiotics can be made easily available.[159,160] Registering them as food supplements may improve access to probiotics, but the poor track record of commercially available probiotic products confirms the consequences of lack of quality control. Defining probiotics as "Foods for Specialized Health Use" (FOSHU), as was done in Japan, may overcome these difficulties.[161,162] Collaboration between all stakeholders is necessary to improve access and to ensure quality of probiotic products. Practical aspects such as tolerance (volume, osmotic load) and safety (probiotic sepsis in the presence of compromised gut integrity) of probiotic supplementation in extremely preterm neonates and those with intrauterine growth restriction are also important. The risk of probiotic sepsis may be higher in conditions associated with compromised gut integrity such as sepsis and NEC. In light of the difficulty involved in differentiating clinical manifestations of ileus of prematurity from those of early stages of sepsis and/or NEC, stopping supplementation may be done in the best interest of the neonate in such situations. Given their thermal sensitivity, the stability of probiotic strains during transport and with storage under fluctuating environmental temperatures needs to be considered. Advances in technology may overcome such issues in the near future.

In summary, current evidence indicates that probiotics significantly reduce the risks of NEC and all-cause mortality in preterm VLBW neonates with no adverse effects. The future of probiotic supplementation for prevention of NEC in preterm neonates depends on interpretation of current evidence by the scientific community. In our opinion, the evidence justifies routine provision of probiotics in this high-risk population if a safe and effective product is available. Provision as a routine, but still as part of continued research, is most appropriate to deal with the unaddressed issues. Most of these can be addressed by studies not involving a placebo arm. Long-term follow-up is essential in light of the potential adverse effects of probiotics in this high-risk population. Continuing research to understand the pathogenesis of NEC is equally important. Given its multifactorial nature, a combination of potentially useful strategies (antenatal glucocorticoids, early preferential feeding with breast milk, prevention and management of sepsis, a cautious approach to enteral feeds, and probiotic supplementation) is the most appropriate approach to the prevention of NEC.

References

1. Lin PW, Stoll BJ. Necrotising enterocolitis. *Lancet*. 2006;368:1271-1283.
2. Stoll BJ. Epidemiology of necrotizing enterocolitis. *Clin Perinatol*. 1994;21:205-218.
3. Wales PW, Christison-Lagay ER. Short bowel syndrome: Epidemiology and etiology. *Semin Pediatr Surg*. 2010;19:3-9.
4. Guarino SG. Neonatal onset intestinal failure: An Italian multicenter study. *J Pediatr*. 2008;153: e674-e676.
5. Rowe MI, Reblock KK, Kurkchubasche AG, et al. Necrotizing enterocolitis in the extremely low birth weight infant. *J Pediatr Surg*. 1994;29:987-990; discussion 990-991.
6. Luig M, Lui K; NSW and ACT NICUS Group. Epidemiology of necrotizing enterocolitis. Part I: Changing regional trends in extremely preterm infants over 14 years. *J Paediatr Child Health*. 2005;41:169-173.

7. Luig M, Lui K, NSW and ACT NICUS Group. Epidemiology of necrotizing enterocolitis. Part II: Risks and susceptibility of premature infants during the surfactant era: A regional study. *J Paediatr Child Health*. 2005;41:174-179.

8. Blakely ML, Lally KP, McDonald S, et al. Postoperative outcomes of extremely low birth-weight infants with necrotizing enterocolitis or isolated intestinal perforation: A prospective cohort study by the NICHD Neonatal Research Network. *Ann Surg*. 2005;241:984-989; discussion 989-994.

9. Wu CH, Tsao PN, Chou HC, et al. Necrotizing enterocolitis complicated with perforation in extremely low birth-weight premature infants. *Acta Paediatr Taiwan*. 2002;43:127-132.

10. Chandler JC, Hebra A. Necrotizing enterocolitis in infants with very low birth weight. *Semin Pediatr Surg*. 2000;9:63-72.

11. Schwartz MZ. Necrotizing enterocolitis. In: O'Neill JA, Grosfeld JL, Fonkalsrud EW, Coran AG, Caldamone AA, eds. *Principles of Pediatric Surgery*. St Louis, Mo: Mosby; 2004:509-517.

12. Hintz S, Kendrick D, Stoll B, et al. Neurodevelopmental and growth outcomes of extremely low birth weight infants after necrotizing enterocolitis. *Pediatrics*. 2005;115:696-703.

13. Schulzke SM, Deshpande GC, Patole SK. Neurodevelopmental outcome of very low birth weight infants with necrotizing enterocolitis: A systematic review of observational studies. *Arch Pediatr Adolesc Med*. 2007;161:583-590.

14. Catlin A. Extremely long hospitalizations of newborns in the United States: Data, descriptions, dilemmas. *J Perinatol*. 2006;26:742-748.

15. Holman RC, Stoll BJ, Curns AT, et al. Necrotising enterocolitis hospitalisations among neonates in the United States. *Paediatr Perinat Epidemiol*. 2006;20:498-506.

16. Cotten CM, Oh W, McDonald S. Prolonged hospital stay for extremely premature infants: Risk factors, center differences, and the impact of mortality on selecting a best-performing center. *J Perinatol*. 2005;25:650-655.

17. Guthrie SO, Gordon PV, Thomas V, et al. Necrotizing enterocolitis among neonates in the United States. *J Perinatol*. 2003;23:278-285.

18. Bisquera JA, Cooper TR, Berseth CL. Impact of necrotizing enterocolitis on length of stay and hospital charges in very low birth weight infants. *Pediatrics*. 2002;109:423-428.

19. Caplan MS. Necrotising Enterocolitis. In: Martin RJ, Fanaroff AA, Walsh MC, eds. *Fanaroff and Martin's Neonatal Perinatal Medicine, Diseases of the Fetus and Infant*. 8th ed. Philadelphia: Elsevier Mosby; 2006:1403-1417.

20. Hsueh W, Caplan MS, Qu XW, et al. Neonatal necrotizing enterocolitis: Clinical considerations and pathogenetic concepts. *Pediatr Dev Pathol*. 2003;6:6-23.

21. Morecroft JA, Spitz L, Hamilton PA, et al. Plasma cytokine levels in necrotizing enterocolitis. *Acta Paediatr Suppl*. 1994;396:18-20.

22. Drenckpohl D. Risk factors that may predispose premature infants to increased incidence of necrotizing enterocolitis. *ICAN: Infant, Child & Adolescent Nutrition*. 2010;2:37-44.

23. Jaattela M. Biologic activities and mechanisms of action of tumor necrosis factor-alpha/cachectin. *Lab Invest*. 1991;64:724-742.

24. Vilcek J, Lee TH. Tumor necrosis factor. New insights into the molecular mechanisms of its multiple actions. *J Biol Chem*. 1991;266:7313-7316.

25. Camussi G, Bussolino F, Salvidio G, et al. Tumor necrosis factor/cachectin stimulates peritoneal macrophages, polymorphonuclear neutrophils, and vascular endothelial cells to synthesize and release platelet-activating factor. *J Exp Med*. 1987;166:1390-1404.

26. Hsueh W, Caplan MS, Sun X, et al. Platelet-activating factor, tumor necrosis factor, hypoxia and necrotizing enterocolitis. *Acta Paediatr Suppl*. 1994;396:11-17.

27. Deitch EA. Role of bacterial translocation in necrotizing enterocolitis. *Acta Paediatr*. 1994;83:33-36.

28. Israel EJ. Neonatal necrotizing enterocolitis, a disease of the immature intestinal mucosal barrier. *Acta Paediatr Suppl*. 1994;396:27-32.

29. Emami CN, Petrosyan M, Giuliani S, et al. Role of the host defense system and intestinal microbial flora in the pathogenesis of necrotizing enterocolitis. *Surg Infect (Larchmt)*. 2009;10:407-417.

30. Hurley BP, McCormick BA. Intestinal epithelial defence systems protect against bacterial threats. *Curr Gastroenterol Rep*. 2004;6:355-361.

31. Taupin D, Podolsky DK. (2003) Trefoil factors: Initiators of mucosal healing. *Nature Rev Mol Cell Biol*. 2003;4:721-734.

32. Shi L, Zhang BH, Yu HG, et al. Intestinal trefoil factor in treatment of neonatal necrotizing enterocolitis in the rat model. *Perinat Med*. 2007;35:443-446.

33. Vieten D, Anthony Corfield A, Carroll D, et al. Impaired mucosal regeneration in neonatal necrotising enterocolitis. *Pediatr Surg Int*. 2005;21:153-160.

34. Leaphart CL, Cavallo J, Gribar SC, et al. A critical role for TLR4 in the pathogenesis of necrotizing enterocolitis by modulating intestinal injury and repair. *J Immunol* 2007, 179; 4808-4820.

35. Neu J. Necrotising enterocolitis. The search for a unifying pathogenic theory leading to prevention. *Pediatr Clin North Am*. 1996;43: 409-432.

36. Patole S. Prevention and treatment of necrotising enterocolitis in preterm neonates. *Early Hum Dev*. 2007;83: 635-642.

37. Björkström MV, Hall L, Söderlund S, et al. Intestinal flora in very low-birth weight infants. *Acta Paediatr*. 2009;98:1762-1767.

38. Schwiertz A, Gruhl B, Löbnitz M, et al. Development of the intestinal bacterial composition in hospitalized preterm infants in comparison with breast-fed, full-term infants. *Pediatr Res*. 2003;54: 393-399.

14

39. Magne F, Abély M, Boyer F, et al. Low species diversity and high interindividual variability in faeces of preterm infants as revealed by sequences of 16S rRNA genes and PCR-temporal temperature gradient gel electrophoresis profiles. *FEMS Microbiol Ecol.* 2006;57:128-138.

40. Butel MJ, Suau A, Campeotto F, et al. Conditions of bifidobacterial colonization in preterm infants: A prospective analysis. *J Pediatr Gastroenterol Nutr.* 2007;44:577-582.

41. Biasucci G, Rubini M, Riboni S, et al. Mode of delivery affects the bacterial community in the newborn gut. *Early Hum Dev.* 2010;86:13-15.

42. Huurre A, Kalliomäki M, Rautava S, et al. Mode of delivery: Effects on gut microbiota and humoral immunity. *Neonatology.* 2008;93:236-240.

43. Hällström M, Eerola E, Vuento R, et al. Effects of mode of delivery and necrotising enterocolitis on the intestinal microflora in preterm infants. *Eur J Clin Microbiol Infect Dis.* 2004;23:463-470.

44. Biasucci G, Benenati B, Morelli L, et al. Cesarean delivery may affect the early biodiversity of intestinal bacteria. *J Nutr.* 2008;138:1796S-1800S.

45. de la Cochetiere MF, Piloquet H, des Robert C, et al. Early intestinal bacterial colonization and necrotizing enterocolitis in premature infants: The putative role of Clostridium. *Pediatr Res.* 2004;56:366-370.

46. Claud EC, Walker WA. Bacterial colonization, probiotics, and necrotizing enterocolitis. *J Clin Gastroenterol.* 2008;42:S46-S52.

47. Martin CR, Walker WA. Probiotics: Role in pathophysiology and prevention in necrotizing enterocolitis. *Semin Perinatol.* 2008;32:127-137.

48. Food and Agriculture Organization of the United Nations (FAO). *Health and Nutritional Properties of Probiotics in Food including Powder Milk with Live Lactic Acid Bacteria.* Rome, Italy: FAO; 2001.

49. Thorpe TE. *A dictionary of applied chemistry, Volume 3.* New York: Longmans, Green and Co.; 1922:159.

50. Genesis 18:8. Scripture quotations taken from the Holy Bible, New International Version, Copyright 1973, 1978, 1984 by International Bible Society, used by permission as checked by a Theologian.

51. Thurmond D. A Handbook of Food Processing in Classical Rome 2006, Brill Leiden, Boston: 193.

52. Metchnikoff E. Études sur la flore intestinale. *Ann Inst Pasteur Paris.* 1908;22:929-955.

53. Renneberg R. Beer, Bread and Cheese—The Tasty Side of Biotechnology. In: Demain A, ed. *Biotechnology for Beginners.* 1st ed. London: Elsevier; 2007:25.

54. Lister J. On the lactic fermentation and its bearing on pathology. *Trans Pathol Soc Lond.* 1878;29:425-467.

55. Tissier H. Recherches sur la flore intestinale des nourrissons (etat normal et pathologique) Paris. *Thèses.* 1900:1-253.

56. Shirota M, Aso K, Iwabuchi A. Study on microflora of human intestine. Alteration of the constitution of intestinal flora by oral administration of L. acidophilus strain Shirota to healthy infants. *Jpn J Bacteriol.* 1966;21:274-283.

57. Lilly DM, Stillwell RH. Probiotics: Growth-promoting factors produced by microorganisms. *Science.* 1965;147:747-748.

58. Parker RB. Probiotics, the other half of the antibiotic story. *Anim Nutr Health.* 1974;29:4-8.

59. Fuller R. A review: Probiotics in man and animals. *J Appl Bacteriol.* 1989;66:365-378.

60. Salminen S, von Wright A, Morelli L, et al. Demonstration of safety of probiotics—a review. *Int J Food Microbiol.* 1998;44:93-106.

61. The Global Probiotic Council. http://www.probioticsresearch.com/gpcouncil.asp accessed 03.10.10

62. Servin AL. Antagonistic activities of lactobacilli and bifidobacteria against microbial pathogens. *FEMS Microbiol Rev.* 2004;28:405-440.

63. Lawton EM, Ross RP, Hill C, et al. Two-peptide lantibiotics: A medical perspective. *Mini Rev Med Chem.* 2007;7:1236-1247.

64. Vanderpool C, Yan F, Polk D. Mechanisms of probiotic action: Implications for therapeutic applications in inflammatory bowel diseases. *Inflamm Bowel Dis.* 2008;14:1585-1596.

65. Makras L, Triantafyllou V, Fayol-Messaoudi D, et al. Kinetic analysis of the antibacterial activity of probiotic lactobacilli towards Salmonella enterica serovar Typhimurium reveals a role for lactic acid and other inhibitory compounds. *Res Microbiol.* 2006;157:241-247.

66. De Keersmaecker SC, Verhoeven TL, Desair J, et al. Strong antimicrobial activity of Lactobacillus rhamnosus GG against Salmonella typhimurium is due to accumulation of lactic acid. *FEMS Microbiol Lett.* 2006;259:89-96.

67. Gotteland M, Brunser O, Cruchet S. Systematic review: Are probiotics useful in controlling gastric colonization by Helicobacter pylori? *Aliment Pharmacol Ther.* 2006;23:1077-1086.

68. Mack DR, Michail S, Wei S, et al. Probiotics inhibit enteropathogenic E. coli adherence in vitro by inducing intestinal mucin gene expression. *Am J Physiol.* 1999;276:G941-G950.

69. Deplancke B, Gaskins HR. Microbial modulation of innate defense: Goblet cells and the intestinal mucus layer. *Am J Clin Nutr.* 2001;73:1131S-1141S.

70. Yu Q-H, Yang Q. Diversity of tight junctions (TJs) between gastrointestinal epithelial cells and their function in maintaining the mucosal barrier. *Cell Biology International.* 2009;33:e78-e82.

71. Madsen K, Cornish A, Soper P, et al. Probiotic bacteria enhance murine and human intestinal epithelial barrier function. *Gastroenterology.* 2001;121:580-591.

72. Kennedy RJ, Kirk SJ, Gardiner KR. Mucosal barrier function and the commensal flora. *Gut.* 2002;50:441-442.

73. Clayburgh DR, Shen L, Turner JR. A porous defense: The leaky epithelial barrier in intestinal disease. *Lab Invest.* 2004;84:282-291.

74. Collado MC, Meriluoto J, Salminen S. Role of commercial probiotic strains against human pathogen adhesion to intestinal mucus. *Lett Appl Microbiol.* 2007;45:454-460.

75. Candela M, Seibold G, Vitali B, et al. Real-time PCR quantification of bacterial adhesion to Caco-2 cells: Competition between bifidobacteria and enteropathogens. *Res Microbiol.* 2005;156:887-895.

76. Roselli M, Finamore A, Britti MS, et al. Probiotic bacteria Bifidobacterium animalis MB5 and Lactobacillus rhamnosus GG protect intestinal Caco-2 cells from the inflammation: Associated response induced by enterotoxigenic Escherichia coli K88. *Br J Nutr.* 2006;95:1177-1184.

77. Zyrek AA, Cichon C, Helms S, et al. Molecular mechanisms underlying the probiotic effects of Escherichia coli Nissie 1917 involve ZO-2 and PKCzeta redistribution resulting in tight junction and epithelial barrier repair. *Cell Microbiol.* 2007;9:804-816.

78. McCormick BA, Parkos CA, Colgan SP, et al. Apical secretion of a pathogen-elicited epithelial chemoattractant activity in response to surface colonization of intestinal epithelia by Samonella typhimurium. *J Immunol.* 1998;160:455-466.

79. Boirivant M, Strober W. The mechanism of action of probiotics. *Curr Opin Gastroenterol.* 2007;23:679-692.

80. Abreu MT, Fukata M, Arditi M. TLR signalling in the gut in health and disease. *J Immunol.* 2005;174:4453-4460.

81. Claud EC. Neonatal necrotizing enterocolitis: Inflammation and intestinal immaturity. *Antiinflamm Antiallergy Agents Med Chem.* 2009;8:248-259.

82. Pagnini C, Saeed R, Bamias G, et al. Probiotics promote gut health through stimulation of epithelial innate immunity. *Proc Natl Acad Sci USA.* 2010;107:454-459.

83. Rakoff-Nahoum S, Paglino J, Eslami-Varzaneh F, et al. Recognition of commensal microflora by toll-like receptors is required for intestinal homeostasis. *Cell.* 2004;118:229-241.

84. Ewaschuk JB, Blacker JL, Churchill TA, et al. Surface expression of Toll-like receptor 9 is upregulated on intestinal epithelial cells in response to pathogenic bacterial DNA. *Infect Immun.* 2007;75:2572-2579.

85. Veckman V, Miettinen M, Pirhonen J, et al. Streptococcus pyogenes and Lactobacillus rhamnosus differentially induce maturation and production of TH1-type cytokines and chemokines in human monocyte-derived dendritic cells. *J Leukoc Biol.* 2004;75:764-771.

86. Lavasani S, Dzhambazov B, Nouri M, et al. A novel probiotic mixture exerts a therapeutic effect on experimental autoimmune encephalomyelitis mediated by IL-10 producing regulatory T cells. *PLoS One.* 2010;5:e9009.

87. O'Donovan DJ, Fernandes CJ. Free radicals and diseases in premature infants. *Antioxid Redox Signal.* 2004;6:169-176.

88. Baker RD, Baker SS, LaRosa K. Polarized Caco-2 cells. Effect of reactive oxygen metabolites on enterocyte barrier function. *Dig Dis Sci.* 1995;40:510-518.

89. Clark DA, Fornabaio DM, McNeill H, et al. Contribution of oxygen-derived free radicals to experimental necrotizing enterocolitis. *Am J Pathol.* 1988;130:537-542.

90. Rogers S, Witz G, Anwar M, et al. Antioxidant capacity and oxygen radical diseases in the preterm newborn. *Arch Pediatr Adolesc Med.* 2000;154:544-548.

91. Viña J, Vento M, García-Sala F, et al. L-cysteine and glutathione metabolism are impaired in premature infants due to cystathionase deficiency. *Am J Clin Nutr.* 1995;61(5):1067-1069. Erratum in: *Am J Clin Nutr.* 2009;89:1951.

92. Sheth PS, Basuroy S, Li C, et al. Role of phosphatidylinositol 3-kinase in oxidative stress-induced disruption of tight junctions. *J Biol Chem.* 2003;278:49239-49245.

93. Rao RK, Polk DB, Seth A, et al. Probiotics the good neighbour: Guarding the gut mucosal barrier. *Am J Infect Dis.* 2009;5:188-192.

94. Spyropoulos B, Misiakos E, Fotiadis C, et al. Antioxidant properties of probiotics and their protective effects in the pathogenesis of radiation-induced enteritis and colitis. *Dig Dis Sci* 2011;56:285-294.

95. Indrio F, Riezzo G, Raimondi F, et al. Effect of probiotic and prebiotic on gastrointestinal motility in newborns. *J Physiol Pharmacol.* 2009;60:S27-S31.

96. Indrio F, Riezzo G, Raimondi F, et al. The effects of probiotics on feeding tolerance, bowel habits, and gastrointestinal motility in preterm newborns. *J Pediatr.* 2008;152:801-806.

97. Hoyos AB. Reduced incidence of necrotising enterocolitis associated with enteral administration of Lactobacillus acidophilus and Bifidobacterium infantis to neonates in an intensive care unit. *Int J Infect Dis.* 1999;3:197-202.

98. Kitajima H, Sumida Y, Tanaka R, et al. Early administration of Bifidobacterium breve to preterm neonates: Randomised control trial. *Arch Dis Child.* 1997;76:F101-F107.

99. Dani C, Biadaioli R, Bertini G, et al. Probiotics feeding in prevention of urinary tract infection, bacterial sepsis and necrotizing enterocolitis in preterm neonates. A prospective double-blind study. *Biol Neonate.* 2002;82:103-108.

100. Costalos C, Skouteri V, Gounaris A, et al. Enteral feeding of premature neonates with Saccharomyces boulardii. *Early Hum Dev.* 2003;74:89-96.

101. Bin-Nun A, Bromiker R, Wilschanski M, et al. Oral probiotics prevent necrotizing enterocolitis in very low birth weight neonates. *J Pediatr.* 2005;147:192-196.

102. Lin HC, Su BH, Chen AC, et al. Oral probiotics reduce the incidence and severity of necrotizing enterocolitis in very low birth weight neonates. *Pediatrics.* 2005;115:1-4.

103. Manzoni P, Mostert M, Leonessa ML, et al. Oral supplementation with Lactobacillus casei Subspecies rhamnosus prevents enteric colonisation by candida species in preterm neonates: A randomised study. *Clin Infect Dis.* 2006;42: 1735-1742.

14

104. Mohan R, Koebnick C, Schildt J, et al. Effects of Bifidobacterium lactis Bb12 supplementation on intestinal microbiota of preterm neonates: A double placebo controlled, randomised study. *J Clin Microbiol.* 2006;44:4025-4031.

105. Stratiki Z, Costalos C, Sevastiadou S, et al. The effect of a bifidobacteria supplemented bovine milk on intestinal permeability of preterm infants. *Early Hum Dev.* 2007;83:575-579.

106. Lin HC, Hsu CH, Chen HL, et al. Oral probiotics prevent necrotizing enterocolitis in very low birth weight preterm infants: A multicenter, randomized, controlled trial. *Pediatrics.* 2008;122:693-700.

107. Samanta M, Sarkar M, Ghosh P, et al. Prophylactic probiotics for prevention of necrotizing enterocolitis in very low birth weight newborns. *J Trop Pediatr.* 2009;55:128-1231.

108. Rougé C, Piloquet H, Butel MJ, et al. Oral supplementation with probiotics in very-low-birth-weight preterm infants: A randomized, double-blind, placebo-controlled trial. *Am J Clin Nutr.* 2009;89: 1828-1835.

109. Mihatsch WA, Vossbeck S, Eikmanns B, et al. Effect of Bifidobacterium lactis on the incidence of nosocomial infections in very-low-birth-weight infants: A randomized controlled trial. *Neonatology.* 2010;98:156-163.

110. Braga TD, da Silva GA, de Lira PI, et al. Efficacy of Bifidobacterium breve and Lactobacillus casei oral supplementation on necrotizing enterocolitis in very-low-birth-weight preterm infants: A double-blind, randomized, controlled trial. *J Clin Nutr* 2010 Oct 27. [Epub ahead of print]

111. Deshpande G, Rao S, Patole S. Probiotics for prevention of necrotising enterocolitis in preterm neonates with very low birthweight: A systematic review of randomised controlled trials. *Lancet.* 2007;369:1614-1620.

112. Alfaleh K, Bassler D. Probiotics for prevention of necrotizing enterocolitis in preterm infants. *Cochrane Database Syst Rev.* 2008;1:CD005496.

113. Barclay AR, Stenson B, Simpson JH, et al. Probiotics for necrotizing enterocolitis: A systematic review. *J Pediatr Gastroenterol Nutr.* 2007;45:569-576.

114. Deshpande G, Rao S, Patole S, et al. Updated meta-analysis of probiotics for preventing necrotizing enterocolitis in preterm neonates. *Pediatrics.* 2010;125:921-930.

115. Soll RF. Probiotics: Are we ready for routine use? *Pediatrics.* 2010;125:1071-1072.

116. Neu J, Shuster J. Nonadministration of routine probiotics unethical-really? *Pediatrics.* 2010;126: e740-e741.

117. Garland SM, Jacobs SE, Tobin JM, et al. A cautionary note on instituting probiotics into routine clinical care for premature infants. *Pediatrics.* 2010;126:e741-e742.

118. Beattie LM, Hansen R, Barclay A. Probiotics for preterm infants: Confounding features warrant caution. *Pediatrics.* 2010;126:e742-e743.

119. Millar M, Wilks M, Fleming P, et al. Should the use of probiotics in the preterm be routine? *Arch Dis Child Fetal Neonatal Ed* 2010 Sep 24. [Epub ahead of print]

120. Deshpande G, Rao S, Patole S, et al. Probiotics for preterm neonates—time to acknowledge the elephant in the room and call the parents. *Pediatrics.* 2010;126:e744-e745.

121. Chou IC, Kuo HT, Chang JS, et al. Lack of effects of oral probiotics on growth and neurodevelopmental outcomes in preterm very low birth weight infants. *J Pediatr.* 2010;156:393-396.

122. Romeo MG, Romeo DM, Trovato L et al. Role of probiotics in the prevention of the enteric colonization by Candida in preterm newborns: Incidence of late-onset sepsis and neurological outcome. *J Perinatol* 31:63-69, 2011.

123. Satoh Y, Shinohara K, Umezaki H, et al. Bifidobacteria prevents necrotising enterocolitis and infection. *Int J Probiot Prebiot.* 2007;2:149-154.

124. Manzoni P, Lista G, Gallo E, et al. Routinary Lactobacillus rhamnosus GG administration in preterm VLBW neonates: A retrospective, 6-Year cohort study from two large tertiary NICUs in Italy E-PAS2009: 2839. Proceedings of PAS/SPR; May 2–5, 2009; Baltimore, MD (Abstract 2839.366)

125. Luoto R, Isolauri E, Lehtonen L. Safety of Lactobacillus GG probiotic in infants with very low birth weight: Twelve years of experience. *Clin Infect Dis.* 2010;50:1327-1378.

126. Newborn. Probiotics for prevention of necrotising enterocolitis in preterm neonates with very low birthweight: A systematic review of randomised controlled trials. In: Stockman JA III, ed. *Yearbook of Pediatrics.* Philadelphia: Elsevier Mosby; 2009:441-443.

127. Tarnow-Mordi WO, Wilkinson D, Trivedi A, et al. Probiotics reduce all-cause mortality and necrotizing enterocolitis: It is time to change practice. *Pediatrics.* 2010;125: 1068-1070.

128. Khailova L, Dvorak K, Arganbright KM, et al. Bifidobacterium bifidum improves intestinal integrity in a rat model of necrotizing enterocolitis. *Am J Physiol Gastrointest Liver Physiol.* 2009;297: G940-G949.

129. Agrawal R, Sharma N, Chaudry R, et al. Effects of oral Lactobacillus GG on enteric microflora in low birth weight neonates. *J Pediatr Gastroenterol Nutr.* 2003;36:397-402.

130. Reuman PD, Duckworth DH, Smith KL, et al. Lack of effect of lactobacillus on gastrointestinal bacterial colonisation in premature neonates. *Pediatr Infect Dis.* 1986;5:663-668.

131. Olivares M, Díaz-Ropero MP, Martín R, et al. Antimicrobial potential of four Lactobacillus strains isolated from breast milk. *J Appl Microbiol.* 2006;101:72-79.

132. Martin R, Olivares M, Marin ML, et al. Probiotic potential of 3 Lactobacilli strains isolated from breast milk. *J Hum Lact.* 2005;21:8-17.

133. Boehm G. Oligosaccharides in milk. *J Nutr.* 2007;137:S847-S849.

134. Su P, Henriksson A, Mitchell H. Prebiotics enhance survival and prolong the retention period of specific probiotic inocula in an in vivo murine model. *J Appl Microbiol.* 2007;103:2392-2400.

135. Panigrahi P, Parida S, Pradhan L, et al. Long-term colonization of a Lactobacillus plantarum synbiotic preparation in the neonatal gut. *J Pediatr Gastroenterol Nutr.* 2008;47:45-53.

14

136. Kataria J, Li N, Wynn JL, Neu J. Probiotic microbes: Do they need to be alive to be beneficial? *Nutr Rev*. 2009;67:546-550.
137. Li N, Russell WM, Douglas-Escobar M, et al. Live and heat-killed Lactobacillus rhamnosus GG: Effects on proinflammatory and anti-inflammatory cytokines/chemokines in gastrostomy-fed infant rats. *Pediatr Res*. 2009;66:203-207.
138. Adams CA. The probiotic paradox: Live and dead cells are biological response modifiers. *Nutr Res Rev*. 2010;23:37-46.
139. Awad H, Mokhtar H, Imam SS, et al. Comparison between killed and living probiotic usage versus placebo for the prevention of necrotizing enterocolitis and sepsis in neonates. *Pak J Biol Sci*. 2010; 13:253-262.
140. Pereira-da-Silva L, Henriques G, Videira-Amaral JM, et al. Osmolality of solutions, emulsions and drugs that may have a high osmolality: Aspects of their use in neonatal care. *J Matern Fetal Neonatal Med*. 2002;11:333-338.
141. Thompson C, McCarter YS, Krause PJ, et al. Lactobacillus acidophilus sepsis in a neonate. *J Perinatol*. 2001;21:258-260.
142. Broughton RA, Gruber WC, Haffar AA, et al. Neonatal meningitis due to lactobacillus. *Pediatr Infect Dis*. 1983;2:382-384.
143. Perapoch J, Planes AM, Querol A, et al. Fungemia with Saccharomyces cerevisiae in two newborns, only one of whom had been treated with ultra-levure. *Eur J Clin Microbiol Infect Dis*. 2000;19: 468-470.
144. Ohishi A, Takahashi S, Ito Y, et al. Bifidobacterium septicemia associated with postoperative probiotic therapy in a neonate with omphalocele. *J Pediatr*. 2010;156:679-681.
145. Egervärn M, Lindmark H, Olsson J, et al. Transferability of a tetracycline resistance gene from probiotic Lactobacillus reuteri to bacteria in the gastrointestinal tract of humans. *Antonie Van Leeuwenhoek*. 2010;97:189-200.
146. Egervärn M, Roos S, Lindmark H. Identification and characterization of antibiotic resistance genes in Lactobacillus reuteri and Lactobacillus plantarum. *J Appl Microbiol*. 2009;107:1658-1668.
147. Liu C, Zhang ZY, Dong K, et al. Antibiotic resistance of probiotic strains of lactic acid bacteria isolated from marketed foods and drugs. *Biomed Environ Sci*. 2009;22:401-412.
148. Toomey N, Monaghan A, Fanning S, et al. Transfer of antibiotic resistance marker genes between lactic acid bacteria in model rumen and plant environments. *Appl Environ Microbiol*. 2009; 75:3146-3152.
149. Hammad AM, Shimamoto T. Towards a compatible probiotic-antibiotic combination therapy: Assessment of antimicrobial resistance in the Japanese probiotics. *J Appl Microbiol*. 2010;109: 1349-1360.
150. Xiao JZ, Takahashi S, Odamaki T, et al. Antibiotic susceptibility of bifidobacterial strains distributed in the Japanese market. *Biosci Biotechnol Biochem*. 2010;74:336-342.
151. Rosander A, Connolly E, Roos S. Removal of antibiotic resistance gene-carrying plasmids from Lactobacillus reuteri ATCC 55730 and characterization of the resulting daughter strain, L. reuteri DSM 17938. *Appl Environ Microbiol*. 2008;74:6032-6040.
152. Rada V, Splichal I, Rockova S, et al. Susceptibility of bifidobacteria to lysozyme as a possible selection criterion for probiotic bifidobacterial strains. *Biotechnol Lett*. 2010;32:451-455.
153. Costeloe K. PiPS: trial of probiotic administered early to prevent infection and necrotising enterocolitis protocol, version 3.1. Available at: www.hta.ac.uk/protocols/200505010004.pdf. Accessed October 20, 2010.
154. Kopp MV, Hennemuth I, Heinzmann A, et al. Randomized, double-blind, placebo-controlled trial of probiotics for primary prevention: No clinical effects of Lactobacillus GG supplementation. *Pediatrics*. 2008;121:e850-e856.
155. Taylor AL, Dunstan JA, Prescott SL. Probiotic supplementation for the first 6 months of life fails to reduce the risk of atopic dermatitis and increases the risk of allergen sensitization in high-risk children: A randomized controlled trial. *Allergy Clin Immunol*. 2007;119:184-191.
156. Taylor AL, Hale J, Wiltschut J, et al. Effects of probiotic supplementation for the first 6 months of life on allergen- and vaccine-specific immune responses. *Clin Exp Allergy*. 2006;36:1227-1235.
157. Hoffman FA. Development of probiotics as biologic drugs. *Clin Infect Dis*. 2008;46:S125-S127, discussion: 144-151.
158. Degnan FH. The US Food and Drug Administration and probiotics: Regulatory categorization. *Clin Infect Dis*. 2008;46:S133-S136; Discussion: S144-S151.
159. Hibberd PL, Davidson L. Probiotic foods and drugs: Impact of US regulatory status on design of clinical trials. *Clin Infect Dis*. 2008;46:S137-S140; discussion S144-151.
160. Henriksson A, Borody T, Clancy R. Probiotics under the regulatory microscope. *Expert Opin Drug Saf*. 2005;4:1135-1143.
161. Amagase H. Current marketplace for probiotics: A Japanese perspective. *Clin Infect Dis*. 2008;46:S73-S75; discussion: S144-S151.
162. Tamayo C. Clinical research on probiotics: The interface between science and regulation. *Clin Infect Dis*. 2008;46:S101-S103.

14

CHAPTER 15

The Ureaplasma Conundrum: Should We Look or Ignore?

Robert L. Schelonka, MD; Peta L. Grigsby, PhD;
Victoria H.J. Roberts, PhD; and Cynthia T. McEvoy, MD

15

- Ureaplasmas as Agents of Human Disease
- *Ureaplasma* spp. Are a Cause of Chorioamnionitis and Preterm Birth
- Vertical Transmission of *Ureaplasma* spp.
- *Ureaplasma* spp. and Fetal and Neonatal Sequelae
- Association of *Ureaplasma* spp. With Development of BPD in Preterm Neonates
- Ureaplasma-Mediated Inflammatory Pathways in the Pathogenesis of Perinatal Lung Injury and Subsequent BPD
- *Ureaplasma* spp. in the Pathogenesis of Bronchopulmonary Dysplasia
- Differential Pathogenicity of *Ureaplasma urealyticum* and *Ureaplasma parvum* in BPD
- Inflammatory Pathways in the Pathogenesis of Cerebral White Matter Injury
- Clinical Association of *Ureaplasma* spp. and Neurologic Sequelae in the Neonate
- Animal Models of Cerebral White Matter Injury: Causal Role of *Ureaplasma* spp.
- Interventional Strategies to Prevent Fetal and Neonatal Sequelae
- Future Research Needed for Treatment of *Ureaplasma* spp.–Infected Infants at Risk for Lung and Brain Injury
- Summary

Today, smaller, more immature infants survive owing to advances in supportive care, antenatal steroids, and exogenous surfactant and ventilator strategies.[1] Increased survival of these vulnerable newborns results in a greater number of infants at risk for morbidity from conditions such as bronchopulmonary dysplasia (BPD) and neurosensory impairment.[2-5] Emerging evidence indicates that intra-amniotic *Ureaplasma* infection may contribute to cerebral white matter injury, as well as to perinatal lung injury; this infection could be a common thread between BPD and neurodevelopmental disability. This review will cover the most recent information on the role of *Ureaplasma* spp. as neonatal pathogens, and will offer insights for clinicians deliberating these organisms as agents of disease and approaching diagnosis and treatment.

Ureaplasmas as Agents of Human Disease

Ureaplasmas and mycoplasmas are eubacteria belonging to the Class Mollicutes. These organisms are unique in that they lack cell walls and are believed to be the smallest and simplest free-living and self-replicating cells.[6] Lack of a rigid cell wall prevents detection by Gram stain, confers a pleomorphic cellular shape, and increases susceptibility to dehydration, limiting these microorganisms to a parasitic existence in association with eukaryotic cells of the host.[7] *Ureaplasma* spp. were first described by Shepard in the 1950s, when they were detected in the urethras of men with urethritis.[8] The genus *Ureaplasma* was designated in view of its use of urea as a metabolic substrate for generation of adenosine triphosphate (ATP). For nearly 30 years, *U. urealyticum* was the only species known to infect humans. However, this species was recently subdivided on the basis of 16S rRNA sequences into two separate species: *U. urealyticum* and *U. parvum*.[7] Fourteen serovars are known; *U. parvum* includes serovars 1, 3, 6, and 14, and *U. urealyticum* includes the remaining 10 serovars—2, 4, 5, 7, 8, 9, 10, 11, 12, and 13. *U. parvum* is isolated more frequently from clinical specimens, although both species may occur simultaneously.[7] Until recently, most clinical studies have not distinguished between *U. urealyticum* and *U. parvum*, because sophisticated nucleic acid amplification tests are necessary to discriminate between the two species.[9,10]

Within a few years following the first descriptions of *Ureaplasma* spp., reports described a possible association of these organisms with adverse pregnancy outcomes and low birth weight in neonates.[11,12] Additional evidence has since accumulated implicating ureaplasmas in a wide array of conditions affecting adult men and women, including infertility, prostatitis, epididymitis, pyelonephritis, cystitis, septic arthritis, subcutaneous abscesses, osteomyelitis, urinary calculi, postpartum endometritis, chorioamnionitis, spontaneous abortion, premature birth, and stillbirth. The body of evidence accumulated since the 1970s strongly points to an important role for ureaplasmas as neonatal pathogens, particularly as mediators of lung disease and other systemic infections.

Ureaplasma spp. Are a Cause of Chorioamnionitis and Preterm Birth

Infection is believed to be a major cause of premature births, especially those occurring before 30 weeks' gestation, and has been the focus of intense investigation in recent years. Uterine contractions may be induced by phospholipases produced by microorganisms, as well as by pro-inflammatory cytokines produced in response to their presence in the amniotic fluid, which in turn trigger prostaglandin synthesis. Isolation of *Ureaplasma* spp. from the chorioamnion has been consistently associated with histologic chorioamnionitis and is inversely related to birth weight, even with adjustments for duration of labor, rupture of fetal membranes, and the presence of other bacteria.[13,14] Ureaplasmas can invade the amniotic fluid early in pregnancy and are the single most common organisms that can be isolated from infected placentas with histologic chorioamnionitis.[13,14] *Ureaplasma* spp. can persist in the amniotic fluid subclinically for up to several weeks, even when fetal membranes are intact, and eventually initiate an intense inflammatory reaction that may or may not be followed by preterm labor.[15-17] *Ureaplasma* spp. can be isolated from the endometrial tissue of healthy, nonpregnant women, indicating that they may be present at the time of implantation and might therefore be involved in early pregnancy losses.[13] One study found that preterm labor and delivery occurred in 58.6% of women who had a positive polymerase chain reaction (PCR) assay for ureaplasmas at 15 to 17 weeks' gestation, but occurred in only 4.4% of women with negative PCR results.[18] In a more recent survey of 1988 singleton pregnancies in Brussels, *Ureaplasma* spp. were detected in 53.6% of patients who delivered before 37 weeks, thus supporting previous studies.[18,19] Logistic regression analyses of demographic and obstetric variables indicate that the presence of *Ureaplasma* alone or with other bacteria in the chorioamnion is independently associated with birth before 37 weeks' gestation, regardless of the duration of labor.[13] The ability of ureaplasmas to invade the amniotic fluid early in gestation and initiate chronic inflammatory processes provides the setting through which they can also produce an intense fetal inflammatory response with increased risk of neonatal sepsis and a higher rate of severe neonatal morbidity.[20-22]

Vertical Transmission of *Ureaplasma* spp.

Evidence of vertical *Ureaplasma* spp. infection comes from observations that urea-plasmas can be isolated from endotracheal secretions in up to 40% of newborn infants within 30 minutes to 24 hours after birth.[23,24] The Alabama Preterm Birth Study[25] reported that 23% of neonates who were born between 23 and 32 weeks' gestation had positive umbilical cord cultures for *U. urealyticum* and/or *Mycoplasma hominis*. These infants had a higher frequency of neonatal sepsis, higher serum interleukin (IL)-6 levels, and more frequent histologic evidence of chorioamnionitis and funisitis than those with negative cultures.[25,26] Infants weighing less than 1000 g appear to be at higher risk of infection when the mother is colonized; the rate of vertical transmission approaches 90% for these infants.[27] The presumed mechanisms of *Ureaplasma* infection include fetal exposure to ascending intra-amniotic infection, passage through an infected birth canal, and hematogenous dissemination through the placenta into umbilical vessels. Ultimately, this exposure leads to colonization of the skin, mucosal membranes, and respiratory tract (via infected amniotic fluid) and sometimes to dissemination into the bloodstream and central nervous system.[7,28-31]

Walsh and associates[32] simulated perinatal vertical transmission by inoculating *U. urealyticum* into the tracheas of prematurely born baboons immediately after hysterotomy delivery. Two of four animals inoculated with *U. urealyticum* developed acute bronchiolitis with epithelial ulceration and neutrophil infiltrates. None of the four control animals (not infected with *U. urealyticum*) developed these lung lesions. Further, *U. urealyticum* were recovered from the trachea, lung, pleural fluid, and blood of infected animals, indicating local and systemic infection with this organism. Yoder and colleagues[33] inoculated the amniotic cavity of 10 pregnant baboons with *U. urealyticum* and then delivered the offspring prematurely. Infant baboons were given comprehensive care that included exogenous surfactant and mechanical ventilation for 14 days. Investigators demonstrated conclusively that vertical transmission can occur in this primate model, and that intra-amniotic exposure to *U. urealyticum* led to elevated tracheal inflammatory cytokines and leukocytes. Histopathologic examination of the lungs in the infected animals showed severe bronchiolitis and interstitial pneumonitis. Animals that remained colonized by *U. urealyticum* in the lower respiratory tract within the first week had greater risk of lung dysfunction and injury than those who eradicated the organisms. Fetal studies in rhesus monkeys support and extend findings in the baboon. Rhesus fetuses infected in utero with *U. parvum* or *M. hominis* demonstrated acute and subacute inflammatory changes in the respiratory tract. With prolonged infection, the acute inflammatory response was partially resolved, but peribronchiolar lymphoid tissue aggregates were conspicuous, as were hyperplastic changes in the overlying epithelium.[34]

Ureaplasma spp. and Fetal and Neonatal Sequelae

Some of the earliest investigations suggestive of a potential role for *Ureaplasma* spp. in neonatal respiratory disease came in the mid-1970s, when Tafari and coworkers[35] described the isolation of these organisms from the lungs of stillborn infants with pneumonitis. Evidence that *Ureaplasma* spp. cause congenital pneumonia includes isolation of the organism in pure culture from amniotic fluid, from the affected lungs of neonates less than 14 hours after birth in the midst of an acute inflammatory response,[28] and from the chorioamnion.[15,16] Further support for the causative role of the ureaplasmas in human disease comes from demonstration of a specific immunoglobulin (Ig)M response in the neonate[36]; radiographic changes indicative of pneumonia in culture-positive infants[37-39]; and demonstration of the organisms in lung tissue by immunofluorescence[40] and electron microscopy.[36] Ureaplasmal bacteremia may accompany severe neonatal pneumonia.[28,41] Accumulating evidence associates the inflammatory cascade induced by *Ureaplasma* spp. colonization of the airways with early dysplastic radiographic changes of the lungs in very low birth weight (VLBW) infants. Crouse and coworkers[37] evaluated the chest radiographs of

15

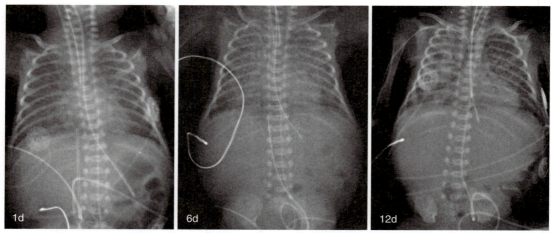

Figure 15-1   Chest radiographs of an infant born at 24 weeks' gestation with *Ureaplasma urealyticum* respiratory tract infection. On day 1, characteristic findings of respiratory distress syndrome (RDS) were noted, and by day 12, early cystic dysplasia was evident. (Reprinted with permission from Schelonka RL, Waites KB. *Ureaplasma* infection and neonatal lung disease. *Semin Perinatol.* 2007;31:2-9.)

44 preterm infants colonized in the lower respiratory tract by *U. urealyticum* in comparison with those who were culture negative and found that pneumonia was twice as common in the ureaplasma-positive group (30% vs. 16%). Precocious dysplastic changes in the lungs within 2 weeks of birth were significantly more common in the ureaplasma-positive group, independent of gestational age, race, and sex.[35] A second cohort study examined 25 ventilated, preterm infants with respiratory tract *U. urealyticum* infection. Although these infants had fewer signs of respiratory distress initially, they were more likely to deteriorate and require later mechanical ventilation.[42] Chest radiographs of ureaplasma-positive infants showed evidence of emphysematous changes as early as 5 days with a pronounced difference by day 10.[40] A subsequent study corroborated the findings in that 9 of 40 (23%) infants with *U. urealyticum* colonization of the airways developed precocious dysplastic radiographic changes as compared with 1 of 42 (2%) who were not *Ureaplasma* colonized.[43] Figure 15-1 demonstrates precocious radiographic evidence of pulmonary dysplasia in an infant who was born at 24 weeks' gestation weighing 585 g at birth. Precocious dysplastic changes on the radiograph prompted an evaluation for ureaplasmal infection at 12 days of age. The infant was found to be culture positive for *U. urealyticum* and then was treated with intravenous azithromycin for 10 days. The classic ground-glass appearance of respiratory distress syndrome was evident on the first postnatal day, with evidence of progression to cystic dysplasia by 12 days.

Association of *Ureaplasma* spp. With Development of BPD in Preterm Neonates

In 1988, three independent groups published results of cohort studies linking the development of BPD with colonization of the airways with *Ureaplasma* spp.[44-46] At least 30 additional studies have since examined this association.[47] A previous meta-analysis of studies completed before 1995 showed a significant association between the presence of *U. urealyticum* colonization in the lower respiratory tract and subsequent development of BPD at 28 postnatal days (BPD28), but available data were insufficient at that time to evaluate *Ureaplasma* spp. colonization and the development of BPD at 36 weeks' corrected age (BPD36).[48] Numerous additional studies have been published since this last review of the literature, several of which provided data with interpretations for BPD36, which is now the preferred diagnostic criterion for this condition.[49] We analyzed 23 cohort studies of VLBW infants colonized/

infected with *Ureaplasma* spp. with an aggregate of 2216 infants in whom BPD was defined as a persisting oxygen requirement at 28 postnatal days, and 751 infants in whom the more rigorous BPD definition of oxygen requirement and consistent radiographic changes at 36 weeks' corrected was used.[13] Our meta-analysis demonstrated a significant association between *Ureaplasma* spp. infection and subsequent development of BPD at 28 days (P <0.001) and 36 weeks (P <.001).[47]

Ureaplasma-Mediated Inflammatory Pathways in the Pathogenesis of Perinatal Lung Injury and Subsequent BPD

Early evidence that *Ureaplasma* spp. can induce a systemic pro-inflammatory response in neonates with *U. urealyticum* colonization of the lower respiratory tract came from three clinical research groups, which found elevated peripheral leukocyte counts, particularly the neutrophil component, in infected neonates.[39,50,51] In addition, Horowitz and associates[24] reported that infants with early *Ureaplasma* spp. colonization were more likely to have neutrophils in their tracheal secretions on day 2 than those who were not colonized. Since the time of these initial studies, multiple investigators have demonstrated that ureaplasmal infection of the respiratory tract promotes a pro-inflammatory cytokine cascade in the lower respiratory tract; neonatal *U. urealyticum* infection is consistently associated with increases in tumor necrosis factor (TNF)-α, IL-1β, and IL-8 in plasma and tracheal aspirates.[52-57] Recently, Viscardi and colleagues[58] examined pathologic specimens from *Ureaplasma* spp.–infected infants and found that transforming growth factor (TGF)-β1 expression was increased compared with control specimens from infants with pneumonia from other causes. Evidence revealed associated myofibroblast proliferation contributing to abnormal septation and interstitial fibrosis, both of which are features of the BPD phenotype.

Li and coworkers[59] demonstrated that human macrophages exposed to *U. urealyticum* antigen will produce TNF-α and IL-6 in vitro. Further, they found that macrophages exposed to *U. urealyticum* antigen release vascular endothelial growth factor (VEGF) and intercellular adhesion molecule-1 (ICAM-1). VEGF is involved in pathologic changes in the lung that occur in BPD through modulation of angiogenesis, whereas ICAM-1 mediates neutrophil activation and transendothelial migration of leukocytes to sites of inflammation.[60]

Apoptosis of type II pneumocytes and pulmonary mesenchymal cells has been shown to occur as part of the pathogenesis of BPD in preterm infants.[61] When lung epithelial cells undergo apoptosis, pulmonary fibrosis can occur as a consequence. Apoptosis of alveolar macrophages may also play a role in the development of BPD because this would influence their ability to phagocytize neutrophils. Unchecked, the proliferation of neutrophils at the site of lung infection will lead to prolonged inflammation by means of pro-inflammatory cytokine production and release of proteases and oxygen free radicals.[62] Using human macrophage and lung epithelial cell lines, Li and associates[61] demonstrated that when these cells are stimulated with *U. urealyticum* antigen, apoptosis will occur in vitro, as evidenced by morphologic evaluation and analysis of DNA fragmentation.[54] Macrophage apoptosis is driven by TNF-α production, because cell death is partially prevented when anti–TNF-α monoclonal antibodies neutralize cytokine production.[54]

Toll-like receptors (TLRs) recognize specific patterns of microbial products and are key components of the innate immune response to microorganisms. Engagement of TLR proteins activates the expression of pro-inflammatory mediators by macrophages, neutrophils, dendritic cells, B cells, endothelial cells, and epithelial cells.[63] Elegant studies of ureaplasmal cellular component extracts show nuclear factor (NF)κB activation through TLR-2 and TLR-4, giving clues to the mechanism of inflammatory induction of these mycoplasma organisms.[64,65] Although human fetal TLR expression is beginning to be characterized, developmental induction of TLR expression is apparent in mice and sheep.[66] It has been hypothesized that low TLR-2 and -4 expression early in gestation may increase the susceptibility of the fetal lung

15

to *Ureaplasma* spp. infection and may delay clearance,[67] but postnatal exposure to mechanical ventilation, oxygen, and other infections may stimulate TLR expression and enhance *Ureaplasma*-mediated inflammatory signaling.[68]

Animal models have contributed substantially to our understanding of the inflammatory potential of *Ureaplasma* spp. in the mammalian respiratory tract. In mouse and primate models, a dysregulated, pro-inflammatory, profibrotic state is induced by ureaplasmal infection.[33,56,69-71] High concentrations of oxygen and mechanical ventilation appear to potentiate the effects of *U. urealyticum*–associated injury to the lungs.[33,71,72] In addition, the infant's age at the time of exposure increases susceptibility to infection.[73] Our group was the first to show that rhesus fetuses infected in utero with *U. parvum* or *M. hominis* demonstrated acute and subacute inflammatory changes in the respiratory tract, depending on the duration of infection before delivery. Among acutely infected fetuses (<5 days), widely scattered alveolar collections of neutrophils reveal little damage to lung parenchyma.[67] However, with prolonged *U. parvum* infection, a diffuse exudative pneumonia was present, characterized by abundant alveolar neutrophils and macrophages and widespread epithelial necrosis in alveoli and terminal airways, accompanied by lymphocytic infiltration of alveolar walls and proliferation of type II pneumocytes. In prolonged ureaplasmal or mycoplasmal infection (>10 days), the acute inflammatory response was partially resolved, but reactive proliferation of epithelial cells and increased collagen gave the appearance of thickened alveolar walls. Peribronchiolar lymphoid tissue aggregates were conspicuous, as were hyperplastic changes in the overlying epithelium of terminal airways.[74]

Ureaplasma spp. in the Pathogenesis of Bronchopulmonary Dysplasia

The cause of BPD is multifactorial and complex, and the pathology of this disease is evolving concomitant with advances in neonatal care.[75] The "old" BPD is characterized by oxidant- and ventilator-induced injury in immature, surfactant-deficient lungs. Pathology of these injured lungs reveals marked airway epithelial lesions and smooth muscle hyperplasia, alternating sites of overinflation and atelectasis, extensive fibrosis, and severe vascular hypertensive lesions.[76] With widespread antenatal corticosteroid use, postnatal exogenous surfactant therapy, and "gentler" ventilator strategies to treat respiratory distress in VLBW infants, a "new BPD" has emerged.[77,78] Lung findings include variable but overall less airway epithelial disease, less airway-associated muscular hyperplasia, reduced vascular disease, varying degrees of interstitial fibrosis, increased elastic fiber deposition in alveolar walls, and simplified air spaces reflecting impaired alveolarization.[79] Common to both "old" and "new" BPD is an alveolar developmental impairment.

Infants who subsequently develop BPD have elevated pro-inflammatory cytokines, IL-1, IL-6, and IL-8. The latter is a potent neutrophil chemoattractant; as a result, these infants have elevated neutrophils in the lungs and increased levels of soluble adhesion molecule ICAM-1. Perinatal infection, particularly with *Ureaplasma* spp., appears to promote the inflammatory cascade in the lung[7,80] and may impair alveolar development directly or in conjunction with oxidant- and ventilator-induced lung injury. Figure 15-2 illustrates a proposed scheme of the complex processes involved in intrauterine or neonatal acquisition of *Ureaplasma* spp. and this organism's potential role in the pathogenesis of BPD.

Differential Pathogenicity of *Ureaplasma urealyticum* and *Ureaplasma parvum* in BPD

The availability of polymerase chain reaction (PCR)-based molecular typing of ureaplasmal organisms improved our ability to diagnose these infections. Several recent studies have described PCR-based assays that allow not only the detection of *Ureaplasma* infection with great accuracy but also the precise determination of biovars and species of ureaplasmal organisms.[81-83] These methods have made it possible to

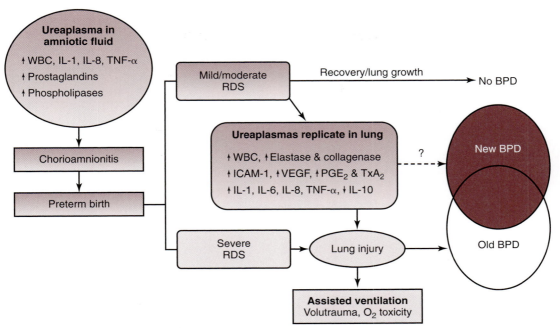

Figure 15-2 Proposed scheme for the role of *Ureaplasma* spp. infection in the pathogenesis of "old" and "new" bronchopulmonary dysplasia (BPD). Overlapping ovals of the "old" and "new" BPD designations represent common features, in particular alveolar developmental impairment. The question mark indicates a potential, yet unproven, direct pathway of ureaplasma-associated inflammatory lung injury impairing alveolar development and remodeling. (Reprinted with permission from Schelonka RL, Waites KB. *Ureaplasma* infection and neonatal lung disease. *Semin Perinatol.* 2007;31:2-9.)

examine the differential pathogenicity and virulence of *U. urealyticum* and *U. parvum* in neonates.

Heggie and associates[84] found no greater risk of developing BPD among 66 *Ureaplasma*-colonized infants, and found no differences between infants harboring *U. parvum* as compared with those with *U. urealyticum*.[75] In contrast, Abele-Horn and colleagues[85] reported that 10 of 18 (56%) infants colonized by *U. urealyticum* developed BPD versus 12 of 48 (25%) infants with *U. parvum* (P <0.05). Katz and colleagues[86] determined rates of BPD in 181 VLBW infants whose endotracheal aspirates were culture positive for *Ureaplasma* spp. No significant differences or trends were noted in the prevalence of BPD in infants harboring *U. urealyticum* or *U. parvum*, although the likelihood of BPD was significantly greater among infants whose endotracheal aspirates were positive for both *U. urealyticum and U. parvum* (odds ratio [OR], 3.02; 95% confidence interval [CI], 1.19 to 7.69; P = 0.012). A limitation of this study was the lack of clearly defined criteria for obtaining endotracheal cultures, which resulted in many infants not being tested for ureaplasmas. Given the limitations of previous studies and conflicting results, more work is needed to determine any differential pathogenicity of the ureaplasmas in neonates.[9]

Inflammatory Pathways in the Pathogenesis of Cerebral White Matter Injury

In humans, the link between the fetal inflammatory response and white matter injury is supported by inferential studies. Elevations in amniotic fluid and cord blood pro-inflammatory cytokines correlate with white matter injury on ultrasound or abnormal neurologic outcome in some but not all studies.[20,87,88] In a meta-analysis of existing cohort and case-control studies, the attributable risk of cerebral palsy secondary to chorioamnionitis was estimated to be 28%.[89] Autopsy results from preterm fetal brains demonstrate elevated expression of TNF-α, IL-1β, and IL-6 at

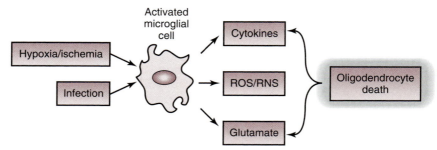

Figure 15-3 Microglia as a convergence point in the pathogenesis of fetal and neonatal white matter brain injury. Infection and inflammation and hypoxia/ischemia together represent the second major upstream mechanism leading to injury or death of pre-oligodendrocytes (pre-OLs). Central to this mechanism is systemic or local upregulation of pro-inflammatory cytokines, reactive oxygen/nitrogen species (ROS/RNS), glutamate, and diffuse activation of microglia within immature white matter. (Adapted from Khwaja O, Volpe JJ. Pathogenesis of cerebral white matter injury of prematurity. *Arch Dis Child Fetal Neonatal Ed.* 2008;93:F153-F161.)

sites of white matter injury, primarily in regions of hypertrophic astrocytes and microglia, although elevation of IL-1β, IL-6, IL-8, and TNF-α in neonatal cord blood provides sensitivity and specificity greater than 88% for the diagnosis of cerebral palsy.[90] Cytokines are toxic in vitro and inhibit oligodendrocyte development. Loss of or injury to premyelinating oligodendrocytes during critical maturational periods can result in profound consequences for later neurodevelopment and function. Taken together, these data support a role for systemic or local upregulation of pro-inflammatory cytokines (fetal inflammatory response) in brain injury. The current conceptual model suggests that pro-inflammatory cytokines act as one final common pathway for central nervous system (CNS) injury initiated by a variety of insults, including infection, hypoxia-ischemia, and reperfusion injury (Fig. 15-3).[91]

Clinical Association of *Ureaplasma* spp. and Neurologic Sequelae in the Neonate

Emerging evidence reveals adverse neonatal outcomes for infants with sepsis associated with positive *U. urealyticum* and *M. hominis* cultures.[14] Other studies have confirmed that these organisms are the causative agents of cerebrospinal fluid (CSF) infection in neonates.[29] Viscardi and colleagues[92] analyzed serum and/or CSF samples from 313 very low birth weight infants and detected ureaplasmal DNA in 24% of the infants studied. Serum *Ureaplasma*-positive infants had a 2.3-fold increased risk of intraventricular hemorrhage. Although epidemiologic data are strong, a causal relationship between *Ureaplasma* spp. infection and brain injury has yet to be clearly established.

Animal Models of Cerebral White Matter Injury: Causal Role of *Ureaplasma* spp.

The relationship between fetal systemic inflammatory response and fetal/neonatal brain injury remains poorly understood. The paucity of mechanistic information in this area of research is, at least in part, related to the limitations in our animal models of cerebral palsy and other forms of neurologic damage. In most animal models of perinatal brain injury, an inflammatory stimulus or infectious agent is administered systemically to pregnant animals.[93] A limitation of these models is that the animals do not uniformly deliver at a premature gestation. Furthermore, systemic administration of inflammatory agents such as lipopolysaccharide to a pregnant animal can cause hypotension in the pregnant animal as well as in the fetus, possibly affecting placental and fetal cerebral blood flow and introducing hypoxia and/or ischemia as a confounding variable.[94]

Ongoing studies on the effects of *Ureaplasma* on the fetal/neonatal brain have shown a variety of brain abnormalities such as increased levels of cytokines, cell death, and white matter damage.[93] In a recent study, Normann and associates[71] used a murine model of intra-amniotic *U. parvum* infection, in which they detected a significant increase in the density of microglial cells, but fewer GABAergic interneurons, in the fetal brain when compared with controls. Oxygen alone had no effect on these parameters and did not exacerbate the *U. parvum* effect. Their findings demonstrated that *U. parvum*–induced perinatal inflammation is sufficient in itself to disturb brain development in mice.

We have developed a nonhuman primate model to investigate the link between *Ureaplasma* intra-amniotic infection, fetal brain inflammation, and neuronal injury. Our preliminary studies indicate that *U. parvum* as a sole pathogen in the amniotic cavity elicits a robust fetal inflammatory response and causes neuropathologic abnormalities that are known antecedents of cerebral white matter injury.[84] We detected extensive inflammatory cell infiltration within the fetal brain periventricular area, microcystic lesions, mononuclear and glial cell infiltration, and microabscesses. Besides microgliosis within the periventricular region, we found foci of reactive astrocytosis within the deep cortical gray matter.[95] Our data support the role of microbial toxins and/or inflammatory factors in the pathogenesis of perinatal brain damage. Further investigation is needed to characterize the inflammatory response in fetal/neonatal cerebral white matter and neuronal injury as a consequence of intra-amniotic *U. parvum* infection during critical periods of fetal brain development, including long-term outcome studies on neurobehavioral and cognitive development.

Interventional Strategies to Prevent Fetal and Neonatal Sequelae

Erythromycin has been the most commonly used antibiotic against *Ureaplasma* spp. with the goal of eradicating the organism from the respiratory tract in neonates.[7] One study in VLBW infants receiving mechanical ventilation showed that 5 or 10 days of treatment with intravenous erythromycin lactobionate failed to eradicate *U. urealyticum* in up to 55% of patients.[96] However, an earlier study demonstrated that 9 of 10 colonized infants were culture negative after 7 or more days of treatment with intravenous erythromycin.[97] Most observational studies have been limited by small sample sizes, varying gestational ages and birth weights at study entry, differences in use and duration of assisted ventilation, wide ranges of postnatal age when treatment was initiated, and lack of documentation of organism eradication following completion of treatment.[31,68,98] Because of these study limitations, the value of erythromycin treatment in eradicating ureaplasmas from the respiratory tract of preterm infants or the impact of treatment on long-term respiratory outcomes remains uncertain.

Two small, randomized, controlled trials of erythromycin therapy aimed at prevention of BPD in preterm infants have been reported. Lyon and coworkers[99] treated infants before culture results were known and found that isolation of *U. urealyticum* was associated with tracheal inflammatory responses, but erythromycin treatment was not associated with a reduction in the incidence or severity of BPD. Jonsson and associates[100] administered erythromycin to infants known to be culture positive for *U. urealyticum* and determined that antibiotic therapy reduced colonization but did not significantly alter length of time that supplemental oxygen was required.

The ORACLE I study[101] evaluated the use of broad-spectrum, antepartum antibiotics for premature rupture of fetal membranes and showed some benefit for infants born to mothers who received erythromycin. Infants of mothers treated with erythromycin had less need for oxygen during the hospital stay and showed a trend toward a reduction in the composite primary outcome of neonatal death, chronic lung disease, or major cerebral abnormality before discharge (12.7% vs. 15.2%; $P = 0.08$). Results from this trial suggest that early antimicrobial treatment could play a role in interrupting the inflammatory cascade to improve neonatal respiratory and other outcomes.[92] However, the recent Oracle II Antibiotic Clinical Trial 7-year follow-up study showed a small increase in the risk of neurologic impairment following prescription of erythromycin during pregnancy.[102] The role of erythromycin therapy remains uncertain, and further evaluation is needed in clinical trials, with careful attention paid to confounding factors such as patient selection bias, misdiagnosis, and late or inappropriate antibiotic therapy.[31,103,104]

In vitro studies with azithromycin, an azalide and subclass of macrolide antibiotics with structural similarity to erythromycin, show good inhibitory activity against the ureaplasmas.[105-107] Pharmacokinetic studies of azithromycin in older children show better tolerance, higher lung tissue concentration, fewer side effects, and fewer drug interactions when compared with erythromycin.[108-111] Although data on the pharmacokinetic profile of azithromycin in low birth weight infants are limited,[112] the clinical pharmacology of this drug suggests several potential therapeutic advantages for the newborn.[109,111] In addition to antimicrobial effects, azithromycin, as well as other macrolides, has multiple anti-inflammatory and immunomodulatory properties.[113] Macrolides accumulate in inflammatory cells, inhibit the release of pro-inflammatory cytokines,[114] and block leukocyte infiltration into tissues by suppressing the expression of adhesion molecules.[115] These anti-inflammatory properties are likely to be mediated via effects on nuclear transcription factors, NFκB, and activator protein 1.[116] This combination of antimicrobial and anti-inflammatory properties makes the macrolide family attractive candidate agents for use in premature infants with ureaplasmal infection.

In a recent randomized controlled trial, azithromycin treatment was associated with a significant reduction in BPD (73% treated vs. 94% control; $P = 0.03$) in infants who were colonized with *U. urealyticum*.[117] The generalizability of this study has been questioned because of the remarkably high rate of BPD (94%) in the control group. No therapeutic trials in human neonates with *U. urealyticum* colonization or infection have demonstrated a reduction in the incidence of BPD,[98] possibly owing to limitations in study design such as small sample size, choice of antibiotic, and the dose and timing of treatment. Although *Ureaplasma* spp. colonization may affect respiratory outcomes, the lack of an effective, proven therapy diminishes the clinical utility of identifying this organism in at-risk infants. These data suggest that routine culture for *Ureaplasma* spp. and treatment of colonization to prevent BPD should still reside in the arena of clinical investigation.

Future Research Needed for Treatment of *Ureaplasma* spp.–Infected Infants at Risk for Lung and Brain Injury

A large, multicenter therapeutic trial is needed to fully evaluate whether a causal relationship exists between colonization of preterm neonates by *Ureaplasma* spp. and development of BPD and adverse neurologic outcomes. Because of the heterogeneity of effect size in previous observational studies, a power analysis based on available observational data is not reliable. Therefore, before a pivotal study is undertaken to examine efficacy of treatment, a smaller pilot study may be needed to establish proof of concept. The antibiotic used for treatment of *Ureaplasma* spp. must be able to eradicate the organism from the respiratory tract and must have an acceptable safety profile.

Erythromycin appears to decrease the rate of colonization with *Ureaplasma* spp. but does not decrease the incidence of BPD or oxygen dependence.[99,118-120] Other macrolides such as azithromycin and clarithromycin may have similar or improved efficacy of eradication of organisms from the airways, but the safety of these antibiotics has not been systematically evaluated in newborn infants. Timing of treatment may be crucial. Because infection with *Ureaplasma* spp. appears to predispose to a pro-inflammatory state, in utero treatment and eradication of the organism may be necessary to interrupt the inflammatory cascade contributing to the development of BPD. Early treatment could include maternally administered antibiotics to combat *Ureaplasma* spp. chorioamnionitis and fetal infection.[32] For some infants, it is possible that postnatal treatment to prevent BPD may be provided too late because the inflammatory process and abnormal airway development and remodeling may already be well established in utero.[34,74,87,121]

Summary

BPD is an important cause of infant mortality and is associated with long-term morbidity, including delayed growth, recurrent respiratory infections, chronic pulmonary dysfunction, and later neurobehavioral impairment.[3-5] Although the pathogenesis of BPD is incompletely understood, a common pathway appears to be inflammation-mediated injury and impaired alveolar development beginning in utero. Available evidence indicates that respiratory infection with *Ureaplasma* spp. contributes to lung inflammation and the subsequent development of BPD. At present, evidence from clinical trials is insufficient to reveal whether postnatal antibiotic treatment of *Ureaplasma* spp. has any influence on the development of BPD and its comorbidities. Future investigation in the context of well-designed, adequately powered, controlled clinical trials should focus on determining whether treatment of *Ureaplasma* spp. infection lessens lung inflammation, decreases rates of BPD, and/or improves long-term pulmonary function and neurodevelopmental outcome. Interventions to reduce the incidence of postnatal infection and to attenuate the systemic inflammatory response could have a significant impact on decreasing the overall rate of neurologic disability among premature survivors[122]; experimental data in the nonhuman primate suggest that this may be best achieved with in utero fetal therapy administered before delivery.[32]

References

1. Stoll BJ, Hansen NI, Bell EF, et al. Neonatal outcomes of extremely preterm infants from the NICHD Neonatal Research Network. *Pediatrics*. 2010 Sep;126(3):443-456.
2. Walsh MC, Szefler S, Davis J, et al. Summary proceedings from the bronchopulmonary dysplasia group. *Pediatrics*. 2006 Mar;117(3 Pt 2):S52-S56.
3. Ehrenkranz RA, Walsh MC, Vohr BR, et al. Validation of the National Institutes of Health consensus definition of bronchopulmonary dysplasia. *Pediatrics*. 2005 Dec;116(6):1353-1360.
4. Short EJ, Klein NK, Lewis BA, et al. Cognitive and academic consequences of bronchopulmonary dysplasia and very low birth weight: 8-year-old outcomes. *Pediatrics*. 2003 Nov;112(5):e359.
5. Vohr BR, Wright LL, Poole WK, et al. Neurodevelopmental outcomes of extremely low birth weight infants <32 weeks' gestation between 1993 and 1998. *Pediatrics*. 2005 Sep;116(3):635-643.
6. Dandekar TB, Snell KC, Razin S, et al. Comparative genome analysis of the Mollicutes. In *Molecular Biology and Pathogenesis of Mycoplasmas*. New York: Kluwer Academic/Plenum Publishers; 2002.
7. Waites KB, Katz B, Schelonka RL. Mycoplasmas and ureaplasmas as neonatal pathogens. *Clin Microbiol Rev*. 2005 Oct;18(4):757-789.
8. Shepard MC. The recovery of pleuropneumonia-like organisms from Negro men with and without nongonococcal urethritis. *Am J Syph Gonorrhea Vener Dis*. 1954;38:113-124.
9. Sung TJ, Xiao L, Duffy L, et al. Frequency of Ureaplasma serovars in respiratory secretions of preterm infants at risk for bronchopulmonary dysplasia. *Pediatr Infect Dis J*. 2011;30(5):Nov 18.
10. Xiao L, Glass JI, Paralanov V, et al. Detection and characterization of human *Ureaplasma* species and serovars by real-time PCR. *J Clin Microbiol*. 2010 Aug;48(8):2715-2723.
11. Klein JO, Buckland D, Finland M. Colonization of newborn infants by mycoplasmas. *N Engl J Med*. 1969 May 8;280(19):1025-1030.
12. Driscoll SG, Kundsin RB, Horne Jr HW, et al. Infections and first trimester losses: Possible role of Mycoplasmas. *Fertil Steril*. 1969 Nov;20(6):1017-1019.
13. Cassell GH, Waites KB, Crouse DT. Mycoplasmal Infections. In: Remington JS, Klein JO, eds. *Infectious diseases of the Fetus and Newborn Infant*. Philadelphia: WB Saunders; 2001:733-767.
14. Cassell GH, Waites KB, Watson HL, et al. *Ureaplasma urealyticum* intrauterine infection: Role in prematurity and disease in newborns. *Clin Microbiol Rev*. 1993 Jan;6(1):69-87.
15. Cassell GH, Davis RO, Waites KB, et al. Isolation of *Mycoplasma hominis* and *Ureaplasma urealyticum* from amniotic fluid at 16-20 weeks of gestation: Potential effect on outcome of pregnancy. *Sex Transm Dis*. 1983 Oct;10(4 Suppl):294-302.
16. Foulon W, Naessens A, Dewaele M, et al. Chronic *Ureaplasma urealyticum* amnionitis associated with abruptio placentae. *Obstet Gynecol*. 1986 Aug;68(2):280-282.
17. Gray DJ, Robinson HB, Malone J, et al. Adverse outcome in pregnancy following amniotic fluid isolation of *Ureaplasma urealyticum*. *Prenat Diagn*. 1992 Feb;12(2):111-117.
18. Gerber S, Vial Y, Hohlfeld P, et al. Detection of *Ureaplasma urealyticum* in second-trimester amniotic fluid by polymerase chain reaction correlates with subsequent preterm labor and delivery. *J Infect Dis*. 2003 Feb 1;187(3):518-521.

15

19. Breugelmans M, Vancutsem E, Naessens A, et al. Association of abnormal vaginal flora and *Ureaplasma* species as risk factors for preterm birth: A cohort study. *Acta Obstet Gynecol Scand*. 2010;89(2): 256-260.
20. Yoon BH, Jun JK, Romero R, et al. Amniotic fluid inflammatory cytokines (interleukin-6, interleukin-1beta, and tumor necrosis factor-alpha), neonatal brain white matter lesions, and cerebral palsy. *Am J Obstet Gynecol*. 1997 Jul;177(1):19-26.
21. Oh KJ, Lee KA, Sohn YK, et al. Intraamniotic infection with genital mycoplasmas exhibits a more intense inflammatory response than intraamniotic infection with other microorganisms in patients with preterm premature rupture of membranes. *Am J Obstet Gynecol*. 2010 Sep;203(3): 211-218.
22. Chaiworapongsa T, Romero R, Kim JC, et al. Evidence for fetal involvement in the pathologic process of clinical chorioamnionitis. *Am J Obstet Gynecol*. 2002 Jun;186(6):1178-1182.
23. Colaizy TT, Kuforiji T, Sklar RS, et al. PCR methods in clinical investigations of human ureaplasmas: A minireview. *Mol Genet Metab*. 2003 Dec;80(4):389-397.
24. Cordero L, Coley BD, Miller RL, et al. Bacterial and *Ureaplasma* colonization of the airway: Radiologic findings in infants with bronchopulmonary dysplasia. *J Perinatol*. 1997 Nov;17(6): 428-433.
25. Goldenberg RL, Andrews WW, Goepfert AR, et al. The Alabama Preterm Birth Study: Umbilical cord blood *Ureaplasma urealyticum* and *Mycoplasma hominis* cultures in very preterm newborn infants. *Am J Obstet Gynecol*. 2008 Jan;198(1):43-45.
26. Kelly VN, Garland SM, Gilbert GL. Isolation of genital mycoplasmas from the blood of neonates and women with pelvic infection using conventional SPS-free blood culture media. *Pathology*. 1987 Jul;19(3):277-280.
27. Sanchez PJ, Regan JA. Vertical transmission of *Ureaplasma urealyticum* from mothers to preterm infants. *Pediatr Infect Dis J*. 1990 Jun;9(6):398-401.
28. Waites KB, Crouse DT, Philips III JB, et al. Ureaplasmal pneumonia and sepsis associated with persistent pulmonary hypertension of the newborn. *Pediatrics*. 1989 Jan;83(1):79-85.
29. Waites KB, Rudd PT, Crouse DT, et al. Chronic *Ureaplasma urealyticum* and *Mycoplasma hominis* infections of central nervous system in preterm infants. *Lancet*. 1988 Jan 2;1(8575-6): 17-21.
30. Waites KB, Duffy LB, Crouse DT, et al. Mycoplasmal infections of cerebrospinal fluid in newborn infants from a community hospital population. *Pediatr Infect Dis J*. 1990 Apr;9(4): 241-245.
31. Waites KB, Schelonka RL, Xiao L, et al. Congenital and opportunistic infections: *Ureaplasma* species and *Mycoplasma hominis*. *Semin Fetal Neonatal Med*. 2009 Aug;14(4):190-199.
32. Walsh WF, Butler J, Coalson J, et al. A primate model of *Ureaplasma urealyticum* infection in the premature infant with hyaline membrane disease. *Clin Infect Dis*. 1993 Aug;17(Suppl 1): S158-S162.
33. Yoder BA, Coalson JJ, Winter VT, et al. Effects of antenatal colonization with *Ureaplasma urealyticum* on pulmonary disease in the immature baboon. *Pediatr Res*. 2003 Dec;54(6):797-807.
34. Novy MJ, Sadowsky DW, Grigsby PL, et al. Maternal Azithromycin (AZI) therapy for Ureaplasma intraamniotic infection (IAI) prevents advanced fetal lung lesions in *Rhesus monkeys*. *Reprod Sci*. 2008;15(Suppl 1):184A.
35. Tafari N, Ross S, Naeye RL, et al. Mycoplasma T strains and perinatal death. *Lancet*. 1976 Jan 17;1(7951):108-109.
36. Quinn PA, Gillan JE, Markestad T, et al. Intrauterine infection with *Ureaplasma urealyticum* as a cause of fatal neonatal pneumonia. *Pediatr Infect Dis*. 1985 Sep;4(5):538-543.
37. Crouse DT, Odrezin GT, Cutter GR, et al. Radiographic changes associated with tracheal isolation of *Ureaplasma urealyticum* from neonates. *Clin Infect Dis*. 1993 Aug;17(Suppl 1):S122-S130.
38. Pacifico L, Panero A, Roggini M, et al. *Ureaplasma urealyticum* and pulmonary outcome in a neonatal intensive care population. *Pediatr Infect Dis J*. 1997 Jun;16(6):579-586.
39. Panero A, Pacifico L, Rossi N, et al. *Ureaplasma urealyticum* as a cause of pneumonia in preterm infants: Analysis of the white cell response. *Arch Dis Child Fetal Neonatal Ed*. 1995 Jul;73(1): F37-F40.
40. Cassell GH, Waites KB, Gibbs RS, et al. Role of *Ureaplasma urealyticum* in amnionitis. *Pediatr Infect Dis*. 1986 Nov;5(6 Suppl):S247-S252.
41. Brus F, van Waarde WM, Schoots C, et al. Fatal ureaplasmal pneumonia and sepsis in a newborn infant. *Eur J Pediatr*. 1991 Sep;150(11):782-784.
42. Theilen U, Lyon AJ, Fitzgerald T, et al. Infection with *Ureaplasma urealyticum*: Is there a specific clinical and radiological course in the preterm infant? *Arch Dis Child Fetal Neonatal Ed*. 2004 Mar;89 (2):F163-F167.
43. Pacifico L, Panero A, Roggini M, et al. *Ureaplasma urealyticum* and pulmonary outcome in a neonatal intensive care population. *Pediatr Infect Dis J*. 1997 Jun;16(6):579-586.
44. Cassell GH, Waites KB, Crouse DT, et al. Association of *Ureaplasma urealyticum* infection of the lower respiratory tract with chronic lung disease and death in very-low-birth-weight infants. *Lancet*. 1988 Jul 30;2(8605):240-245.
45. Wang EE, Frayha H, Watts J, et al. Role of *Ureaplasma urealyticum* and other pathogens in the development of chronic lung disease of prematurity. *Pediatr Infect Dis J*. 1988 Aug;7(8): 547-551.
46. Sanchez PJ, Regan JA. *Ureaplasma urealyticum* colonization and chronic lung disease in low birth weight infants. *Pediatr Infect Dis J*. 1988 Aug;7(8):542-546.

47. Schelonka RL, Katz B, Waites KB, et al. Critical appraisal of the role of *Ureaplasma* in the development of bronchopulmonary dysplasia with metaanalytic techniques. *Pediatr Infect Dis J*. 2005 Dec; 24(12):1033-1039.

48. Wang EE, Ohlsson A, Kellner JD. Association of *Ureaplasma urealyticum* colonization with chronic lung disease of prematurity: Results of a metaanalysis. *J Pediatr*. 1995 Oct;127(4):640-644.

49. Jobe AH, Bancalari E. Bronchopulmonary dysplasia. *Am J Respir Crit Care Med*. 2001 Jun;163(7): 1723-1729.

50. Ohlsson A, Wang E, Vearncombe M. Leukocyte counts and colonization with *Ureaplasma urealyticum* in preterm neonates. *Clin Infect Dis*. 1993 Aug;17(Suppl 1):S144-S147.

51. Ollikainen J, Heiskanen-Kosma T, Korppi M, et al. Clinical relevance of *Ureaplasma urealyticum* colonization in preterm infants. *Acta Paediatr*. 1998 Oct;87(10):1075-1078.

52. De Dooy JJ, Mahieu LM, Van Bever HP. The role of inflammation in the development of chronic lung disease in neonates. *Eur J Pediatr*. 2001 Aug;160(8):457-463.

53. Groneck P, Schmale J, Soditt V, et al. Bronchoalveolar inflammation following airway infection in preterm infants with chronic lung disease. *Pediatr Pulmonol*. 2001 May;31(5): 331-338.

54. Patterson AM, Taciak V, Lovchik J, et al. *Ureaplasma urealyticum* respiratory tract colonization is associated with an increase in interleukin 1-beta and tumor necrosis factor alpha relative to interleukin 6 in tracheal aspirates of preterm infants. *Pediatr Infect Dis J*. 1998 Apr;17(4):321-328.

55. Viscardi RM, Manimtim WM, Sun CC, et al. Lung pathology in premature infants with *Ureaplasma urealyticum* infection. *Pediatr Dev Pathol*. 2002 Mar;5(2):141-150.

56. Viscardi RM, Muhumuza CK, Rodriguez A, et al. Inflammatory markers in intrauterine and fetal blood and cerebrospinal fluid compartments are associated with adverse pulmonary and neurologic outcomes in preterm infants. *Pediatr Res*. 2004 Jun;55(6):1009-1017.

57. Manimtim WM, Hasday JD, Hester L, et al. *Ureaplasma urealyticum* modulates endotoxin-induced cytokine release by human monocytes derived from preterm and term newborns and adults. *Infect Immun*. 2001 Jun;69(6):3906-3915.

58. Viscardi R, Manimtim W, He JR, et al. Disordered pulmonary myofibroblast distribution and elastin expression in preterm infants with *Ureaplasma urealyticum* pneumonitis. *Pediatr Dev Pathol*. 2006 Mar;9(2):143-151.

59. Li YH, Brauner A, Jonsson B, et al. *Ureaplasma urealyticum*-induced production of proinflammatory cytokines by macrophages. *Pediatr Res*. 2000 Jul;48(1):114-119.

60. Li YH, Brauner A, Jensen JS, et al. Induction of human macrophage vascular endothelial growth factor and intercellular adhesion molecule-1 by *Ureaplasma urealyticum* and downregulation by steroids. *Biol Neonate*. 2002;82(1):22-28.

61. Li YH, Chen M, Brauner A, et al. *Ureaplasma urealyticum* induces apoptosis in human lung epithelial cells and macrophages. *Biol Neonate*. 2002;82(3):166-173.

62. Greenhalgh DG. The role of apoptosis in wound healing. *Int J Biochem Cell Biol*. 1998 Sep;30(9): 1019-1030.

63. Kaisho T, Akira S. Toll-like receptor function and signaling. *J Allergy Clin Immunol*. 2006 May;117(5): 979-987.

64. Peltier MR, Freeman AJ, Mu HH, et al. Characterization of the macrophage-stimulating activity from *Ureaplasma urealyticum*. *Am J Reprod Immunol*. 2007 Mar;57(3):186-192.

65. Shimizu T, Kida Y, Kuwano K. *Ureaplasma parvum* lipoproteins, including MB antigen, activate NF-κB through TLR1, TLR2 and TLR6. *Microbiology*. 2008 May;154(Pt 5):1318-1325.

66. Koga K, Mor G. Toll-like receptors at the maternal-fetal interface in normal pregnancy and pregnancy disorders. *Am J Reprod Immunol*. 2010 Jun;63(6):587-600.

67. Harju K, Glumoff V, Hallman M. Ontogeny of Toll-like receptors Tlr2 and Tlr4 in mice. *Pediatr Res*. 2001 Jan;49(1):81-83.

68. Viscardi RM, Hasday JD. Role of *Ureaplasma* species in neonatal chronic lung disease: Epidemiologic and experimental evidence. *Pediatr Res*. 2009 May;65(5 Pt 2):84R-90R.

69. Viscardi RM, Kaplan J, Lovchik JC, et al. Characterization of a murine model of *Ureaplasma urealyticum* pneumonia. *Infect Immun*. 2002 Oct;70(10):5721-5729.

70. Viscardi RM, Atamas SP, Luzina IG, et al. Antenatal *Ureaplasma urealyticum* respiratory tract infection stimulates proinflammatory, profibrotic responses in the preterm baboon lung. *Pediatr Res*. 2006 Aug;60(2):141-146.

71. Normann E, Lacaze-Masmonteil T, Eaton F, et al. A novel mouse model of *Ureaplasma*-induced perinatal inflammation: Effects on lung and brain injury. *Pediatr Res*. 2009 Apr;65(4):430-436.

72. Crouse DT, Cassell GH, Waites KB, et al. Hyperoxia potentiates *Ureaplasma urealyticum* pneumonia in newborn mice. *Infect Immun*. 1990 Nov;58(11):3487-3493.

73. Rudd PT, Cassell GH, Waites KB, et al. *Ureaplasma urealyticum* pneumonia: Experimental production and demonstration of age-related susceptibility. *Infect Immun*. 1989 Mar;57(3): 918-925.

74. Novy MJ, Duffy L, Axthelm MK, et al. *Ureaplasma parvum* or *Mycoplasma hominis* as sole pathogens cause chorioamnionitis, preterm delivery, and fetal pneumonia in rhesus macaques. *Reprod Sci*. 2009 Jan;16(1):56-70.

75. Bancalari E, Claure N, Sosenko IR. Bronchopulmonary dysplasia: Changes in pathogenesis, epidemiology and definition. *Semin Neonatol*. 2003 Feb;8(1):63-71.

76. Northway Jr WH, Rosan RC, Porter DY. Pulmonary disease following respirator therapy of hyaline-membrane disease. Bronchopulmonary dysplasia. *N Engl J Med*. 1967 Feb 16;276(7): 357-368.

15

77. Jobe AJ. The new BPD: An arrest of lung development. *Pediatr Res.* 1999 Dec;46(6):641-643.

78. Coalson JJ. Pathology of new bronchopulmonary dysplasia. *Semin Neonatol.* 2003 Feb;8(1):73-81.

79. Coalson JJ. Pathology of bronchopulmonary dysplasia. *Semin Perinatol.* 2006 Aug;30(4):179-184.

80. Lyon A. Chronic lung disease of prematurity. The role of intra-uterine infection. *Eur J Pediatr.* 2000 Nov;159(11):798-802.

81. Kong F, James G, Ma Z, et al. Phylogenetic analysis of *Ureaplasma urealyticum*—support for the establishment of a new species, *Ureaplasma parvum. Int J Syst Bacteriol.* 1999 Oct;49 (Pt 4):1879-1889.

82. Pitcher D, Sillis M, Robertson JA. Simple method for determining biovar and serovar types of *Ureaplasma urealyticum* clinical isolates using PCR-single-strand conformation polymorphism analysis. *J Clin Microbiol.* 2001 May;39(5):1840-1844.

83. Robertson JA, Vekris A, Bebear C, et al. Polymerase chain reaction using 16S rRNA gene sequences distinguishes the two biovars of Ureaplasma urealyticum. *J Clin Microbiol.* 1993 Apr;31(4): 824-830.

84. Heggie AD, Bar-Shain D, Boxerbaum B, et al. Identification and quantification of ureaplasmas colonizing the respiratory tract and assessment of their role in the development of chronic lung disease in preterm infants. *Pediatr Infect Dis J.* 2001 Sep;20(9):854-859.

85. Abele-Horn M, Wolff C, Dressel P, et al. Association of *Ureaplasma urealyticum* biovars with clinical outcome for neonates, obstetric patients, and gynecological patients with pelvic inflammatory disease. *J Clin Microbiol.* 1997 May;35(5):1199-1202.

86. Katz B, Patel P, Duffy L, et al. Characterization of ureaplasmas isolated from preterm infants with and without bronchopulmonary dysplasia. *J Clin Microbiol.* 2005 Sep;43(9):4852-4854.

87. Yoon BH, Romero R, Jun JK, et al. Amniotic fluid cytokines (interleukin-6, tumor necrosis factor-alpha, interleukin-1 beta, and interleukin-8) and the risk for the development of bronchopulmonary dysplasia. *Am J Obstet Gynecol.* 1997 Oct;177(4):825-830.

88. Dammann O, Allred EN, Genest DR, et al. Antenatal mycoplasma infection, the fetal inflammatory response and cerebral white matter damage in very-low-birthweight infants. *Paediatr Perinat Epidemiol.* 2003 Jan;17(1):49-57.

89. Wu YW, Colford Jr JM. Chorioamnionitis as a risk factor for cerebral palsy: A meta-analysis. *JAMA.* 2000 Sep 20;284(11):1417-1424.

90. Jeohn GH, Kong LY, Wilson B, et al. Synergistic neurotoxic effects of combined treatments with cytokines in murine primary mixed neuron/glia cultures. *J Neuroimmunol.* 1998 May 1;85(1): 1-10.

91. Khwaja O, Volpe JJ. Pathogenesis of cerebral white matter injury of prematurity. *Arch Dis Child Fetal Neonatal Ed.* 2008 Mar;93(2):F153-F161.

92. Viscardi RM, Hashmi N, Gross GW, et al. Incidence of invasive ureaplasma in VLBW infants: Relationship to severe intraventricular hemorrhage. *J Perinatol.* 2008 Nov;28(11):759-765.

93. Kramer BW, Kramer S, Ikegami M, et al. Injury, inflammation, and remodeling in fetal sheep lung after intra-amniotic endotoxin. *Am J Physiol Lung Cell Mol Physiol.* 2002 Aug;283(2): L452-L459.

94. Elovitz MA, Mrinalini C. Animal models of preterm birth. *Trends Endocrinol Metab.* 2004 Dec;15(10): 479-487.

95. Coksaygan T, Viscardi RM, Waites KB, et al. Periventricular neuronal damage associated with ureaplasma intra-amniotic infection is diminished by maternal azithromycin (AZI) treatment. *Reprod Sci.* 2010;17:178A.

96. Baier RJ, Loggins J, Kruger TE. Failure of erythromycin to eliminate airway colonization with *Ureaplasma urealyticum* in very low birth weight infants. *BMC Pediatr.* 2003;3:10.

97. Waites KB, Sims PJ, Crouse DT, et al. Serum concentrations of erythromycin after intravenous infusion in preterm neonates treated for *Ureaplasma urealyticum* infection. *Pediatr Infect Dis J.* 1994 Apr;13(4):287-293.

98. Mabanta CG, Pryhuber GS, Weinberg GA, et al. Erythromycin for the prevention of chronic lung disease in intubated preterm infants at risk for, or colonized or infected with *Ureaplasma urealyticum. Cochrane Database Syst Rev.* 2003;(4):CD003744.

99. Lyon AJ, McColm J, Middlemist L, et al. Randomised trial of erythromycin on the development of chronic lung disease in preterm infants. *Arch Dis Child Fetal Neonatal Ed.* 1998 Jan;78(1):F10-F14.

100. Jonsson B, Karell AC, Ringertz S, et al. Neonatal Ureaplasma urealyticum colonization and chronic lung disease. *Acta Paediatr.* 1994 Sep;83(9):927-930.

101. Kenyon SL, Taylor DJ, Tarnow-Mordi W. Broad-spectrum antibiotics for preterm, prelabour rupture of fetal membranes: The ORACLE I randomised trial. ORACLE Collaborative Group. *Lancet.* 2001 Mar 31;357(9261):979-988.

102. Kenyon S, Pike K, Jones DR, et al. Childhood outcomes after prescription of antibiotics to pregnant women with spontaneous preterm labour: 7-year follow-up of the ORACLE II trial. *Lancet.* 2008 Oct 11;372(9646):1319-1327.

103. King J, Flenady V. Prophylactic antibiotics for inhibiting preterm labour with intact membranes. *Cochrane Database Syst Rev.* 2002;(4):CD000246.

104. Stetzer BP, Mercer BM. Antibiotics and preterm labor. *Clin Obstet Gynecol.* 2000 Dec;43(4): 809-817.

105. Rylander M, Hallander HO. In vitro comparison of the activity of doxycycline, tetracycline, erythromycin and a new macrolide, CP 62993, against *Mycoplasma pneumoniae, Mycoplasma hominis* and *Ureaplasma urealyticum. Scand J Infect Dis Suppl.* 1988;53:12-17.

15

106. Rumpianesi F, Morandotti G, Sperning R, et al. In vitro activity of azithromycin against *Chlamydia trachomatis, Ureaplasma urealyticum* and *Mycoplasma hominis* in comparison with erythromycin, roxithromycin and minocycline. *J Chemother*. 1993 Jun;5(3):155-158.

107. Matlow A, Th'ng C, Kovach D, et al. Susceptibilities of neonatal respiratory isolates of *Ureaplasma urealyticum* to antimicrobial agents. *Antimicrob Agents Chemother*. 1998 May;42(5):1290-1292.

108. Hopkins S. Clinical toleration and safety of azithromycin. *Am J Med*. 1991 Sep 12;91(3A):40S-45S.

109. Luke DR, Foulds G, Cohen SF, et al. Safety, toleration, and pharmacokinetics of intravenous azithromycin. *Antimicrob Agents Chemother*. 1996 Nov;40(11):2577-2581.

110. Langtry HD, Balfour JA. Azithromycin. A review of its use in paediatric infectious diseases. *Drugs*. 1998 Aug;56(2):273-297.

111. Rapp RP. Pharmacokinetics and pharmacodynamics of intravenous and oral azithromycin: Enhanced tissue activity and minimal drug interactions. *Ann Pharmacother*. 1998 Jul;32(7-8):785-793.

112. Hassan HE, Othman AA, Eddington ND, et al. Pharmacokinetics, safety, and biologic effects of azithromycin in extremely preterm infants at risk for Ureaplasma colonization and bronchopulmonary dysplasia. *J Clin Pharmacol*. 2011;51:1264-1275.

113. Tamaoki J, Kadota J, Takizawa H. Clinical implications of the immunomodulatory effects of macrolides. *Am J Med*. 2004 Nov 8;117(Suppl 9A):5S-11S.

114. Ivetic TV, Bosnjak B, Hrvacic B, et al. Anti-inflammatory activity of azithromycin attenuates the effects of lipopolysaccharide administration in mice. *Eur J Pharmacol*. 2006 Jun 6;539(1-2):131-138.

115. Sanz MJ, Nabah YN, Cerda-Nicolas M, et al. Erythromycin exerts in vivo anti-inflammatory activity downregulating cell adhesion molecule expression. *Br J Pharmacol*. 2005 Jan;144(2):190-201.

116. Kikuchi T, Hagiwara K, Honda Y, et al. Clarithromycin suppresses lipopolysaccharide-induced interleukin-8 production by human monocytes through AP-1 and NF-kappa B transcription factors. *J Antimicrob Chemother*. 2002 May;49(5):745-755.

117. Ballard HO, Shook LA, Bernard P, et al. Use of azithromycin for the prevention of bronchopulmonary dysplasia in preterm infants: A randomized, double-blind, placebo-controlled trial. *Pediatr Pulmonol*. 2011;46:111-118.

118. Bowman ED, Dharmalingam A, Fan WQ, et al. Impact of erythromycin on respiratory colonization of *Ureaplasma urealyticum* and the development of chronic lung disease in extremely low birth weight infants. *Pediatr Infect Dis J*. 1998 Jul;17(7):615-620.

119. Jonsson B, Rylander M, Faxelius G. *Ureaplasma urealyticum,* erythromycin and respiratory morbidity in high-risk preterm neonates. *Acta Paediatr*. 1998 Oct;87(10):1079-1084.

120. Buhrer C, Hoehn T, Hentschel J. Role of erythromycin for treatment of incipient chronic lung disease in preterm infants colonised with *Ureaplasma urealyticum*. *Drugs*. 2001;61(13):1893-1899.

121. Yoon BH, Romero R, Kim KS, et al. A systemic fetal inflammatory response and the development of bronchopulmonary dysplasia. *Am J Obstet Gynecol*. 1999 Oct;181(4):773-779.

122. Chapman I, Stoll BJ. Neonatal infection and long-term neurodevelopmental outcome in the preterm infant. *Curr Opin Infect Dis*. 2006 Jun;19(3):290-297.

15

CHAPTER 16

Control of Antibiotic-Resistant Bacteria in the Neonatal Intensive Care Unit

Philip Toltzis, MD

- Epidemiology of MRSA in the NICU
- Epidemiology of MDR-GNR in the NICU
- Control Strategies for Nonepidemic MRSA and MDR-GNR
- Control Strategies for NICU Outbreaks of MRSA and MDR-GNR

The neonatal intensive care unit (NICU) harbors many microorganisms expressing antibiotic resistance. Three ICU-related resistance phenotypes have generated particular concern over the recent past, namely, methicillin-resistant *Staphylococcus aureus* (MRSA), vancomycin-resistant enterococci (VRE), and multiple-drug resistant Gram-negative rods (MDR-GNR). Studies in adult patients indicate that infections by resistant organisms prolong hospitalization and increase health care costs, and that they are associated with higher mortality compared with infection by susceptible bacteria.[1] Mortality is increased in part because resistance limits the choice of antibiotics, forcing the use of agents that have poor tissue penetration (e.g., vancomycin for MRSA) or that are bacteriostatic rather than bactericidal (e.g., trimethoprim-sulfamethoxazole for multiple-drug resistant *Stenotrophomonas*). Furthermore, the expression of resistance may lead to delays in prescribing the most effective therapies for the first 2 to 3 days of illness—the time required to complete drug susceptibility testing.[1] In the NICU, an additional consequence of antibiotic resistance is that it may obligate the clinician to use an antimicrobial agent for which few or no data are available regarding pharmacokinetics, distribution, or toxicity in premature infants.

Given the alarming consequences of infection by antibiotic-resistant organisms, it is imperative to understand and apply strategies to contain their spread, particularly among vulnerable populations such as those admitted to the NICU. VRE has only occasionally been problematic in the intensive care nursery, despite its high prevalence in non-neonatal ICUs. This article, therefore, will review the epidemiology of MRSA and MDR-GNR in the NICU setting and will discuss strategies to contain them.

Epidemiology of MRSA in the NICU

MRSA appeared in NICUs beginning in the early 1980s, soon after its discovery elsewhere, and it has persisted in intensive care nurseries ever since.[2-8] This phenotype is mediated through the expression of an altered penicillin-binding protein, resulting in diminished affinity of all β-lactams for their target molecule on the bacterial cell wall.[9] The abnormal penicillin-binding protein is encoded by the gene *mecA,* which is included on a cassette inserted into the bacterial chromosome. The de novo acquisition of *mecA* is an infrequent event, and most MRSA isolates are derived from a finite number of international clones. Investigators at the Centers for Disease Control and Prevention (CDC) have categorized American MRSA isolates on the basis of DNA restriction fragment polymorphisms as defined by pulsed field gel electrophoresis (PFGE),[10] a technique commonly used to establish clonal relationships between bacteria of the same species. More than 93% of their sample of 957 American isolates belonged to one of only eight major clones as defined by PFGE. These observations indicate that, in a given patient, MRSA is virtually never derived from a susceptible staphylococcus that emerges resistant under antibiotic pressure; rather, the organism is always acquired from an external source, particularly other patients via the hands of caregivers and inanimate hospital surfaces.[11] Control of MRSA therefore focuses on interrupting its spread from those external sources.

Almost all data regarding MRSA in the nursery are derived from outbreak reports.[2,4-8,12] Less is known about endemic colonization and disease in the NICU, although certainly sporadic cases of MRSA occur. Once introduced into the NICU environment, however, MRSA may spread rapidly, and the identification of any case of MRSA in a hospitalized newborn should be considered a sentinel event of a potential outbreak. Once an epidemic is established, frequently 20% to 50% of all infants become colonized or infected.[4,5,7,13] MRSA characteristically is difficult to eradicate from the NICU using conventional infection control measures after an outbreak has started.[2,4,5,8] Consequently, the duration of published MRSA nursery epidemics is long, ranging from 2 months to over 4 years.[2,4-7,12-15]

As in older patients, infants become colonized with MRSA antecedent to their infection.[16-18] In newborns, the organism most commonly colonizes the anterior nares, similar to patients outside the newborn period, but MRSA also may be isolated from the umbilicus, the axillary and groin skin folds, and the rectum. The duration of MRSA colonization in the neonate is variable. Some infants are colonized transiently, but in others, colonization may persist for weeks or months, resulting in clinical infection after discharge from the nursery and allowing spread of the organism to household contacts.[4,19]

MRSA colonization and infection in the newborn usually is a nosocomial event, appearing typically on days of life 15 to 30.[3,5,7,12] The organism affects infants at high risk of a complicated NICU course, particularly those of low birth weight and gestational age, requiring indwelling catheters and mechanical ventilation.[3,7,12,13,16,20] Other predisposing factors for MRSA colonization and infection include multiple gestation, prior surgery, and prolonged exposure to antibiotics[12-14]—all of which are confounders of a prolonged, complicated course.

Older reports of MRSA in the NICU documented the presence of multiple-antibiotic resistant hospital-associated MRSA (HA-MRSA) strains, similar to those found in adult ICUs. Over the past decade, *community-associated MRSA* (CA-MRSA) has become prominent both in and out of the hospital setting. Cases of CA-MRSA were initially identified in 1998 among healthy children with no prior hospital exposure. The strains implicated in these cases were molecularly unrelated to previously studied hospital-associated MRSA.[21] In particular, the *mecA* gene was included on cassettes distinct from hospital-associated strains, and the organisms remained susceptible to many antibiotics, including clindamycin, to which HA-MRSA organisms were resistant.[21] Moreover, they replicated very rapidly and frequently expressed exotoxins that were unusual in hospital-associated isolates. Chief among these is Panton-Valentine leukocidin (PVL), a molecule that lyses white blood cells and fosters the development of tissue necrosis.[22] The past several years have witnessed the alarmingly rapid geographic dissemination of CA-MRSA throughout North America and Europe, presumably reflecting biological characteristics that especially promote person-to-person transmission.

CA-MRSA has been implicated in infections affecting both the mother and her full-term newborn. Mother-to-child transmission of CA-MRSA may occur after maternal peripartum sepsis or maternal mastitis.[7,14,23,24] Most of the infants in these reports suffered from bacteremia or skin and soft tissue infection.[7,14,15,24] More worrisome is the occurrence of nosocomially acquired CA-MRSA among premature NICU residents.[25] A sentinel report from Houston, a metropolitan area with a particularly high prevalence of CA-MRSA, described six NICU infants within a year who acquired CA-MRSA after admission to the unit. Similar to the typical experience with HA-MRSA, patients were of low birth weight, and onset of infection occurred several weeks after gestation. Unlike prior experience with hospital-associated strains, however, patients typically suffered from fulminant septic shock, necrotizing pneumonia, and severe central nervous system infection,[25] raising concern that PVL-positive CA-MRSA strains may be particularly virulent if introduced into the tertiary care nursery. Since that time, CA-MRSA has been documented in multiple other nurseries.[14,26,27] In these latter reports, isolation of CA-MRSA strains became increasingly more frequent throughout the first decade of the 2000s, reflecting their burgeoning presence in the community and in other areas of the hospital.

Epidemiology of MDR-GNR in the NICU

As with MRSA, the epidemiology of MDR-GNR can be best appreciated by reviewing the mechanisms of resistance.[9] The phenotypes for MDR-GNR are varied, encompassing resistance to all classes of β-lactam agents, to the aminoglycosides, and to the quinolones. Many of the resistance determinants to the β-lactams and aminoglycosides—phenotypes relevant to the NICU—are encoded on transmissible genetic elements such as transposons or plasmids. Those resistance genes that are encoded on the bacterial genome usually are controlled by upstream sequences that turn on production of the resistance molecule in the presence of antibiotic or, alternatively, that spontaneously mutate to generate constitutively resistant subpopulations that then expand under antibiotic pressure. In all these cases, resistance is promoted by antibiotic exposure, so that the association between prior antibiotic administration and colonization or infection by MDR-GNR is much stronger than with MRSA. Once resistance is selected, the organisms primarily colonize the gastrointestinal tract and in most cases are asymptomatically excreted in the stool. Hand contamination by caregivers during routine care can result in transfer to the NICU environment or direct horizontal transmission to a noncolonized infant. In sum, then, the infant can acquire an MDR-GNR through several different mechanisms, namely, by exposure to an antibiotic that selects or induces a resistant subpopulation, by acquisition from a contaminated external source, or both.

Epidemiology of MDR-GNR During Non-Outbreak Periods

Unlike MRSA, some aspects of the epidemiology of MDR-GNR during non-outbreak periods in the nursery have been defined (Fig. 16-1). Under normal circumstances, fetal development occurs in the sterile intrauterine environment, and the infant is born uncolonized. The gastrointestinal ecology of the healthy, nonhospitalized infant rapidly assumes substantial complexity, involving many different anaerobic and facultative species, including but not limited to *Bifidobacteria, Bacteroides, Clostridia,* enteric streptococci, *Veillonella, Bacillus,* and *Lactobacillus.* This gastrointestinal ecology is essentially established by the fifth day of life and remains stable over the next several months.[28-33] It is likely that the normal flora at least partially prevents sustained colonization by pathogenic species such as those represented by MDR-GNRs.

Initial Colonization by Gram-Negative Bacilli in the NICU

(Fig. 16-1, *A* and *B*)
The newborn admitted to the NICU does not have the opportunity to acquire normal colonizing flora through postnatal maternal contact, and acquisition is not mediated by breast milk or formula in the newborn too ill to feed. The colonizing flora of the infant admitted to the NICU, therefore, is primarily influenced by organisms present in that environment and by exposure to antibiotics. It is assumed that Gram-negative bacilli, both antibiotic-susceptible and -resistant, initially are acquired by the patient via the contaminated hands of caregivers, because besides the mother's vaginal tract, few other conceivable sources for these organisms are known. Studies performed decades ago indicated that the hands of hospital caregivers frequently are positive for Gram-negative bacilli.[34,35] Hand cultures performed on NICU nurses in the early 1970s, for example, revealed bacillary contamination in more than 86% of samples.[35]

Goldmann and colleagues[36] were among the first to describe the ontogeny of bacterial colonization in the critically ill newborn. In their study, approximately 50%

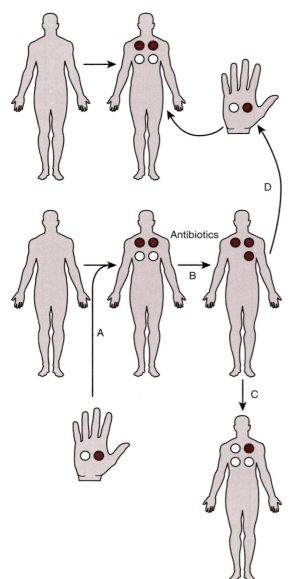

Figure 16-1 Descriptive epidemiology of multiple-drug resistant Gram-negative rods (MDR-GNR) in the neonatal intensive care unit (NICU) during a non-outbreak period. **A,** Infants are born noncolonized by Gram-negative bacilli and acquire their Gram-negative flora, both antibiotic-susceptible *(open circles)* and antibiotic-resistant *(closed circles)*, from the NICU environment, largely through the hands of caregivers. **B,** Antibiotic exposure reduces susceptible bacilli while selecting resistant ones, increasing the density of the latter. **C,** In most infants, colonization by the resistant organism is transient and is quickly replaced by susceptible and other resistant Gram-negative bacilli, but **(D)** in some instances, the resistant organism contaminates the hands of caregivers, who then transmit it to another infant.

of rectal and nasal swab specimens demonstrated no growth of any organism on admission to the NICU, and 16% to 30% of samples were still negative for growth by the third NICU day. Slow acquisition of colonizing flora appeared to be the consequence of nearly uniform exposure to antibiotics upon admission to the NICU and of the relative paucity of contact with humans who were not hospital personnel.[36] When colonization ultimately did occur, more than half of infants became colonized with *Klebsiella, Enterobacter,* or *Citrobacter* species, and once such organisms appeared, they grew to high density.[36] This abnormal ontogeny of stool flora among NICU residents compared with healthy infants has been confirmed by many subsequent studies.[37-41]

Gain and Loss of MDR-GNR While in the NICU

(Fig. 16-1, *C*)
Once the NICU resident becomes colonized by a resistant Gram-negative organism, usually colonization is inconsequential and short-lived. We studied the acquisition

of MDR-GNR in a tertiary care NICU in Cleveland, Ohio, over a 12-month period.[42] Nasopharyngeal and rectal swab specimens were obtained three times a week and were screened for Gram-negative bacilli resistant to gentamicin, piperacillin-tazobactam, or ceftazidime. A total of 8.6% of infants in the Cleveland NICU became colonized before discharge with a Gram-negative bacillus resistant to at least one of these agents. Antibiotic-resistant organisms were acquired from the first NICU day; acquisition then continued gradually and cumulatively throughout the infant's NICU course. When colonization with a resistant organism did occur, it frequently was cleared rapidly, however, with a median duration less than a week,[42] reflecting a particularly unstable microflora in this population. Small proportions of infants, however, may become persistently colonized by MDR-GNR. In a study conducted at two NICUs in London,[43] 26% of infants colonized by a drug-resistant *Escherichia coli* at hospital discharge, and 7% of those colonized by *Klebsiella*, were colonized by genetically indistinguishable organisms at 6-month follow-up.

Horizontal Transmission of MDR-GNR to Other NICU Patients

(Fig. 16-1, *D*)
The degree of direct infant-to-infant transmission of antibiotic-resistant Gram-negative bacilli during non-outbreak periods has been addressed by several studies.[41,42,44,45] In most of these reports, regularly collected rectal swab cultures were obtained on large numbers of NICU patients.[41,42] The isolated organisms then were subjected to PFGE analysis to determine the proportion of PFGE types that were present in more than one infant, suggesting person-to-person spread. The frequency of horizontal transmission has varied widely from unit to unit, presumably reflecting local factors such as the physical design of the nursery, adherence to hand hygiene, nurse-to-infant ratios, acuity, and crowding. In a survey in Cleveland, approximately 12% of 154 genetically distinct resistant bacilli were shared[42] versus more than 21% of organisms cultured from infants hospitalized in New Haven, Connecticut,[45] 34% in New York City,[44] and nearly three quarters of resistant organisms colonizing infants in Palermo, Italy.[41] In these reports, horizontal transmission typically was detected among infants housed in the same room during overlapping periods. Most clusters of infants colonized by horizontally transmitted organisms have involved 10 or fewer infants, although two clusters including 21 patients were noted in the Italian study.[41,42,45] In almost all circumstances, clustering of organisms would have been undetected by routine clinical practice, and horizontal transmission ceased without intervention. These data suggest that undetected mini-epidemics of antibiotic-resistant Gram-negative bacilli probably occur routinely in busy referral NICUs, but that they are small and self-limiting.

Epidemiology of MDR-GNR During Outbreaks

NICU outbreaks with antibiotic-resistant bacilli have been reported throughout the era of modern infant intensive care.[46] Resistant organisms causing outbreaks have evolved over time, encompassing ever greater varieties of genera and resistance phenotypes. Recently reported NICU outbreaks have been caused primarily by *Enterobacter*,[47-51] *Klebsiella*,[52-54] and *Serratia*[55-57] that typically express resistance to one or more parenteral antibiotics commonly employed in the NICU. In some instances, outbreaks caused by more than one MDR-GNR have occurred simultaneously[58,59]; these latter epidemics may be due to the cross-species transfer of a single transmissible genetic element containing the resistance determinants.[60] Over the past several years, NICU outbreak reports have emphasized the importance of organisms expressing extended-spectrum β-lactamases (ESBLs).[50,61-65]

The epidemiologic characteristics of outbreaks of Gram-negative bacilli differ from those noted during endemic periods. After introduction of the epidemic strain into the unit, the clone spreads rapidly from infant to infant. Cross-sectional surveillance frequently reveals previously undetected colonization in a large proportion of infants. The strain characteristically persists in the individual patient, and especially in the unit, over long periods; similar to MRSA, it is not unusual for colonization and infection by the epidemic strain to occur over months or even years. In outbreaks

16

due to antibiotic-resistant organisms, acquisition of the epidemic clone is strongly associated with exposure to the antibiotic to which the bacillus is resistant.

Contrary to the endemic situation, in which environmental contamination by Gram-negative bacilli is of low density, outbreak clones are readily cultured from one or more environmental sources that then may serve to perpetuate the epidemic. NICU outbreaks of Gram-negative bacilli have isolated the epidemic strain from rectal thermometers,[51,54] incubator doors,[66] pulse oximeter probes,[54] reused suction catheters and laryngoscope blades,[67,68] breast pumps,[67] hand washing disinfectants,[57] and heparin flushes.[69] Additionally, outbreak clones have been identified from nutritional sources, including contaminated parenteral nutrition solutions[70] and formulas.[71]

Control Strategies for Nonepidemic MRSA and MDR-GNR

Few reports outside NICU outbreak descriptions address the containment of MRSA and MDR-GNR in the NICU. Some potential strategies to control resistant organisms during endemic periods can be derived from expert opinion and experience in non-neonatal ICUs, however. Given the differences in their epidemiology, not all potential measures are applicable to both MRSA and MDR-GNR; each measure listed here (summarized in Table 16-1) is denoted accordingly.

Prevention of All Infections Through Promotion of Hand Hygiene (MRSA and MDR-GNR)

The most effective strategy to prevent infections with antibiotic-resistant bacteria is to adopt interventions likely to prevent all infections. Hand hygiene is thus central to any such program. Indeed, because newborns rapidly acquire their colonizing flora through exposure to their environment, hand disinfection is particularly important in the NICU.

Bacteria occupying the hands of health care workers are composed of two populations. The resident flora is relatively permanent and is made up of organisms of low pathogenic potential, particularly coagulase-negative staphylococci, diptheroids, and viridans streptococci.[72] The transient population, composed of more dangerous microbes, colonizes the superficial layers of the dermis.[72] Although contamination of caregiver hands by potentially pathogenic bacteria and fungi can occur with virtually

Table 16-1   MEASURES TO REDUCE MRSA AND MDR-GNR COLONIZATION AND INFECTION IN THE NICU

Endemic
Prevent infection through promotion of hand hygiene
Prevent infection through quality improvement initiatives
Apply barrier isolation to identified infants
Reserve equipment and decontaminate surfaces
Develop antibiotic policies (MDR-GNR)
Perform preemptive surveillance (MRSA)

Epidemic
Strictly enforce and police hand hygiene
Cohort identified infants
Enforce strict barrier isolation
Assign all equipment to colonized versus noncolonized patients
Screen health care workers (MRSA)
Perform environmental cultures (MDR-GNR)
Restrict antibiotics (MDR-GNR)
Close the unit to new admissions

MDR-GNR, Multiple-drug resistant Gram-negative rods; *MRSA,* methicillin-resistant *Staphylococcus aureus; NICU,* neonatal intensive care unit.

any aspect of patient care, including contact with the patient's inanimate environment, selected frequently encountered activities, especially contact with respiratory secretions and diapers, are particularly prone to cause such contamination.[73,74]

Unlike the resident flora, bacteria composing the transient flora can be readily removed by hand hygiene. Even hand washing with nondisinfectant soap at least partially removes elements of the transient flora, probably largely through mechanical action. Use of a disinfectant, however, is required to reliably eradicate most of the transient flora. The compounds most commonly used for hospital disinfection are iodophors, chlorhexidine, and alcohol. All three agents have broad activity against Gram-positive and Gram-negative bacteria, fungi, and many viruses.[72,75] Disinfectant-containing scrub brushes, traditionally employed in the past, are no longer recommended, because they promote skin breakdown, which, in turn, results in heavy bacterial growth on the hands. Iodophor and chlorhexidine hand disinfectants have a residual antibacterial effect that can last many hours when allowed to dry, but this requirement, if strictly applied, would occupy an inordinate amount of caregiver time.[76] Alcohol-based disinfectants provide less residual activity, but they reduce hand bacterial concentrations rapidly,[75] and they can be applied without a sink. These properties have rendered alcohol-based hand products the preferred agents for hand hygiene and prevention of nosocomial infections (NIs) in all areas of the hospital.[72] Indeed, in a recent report from a Japanese NICU, promotion and use of alcohol-based hand disinfectant was the only intervention among several that was effective in reducing the presence of MRSA in the unit.[18]

Current standards require hand disinfection before and after contact with the patient or his or her immediate environment. Long nails (both artificial and natural) and hand jewelry should be avoided, because both can harbor a broad spectrum of potentially pathogenic microorganisms. Long nails in particular have been implicated in perpetuating nursery epidemics.[77,78] Some authorities accept the use of gloves as a substitute for hand disinfection.[74,79,80] Studies in the care of adults patients, however, have demonstrated that hands frequently can become contaminated during de-gloving,[81] emphasizing the need to employ hand disinfection even with the use of gloves.

Despite the compelling logic underlying hand disinfection in the hospital setting, adherence to hand hygiene standards by health care workers generally has been abysmal, and surveys performed specifically in the NICU have recorded compliance rates as low as 22% to 28%.[80,82] Recent experience both in and out of the NICU has made it clear that sustained improvement in hand hygiene among hospital workers will not occur unless a prolonged, ambitious, multifaceted effort is made.[75] Uniformly, the most effective programs have been supported both administratively and financially by hospital officials and policy makers who have made it a visible, sustained priority for their institution. Personal investment and role modeling by attending staff are critical. Virtually every published program has incorporated regular hand hygiene audits over many months, frequently completed surreptitiously by unidentified observers, with immediate feedback to the staff in the targeted unit.[75,83-86]

Several recent studies have reported programs that have attempted to improve hand hygiene in the NICU setting and, secondarily, to reduce the incidence of NIs. Lam and colleagues[83] instituted an aggressive program in a Hong Kong nursery in which step-by-step protocols were designed to improve hand hygiene during hands-on interventions. Adherence to hand hygiene was significantly improved and the incidence of NIs was reduced nearly in half, from 17.2 infections/100 admissions before the intervention to 9.0 infections/100 admissions afterward. A second program, in Geneva, Switzerland, employed an ambitious series of in-services and focus groups to similarly develop protocols regarding practices during direct patient care.[84] Proper hand hygiene increased from 42% of opportunities to 55%, and the incidence of NIs among very low birth weight (VLBW) infants was reduced by one third—a benefit that persisted over a 9-month follow-up period. Taiwanese investigators[86] achieved similar improvement in hand hygiene compliance and nosocomial infection rates by instituting a program using many of the same features, additionally establishing a schedule of financial penalties and awards for nursing staff according to their hand hygiene performance.

Prevention of All Infections Through Quality Improvement Initiatives (MRSA and MDR-GNR)

Hand hygiene practice has been folded into larger, broader interventions (called "bundles") designed to reduce NIs in the NICU and elsewhere in the hospital. In neonatology, the Vermont Oxford Network (VON) Collaborative for Quality Improvement pioneered projects using a collaborative improvement model, reflecting many of the methods promulgated by the Institute for Healthcare Improvement.[87] In this model, collaboratives are built from similar institutions that share a common goal of improving a specified health care outcome. Improvement is achieved through *benchmarking,* by which members of the collaborative emulate the practices of the institutions enjoying the best outcomes at baseline. Benchmarking began as a method employed by industry when it was noted that some facilities produced superior products compared with others within the same company that were performing apparently nearly identical tasks. Health care organizations, faced with increasing pressure to control costs and to improve patient outcomes, soon saw the potential benefit of using similar analyses in targeting care practices to improve the outcomes of patients.[88] The collaborative improvement models recognize that NIs, similar to many untoward health care events, result from complex, interacting systems that are strongly influenced by the local culture in which they occur,[89,90] and that these outcomes are unlikely to improve until the culture is changed.

Member institutions within a collaborative begin the process by building multidisciplinary teams led by a physician champion. Multicenter focus groups derived from these teams develop the bundles whose components are selected from well-designed clinical trials, expert opinion, and interventions practiced at the benchmark institutions. Individual hospitals within the collaborative then choose from a package of available interventions, with selection biased toward those practiced at the better-performing sites.[91,92] Each component of the selected bundle is initially integrated at each member hospital through small-scale, short-duration trials termed *PDSA (Plan, Do, Study, Act) cycles.* The PDSA method allows the team to determine the adaptability of a particular intervention by applying it to a limited sample size over a contracted period, after which team members reflect on the effect and apply the intervention on a larger scale, modify it to better fit the workings of their institution, or reject it. Members of the collaborative then relate their experiences in changing local processes to each other through regular meetings, so that the entire group can take advantage of a collective wisdom.

The goal of the first VON project was to reduce nosocomial bacteremias in the NICU among a group of six self-selected NICUs. The overall rate of nosocomial bacteremia at those units declined from 26.3% in 1994 to 20.9% in 1996 ($P = 0.007$).[93] Although significant variation was noted among NICUs with respect to the magnitude of improvement achieved, as a whole their outcomes were substantially better than those observed at the 66 other VON centers that did not participate in the infection reduction project. Nosocomial bacteremia rates continued to decrease among the six test centers during an additional year of follow-up, compared with static incidence rates recorded at the comparison institutions.[94] In a companion analysis, Rogowski and coauthors demonstrated statistically significant decreases in average health care costs for infants cared for at the six collaborative sites, from $57,606 to $46,674, for an estimated annual per-hospital savings of $2.3 million.[95] The estimated per-hospital cost of the nosocomial bacteremia reduction program itself was less than $80,000 over 2 years. Subsequent VON collaborative groups have refined the methods to reduce nosocomial bacteremia and have demonstrated further reductions, from 24.6% in 1997 to 16.4% in 2000.[96]

The VON infection reducing bundle has been described in detail.[97] Components of this bundle were termed *possible best practices,* conceding that many of the interventions have never been directly tested in neonates. In addition to the hand hygiene practices noted earlier, key components of the bundle include the following:

1. *Standard assessment of blood culture results:* This component resulted from the recognition that overreaction to a single positive blood culture, especially for skin commensals such as coagulase-negative staphylococci, resulted in unnecessary antibiotic exposure and promotion of colonization and infection by resistant organisms. Member institutions embraced a standard of obtaining two cultures at separate sites, each composed of 1 mL; applying antiseptic rigorously to the skin before sampling; and encouraging the collection of corroborative laboratory results (C-reactive protein, total white blood cell count, and assessment of immature cells) to inform the decision to start or continue antibiotics.
2. Enforcing maximum barriers (sterile gowns and gloves plus surgical mask) among personnel inserting central catheters.
3. Adopting closed catheter systems.
4. Minimizing line entry by reducing unnecessary sampling.
5. Applying a sterile field under the port whenever the catheter was entered.
6. Reducing the duration of parenteral nutrition through aggressive institution of enteral feeds, thereby limiting the duration of central catheterization.

The successes of collaborative models in reducing nosocomial bacteremia have been shared by other groups. The California Perinatal Quality Care Collaborative (CPQCC) has adapted the VON method to allow large numbers of sites to participate simultaneously using webinars and online tool kits (available at www.cpqcc.org). This collaborative has the advantage of partnering with the State of California to encourage and ultimately financially reward participation and improved outcomes. Similar collaborative programs have been adopted by the New York State Regional Perinatal Centers (NYS RPC),[98] the National Initiative for Child Health Quality (NICHQ), the Children's Hospital Association (CHA), the National Association for Children's Hospitals and Related Institutions (NACHRI), and the Ohio Perinatal Quality Collaborative (OPQC). Additionally, similar collaborative methods have been used with dramatic results to reduce central venous catheter infections in adult ICUs[99] and pediatric ICUs.[100]

Instituting and Enforcing Maximal Barrier Protection (MRSA and MDR-GNR)

This includes gloves, gowns, and, for MRSA, masks when caring for infants identified with colonization or infection by antibiotic-resistant organisms (MRSA and MDR-GNR). Most patient acquisition of MRSA in the hospital is the result of transmission from a colonized health care worker, and at least some acquisition of MDR-GNR is acquired in the same fashion. The hands and possibly the clothing of the health care worker[101] are the likely culprits in most circumstances, underlining the requirement for glove and gown use when caring for a patient with established resistant-organism colonization or infection. At our hospital, barrier isolation is initiated for all patients colonized or infected with MRSA or Gram-negative bacteria resistant to three or more classes of antibiotic.

Decontamination of Environmental Surfaces (MRSA and MDR-GNR)

The role of MRSA- and MDR-GNR–contaminated medical equipment and environmental surfaces in promoting transmission has not been well studied, but it is certain that such contamination occurs. Boyce and colleagues documented contamination of inanimate surfaces in more than two thirds of rooms occupied by MRSA-colonized adult patients.[101] The health care worker may acquire MRSA on his or her ungloved hand after contact with such contaminated surfaces, resulting in transmission to an unaffected patient. Even in the absence of clear evidence implicating contaminated fomites in the spread of MRSA and MDR-GNR in the nursery, it is prudent to assign medical equipment for exclusive use in the MRSA- and MDR-GNR–colonized infant, and to thoroughly disinfect the immediate area once the patient has been discharged.

Antibiotic Control (MDR-GNR)

No compelling data suggest that antibiotic control limits the presence of MRSA. However, a portion of antibiotic resistance in MDR-GNR emerges under antibiotic pressure, suggesting that manipulation of antibiotics in the NICU may afford some benefit.

Some data document the relative propensity of selected classes of antibiotics to promote bacillary resistance in the NICU. Many centers have used gentamicin in combination with ampicillin and vancomycin for well over a decade, for example, and have had few if any problems with resistance to aminoglycosides.[102] Tullus and colleagues surveyed rectal swab samples from 22 Swedish nurseries through the late 1980s[103]; none of 1369 isolates of E. coli, Klebsiella, and Enterobacter screened during the course of this study were resistant to gentamicin, despite the routine use of this drug by many participating centers. The use of third-generation cephalosporins, on the other hand, may be especially associated with the promotion of autologous resistance among Gram-negative species in the NICU. Indeed, it is well established that exposure to this class of antibiotics among seriously ill adults may rapidly select β-lactam–resistant Enterobacteriaceae, especially among Enterobacter[104] and ESBL-producing bacteria.[63,105] When cefotaxime was substituted for gentamicin in an NICU experiencing an outbreak of gentamicin-resistant Klebsiella pneumoniae, a high frequency of colonization with cephalosporin-resistant Enterobacter cloacae appeared after just 10 weeks.[102] De Man and colleagues[106] studied the relative propensity of penicillin-tobramycin use and ampicillin-cefotaxime in promoting resistance in a Dutch NICU, employing a 6-month crossover design, during which each regimen was used as the preferred first-line antibiotic choice in side-by-side nurseries. Investigators found a marked increase in colonization and infection by cephalosporin-resistant E. cloacae during the period of ampicillin-cefotaxime use versus little aminoglycoside resistance during the penicillin-tobramycin period. These experiences caution against routine sustained use of third-generation cephalosporins in the NICU during non-outbreak periods. The relative propensity of most other antibiotic classes to promote resistance is not known, but concern is increasing that overuse of the carbapenems in adult patients may result in colonization or infection with carbapenem-resistant Pseudomonas[107] and carbapenemase-expressing Klebsiella.[108]

Stopping antibiotics in a patient in whom infection appears unlikely is probably effective in reducing colonization and infection with resistant organisms in all ICU settings. In the study by Singh and colleagues,[109] adult ICU patients in whom a diagnosis of ventilator-associated pneumonia was suspected were evaluated by a pneumonia infection score when therapy was initiated, and again 3 days later. Investigators used a persistently low score to identify patients in whom the diagnosis of pulmonary infection was unlikely, recognizing that in common practice, such patients regularly are treated with a prolonged course of antibiotics anyway. This trial demonstrated that stopping antibiotics in low-risk patients at day 3 of therapy resulted in significantly lower acquisition of antibiotic-resistant organisms without adversely affecting patient mortality and length of stay in the ICU, when compared with similar patients in whom antibiotic stoppage was not required.[109]

Another strategy involving antibiotic control that has been proposed to reduce the prevalence of MDR-GNR in the ICU setting is antibiotic cycling. This strategy mandates a regular, scheduled rotation of antibiotic preference within the ICU. We tested the benefit of antibiotic cycling in our NICU in Cleveland.[110] A monthly rotation of gentamicin, piperacillin-tazobactam, and ceftazidime was compared with unrestricted antibiotic use in side-by-side NICU populations. Pharyngeal and rectal samples were obtained three times a week and were tested for Gram-negative bacilli resistant to each of the antibiotics in the rotation schedule. Over a 1-year trial, cycling failed to reduce the prevalence of colonization by resistant Gram-negative rods: 10.7% of infants in the population assigned to the antibiotic cycling schedule were colonized with an organism resistant to one or more of the rotation antibiotics versus 7.7% of the control population ($P < 0.09$).[110] The incidences of nosocomial infection and mortality also were similar between study populations. Although some trials of antibiotic cycling in adult ICUs have been positive,[111] more recent data in non-NICU patients have been less optimistic.[112] Unfortunately, coresistance to agents of different antibiotic classes is common among hospital-acquired Gram-negative bacilli; consequently, changing from one broad-spectrum agent to another may not relieve antibiotic pressure. Additionally, some resistance determinants in MDR-GNRs are linked to other factors that confer survival advantage, such as those improving adherence to epithelial surfaces or resulting in resistance to disinfectants[113,114]— properties that will not be easily surrendered in the face of antibiotic cycling. As a result, it is unlikely that this strategy will have a major impact in reducing the endemic presence of MDR-GNRs in the NICU.

Antibiotic control in the NICU ultimately may be best achieved through antibiotic stewardship programs (ASPs). These programs are led by a team of experts in anti-infective therapy who provide real-time assistance to practitioners in selecting the most appropriate antibiotic for a given situation. The goals of ASPs are to reduce costs, lessen adverse drug events, and ensure that the chosen antibiotic is active against the offending organism and is administered according to evidence-based guidelines. Reports of ASPs in adult patients document their ability to reduce the institutional prevalence of resistant organisms by limiting the use of unnecessarily broad-spectrum agents and of all agents for longer than they are needed.[115] A growing number of pediatric institutions are developing antibiotic stewardship programs.[116-118] Although few published data have examined the effectiveness of ASPs specifically in the NICU, the success of a vancomycin-use algorithm in safely reducing two tertiary care NICUs exposure to that drug[119] supports the contention that carefully conceived stewardship programs can be relevant and effective in intensive care nurseries.

Preemptive Surveillance and Isolation of All Patients for MRSA Colonization (MRSA)

Perhaps the most controversial potential strategy to control endemic MRSA currently debated among non-neonatologists is the routine performance of surveillance cultures in all patients upon hospital admission and at fixed intervals thereafter. Most authorities have estimated that the risk of MRSA transmission in adult ICUs is reduced 3- to 16-fold if the colonized subject is in isolation rather than on the open ward.[11,120,121] Mathematical models of MRSA transmission in the hospital have implicated the unidentified, and therefore nonisolated, MRSA-colonized patient as being the most influential factor in the spread of resistant staphylococci.[120,121]

In response to these observations, some European countries, most notably the Netherlands, have adapted a very aggressive National Health Institute–mandated policy for preemptive screening for MRSA. Hospital-wide, all patients are regularly screened for MRSA colonization upon admission, and those falling into predefined high-risk categories are isolated immediately with full barrier protection until proven MRSA free. Patients at lesser risk similarly are isolated if colonization is subsequently identified. Identification of colonization in a patient who had not been isolated triggers immediate screening of all nearby patients and all exposed health care workers. The identification of secondary cases generates further screening. Identified health care workers are furloughed with pay until their colonization disappears. The results are compelling: the incidence of nosocomial MRSA infection in Dutch facilities remains minuscule compared with that measured in North American hospitals.

On the other hand, preemptive surveillance is expensive and burdensome, and institution of isolation precautions may interfere with caregiver tasks. Consequently, there is a pressing need to establish empiric, scientifically derived evidence of its effectiveness. Observational data regarding the value of preemptive surveillance recently generated in American adult ICUs have been inconsistent. Huang and colleagues,[122] for example, applied four infection control interventions designed to reduce MRSA colonization and infection in a step-wise fashion at a large hospital in Boston over a 9-year period; institution of routine surveillance nares cultures for MRSA was the only intervention that was followed by a statistically detectable reduction in MRSA bacteremia. By contrast, little MRSA transmission occurred in a Chicago adult ICU[123] where surveillance cultures were obtained as a research tool, but results were not reported to bedside staff. In the only side-by-side trial comparing the value of preemptive screening for MRSA in adults,[124] 18 ICUs were assigned to a preemptive surveillance strategy, and 10 control units followed their existing practice. No differences in MRSA colonization were detectable between the two groups of ICUs.[124]

Although many NICUs employ preemptive screening to detect MRSA colonization,[16-18,125] the effectiveness of this strategy has not been well established empirically in the nursery setting. The most pressing argument against implementing preemptive screening in the NICU is that it is likely to have little impact unless the policy is applied hospital-wide. Without this universal application, a portion of the personnel who routinely work outside the NICU (e.g., surgical staff and other non-neonatology consultants) may import the organism from other parts of the hospital where the control of MRSA is more lax.[8] Perhaps a stronger rationale may pertain to preemptive screening of infants transferred from another hospital for MRSA colonization if they have been hospitalized at the referring unit for longer than a few hours. Indeed, in some circumstances, preemptive screening of transferred infants for MDR-GNR has proved useful.[56]

Control Strategies for NICU Outbreaks of MRSA and MDR-GNR

In many ways, control of a nursery outbreak of an antibiotic-resistant organism is more straightforward than control of endemic disease. For both MRSA and MDR-GNR, accumulated experience has recommended several maneuvers to contain an epidemic (see Table 16-1).[46,126] These measures usually are instituted simultaneously or in rapid succession, so the independent contribution of each is unknown. It may be that no one intervention can succeed on its own, and that successful containment requires application of a package of measures, including the following:

1. Reinforce strict hand hygiene practices, including presentation of in-services and policing of adherence through overt and covert observation.
2. Cohort colonized and infected patients. This measure usually requires that cross-sectional prevalence of colonization should be defined by culturing at frequent and regular intervals (e.g., once or twice a week).[13,127,128] Culture-positive subjects then are moved to a geographically distinct area of the nursery. When staffing allows, nursing should be segregated so that each person cares only for colonized infants or for noncolonized infants. Segregation of physician and ancillary staff may be required as well.
3. Establish and enforce strict barrier isolation precautions for all contact with a colonized or infected patient. This includes wearing gowns and gloves and, for MRSA, a mask, and changing protective gear with each new patient contact. Hand hygiene should be applied between all patient contacts, that is, gloving and gowning does not preclude hand washing or use of alcohol-based hand gels. In the face of a rapidly progressive outbreak, barrier isolation may need to be applied to every infant in the NICU, regardless of colonization status, because cross-sectional prevalence audits may miss a small proportion of colonized infants.
4. Assign medical equipment to individual colonized or infected patients, or, if sharing cannot be avoided, segregate equipment to colonized versus non-colonized groups.
5. If these measures fail, close the unit to new admissions until the outbreak is contained.

Additional measures may be applied specifically to MRSA and MRD-GNR outbreaks, respectively. For MRSA epidemics:

6. Screen health care workers for nasal colonization with MRSA and decolonize when possible. The role of colonization of health care workers' nares in sustaining an MRSA outbreak is uncertain, but the opinion that it is important is growing.[11] In the ideal situation, colonized health care workers are relieved of duties until colonization spontaneously disappears or is eradicated.

Anecdotal success has been achieved by using the following regimen for MRSA decolonization in the adult: mupirocin ointment to the nares 2 to 3 times/day for 5 to 7 days, chlorhexidine baths once a day for 3 to 5 successive days, and a course of systemic antibiotics, including rifampin and another agent to which the isolate is susceptible.[11] Attempts to decolonize infants during an MRSA epidemic are of uncertain utility, but some investigators have applied mupirocin to the nares of colonized infants as part of a comprehensive strategy to end the outbreak.[129,130]

For MDR-GNR epidemics:

7. Perform environmental cultures to determine whether there is a common source for the outbreak strain. The need for these cultures depends to some extent on the organism. *Serratia marcescens* in particular has frequently been implicated in common-source epidemics.

8. Restrict the use of antibiotics to which the outbreak strain is resistant.

16

References

1. Cosgrove SE. The relationship between antimicrobial resistance and patient outcomes: Mortality, length of hospital stay, and health care costs. *Clin Infect Dis*. 2006;42(Suppl 2):S82-S89.
2. Back NA, Linnemann Jr CC, Staneck JL, et al. Control of methicillin-resistant *Staphylococcus aureus* in a neonatal intensive-care unit: Use of intensive microbiologic surveillance and mupirocin. *Infect Control Hosp Epidemiol*. 1996;17(4):227-231.
3. Campbell JR, Zaccaria E, Mason Jr EO, et al. Epidemiological analysis defining concurrent outbreaks of *Serratia marcescens* and methicillin-resistant *Staphylococcus aureus* in a neonatal intensive-care unit. *Infect Control Hosp Epidemiol*. 1998;19(12):924-928.
4. Haddad Q, Sobayo EI, Basit OB, et al. Outbreak of methicillin-resistant *Staphylococcus aureus* in a neonatal intensive care unit. *J Hosp Infect*. 1993;23(3):211-222.
5. Haley RW, Cushion NB, Tenover FC, et al. Eradication of endemic methicillin-resistant *Staphylococcus aureus* infections from a neonatal intensive care unit. *J Infect Dis*. 1995;171(3):614-624.
6. Karchmer TB, Durbin LJ, Simonton BM, et al. Cost-effectiveness of active surveillance cultures and contact/droplet precautions for control of methicillin-resistant *Staphylococcus aureus*. *J Hosp Infect*. 2002;51(2):126-132.
7. Regev-Yochay G, Rubinstein E, Barzilai A, et al. Methicillin-resistant *Staphylococcus aureus* in neonatal intensive care unit. *Emerg Infect Dis*. 2005;11(3):453-456.
8. Saiman L, Cronquist A, Wu F, et al. An outbreak of methicillin-resistant *Staphylococcus aureus* in a neonatal intensive care unit. *Infect Control Hosp Epidemiol*. 2003;24(5):317-321.
9. Toltzis P, Blumer JL. Antibiotic resistance. In: Feigin RD, Cherry JD, Demmler-Harrison GJ, Kaplan SL, eds. *Textbook of Pediatric Infectious Diseases*. Philadelphia: Elsevier; 2009:3132-3155.
10. McDougal LK, Steward CD, Killgore GE, et al. Pulsed-field gel electrophoresis typing of oxacillin-resistant *Staphylococcus aureus* isolates from the United States: Establishing a national database. *J Clin Microbiol*. 2003;41(11):5113-5120.
11. Muto CA, Jernigan JA, Ostrowsky BE, et al. SHEA guideline for preventing nosocomial transmission of multidrug-resistant strains of *Staphylococcus aureus* and enterococcus. *Infect Control Hosp Epidemiol*. 2003;24(5):362-386.
12. Graham DR, Correa-Villasenor A, Anderson RL, et al. Epidemic neonatal gentamicin-methicillin–resistant *Staphylococcus aureus* infection associated with nonspecific topical use of gentamicin. *J Pediatr*. 1980;97(6):972-978.
13. Khoury J, Jones M, Grim A, et al. Eradication of methicillin-resistant *Staphylococcus aureus* from a neonatal intensive care unit by active surveillance and aggressive infection control measures. *Infect Control Hosp Epidemiol*. 2005;26(7):616-621.
14. Bratu S, Eramo A, Kopec R, et al. Community-associated methicillin-resistant *Staphylococcus aureus* in hospital nursery and maternity units. *Emerg Infect Dis* 2005;11(6):808-813.
15. Saiman L, O'Keefe M, Graham 3rd PL, et al: Hospital transmission of community-acquired methicillin-resistant *Staphylococcus aureus* among postpartum women. *Clin Infect Dis*. 2003;37(10):1313-1319.
16. Huang YC, Chou YH, Su LH, et al. Methicillin-resistant *Staphylococcus aureus* colonization and its association with infection among infants hospitalized in neonatal intensive care units. *Pediatrics*. 2006;118(2):469-474.
17. Maraqa NF, Aigbivbalu L, Masnita-Iusan C, et al. Prevalence of and risk factors for methicillin-resistant *Staphylococcus aureus* colonization and infection among infants at a level III neonatal intensive care unit. *Am J Infect Control*. 2011;39(1):35-41.
18. Sakamoto F, Yamada H, Suzuki C, et al. Increased use of alcohol-based hand sanitizers and successful eradication of methicillin-resistant *Staphylococcus aureus* from a neonatal intensive care unit: A multivariate time series analysis. *Am J Infect Control*. 2010;38(7):529-534.
19. Hollis RJ, Barr JL, Doebbeling BN, et al. Familial carriage of methicillin-resistant *Staphylococcus aureus* and subsequent infection in a premature neonate. *Clin Infect Dis*. 1995;21(2):328-332.

20. Sakaki H, Nishioka M, Kanda K, et al. An investigation of the risk factors for infection with methicillin-resistant *Staphylococcus aureus* among patients in a neonatal intensive care unit. *Am J Infect Control*. 2009;37(7):580-586.
21. Deresinski S. Methicillin-resistant *Staphylococcus aureus*: An evolutionary, epidemiologic, and therapeutic odyssey. *Clin Infect Dis*. 2005;40(4):562-573.
22. Lina G, Piemont Y, Godail-Gamot F, et al. Involvement of Panton-Valentine leukocidin-producing *Staphylococcus aureus* in primary skin infections and pneumonia. *Clin Infect Dis*. 1999;29(5):1128-1132.
23. Behari P, Englund J, Alcasid G, et al. Transmission of methicillin-resistant *Staphylococcus aureus* to preterm infants through breast milk. *Infect Control Hosp Epidemiol*. 2004;25(9):778-780.
24. Eckhardt C, Halvosa JS, Ray SM, et al. Transmission of methicillin-resistant *Staphylococcus aureus* in the neonatal intensive care unit from a patient with community-acquired disease. *Infect Control Hosp Epidemiol*. 2003;24(6):460-461.
25. Healy CM, Hulten KG, Palazzi DL, et al. Emergence of new strains of methicillin-resistant *Staphylococcus aureus* in a neonatal intensive care unit. *Clin Infect Dis*. 2004;39(10):1460-1466.
26. Carey AJ, Della-Latta P, Huard R, et al. Changes in the molecular epidemiological characteristics of methicillin-resistant *Staphylococcus aureus* in a neonatal intensive care unit. *Infect Control Hosp Epidemiol*. 2010;31(6):613-619.
27. Gregory ML, Eichenwald EC, Puopolo KM. Seven-year experience with a surveillance program to reduce methicillin-resistant *Staphylococcus aureus* colonization in a neonatal intensive care unit. *Pediatrics*. 2009;123(5):e790-e796.
28. Balmer SE, Scott PH, Wharton BA. Diet and faecal flora in the newborn: Lactoferrin. *Arch Dis Child*. 1989;64(12):1685-1690.
29. Balmer SE, Wharton BA. Diet and faecal flora in the newborn: Breast milk and infant formula. *Arch Dis Child*. 1989;64(12):1672-1677.
30. Benno Y, Sawada K, Mitsuoka T. The intestinal microflora of infants: Composition of fecal flora in breast-fed and bottle-fed infants. *Microbiol Immunol*. 1984;28(9):975-986.
31. Hokama T, Imamura T. Members of the throat microflora among infants with different feeding methods. *J Trop Pediatr*. 1998;44(2):84-86.
32. Biasucci G, Rubini M, Riboni S, et al. Mode of delivery affects the bacterial community in the newborn gut. *Early Hum Dev*. 2010;86(Suppl 1):13-15.
33. Palmer C, Bik EM, DiGiulio DB, et al. Development of the human infant intestinal microbiota. *PLoS Biol*. 2007;5(7):e177.
34. Casewell M, Phillips I. Hands as route of transmission for *Klebsiella* species. *BMJ*. 1977;2(6098):1315-1317.
35. Knittle MA, Eitzman DV, Baer H. Role of hand contamination of personnel in the epidemiology of gram-negative nosocomial infections. *J Pediatr*. 1975;86(3):433-437.
36. Goldmann DA, Leclair J, Macone A. Bacterial colonization of neonates admitted to an intensive care environment. *J Pediatr*. 1978;93(2):288-293.
37. Eriksson M, Melen B, Myrback KE, et al. Bacterial colonization of newborn infants in a neonatal intensive care unit. *Acta Paediatr Scand*. 1982;71(5):779-783.
38. Finelli L, Livengood JR, Saiman L. Surveillance of pharyngeal colonization: Detection and control of serious bacterial illness in low birth weight infants. *Pediatr Infect Dis J*. 1994;13(10):854-859.
39. Savey A, Fleurette J, Salle BL. An analysis of the microbial flora of premature neonates. *J Hosp Infect*. 1992;21(4):275-289.
40. Tullus K, Fryklund B, Berglund B, et al. Influence of age on faecal carriage of P-fimbriated *Escherichia coli* and other gram-negative bacteria in hospitalized neonates. *J Hosp Infect*. 1988;11(4):349-356.
41. Mammina C, Di Carlo P, Cipolla D, et al. Surveillance of multidrug-resistant gram-negative bacilli in a neonatal intensive care unit: Prominent role of cross transmission. *Am J Infect Control*. 2007;35(4):222-230.
42. Toltzis P, Dul MJ, Hoyen C, et al. Molecular epidemiology of antibiotic-resistant gram-negative bacilli in a neonatal intensive care unit during a nonoutbreak period. *Pediatrics*. 2001;108(5):1143-1148.
43. Millar M, Philpott A, Wilks M, et al. Colonization and persistence of antibiotic-resistant Enterobacteriaceae strains in infants nursed in two neonatal intensive care units in East London, United Kingdom. *J Clin Microbiol*. 2008;46(2):560-567.
44. Waters V, Larson E, Wu F, et al. Molecular epidemiology of gram-negative bacilli from infected neonates and health care workers' hands in neonatal intensive care units. *Clin Infect Dis*. 2004;38(12):1682-1687.
45. Almuneef MA, Baltimore RS, Farrel PA, et al. Molecular typing demonstrating transmission of gram-negative rods in a neonatal intensive care unit in the absence of a recognized epidemic. *Clin Infect Dis*. 2001;32(2):220-227.
46. Toltzis P, Blumer JL. Antibiotic-resistant gram-negative bacteria in the critical care setting. *Pediatr Clin N Am*. 1995;42(3):687-702.
47. Fernandez-Baca V, Ballesteros F, Hervas JA, et al. Molecular epidemiological typing of *Enterobacter cloacae* isolates from a neonatal intensive care unit: Three-year prospective study. *J Hosp Infect*. 2001;49(3):173-182.
48. Kartali G, Tzelepi E, Pournaras S, et al. Outbreak of infections caused by *Enterobacter cloacae* producing the integron-associated beta-lactamase IBC-1 in a neonatal intensive care unit of a Greek hospital. *Antimicrobiol Agents Chemother*. 2002;46(5):1577-1580.

49. Liu SC, Leu HS, Yen MY, et al. Study of an outbreak of *Enterobacter cloacae* sepsis in a neonatal intensive care unit: The application of epidemiologic chromosome profiling by pulsed-field gel electrophoresis. *Am J Infect Control*. 2002;30(7):381-385.

50. Talon D, Menget P, Thouverez M, et al. Emergence of *Enterobacter cloacae* as a common pathogen in neonatal units: Pulsed-field gel electrophoresis analysis. *J Hosp Infect*. 2004;57(2):119-125.

51. v Dijk Y, Bik EM, Hochstenbach-Vernooij S, et al. Management of an outbreak of *Enterobacter cloacae* in a neonatal unit using simple preventive measures. *J Hosp Infect*. 2002;51(1):21-26.

52. Berthelot P, Grattard F, Patural H, et al. Nosocomial colonization of premature babies with *Klebsiella oxytoca*: Probable role of enteral feeding procedure in transmission and control of the outbreak with the use of gloves. *Infect Control Hosp Epidemiol*. 2001;22(3):148-151.

53. Jeong SH, Kim WM, Chang CL, et al. Neonatal intensive care unit outbreak caused by a strain of *Klebsiella oxytoca* resistant to aztreonam due to overproduction of chromosomal beta-lactamase. *J Hosp Infect*. 2001;48(4):281-288.

54. Macrae MB, Shannon KP, Rayner DM, et al. A simultaneous outbreak on a neonatal unit of two strains of multiply antibiotic resistant *Klebsiella pneumoniae* controllable only by ward closure. *J Hosp Infect*. 2001;49(3):183-192.

55. Assadian O, Berger A, Aspock C, et al. Nosocomial outbreak of *Serratia marcescens* in a neonatal intensive care unit. *Infect Control Hosp Epidemiol*. 2002;23(8):457-461.

56. Fleisch F, Zimmermann-Baer U, Zbinden R, et al. Three consecutive outbreaks of *Serratia marcescens* in a neonatal intensive care unit. *Clin Infect Dis*. 2002;34(6):767-773.

57. Villari P, Crispino M, Salvadori A, et al. Molecular epidemiology of an outbreak of *Serratia marcescens* in a neonatal intensive care unit. *Infect Control Hosp Epidemiol*. 2001;22(10):630-634.

58. Casolari C, Pecorari M, Fabio G, et al. A simultaneous outbreak of *Serratia marcescens* and *Klebsiella pneumoniae* in a neonatal intensive care unit. *J Hosp Infect*. 2005;61(4):312-320.

59. Crivaro V, Bagattini M, Salza MF, et al. Risk factors for extended-spectrum beta-lactamase-producing *Serratia marcescens* and *Klebsiella pneumoniae* acquisition in a neonatal intensive care unit. *J Hosp Infect*. 2007;67(2):135-141.

60. Bagattini M, Crivaro V, Di Popolo A, et al. Molecular epidemiology of extended-spectrum beta-lactamase-producing *Klebsiella pneumoniae* in a neonatal intensive care unit. *J Antimicrob Chemother*. 2006;57(5):979-982.

61. Conte MP, Venditti M, Chiarini F, et al. Extended spectrum beta-lactamase-producing *Klebsiella pneumoniae* outbreaks during a third generation cephalosporin restriction policy. *J Chemother*. 2005;17(1):66-73.

62. Lebessi E, Dellagrammaticas H, Tassios PT, et al. Extended-spectrum beta-lactamase-producing *Klebsiella pneumoniae* in a neonatal intensive care unit in the high-prevalence area of Athens, Greece. *J Clin Microbiol*. 2002;40(3):799-804.

63. Linkin DR, Fishman NO, Patel JB, et al. Risk factors for extended-spectrum beta-lactamase-producing Enterobacteriaceae in a neonatal intensive care unit. *Infect Control Hosp Epidemiol*. 2004;25(9):781-783.

64. Otman J, Cavassin ED, Perugini ME, et al. An outbreak of extended-spectrum beta-lactamase-producing *Klebsiella* species in a neonatal intensive care unit in Brazil. *Infect Control Hosp Epidemiol*. 2002;23(1):8-9.

65. Kristof K, Szabo D, Marsh JW, et al. Extended-spectrum beta-lactamase-producing *Klebsiella* spp. in a neonatal intensive care unit: Risk factors for the infection and the dynamics of the molecular epidemiology. *Eur J Clin Microbiol Infect Dis*. 2007;26(8):563-570.

66. Jang TN, Fung CP, Yang TL, Shen SH, Huang CS, Lee SH. Use of pulsed-field gel electrophoresis to investigate an outbreak of *Serratia marcescens* infection in a neonatal intensive care unit. *J Hosp Infect*. 2001;48(1):13-19.

67. Jones BL, Gorman LJ, Simpson J, et al. An outbreak of *Serratia marcescens* in two neonatal intensive care units. *J Hosp Infect*. 2000;46(4):314-319.

68. Pillay T, Pillay DG, Adhikari M, Pillay A, Sturm AW. An outbreak of neonatal infection with *Acinetobacter* linked to contaminated suction catheters. *J Hosp Infect*. 1999;43(4):299-304.

69. Kimura AC, Calvet H, Higa JI, et al. Outbreak of *Ralstonia pickettii* bacteremia in a neonatal intensive care unit. *Pediatr Infect Dis J*. 2005;24(12):1099-1103.

70. Tresoldi AT, Padoveze MC, Trabasso P, et al. *Enterobacter cloacae* sepsis outbreak in a newborn unit caused by contaminated total parenteral nutrition solution. *Am J Infect Control*. 2000;28(3):258-261.

71. van Acker J, de Smet F, Muyldermans G, et al. Outbreak of necrotizing enterocolitis associated with *Enterobacter sakazakii* in powdered milk formula. *J Clin Microbiol*. 2001;39(1):293-297.

72. Boyce JM, Pittet D. Guideline for Hand Hygiene in Health-Care Settings. Recommendations of the Healthcare Infection Control Practices Advisory Committee and the HICPAC/SHEA/APIC/IDSA Hand Hygiene Task Force. Society for Healthcare Epidemiology of America/Association for Professionals in Infection Control/Infectious Diseases Society of America. *MMWR Recomm Rep*. 2002;51(RR-16):1-45.

73. Pessoa-Silva CL, Dharan S, Hugonnet S, et al. Dynamics of bacterial hand contamination during routine neonatal care. *Infect Control Hosp Epidemiol*. 2004;25(3):192-197.

74. Pittet D, Dharan S, Touveneau S, et al. Bacterial contamination of the hands of hospital staff during routine patient care. *Arch Intern Med*. 1999;159(8):821-826.

75. Pittet D. Improving adherence to hand hygiene practice: A multidisciplinary approach. *Emerg Infect Dis*. 2001;7(2):234-240.

16

76. Voss A, Widmer AF. No time for handwashing!? Handwashing versus alcoholic rub: Can we afford 100% compliance? *Infect Control Hosp Epidemiol.* 1997;18(3):205-208.

77. Hedderwick SA, McNeil SA, Lyons MJ, et al. Pathogenic organisms associated with artificial fingernails worn by healthcare workers. *Infect Control Hosp Epidemiol.* 2000;21(8):505-509.

78. Moolenaar RL, Crutcher JM, San Joaquin VH, et al. A prolonged outbreak of *Pseudomonas aeruginosa* in a neonatal intensive care unit: Did staff fingernails play a role in disease transmission? *Infect Control Hosp Epidemiol.* 2000;21(2):80-85.

79. Brown SM, Lubimova AV, Khrustalyeva NM, et al. Use of an alcohol-based hand rub and quality improvement interventions to improve hand hygiene in a Russian neonatal intensive care unit. *Infect Control Hosp Epidemiol.* 2003;24(3):172-179.

80. Harbarth S, Pittet D, Grady L, et al. Interventional study to evaluate the impact of an alcohol-based hand gel in improving hand hygiene compliance. *Pediatr Infect Dis J.* 2002;21(6):489-495.

81. Tenorio AR, Badri SM, Sahgal NB, et al. Effectiveness of gloves in the prevention of hand carriage of vancomycin-resistant enterococcus species by health care workers after patient care. *Clin Infect Dis.* 2001;32(5):826-829.

82. Cohen B, Saiman L, Cimiotti J, et al. Factors associated with hand hygiene practices in two neonatal intensive care units. *Pediatr Infect Dis J.* 2003;22(6):494-499.

83. Lam BC, Lee J, Lau YL. Hand hygiene practices in a neonatal intensive care unit: A multimodal intervention and impact on nosocomial infection. *Pediatrics.* 2004;114(5):e565-e571.

84. Pessoa-Silva CL, Hugonnet S, Pfister R, et al. Reduction of health care associated infection risk in neonates by successful hand hygiene promotion. *Pediatrics.* 2007;120(2):e382-e390.

85. Pittet D, Hugonnet S, Harbarth S, et al. Effectiveness of a hospital-wide programme to improve compliance with hand hygiene. Infection Control Programme. *Lancet.* 2000;356(9238):1307-1312.

86. Won SP, Chou HC, Hsieh WS, et al. Handwashing program for the prevention of nosocomial infections in a neonatal intensive care unit. *Infect Control Hosp Epidemiol.* 2004;25(9):742-746.

87. Berwick DM. Developing and testing changes in delivery of care. *Ann Intern Med.* 1998;128(8):651-656.

88. Laffel G, Blumenthal D. The case for using industrial quality management science in health care organizations. *JAMA.* 1989;262(20):2869-2873.

89. Berwick DM. The science of improvement. *JAMA.* 2008;299(10):1182-1184.

90. Schulman J, Wirtschafter DD, Kurtin P. Neonatal intensive care unit collaboration to decrease hospital-acquired bloodstream infections: From comparative performance reports to improvement networks. *Pediatr Clin N Am.* 2009;56(4):865-892.

91. Plsek P. Innovative thinking for the improvement of medical systems. *Ann Intern Med.* 1999;131(6):438-444.

92. Plsek PE. Quality improvement methods in clinical medicine. *Pediatrics.* 1999;103(1 Suppl E):203-214.

93. Horbar JD. The Vermont Oxford Network: Evidence-based quality improvement for neonatology. *Pediatrics.* 1999;103(1 Suppl E):350-359.

94. Horbar JD, Rogowski J, Plsek PE, et al. Collaborative quality improvement for neonatal intensive care. NIC/Q Project Investigators of the Vermont Oxford Network. *Pediatrics.* 2001;107(1):14-22.

95. Rogowski JA, Horbar JD, Plsek PE, et al. Economic implications of neonatal intensive care unit collaborative quality improvement. *Pediatrics.* 2001;107(1):23-29.

96. Kilbride HW, Wirtschafter DD, Powers RJ, Sheehan MB. Implementation of evidence-based potentially better practices to decrease nosocomial infections. *Pediatrics.* 2003;111(4 Pt 2):e519-e533.

97. Kilbride HW, Powers R, Wirtschafter DD, et al. Evaluation and development of potentially better practices to prevent neonatal nosocomial bacteremia. *Pediatrics.* 2003;111(4 Pt 2):e504-e518.

98. Schulman J, Stricof RL, Stevens TP, et al. Development of a statewide collaborative to decrease NICU central line-associated bloodstream infections. *J Perinatol.* 2009;29(9):591-599.

99. Pronovost P, Needham D, Berenholtz S, et al. An intervention to decrease catheter-related bloodstream infections in the ICU. *N Engl J Med.* 2006;355(26):2725-2732.

100. Miller MR, Griswold M, Harris JM, et al. Decreasing PICU catheter-associated bloodstream infections: NACHRI's quality transformation efforts. *Pediatrics.* 2010;125(2):206-213.

101. Boyce JM, Potter-Bynoe G, Chenevert C, et al. Environmental contamination due to methicillin-resistant *Staphylococcus aureus*: Possible infection control implications. *Infect Control Hosp Epidemiol.* 1997;18(9):622-627.

102. Bryan CS, John Jr JF, Pai MS, et al. Gentamicin vs cefotaxime for therapy of neonatal sepsis. Relationship to drug resistance. *Am J Dis Child (1960).* 1985;139(11):1086-1089.

103. Tullus K, Burman LG. Ecological impact of ampicillin and cefuroxime in neonatal units. *Lancet.* 1989;1(8652):1405-1407.

104. Chow JW, Fine MJ, Shlaes DM, et al. *Enterobacter* bacteremia: Clinical features and emergence of antibiotic resistance during therapy. *Ann Intern Med.* 1991;115(8):585-590.

105. Zaoutis TE, Goyal M, Chu JH, et al. Risk factors for and outcomes of bloodstream infection caused by extended-spectrum beta-lactamase-producing *Escherichia coli* and *Klebsiella* species in children. *Pediatrics.* 2005;115(4):942-949.

106. de Man P, Verhoeven BA, Verbrugh HA, et al. An antibiotic policy to prevent emergence of resistant bacilli. *Lancet.* 2000;355(9208):973-978.

107. Pakyz AL, Oinonen M, Polk RE. Relationship of carbapenem restriction in 22 university teaching hospitals to carbapenem use and carbapenem-resistant Pseudomonas aeruginosa. *Antimicrob Agents Chemother.* 2009;53(5):1983-1986.

16

108. Gupta N, Limbago BM, Patel JB, et al. Carbapenem-resistant Enterobacteriaceae: Epidemiology and prevention. *Clin Infect Dis.* 2011;53(1):60-67.

109. Singh N, Rogers P, Atwood CW, et al. Short-course empiric antibiotic therapy for patients with pulmonary infiltrates in the intensive care unit. A proposed solution for indiscriminate antibiotic prescription. *Am J Respir Crit Care Med.* 2000;162(2 Pt 1):505-511.

110. Toltzis P, Dul MJ, Hoyen C, et al. The effect of antibiotic rotation on colonization with antibiotic-resistant bacilli in a neonatal intensive care unit. *Pediatrics.* 2002;110(4):707-711.

111. Gruson D, Hilbert G, Vargas F, et al. Strategy of antibiotic rotation: Long-term effect on incidence and susceptibilities of Gram-negative bacilli responsible for ventilator-associated pneumonia. *Crit Care Med.* 2003;31(7):1908-1914.

112. Warren DK, Hill HA, Merz LR, et al. Cycling empirical antimicrobial agents to prevent emergence of antimicrobial-resistant Gram-negative bacteria among intensive care unit patients. *Crit Care Med.* 2004;32(12):2450-2456.

113. Fierer J, Guiney D. Extended-spectrum beta-lactamases: A plague of plasmids. *JAMA.* 1999;281(6):563-564.

114. Timmis KN, Gonzalez-Carrero MI, Sekizaki T, et al. Biological activities specified by antibiotic resistance plasmids. *J Antimicrob Chemother.* 1986;18(Suppl C):1-12.

115. Carling P, Fung T, Killion A, et al. Favorable impact of a multidisciplinary antibiotic management program conducted during 7 years. *Infect Control Hosp Epidemiol.* 2003;24(9):699-706.

116. Metjian TA, Prasad PA, Kogon A, et al. Evaluation of an antimicrobial stewardship program at a pediatric teaching hospital. *Pediatr Infect Dis J.* 2008;27(2):106-111.

117. Newland JG, Hersh AL. Purpose and design of antimicrobial stewardship programs in pediatrics. *Pediatr Infect Dis J.* 2010;29(9):862-863.

118. Patel SJ, Larson EL, Kubin CJ, et al. A review of antimicrobial control strategies in hospitalized and ambulatory pediatric populations. *Pediatr Infect Dis J.* 2007;26(6):531-537.

119. Chiu CH, Michelow IC, Cronin J, et al. Effectiveness of a guideline to reduce vancomycin use in the neonatal intensive care unit. *Pediatr Infect Dis J.* 2011;30(4):273-278.

120. Forrester M, Pettitt AN. Use of stochastic epidemic modeling to quantify transmission rates of colonization with methicillin-resistant *Staphylococcus aureus* in an intensive care unit. *Infect Control Hosp Epidemiol.* 2005;26(7):598-606.

121. Raboud J, Saskin R, Simor A, et al. Modeling transmission of methicillin-resistant *Staphylococcus aureus* among patients admitted to a hospital. *Infect Control Hosp Epidemiol.* 2005;26(7):607-615.

122. Huang SS, Yokoe DS, Hinrichsen VL, et al. Impact of routine intensive care unit surveillance cultures and resultant barrier precautions on hospital-wide methicillin-resistant *Staphylococcus aureus* bacteremia. *Clin Infect Dis.* 2006;43(8):971-978.

123. Nijssen S, Bonten MJ, Weinstein RA. Are active microbiological surveillance and subsequent isolation needed to prevent the spread of methicillin-resistant *Staphylococcus aureus*? *Clin Infect Dis.* 2005;40(3):405-409.

124. Huskins WC, Huckabee CM, O'Grady NP, et al. Intervention to reduce transmission of resistant bacteria in intensive care. *N Engl J Med.* 2011;364(15):1407-1418.

125. Sarda V, Molloy A, Kadkol S, et al. Active surveillance for methicillin-resistant Staphylococcus aureus in the neonatal intensive care unit. *Infect Control Hosp Epidemiol.* 2009;30(9):854-860.

126. Gerber SI, Jones RC, Scott MV, et al. Management of outbreaks of methicillin-resistant Staphylococcus aureus infection in the neonatal intensive care unit: A consensus statement. *Infect Control Hosp Epidemiol.* 2006;27(2):139-145.

127. Heinrich N, Mueller A, Bartmann P, et al. Successful management of an MRSA outbreak in a neonatal intensive care unit. *Eur J Clin Microbiol Infect Dis.* 2011;30(7):909-913.

128. Song X, Cheung S, Klontz K, et al. A stepwise approach to control an outbreak and ongoing transmission of methicillin-resistant *Staphylococcus aureus* in a neonatal intensive care unit. *Am J Infect Control.* 2010;38(8):607-611.

129. Bertin ML, Vinski J, Schmitt S, et al. Outbreak of methicillin-resistant *Staphylococcus aureus* colonization and infection in a neonatal intensive care unit epidemiologically linked to a healthcare worker with chronic otitis. *Infect Control Hosp Epidemiol.* 2006;27(6):581-585.

130. Lepelletier D, Corvec S, Caillon J, et al. Eradication of methicillin-resistant *Staphylococcus aureus* in a neonatal intensive care unit: Which measures for which success? *Am J Infect Control.* 2009;37(3):195-200.

16

CHAPTER 17

Neonatal Fungal Infections

Misti Ellsworth, DO; Charles R. Sims, MD; and
Luis Ostrosky-Zeichner, MD, FACP, FIDSA

17

- ● **Candidiasis**
- ● **Aspergillosis**
- ● **Zygomycosis (Mucormycosis)**
- ● **Other Fungi**
- ● **Summary**

Fungal infections are common in the neonate and present with a variety of clinical syndromes ranging from trivial mucocutaneous infection to life-threatening fungemia and deeply invasive mycoses. Fungi are ubiquitous environmental organisms that can be found free-living in the soil, on bird and mammalian feces, and in decaying organic matter. They are also frequently found in the hospital environment. Some species, such as *Candida,* are commensal organisms in the human oral cavity, gastrointestinal tract, genitourinary tract, and moist intertriginous skin folds. Neonates often acquire the organisms from their mother during passage through the birth canal and in utero from hematogenous spread or ascending vaginal infection. They can also acquire the infections post-partum through inhalation, ingestion, direct inoculation into the skin, and exposure to the hospital environment. Most of the specific defects in the immune response allowing susceptibility to fungal infections in certain individual are unknown and are under investigation. Risk factors, clinical presentation, diagnosis, therapy, and prognosis vary with each species of fungus and will be discussed later. Data for neonates are limited, and guidelines have been extrapolated from adult and pediatric data.

Candidiasis

Epidemiology

The reported frequency of *Candida* infections has increased, and candidemia now represents the fourth most common cause of nosocomial bloodstream infection in adults and children younger than 16 years of age in the United States.[1,2] *Candida* is the third most common pathogen isolated in nosocomial bloodstream infections of premature infants.[3] The reported incidence of neonatal sepsis due to *Candida* varies between 0.57% and 1.28% of all neonatal intensive care admissions and between 4.8% and 7.0% of neonates weighing less than 1500 g.[4-6] Neonatal age and birthweight have been linked to increased risk of invasive candidal infections. One prospective analysis reported an incidence of 0.26% for infants weighing more than 2500 g, 3.1% for infants weighing more than 1500 g, and 5.5% for extremely low birth weight infants over a 3-year period.[3] In addition, extreme prematurity increases the risk of developing invasive candidiasis; one study found that a gestational age of less than 25 weeks led to an odds ratio of 4.15 for developing candidiasis when compared with infants greater than 28 weeks.[2] The cost of candidemia is enormous in terms of loss of life. Attributable mortality in neonates weighing less than 1500 g varies from 10.2% to 43%.[7,8] The specific species causing the infection appears to

Table 17-1   RISK FACTORS AND CONDITIONS ASSOCIATED WITH INVASIVE CANDIDIASIS

Primary Risk Factors	Associated Conditions
Prolonged antibiotic use	Birth weight less than 1000 g
Central venous catheter	Gestational age less than 32 weeks
ICU stay longer than 7 days	5 minute Apgar <5
Abdominal surgery	Gastrointestinal *Candida* colonization
Hyperalimentation	Nasogastric tubes
Acid-suppressing medications	Vaginal birth

ICU, Intensive care unit.
Modified from Saiman et al.[7] and Shetty et al.[133]

affect mortality, as demonstrated in a recent study of adult candidemia showing a mortality rate of 44% in all patients, and increased mortality in *C. glabrata* (60%) and *C. tropicalis* (75%) infections.[9] The estimated costs in the United States of treating a single adult episode of nosocomial candidemia are $34,123 per Medicare patient and $44,536 per private insurance patient.[10] In children, candidemia can increase the hospital stay by up to 21 days and the cost by nearly $100,000 (U.S.).[3] The current annual monetary cost of candidemia in the United States may be approaching $1 billion,[11] taking into account that these figures were calculated just after the introduction of fluconazole and before the widespread use of lipid preparations of amphotericin or the echinocandins.

Colonization of *Candida* may be acquired by the fetus during gestation or at delivery while passing through the birth canal.[12] Although as many as 25% of pregnant women experience vaginal candidiasis late in gestation, congenital candidiasis is rare. The literature contains many case reports and short series of congenitally acquired candidiasis (cutaneous and disseminated) with intact or ruptured membranes, placental involvement, and umbilical cord involvement.[13-15] Many of these cases are associated with uterine foreign bodies, including intrauterine contraceptive devices and cervical cerclage sutures.[16] In addition to maternal–fetal transmission, *Candida* species are found in the hospital environment in the air; on food, floors, and other surfaces and objects; and on the hands of hospital personnel.[17] Nosocomial spread among patients has been traced to hand carriage and to artificial nails.[18-20] General risk factors for candidiasis are related to the specific site of infection and to the disease process and are summarized in Table 17-1.

Of the more than 100 species of *Candida,* seven are well-known pathogens in humans, and many other species are described infrequently in epidemiologic surveys, case reports, or short case series. Table 17-2 summarizes the overall

Table 17-2   SPECIES DISTRIBUTION (%) OF *CANDIDA* BLOODSTREAM ISOLATES IN NEONATES AND GENERAL SUSCEPTIBILITY OF *CANDIDA* SPECIES TO ANTIFUNGAL AGENTS

Species	Frequency (%)	Fluc	Itra	Vori	5FC	Ampho	Caspo
C. albicans	53–70	S	S	S	S	S	S
C. parapsilosis	15–39	S	S	S	S	S	S (to I?)
C. glabrata	0–14	S-DD to R	S-DD to R	S to S-DD	S	S to I	S
C. tropicalis	0–16	S	S	S	S	S	S
C. krusei	0–3	R	S-DD to R	S to S-DD	I to R	S to I	S
Other *Candida* spp.	0–3	V	V	V	V	V	V

Adapted from Pappas PG, Rex JH, Sobel JD, et al. Guidelines for treatment of candidiasis. *Clin Infect Dis.* 2004;38(2):161-189.
Ampho, Amphotericin B; *Caspo,* caspofungin; *5FC,* flucytosine; *Fluc,* fluconazole; *I,* intermediate; *Itra,* itraconazole; *R,* resistant; *S,* susceptible; *S-DD,* susceptible dose-dependent; *V,* variable; *Vori,* voriconazole.
Frequency data from different surveillance studies.[3-5,133-136]

frequency distribution of *Candida* species causing fungemia in neonates. Most neonatal series note a higher percentage of *C. parapsilosis* (up to 36%[21]) than adult series. Although *Candida albicans* remains the most common isolate, non-*albicans Candida* have greatly increased in frequency as the cause of invasive disease.[22-24] Studies in neonates have shown non-*albicans* rates between 35% and 79%.[5,25]

Diagnosis

Multiple direct and indirect methods of diagnosing *Candida* infections are currently available.[26] The indirect methods, unfortunately, have not yet been widely accepted for clinical use, and current direct diagnostic methods have exhibited substandard performance. Although *Candida* will grow in standard blood culture bottles, detection and growth can be enhanced by pretreating blood specimens with lysis and centrifugation.[27,28] Still, in the best of circumstances, cultures are negative in the presence of disseminated candidiasis in at least one quarter to one third of cases.[27] After isolation, *C. albicans* can be presumptively identified in 90 minutes by germ tube formation. Other species may require 72 hours to be identified by morphology and carbohydrate metabolism using many available commercial kits. Indirect methods for diagnosing *Candida* infections include detection of serologic markers and DNA.[29] In adults, the most promising methods involve measuring serum mannan[30] and 1-3-beta-D-glucan (two cell wall components),[31] enolase (a cytoplasmic enzyme),[32] antibodies against enolase and hsp90 (a stress protein),[33] and fungal metabolites such as D-arabinitol.[34] Methods for detecting candidal DNA are also being investigated but have not yet reached the clinical stage.[35]

The clinician may be forced to treat empirically for candidiasis based on clinical suspicion and risk factors. The gold standard for the diagnosis of *Candida* infection is a positive culture from normally sterile body sites such as blood, cerebrospinal fluid, urine, joint aspirate, sterilely drained abscess, or other sterile surgical specimens. In neonates with a sterile body fluid culture or urine culture positive for *Candida*, lumbar puncture and a dilated retinal examination should be performed. If sterile body fluid cultures persist as positive, imaging of the genitourinary tract, liver, and spleen should be performed.[3] Culture from tracheal aspirates, bronchoalveolar lavage fluid, exposed wounds, abdominal drains, epithelium, or other mucocutaneous sources is not diagnostic and cannot differentiate colonization from infection.[36,37] Heavy colonization is an important risk factor for the development of deep candidiasis,[38] but it must be interpreted with the rest of the clinical information in the individual patient and should not be the sole reason for treating with antifungal agents.

Clinical Manifestations

Congenital Candidiasis

Congenital candidiasis is a rare complication caused by intrauterine *Candida* infection; it presents with a spectrum of diseases depending on the maturity of the infant. In neonates weighing more than 1000 g, the disease usually presents solely with cutaneous manifestations of erythematous macules, papules, and pustules that occasionally can form vesicles and bullae. Mortality is low (8%) in isolated cutaneous disease. Systemic disease, characterized by respiratory distress, leukocytosis, and positive blood, urine, or cerebrospinal fluid (CSF) culture, will occur in 10% of these infants and carries a high associated mortality. In neonates weighing less than 1000 g, the disease presents with widespread desquamation, systemic disease is common (67%), and mortality is high.[13] Risk factors include intrauterine foreign bodies such as intrauterine contraceptive devices and cervical cerclage sutures, as well as *Candida* chorioamnionitis, funisitis, or placental infection.[15,39] Congenital candidiasis develops in 16% of cases in which examination of the placenta of infants shows evidence of *Candida* infection. These placental findings should prompt close neonatal evaluation.

Hematogenous Candidiasis

Hematogenous candidiasis may occur at the time of delivery or over the first few days of life in severe congenital candidiasis, or it may develop later as an acquired infection. The clinical presentation of hematogenous candidiasis is similar to that of bacterial sepsis, with respiratory distress and apnea being the prominent clinical signs. Fever, hypotension, and thrombocytopenia are common. Hematogenous spread to multiple organs is commonly seen; the skin (66%), central nervous system (CNS) (64%), and retina (54%) are the most frequently affected areas.[40] Persistence of candidemia longer than 24 hours after adequate antifungal dosing is achieved is associated with higher rates of end-organ disease and with higher mortality.[41]

The routes of invasion of *Candida* can be divided into endogenous and exogenous routes. The endogenous route is the most important, in that *Candida* infections originate predominantly from the patient's own colonizing organisms from the gastrointestinal tract and skin.[24,42] Infection, however, requires some defect in the normal host immunity. Breakdowns in mucosal barriers related to surgery, gastrointestinal injury in enterocolitis, and total parenteral nutrition[43] are examples. Cutaneous barriers are not well established in the fetus, allowing translocation (the likely mechanism in congenital candidiasis), and are disrupted in the neonate by central venous catheters, surgical wounds, and trauma. Cell-mediated immunity is not well developed in the neonatal period and is further inhibited by hyperglycemia and corticosteroids. Overgrowth of *Candida* in the gastrointestinal and genitourinary tracts occurs with antibiotic use and urinary catheterization. Critically ill neonates may have several of these defects at any given time.

Two main theories have been put forth regarding the mechanisms responsible for candidemia. The first is translocation of colonizing *Candida* organisms across the gut epithelium. This theory is supported by multiple adult studies showing a relationship between the presence and density of colonization and increased rates of candidemia, and correlation between the colonizing *Candida* strain and the strain isolated from the blood.[42,44-46] The second mechanism relates to the presence of intravenous catheters.[47] Infection could be initiated by contamination of the catheter hub at the skin, resulting in catheter infection, or by transient candidemia from another source, resulting in secondary catheter colonization/infection.[42,48] Less evidence is available for catheters than for gut translocation as the primary source of candidemia, and the presence of central venous catheters may only serve as a marker for severity of illness. However, whether via primary or secondary infection, venous catheters are the prominent final site of *Candida* infection and can lead to longer candidemia, thrombophlebitis with seeding of organisms into the clot, and increased risk of disseminated disease.[49,50] Failure to promptly remove lines in candidemic neonates has been shown to lead to significantly higher mortality.[51]

Exogenous routes of infection are infrequent but can be important, depending on the site of contamination. Multiple related diseases have been described, including candidemia resulting from contaminated blood pressure transducers, from contaminated parenteral nutrition solutions and fluids,[52,53] and from health care workers' hands.[18,54]

Urinary Candidiasis

Urinary candidiasis in the neonate can be the result of a primary urinary tract infection or spread from a disseminated candidal infection. Among candidemic neonates, secondary candiduria is seen in 40% to 70% and renal abscess in 0% to 14%.[55] Primary urinary candidiasis is related to the presence of indwelling catheters, urinary tract instrumentation, diabetes, and steroid and antibiotic use. Clinical manifestations are varied, with a spectrum including benign colonization, urethritis, cystitis, pyelitis, fungus ball from papillary necrosis and sloughing, and perinephric or renal abscess.[56]

Abdominal Candidiasis

Candida peritonitis is caused by two distinct clinical entities in the neonate: focal intestinal perforation and necrotizing enterocolitis. Although the clinical presentations may be similar, focal perforation lacks the X-ray findings and extensive bowel disease of necrotizing enterocolitis and is associated with lower birth weight infants. *Candida* is isolated from 44% of focal perforation cases as opposed to only 15% of necrotizing enterocolitis cases.[57] *Candida* accounts for 8% of dialysis-related peritonitis in adults and is reported in infants undergoing peritoneal dialysis. *C. albicans* is the most commonly isolated species.[58] Patients with dialysis-related *Candida* peritonitis usually present with fever, abdominal tenderness, cloudy dialysate, and peritoneal fluid neutrophil count greater than 100 cells/mL. If left untreated, patients may develop candidemia.[59]

Endocarditis

Endocarditis involving the vena cava or cardiac valves occurs in approximately 5% of cases of candidemia,[55] with reports of occurrence as high as 13%.[60] *C. albicans* accounts for one half of the *Candida* species.[61] The mortality rate is lower than with other fungal causes of endocarditis, but it is reported at up to 60%. Patients usually present with fever, respiratory distress, thrombocytopenia, and a cardiac murmur.[60] Risk factors include the presence of a central venous catheter and previous antibiotic therapy,[62] although cases without risk factors have been described.[63] Late development after fungemia has been described in adults after 22 months and has recently been described in neonatal endocarditis as well.[64] Embolization is more common in *Candida* endocarditis than in bacterial disease, occurring in two thirds of cases.[61]

Ocular Candidiasis

Ocular *Candida* infection can present as keratoconjunctivitis due to topical steroids, local trauma[65] or, more important, as chorioretinitis and endophthalmitis due to hematogenous seeding. Although retina involvement in candidemia is reported in 10% to 45% of adults,[66-68] and in 50% of neonates in older studies,[69] more recent, large series have reported much lower rates of 0% to 17% in neonates.[55,70,71] The lower rate may be due to earlier, more aggressive treatment of candidemia because end-organ involvement is associated with more prolonged candidemia.[72] Ocular presentations may be the first manifestations of hematogenous disease or may develop after the diagnosis of candidemia,[73,74] and may lead to permanent blindness if not identified.[75] The most common signs and symptoms are eye redness, hazy vitreous, pain, and diminished or blurry vision. Premature infants may be at higher risk of developing complicated ocular candidiasis (such as lens abscess) if candidemia occurs around 29 weeks post conception as the lens structures lose their developmental arterial supply and become avascular and less likely to respond to systemic treatment.[76] Endophthalmitis can present up to 2 weeks after the diagnosis of candidemia, and some authors have suggested that patients should have a dilated retinal examination at baseline and 2 weeks after documentation of candidemia.[73,77] A recent consensus document, however, recommends that all patients with candidemia should have at least one careful retinal examination.[78]

Central Nervous System Candidiasis

Candida infection of the CNS is usually secondary to hematogenous disease and presents as meningitis or brain abscess.[79] Primary CNS disease is most commonly due to iatrogenic causes, including ventriculoperitoneal shunt placement.[80] The rate of secondary *Candida* meningitis during candidemia is approximately 15%, with a range of 3% to 23% in the literature[55] and an overall rate of 0.4% of all neonatal intensive care unit (ICU) admissions.[81] Symptoms of *Candida* meningitis are similar to those of bacterial meningitis and include fever, confusion, nuchal rigidity, and respiratory distress.[82] In neonates, symptoms are often nonspecific and may include apnea, hypotension, poor feeding, and temperature instability. CSF analysis generally shows hypoglycorrhachia. Pleocytosis and protein elevation are often mild or absent, and in one series, only 25% of patients revealed any abnormality on CSF analysis.[83] Another series confirmed the lack of CSF abnormalities and further reported a negative Gram stain in 100% of cases and culture positive for *Candida* in only 74%.[81] *Candida* brain abscess and ventriculitis have been reported in 4% of neonates with candidemia.[55] Among adult patients who died of disseminated candidiasis, 50%

were found to have *Candida* brain microabscesses at autopsy.[84] These abscesses generally were not symptomatic, so the rate of brain microabscesses may be significantly higher than diagnosed.

Bone and Joint Candidiasis

Osteomyelitis and septic arthritis caused by *Candida* are usually the result of hematogenous spread, with primary disease being extremely rare and occurring in adults with inoculation of organisms into the area by trauma, during steroid injection into the joint, and during surgery (i.e., sternotomy or arthrotomy).[85-87] *Candida* accounts for 7% to 17% of cases of septic arthritis and osteomyelitis in neonates.[88,89] The literature consists mostly of case reports and small series showing *C. albicans* followed by *C. tropicalis* as the main isolates involved.[90,91] The most common symptom is localized pain, but soft tissue swelling with erythema, adjacent abscess, and arthritis is also described. Fever and leukocytosis are usually absent. Large joints are most commonly affected, with at least one knee joint involved in 71% of cases of polyarticular disease. In adults, synovial fluid microscopic analysis shows high white blood cells (15,000 to 100,000/mm^3) with polymorphonuclear cell predominance and visualization of the organisms in 20% of cases.[26] Synovial fluid culture is positive in nearly 100% of cases.[88] No data are available for neonates. Onset of symptoms of osteomyelitis may be concurrent with candidemia or may present many months later. One case of neonatal *C. albicans* osteomyelitis has been described 1 year after completion of presumed adequate therapy for candidemia.[92]

Pulmonary Candidiasis

Although *Candida* is frequently isolated from multiple respiratory specimens, including sputum, bronchoalveolar lavage fluid, and endotracheal tube secretions, it is more commonly a colonizer than a pathogen in the seriously ill patient. Definitive diagnosis is made by demonstrating fungal elements invading the lung tissue. An adult study comparing various sampling modalities versus autopsy in ICU patients showed a 40% colonization rate with only an 8% rate of *Candida* bronchopneumonia. The study also found no correlation between the type of sampling and the diagnosis of true pneumonia.[36] The vast majority of true infection results from disseminated candidiasis causing seeding of the lungs. Notable exceptions are the rare cases of severe congenital candidiasis in which alveolitis is common[14] and of direct lung exposure to *Candida*-infected amniotic fluid.[93]

Mucocutaneous Candidiasis

Candida colonization occurs in 27% of neonates within the first week of life; approximately 8% will develop mucocutaneous candidiasis.[12] Oropharyngeal infection (thrush) and axillary, intertriginous, perineal, and periumbilical dermatitis are the most common presentations. These diseases are usually self-limited and do not require therapy. Topical therapy is effective in clearing these sites of infection within 1 week; however, infection commonly recurs after cessation of therapy. The importance of these mild forms of candidiasis lies in the fact that the rate of invasive candidiasis (of any type) is significantly higher in neonates with mucocutaneous disease. Rates may be as high as 32% in neonates weighing less than 1000 g and do not decrease with topical treatment.[40]

One severe form of mucocutaneous disease is invasive fungal dermatitis, which occurs in the smallest, most premature infants. Presentation occurs from 6 to 14 days of life, with erosive, crusting lesions demonstrating fungal invasion beyond the stratum corneum on pathology. *C. albicans* is the most common source, but other *Candida* species, as well as other fungi, can cause the disease. Risk factors include prematurity, postnatal steroid administration, and hyperglycemia; dissemination occurs in 69% of *Candida* cases.[94]

Treatment

The decision of whether to treat candidiasis and with what agent depends on multiple factors, including the site of the infection, the clinical status of the patient, the toxicity of the medications, and the species of *Candida* isolated. Empiric therapy is warranted in some situations, and identification to the species level is critical in others. The Infectious Disease Society of America (IDSA) has recently issued guidelines based on the supporting evidence for the treatment of candidemia and invasive candidiasis,[78] but only a small number of recommendations involve neonates because only a few small trials have focused on this population. The most commonly used therapy is amphotericin B owing to its long history of use and relative safety in the neonatal population. A significant quantity of data is accumulating for fluconazole; most recently, studies involving the echinocandins and lipid preparations of amphotericin B are being reported. Table 17-3 presents specific treatment recommendations for forms of invasive candidiasis.

17

Table 17-3 RECOMMENDED TREATMENT FOR SPECIFIC FORMS OF INVASIVE CANDIDIASIS

Condition	Specific Comments
Candidemia and disseminated candidiasis	Candidemia and disseminated diseases are treated in a similar manner; options include amphotericin B deoxycholate (0.7–1.0 mg/kg/day), lipid preparations of amphotericin B (3–5 mg/kg/day), fluconazole (12 mg/kg/day),[143,144] or a combination of fluconazole and amphotericin B. Treatment should continue for 14 days after sterilization of blood cultures in candidemia. All central venous catheters should be removed.
Abdominal candidiasis	*Candida* peritonitis should be treated with surgical drainage and intravenous amphotericin B or oral/intravenous fluconazole (12 mg/kg/day)[145,146] for 2 to 6 weeks or until resolution of abscesses. Use of intraperitoneal amphotericin B is not recommended owing to chemical peritonitis, pain, and fibrosis.[147,148] Most authorities recommend removal of peritoneal dialysis catheters.[149]
Endocarditis	*Candida* endocarditis requires a combination of surgery and systemic antifungal therapy. The recommended antifungal regimen consists of amphotericin B (deoxycholate or lipid formulation) for 1 to 2 weeks before and 6 to 8 weeks after surgery, followed by fluconazole suppression for up to 2 years, although the doses and duration have not yet been established. Long-term flucytosine may be added to the regimen. Removal of pacemakers is almost always required.
Endophthalmitis	Ocular candidiasis requires immediate treatment to prevent blindness. Treatment options include systemic amphotericin B (1.0 mg/kg/day) with or without flucytosine; intravitreal amphotericin B (0.005 mg/0.01 mL) with or without pars plana vitrectomy[75,150,151]; and fluconazole (12 mg/kg/day). Experiences with voriconazole and caspofungin are encouraging.[152]
Osteomyelitis and arthritis	*Candida* osteomyelitis requires surgical drainage and debridement of devitalized bone.[87] Therapy consists of fluconazole or amphotericin B with or without flucytosine for 6 weeks to 6 months.[87,91,153,154]
Central nervous system	Recommended treatment for *Candida* meningitis includes systemic amphotericin B (1.0 mg/kg/day) ± flucytosine (100–200 mg/kg/day).[79,155] An alternate therapeutic regimen consists of fluconazole (12 mg/kg/day) ± flucytosine. Case reports have described refractory meningitis treated successfully with caspofungin.[155] Treatment should continue until all signs and symptoms of meningitis have resolved. Brain abscess is associated with hematogenous disease and should be treated in a similar manner. If the brain abscess is large and is causing focal symptoms, drainage may be indicated.
Urinary candidiasis	Asymptomatic candiduria in a catheterized patient is usually a transient, benign condition that does not require antifungal therapy. Clearance of candiduria can be seen in 40% of patients simply by removing the urinary catheter and stopping antibiotics.[54] The risk of invasive candidiasis is low in this setting, with the exception of candiduria after renal transplantation[37] and situations in which urologic instrumentation or surgery is planned. Treatment can consist of amphotericin B bladder irrigation or systemic amphotericin B or fluconazole.[157] Keep in mind that in a high-risk host, candiduria may be the only manifestation of disseminated candidiasis.

As was discussed earlier, the emergence of non-*albicans* species and the development of acquired resistance may change the selection of antifungal agents for empiric treatment. Antifungal susceptibility testing is now an important piece of microbiological data to guide therapy. Clinical interpretive breakpoint minimum inhibitory concentrations (MICs) are available for fluconazole, itraconazole, voriconazole, and flucytosine.[78] No interpretive breakpoints have been established for amphotericin B and its lipid preparations, the echinocandins, or the newer triazoles (posaconazole), but MIC data are available for these compounds for the pathologic *Candida* species.[95] Table 17-2 summarizes the general susceptibility patterns of the most common pathologic species of *Candida*. Although susceptibility usually can be predicted when the species of the organism is known, one recent study has recommended susceptibility testing for *Candida* bloodstream isolates in the setting of previous azole use and recurrent mucosal disease in deep infections requiring prolonged therapy (i.e., osteomyelitis, endocarditis, abscess), and in establishing local antibiograms to guide therapy in specific institutions.[96]

Candidemia and General Guidelines

Initial management options in candidemia include amphotericin B deoxycholate (0.6 to 1.0 mg/kg/day), lipid preparations of amphotericin B (3 to 5 mg/kg/day), fluconazole (5 to 12 mg/kg/day), or a combination of fluconazole and amphotericin B. Echinocandins may be used with caution when no other options exist. Selection of therapy should depend on the presence of organ dysfunction affecting drug clearance, relative drug toxicity, previous exposure to antifungal agents for therapy or prophylaxis, and the physician's knowledge of the species and the potential susceptibility pattern of the isolate.

For a clinically unstable patient with an unknown isolate, many authorities recommend amphotericin B deoxycholate[97,98] or lipid preparation,[5] or an echinocandin in circumstances when no other appropriate therapy exists. CSF penetration of amphotericin is greater in neonates (up to 40%) than in adults.[99] Echinocandins have not been widely studied in the neonatal population, and available data have been derived from small retrospective studies and case reports. Among the echinocandins, the pharmacokinetics of micafungin in neonates is most often described. Micafungin has a shorter half-life and an increased rate of clearance in neonates.[105] Small studies in premature infants have shown micafungin levels similar to those of adults at doses of 7 to 15 mg/kg/day.[100,101] Few data are available for caspofungin, which has been safe and effective in clearing fungemia in amphotericin-refractory disease from multiple sources.[102] Although caspofungin is a good first-line agent in this setting, long-term use has resulted in resistance in *C. parapsilosis*.[103] Neonates have been shown to clear all echinocandins more quickly than children and adults,[104,105] and so the doses used must be higher for neonates. High-dose fluconazole has also been shown to be effective in this clinical setting,[106] although it is a fungistatic agent. For neonates with previous azole treatment or prophylaxis, or for patients whose mother received azoles for vaginal candidiasis in pregnancy, another class of agents should be considered. Voriconazole was recently approved by the Food and Drug Administration (FDA) for the treatment of candidemia in immunocompetent adults after a large clinical trial using amphotericin B as the comparator showed similar efficacy.[107] A single case report has described successful use of voriconazole (6 mg/kg every 8 hours) in combination with liposomal amphotericin for a neonate with refractory candidemia.[108] No pharmacodynamic information is available for voriconazole in neonates, and appropriate dosing is not known. Owing to concern for possible toxicity to the developing retina, it should be used with caution in neonates.[99]

Refractory candidemia should prompt clinicians to evaluate several possibilities. Ensuring the accuracy of the diagnosis is the critical first step in evaluating refractory disease. Next, the dose of medication should be examined because underdosing, particularly with azoles, is responsible for refractory disease and the development of resistance. Few data are available on the pharmacokinetics of antifungals other than fluconazole in neonates, but data that are available generally show shorter half-lives as compared with traditional doses in adults. Once the previous factors have been considered, a new drug regimen can be developed. Combination therapy with agents that have different mechanisms of activity can also be considered in cases refractory to monotherapy. Combinations of flucytosine-amphotericin, flucytosine-azole, amphotericin-azole, and azole-echinocandin have been tried in adults with varying results.[109] The only large-scale trial of combination therapy showed that fluconazole (12 mg/kg/day) plus amphotericin B (0.7 mg/kg/day) was not antagonistic compared with fluconazole alone. The combination showed a trend toward more rapid clearance of candidemia and successful treatment ($P = 0.043$), particularly in patients who were not at the extremes of the severity scores.[110] All neonatal data on combination therapy have been derived from single case reports.

In addition to antifungal chemotherapy, several other issues should be considered in the management of fungemia. Intravenous catheters and other implants should be removed as soon as clinically possible, because their removal has been associated with lower mortality.[51] A dilated ophthalmologic examination should be performed to exclude endophthalmitis,[73,74] because this diagnosis would alter the duration of therapy.

Prevention

Infection Control

Candida colonization of the hands and fingernails of health care workers, transmission of *Candida* from health care workers to patients, and transmission from patient to patient via health care workers' hands have all been documented, as was discussed previously. Hand hygiene, via washing with soap and water[111] or use of alcohol gels, can reduce health care worker carriage and transmission to patients. Furthermore, outbreaks have been linked to the use of artificial nails[112]; therefore wearing of artificial nails should be restricted in the neonatal ICU. Transmission of *Candida* to patients has been described via infusion of intravenous fluids and total parenteral nutrition solutions, and via intravascular devices and surgical instruments. Proper handling of instruments and proper techniques in sterilizing and preparing these instruments and fluids can reduce nosocomial infection.

Chemoprophylaxis

Ill neonates have multiple risk factors associated with invasive fungal infections and colonization. Fluconazole prophylaxis has been suggested and studied as a possible agent to reduce both colonization and infection rates among neonatal intensive care unit (NICU) patients. In a few retrospective cohort studies and in prospective randomized trials, fluconazole appears to reduce the rates of invasive infection and colonization; however, long-term effects on morbidity and mortality are unknown.[113] Research is needed to evaluate for adverse outcomes associated with prolonged exposure to fluconazole therapy.[113]

Antifungal chemoprophylaxis should be considered for premature infants (<32 weeks) with any additional risk factor for invasive candidiasis, including central venous catheter, broad-spectrum antibiotics (especially third-generation cephalosporins), postnatal steroids, abdominal surgery, enterocolitis, total parenteral nutrition, and skin/mucosal defects.[114] Additional research is needed before widespread fluconazole prophylaxis is recommended.

Aspergillosis

Epidemiology

Aspergillosis is a rare infection of the neonate, but it appears to be an emerging clinical entity as medical advances allow for the survival of more immature neonates.[115] The organism is found throughout the world in grains and decaying organic matter. Many species exist, but only eight have been found to be pathogens in humans. *Aspergillus fumigatus* and *A. flavus* are the most common. The disease ranges from isolated cutaneous disease to invasive pulmonary disease to disseminated aspergillosis. Most cases appear to be nosocomial in origin; contact with contaminated medical equipment[116] and inhalation of spores[117] have been identified as sources. Risk factors include prematurity, chronic granulomatous disease, postnatal steroid administration, neutropenia, and environmental exposure (such as construction in the NICU).[118]

Clinical Manifestations

Primary cutaneous aspergillosis can develop as a maculopapular rash at the site of inoculation or contamination, which later becomes scaling and pustular. Neonates with invasive pulmonary disease may have nasal sinusitis or nodular infiltrates on chest radiographs, along with a clinical picture of pneumonia that does not respond to antibiotic therapy. Hepatosplenomegaly, jaundice, and skin lesions are common findings in disseminated disease. These skin lesions tend to be nodular and hyperpigmented to purple, and they tend to ulcerate.

Diagnosis

Diagnosis is made by culturing the organism from a sterile site or by demonstrating invading fungal elements on tissue biopsy. Simply culturing *Aspergillus* from the skin or a pulmonary sample is not diagnostic because this is a common environmental pathogen. Blood cultures are usually negative. In adults, serologic testing for galactomannan can be helpful in diagnosis, but data gathered from neonates show an extremely high false-positive rate, making this test unhelpful for diagnosis.[119,120]

Treatment

Treatment for primary cutaneous disease consists of surgical debridement along with systemic antifungal therapy, and the prognosis is good. Case reports have described cure with medical therapy alone.[121] Invasive pulmonary aspergillosis and disseminated aspergillosis require systemic antifungal therapy. The prognosis in adults is poor, with survival between 14% and 71% depending on the underlying comorbidity. The prognosis in neonates may be better; the largest review reports survival of 73% to 88%.[118,122] Traditionally, amphotericin B deoxycholate has been the treatment of choice. Few neonatal data pertain to lipid preparations of amphotericin in neonates, but some pediatric data show lower toxicity.[122] Presumably these preparations should be as effective and potentially more effective owing to lower toxicity and the ability to treat at higher doses and for a longer duration in this severe, refractory disease. Recently, voriconazole and caspofungin have been approved for the treatment of aspergillosis in adults for primary and salvage therapy. Voriconazole was found to be superior to amphotericin B in one study in immunocompromised patients[123] and has been used successfully in combination with amphotericin in the pediatric population.[124] No data are available on the use of caspofungin in neonates with aspergillosis.

No controlled clinical trials have supported combination therapy in invasive aspergillosis.

Zygomycosis (Mucormycosis)

Epidemiology

Infection caused by *Zygomycetes* is a rare but emerging infection in the neonate.[112] Organisms are found throughout the world in the soil, on animal feces, and on fruits. Most infections in the neonate are nosocomial and arise from ingestion or contact with contaminated objects. Cutaneous cases have been described from elastic tape used to secure umbilical catheters and monitoring devices[125] and from wooden tongue depressors used as arm boards[126]; disseminated cases have been described from infusion of contaminated fluids.[127] Other sporadic cases of neonatal cutaneous zygomycosis have been reported without a specific cause. In addition to traumatic inoculation or contact with contaminated materials, risk factors include prematurity, diabetes mellitus especially with ketoacidosis, immunosuppression, and neutropenia. Cases have been seen in neonates with acidosis caused by conditions other than diabetes.[128,129]

Clinical Manifestations

Cutaneous zygomycosis manifests as a rapidly progressive cellulitis with black, necrotic ulceration. Destruction of deep tissue is rapid, and sepsis can develop if not treated aggressively. Another disease manifestation in neonates is colonic zygomycosis, in which infants present with sepsis and peritonitis. Necrotic colon with perforation is found during surgery, with fungal elements invading the tissues on histopathology. The diagnosis is difficult to make preoperatively, and mortality is very high.[130] Disseminated disease occurs in neonates, but the rhinocerebral presentation most often associated with zygomycosis in adults has not been reported in any patient younger than 8 months of age.[131]

Treatment

Aggressive surgical debridement is the cornerstone of therapy for isolated cutaneous disease. Systemic amphotericin in combination with surgery has shown the highest survival rates for this disease in adults,[132] but case reports have described successful treatment of cutaneous disease in the neonate with medical management alone.[133] Colonic and disseminated infections require systemic antifungal therapy. Recent literature on adults shows lipid formulations of amphotericin to be successful for treatment. Because they have less toxicity than amphotericin B, these preparations can be used for longer periods of time.[134] Voriconazole should not be used in this infection because it has little activity against *Zygomycetes,* and the disease has been repeatedly described in adult patients as a breakthrough mycosis on voriconazole prophylaxis.[135]

Other Fungi

Several other fungi, including *Cryptococcus, Blastomycetes,* and *Histoplasma,* have been described in a few case reports of neonates. Among these, *Cryptococcus* most frequently caused severe infection in pregnant women. In these cases of pneumonia and meningitis, no evidence of transplacental spread to the neonate was found.[136] Although they are less common, cases of transplacental spread have been reported during maternal histoplasmosis[137] and blastomycosis.[138]

Summary

The incidence of neonatal mycosis is rising and will continue to rise as advances in medical therapies lead to increased numbers of surviving premature infants requiring prolonged ICU care and increased use of invasive devices and catheters. Several agents are available to treat mycoses; each will probably have a role in specific scenarios. The role of combination drug therapy is still being evaluated, but it may improve outcomes, especially in breakthrough and refractory infections. The role of fluconazole for prophylaxis is still under investigation, and it should be used in select patients. Use of serologic markers in earlier diagnosis will lead to the development of pre-emptive strategies, resulting in lower utilization of drugs, lower toxicity, and less resistance.

References

1. Pfaller MA, Jones RN, Messer SA, et al. National surveillance of nosocomial blood stream infection due to *Candida albicans:* Frequency of occurrence and antifungal susceptibility in the SCOPE Program. *Diagn Microbiol Infect Dis.* 1998;31(1):327-332.
2. Steinbach, WJ. Epidemiology of invasive fungal infections in neonates and children. *Clin Microbiol Infect.* 2010;16(9):1321-1327.
3. Morgan C, Benjamin D. Treatment of neonatal fungal infections. In *Hot Topics in Infection and Immunity in Children IV, Advances in Experimental Medicine and Biology.* New York: Springer Science + Business Media; 2010.
4. Healy CM, Baker CJ, Zaccaria E, et al. Impact of fluconazole prophylaxis on incidence and outcome of invasive candidiasis in a neonatal intensive care unit. *J Pediatr.* 2005;147(2):166-171.

5. Lopez Sastre JB, Coto GD, Cotallo F, et al. Neonatal invasive candidiasis: A prospective multicenter study of 118 cases. *Am J Perinatol*. 2003;20(3):153-163.

6. Roilides E, Farmaki E, Evdoridou J, et al. Neonatal candidiasis: Analysis of epidemiology, drug susceptibility, and molecular typing of causative isolates. *Eur J Clin Microbiol Infect Dis*. 2004;23(10): 745-750.

7. Saiman L, Ludington E, Pfaller M, et al. Risk factors for candidemia in Neonatal Intensive Care Unit patients. The National Epidemiology of Mycosis Survey study group. *Pediatr Infect Dis J*. 2000;19(4): 319-324.

8. Rønnestad A, Abrahamsen TG, Medbø S, et al. Late-onset septicemia in a Norwegian national cohort of extremely premature infants receiving very early full human milk feeding. *Pediatrics*. 2005;115(3): e269-e276.

9. Safdar A, Bannister TW, Safdar Z. The predictors of outcome in immunocompetent patients with hematogenous candidiasis. *Int J Infect Dis*. 2004;8(3):180-186.

10. Rentz AM, Halpern MT, Bowden R. The impact of candidemia on length of hospital stay, outcome, and overall cost of illness. *Clin Infect Dis*. 1998;27(4):781-788.

11. Miller LG, Hajjeh RA, Edwards JE. Estimating the cost of nosocomial candidemia in the United States. *Clin Infect Dis*. 2001;32(7):1110.

12. Baley JE, Kliegman RM, Boxerbaum B, et al. Fungal colonization in the very low birth weight infant. *Pediatrics*. 1986;78(2):225-232.

13. Darmstadt GL, Dinulos JG, Miller Z. Congenital cutaneous candidiasis: Clinical presentation, pathogenesis, and management guidelines. *Pediatrics*. 2000;105(2):438-444.

14. Baud O, Boithias C, Lacaze-Masmonteil T, et al. Maternofetal disseminated candidiasis and high-grade prematurity. *Arch Pediatr*. 1997;4(4):331-334.

15. Qureshi F, Jacques SM, Bendon RW, et al. Candida funisitis: A clinicopathologic study of 32 cases. *Pediatr Dev Pathol*. 1998;1(2):118-124.

16. Baley JE, Silverman RA. Systemic candidiasis: Cutaneous manifestations in low birth weight infants. *Pediatrics*. 1988;82(2):211-215.

17. Saiman L, Ludington E, Dawson JD, et al. Risk factors for *Candida* species colonization of neonatal intensive care unit patients. *Pediatr Infect Dis J*. 2001;20(12):1119-1124.

18. Finkelstein R, Reinhertz G, Hashman N, et al. Outbreak of *Candida tropicalis* fungemia in a neonatal intensive care unit. *Infect Control Hosp Epidemiol*. 1993;14(10):587-590.

19. Saxen H, Virtanen M, Carlson P, et al. Neonatal *Candida parapsilosis* outbreak with a high case fatality rate. *Pediatr Infect Dis J*. 1995;14(9):776-781.

20. Huang YC, Lin TY, Leu HS, et al. Outbreak of *Candida parapsilosis* fungemia in neonatal intensive care units: Clinical implications and genotyping analysis. *Infection*. 1999;27(2):97-102.

21. Giusiano GE, Mangiaterra M, Rojas F, Gomez V. Yeasts species distribution in Neonatal Intensive Care Units in northeast Argentina. *Mycoses*. 2004;47(7):300-303.

22. Abi-Said D, Anaissie E, Uzun O, et al. The epidemiology of hematogenous candidiasis caused by different *Candida* species. *Clin Infect Dis*. 1997;24(6):1122-1128.

23. Krcmery V, Barnes AJ. Non-*albicans Candida* spp. causing fungaemia: Pathogenicity and antifungal resistance. *J Hosp Infect*. 2002;50(4):243-260.

24. Pfaller MA. Epidemiology of candidiasis. *J Hosp Infect*. 1995;30(Suppl):329-338.

25. Gupta N, Mittal N, Sood P, et al. Candidemia in neonatal intensive care unit. *Indian J Pathol Microbiol*. 2001;44(1):45-48.

26. Anaissie E, McGinnis MR, Pfaller MA, eds. *Clinical Mycology*, 1st ed. Philadelphia: Elsevier Science; 2003:195-239.

27. Berenguer J, Buck M, Witebsky F, et al. Lysis-centrifugation blood cultures in the detection of tissue-proven invasive candidiasis. Disseminated versus single-organ infection. *Diagn Microbiol Infect Dis* 1993;17(2):103-109.

28. Noda T, Kohno S, Mitsutake K, et al. (Basic and clinical evaluation of lysis centrifugation in candidemia). *Kansenshogaku Zasshi*. 1995;69(2):145-150.

29. Yamaguchi H. Advances in serological systems for diagnosis of systemic fungal infections, particularly those caused by Candida and Aspergillus. *Nippon Ishinkin Gakkai Zasshi*. 2002;43(4): 215-231.

30. Rimek D, Redetzke K, Singh J, et al. Performance of the Candida mannan antigen detection in patients with fungemia. *Mycoses*. 2004;47(Suppl 1):23-26.

31. Miyazaki T, Kohno S, Mitsutake K, et al. Plasma (1–>3)-beta-D-glucan and fungal antigenemia in patients with candidemia, aspergillosis, and cryptococcosis. *J Clin Microbiol*. 1995;33(12): 3115-3118.

32. Walsh TJ, Hathorn JW, Sobel JD, et al. Detection of circulating candida enolase by immunoassay in patients with cancer and invasive candidiasis. *N Engl J Med*. 1991;324(15):1026-1031.

33. Reiss E, Obayashi T, Orle K, et al. Non-culture based diagnostic tests for mycotic infections. *Med Mycol*. 2000;38(Suppl 1):147-159.

34. Walsh TJ, Merz WG, Lee JW, et al. Diagnosis and therapeutic monitoring of invasive candidiasis by rapid enzymatic detection of serum D-arabinitol. *Am J Med*. 1995;99(2):164-172.

35. Alexander BD. Diagnosis of fungal infection: New technologies for the mycology laboratory. *Transpl Infect Dis*. 2002;4(Suppl 3):32-37.

36. el-Ebiary M, Torres A, Fabregas N, et al. Significance of the isolation of Candida species from respiratory samples in critically ill, non-neutropenic patients. An immediate postmortem histologic study. *Am J Respir Crit Care Med*. 1997;156(2 Pt 1):583-590.

37. Cornwell EE, Belzberg H, Offne TV, et al. The pattern of fungal infections in critically ill surgical patients. *Am Surg*. 1995;61(10):847-850.

17

38. Safdar A, Armstrong D. Prospective evaluation of *Candida* species colonization in hospitalized cancer patients: Impact on short-term survival in recipients of marrow transplantation and patients with hematological malignancies. *Bone Marrow Transplant.* 2002;30(12):931-935.

39. Delprado WJ, Baird PJ, Russell P. Placental candidiasis: Report of three cases with a review of the literature. *Pathology.* 1982;14(2):191-195.

40. Faix RG, Kovarik SM, Shaw TR, et al. Mucocutaneous and invasive candidiasis among very low birth weight (less than 1,500 grams) infants in intensive care nurseries: A prospective study. *Pediatrics.* 1989;83(1):101-107.

41. Chapman RL, Faix RG. Persistently positive cultures and outcome in invasive neonatal candidiasis. *Pediatr Infect Dis J.* 2000;19(9):822-827.

42. Krause W, Matheis H, Wulf K. Fungaemia and funguria after oral administration of *Candida albicans.* *Lancet.* 1969;1(7595):598-599.

43. Pappo I, Polacheck I, Zmora O, et al. Altered gut barrier function to *Candida* during parenteral nutrition. *Nutrition.* 1994;10(2):151-154.

44. Uzun O, Anaissie EJ. Antifungal prophylaxis in patients with hematologic malignancies: A reappraisal. *Blood.* 1995;86(6):2063-2072.

45. Voss A, Hollis RJ, Pfaller MA, et al. Investigation of the sequence of colonization and candidemia in nonneutropenic patients. *J Clin Microbiol.* 1994;32(4):975-980.

46. Pfaller M, Cabezudo I, Koontz F, et al. Predictive value of surveillance cultures for systemic infection due to *Candida* species. *Eur J Clin Microbiol.* 1987;6(6):628-633.

47. Wey SB, Mori M, Pfaller MA, et al. Risk factors for hospital-acquired candidemia. A matched case-control study. *Arch Intern Med.* 1989;149(10):2349-2353.

48. Anaissie EJ, Rex JH, Uzun O, et al. Predictors of adverse outcome in cancer patients with candidemia. *Am J Med.* 1998;104(3):238-245.

49. Rex JH, Bennett JE, Sugar AM, et al. Intravascular catheter exchange and duration of candidemia. NIAID Mycoses Study Group and the Candidemia Study Group. *Clin Infect Dis.* 1995;21(4):994-996.

50. Benoit D, Decruyenaere J, Vandewoude K, et al. Management of candidal thrombophlebitis of the central veins: Case report and review. *Clin Infect Dis.* 1998;26(2):393-397.

51. Karlowicz MG, Hashimoto LN, Kelly RE, Buescher ES. Should central venous catheters be removed as soon as candidemia is detected in neonates? *Pediatrics.* 2000;106(5):E63.

52. Weems JJ, Chamberland ME, Ward J, et al. *Candida parapsilosis* fungemia associated with parenteral nutrition and contaminated blood pressure transducers. *J Clin Microbiol.* 1987;25(6):1029-1032.

53. Plouffe JF, Brown DG, Silva J, et al. Nosocomial outbreak of *Candida parapsilosis* fungemia related to intravenous infusions. *Arch Intern Med.* 1977;137(12):1686-1689.

54. Voss A, Pfaller MA, Hollis RJ, et al. Investigation of *Candida albicans* transmission in a surgical intensive care unit cluster by using genomic DNA typing methods. *J Clin Microbiol.* 1995;33(3):576-580.

55. Benjamin DK, Poole C, Steinbach WJ, et al. Neonatal candidemia and end-organ damage: A critical appraisal of the literature using meta-analytic techniques. *Pediatrics.* 2003;112(3 Pt 1):634-640.

56. Fisher JF, Chew WH, Shadomy S, et al. Urinary tract infections due to *Candida albicans.* *Rev Infect Dis.* 1982;4(6):1107-1118.

57. Coates EW, Karlowicz MG, Croitoru DP, et al. Distinctive distribution of pathogens associated with peritonitis in neonates with focal intestinal perforation compared with necrotizing enterocolitis. *Pediatrics.* 2005;116(2):e241-e246.

58. Echeverria MJ, Ayarza R, Lopez de Goicoechea MJ, et al. Microbiological diagnosis of peritonitis in patients undergoing continuous ambulatory peritoneal dialysis. Review of 5 years at the Hospital de Galdakao. *Enferm Infecc Microbiol Clin.* 1993;11(4):178-181.

59. Solomkin JS, Flohr AB, Quie PG, et al. The role of *Candida* in intraperitoneal infections. *Surgery.* 1980;88(4):524-530.

60. Pacheco-Rios A, Araujo-Hernandez L, Cashat-Cruz M, et al. *Candida* endocarditis in the first year of life. *Bol Med Hosp Infant Mex.* 1993;50(3):157-161.

61. Ellis ME, Al-Abdely H, Sandridge A, et al. Fungal endocarditis: Evidence in the world literature, 1965–1995. *Clin Infect Dis.* 2001;32(1):50-62.

62. Tissieres P, Jaeggi ET, Beghetti M, et al. Increase of fungal endocarditis in children. *Infection.* 2005;33(4):267-272.

63. Mogyorosy G, Soos G, Nagy A. *Candida* endocarditis in a premature infant. *J Perinat Med.* 2000;28(5):407-411.

64. Divekar A, Rebekya IM, Soni R. Late onset *Candida parapsilosis* endocarditis after surviving nosocomial candidemia in an infant with structural heart disease. *Pediatr Infect Dis J.* 2004;23(5):472-475.

65. Ainbinder DJ, Parmley VC, Mader TH, et al. Infectious crystalline keratopathy caused by *Candida guilliermondii.* *Am J Ophthalmol.* 1998;125(5):723-725.

66. Parke DW, Jones DB, Gentry LO. Endogenous endophthalmitis among patients with candidemia. *Ophthalmology.* 1982;89(7):789-796.

67. Brooks RG. Prospective study of *Candida* endophthalmitis in hospitalized patients with candidemia. *Arch Intern Med.* 1989;149(10):2226-2228.

68. Henderson DK, Edwards JE, Montgomerie JZ. Hematogenous candida endophthalmitis in patients receiving parenteral hyperalimentation fluids. *J Infect Dis.* 1981;143(5):655-661.

69. Baley JE, Annable WL, Kliegman RM. *Candida* endophthalmitis in the premature infant. *J Pediatr.* 1981;98(3):458-461.

70. Fisher RG, Karlowicz MG, Lall-Trail J. Very low prevalence of endophthalmitis in very low birthweight infants who survive candidemia. *J Perinatol.* 2005;25(6):408-411.

17

71. Donahue SP, Hein E, Sinatra RB. Ocular involvement in children with candidemia. *Am J Ophthalmol.* 2003;135(6):886-887.

72. Baley JE, Ellis FJ. Neonatal candidiasis: Ophthalmologic infection. *Semin Perinatol.* 2003;27(5): 401-405.

73. Krishna R, Amuh D, Lowder CY, et al. Should all patients with candidaemia have an ophthalmic examination to rule out ocular candidiasis? *Eye.* 2000;14(Pt 1):30-34.

74. Rodriguez-Adrian LJ, King RT, Tamayo-Derat LG, et al. Retinal lesions as clues to disseminated bacterial and candidal infections: Frequency, natural history, and etiology. *Medicine (Baltimore).* 2003;82(3):187-202.

75. Edwards JE, Foos RY, Montgomerie JZ, Guze LB. Ocular manifestations of *Candida* septicemia: Review of seventy-six cases of hematogenous *Candida* endophthalmitis. *Medicine (Baltimore).* 1974;53(1):47-75.

76. Drohan L, Colby CE, Brindle ME, et al. *Candida* (amphotericin-sensitive) lens abscess associated with decreasing arterial blood flow in a very low birth weight preterm infant. *Pediatrics.* 2002; 110(5):e65.

77. Arroyo JG, Bula DV, Grant CA, et al. Bilateral *Candida albicans* endophthalmitis associated with an infected deep venous thrombus. *Jpn J Ophthalmol.* 2004;48(1):30-33.

78. Pappas PG, Rex JH, Sobel JD, et al. Guidelines for treatment of candidiasis. *Clin Infect Dis.* 2004;38(2):161-189.

79. Sanchez-Portocarrero J, Perez-Cecilia E, Corral O, et al. The central nervous system and infection by *Candida* species. *Diagn Microbiol Infect Dis.* 2000;37(3):169-179.

80. Montero A, Romero J, Vargas JA, et al. *Candida* infection of cerebrospinal fluid shunt devices: Report of two cases and review of the literature. *Acta Neurochir (Wien).* 2000;142(1):67-74.

81. Fernandez M, Moylett EH, Noyola DE, et al. Candidal meningitis in neonates: A 10-year review. *Clin Infect Dis.* 2000;31(2):458-463.

82. Moylett EH. Neonatal *Candida* meningitis. *Semin Pediatr Infect Dis.* 2003;14(2):115-122.

83. Doctor BA, Newman N, Minich NM, et al. Clinical outcomes of neonatal meningitis in very-low birth-weight infants. *Clin Pediatr (Phila).* 2001;40(9):473-480.

84. Salaki JS, Louria DB, Chmel H. Fungal and yeast infections of the central nervous system. A clinical review. *Medicine (Baltimore).* 1984;63(2):108-132.

85. Gathe JC, Harris RL, Garland B, et al. *Candida* osteomyelitis. Report of five cases and review of the literature. *Am J Med.* 1987;82(5):927-937.

86. Campen DH, Kaufman RL, Beardmore TD. *Candida* septic arthritis in rheumatoid arthritis. *J Rheumatol.* 1990;17(1):86-88.

87. Malani PN, McNeil SA, Bradley SF, et al. *Candida albicans* sternal wound infections: A chronic and recurrent complication of median sternotomy. *Clin Infect Dis.* 2002;35(11):1316-1320.

88. Dan M. Neonatal septic arthritis. *Isr J Med Sci.* 1983;19(11):967-971.

89. Deshpande SS, Taral N, Modi N, Singrakhia M. Changing epidemiology of neonatal septic arthritis. *J Orthop Surg (Hong Kong).* 2004;12(1):10-13.

90. Evdoridou J, Roilides E, Bibashi E, et al. Multifocal osteoarthritis due to *Candida albicans* in a neonate: Serum level monitoring of liposomal amphotericin B and literature review. *Infection.* 1997;25(2):112-116.

91. Weisse ME, Person DA, Berkenbaugh JT. Treatment of *Candida* arthritis with flucytosine and amphotericin B. *J Perinatol.* 1993;13(5):402-404.

92. Swanson H, Hughes PA, Messer SA, et al. *Candida albicans* arthritis one year after successful treatment of fungemia in a healthy infant. *J Pediatr.* 1996;129(5):688-694.

93. Mamlok RJ, Richardson CJ, Mamlok V, et al. A case of intrauterine pulmonary candidiasis. *Pediatr Infect Dis.* 1985;4(6):692-693.

94. Rowen JL, Atkins JT, Levy ML, et al. Invasive fungal dermatitis in the < or = 1000-gram neonate. *Pediatrics.* 1995;95(5):682-687.

95. Ostrosky-Zeichner L, Rex JH, Pappas PG, et al. Antifungal susceptibility survey of 2,000 bloodstream *Candida* isolates in the United States. *Antimicrob Agents Chemother.* 2003;47(10): 3149-3154.

96. Hospenthal DR, Murray CK, Rinaldi MG. The role of antifungal susceptibility testing in the therapy of candidiasis. *Diagn Microbiol Infect Dis.* 2004;48(3):153-160.

97. Edwards JE, Bodey GP, Bowden RA, et al. International Conference for the Development of a Consensus on the Management and Prevention of Severe Candidal Infections. *Clin Infect Dis.* 1997;25(1):43-59.

98. Buchner T, Fegeler W, Bernhardt H, et al. Treatment of severe *Candida* infections in high-risk patients in Germany: Consensus formed by a panel of interdisciplinary investigators. *Eur J Clin Microbiol Infect Dis.* 2002;21(5):337-352.

99. Cohen-Wolkowiez M, Moran C, Benjamin D, et al. Pediatric antifungal agents. *Curr Opin Infect Dis* 2009;22:553-558.

100. Smith PB, Walsh TJ, Hope W, et al. Pharmacokinetics of an elevated dosage of Micafungin in premature neonates. *Pediatr Infect Dis J.* 2009;28:412-415.

101. Benjamin Jr DK, Smith P, Arrieta A, et al. Safety and pharmacokinetics of repeat-dose micafungin in neonates. In: *Program and Abstracts of the 48th Annual Interscience Conference on Antimicrobial Agents and Chemotherapy.* Washington D.C.: American Society for Microbiology; 2008.

102. Odio CM, Araya R, Pinto LE, et al. Caspofungin therapy of neonates with invasive candidiasis. *Pediatr Infect Dis J.* 2004;23(12):1093-1097.

17

103. Moudgal V, Little T, Boikov D, et al. Multiechinocandin- and multiazole-resistant *Candida parapsilosis* isolates serially obtained during therapy for prosthetic valve endocarditis. *Antimicrob Agents Chemother*. 2005;49(2):767-769.

104. Steinbach WJ, Benjamin DK. New antifungal agents under development in children and neonates. *Curr Opin Infect Dis*. 2005;18(6):484-489.

105. Heresi G, Gerstmann DR, Blumer JL. Pharmacokinetic, safety, and tolerance study of micafungin (FK463) in premature infants. Presented at Pediatric Academic Society Annual Meeting, Abstract 1808. Seattle, WA: May 3-6; 2003.

106. Driessen M, Ellis JB, Cooper PA, et al. Fluconazole vs. amphotericin B for the treatment of neonatal fungal septicemia: A prospective randomized trial. *Pediatr Infect Dis J*. 1996;15(12):1107-1112.

107. Kullberg BJ. Voriconazole compared with a strategy of amphotericin B followed by fluconazole for treatment of candidaemia in non-neutropenic patients. Abstract No. O245. Presented at 14th European Conference of Clinical Microbiology and Infectious Diseases. Prague, Czech Republic: May 1-4; 2004.

108. Muldrew KM, Maples HD, Stowe CD, et al. Intravenous voriconazole therapy in a preterm infant. *Pharmacotherapy*. 2005;25(6):893-898.

109. Johnson MD, MacDougall C, Ostrosky-Zeichner L, et al. Combination antifungal therapy. *Antimicrob Agents Chemother*. 2004;48(3):693-715.

110. Rex JH, Pappas PG, Karchmer AW, et al. A randomized and blinded multicenter trial of high-dose fluconazole plus placebo versus fluconazole plus amphotericin B as therapy for candidemia and its consequences in nonneutropenic subjects. *Clin Infect Dis*. 2003;36(10):1221-1228.

111. Albert RK, Condie F. Hand-washing patterns in medical intensive-care units. *N Engl J Med*. 1981;304(24):1465-1466.

112. Parry MF, Grant B, Yukna M, et al. *Candida* osteomyelitis and diskitis after spinal surgery: An outbreak that implicates artificial nail use. *Clin Infect Dis*. 2001;32(3):352-357.

113. Reed BN, Cuadle KE, Rogers PD. Fluconazole prophylaxis in high-risk neonates. *Ann Pharmacother*. 2010;44(1):178-184.

114. Kaufman D. Strategies for prevention of neonatal invasive candidiasis. *Semin Perinatol*. 2003;27(5):414-424.

115. Smolinski KN, Shah SS, Honig PJ, Yan AC. Neonatal cutaneous fungal infections. *Curr Opin Pediatr*. 2005;17(4):486-493.

116. James MJ, Lasker BA, McNeil MM, et al. Use of a repetitive DNA probe to type clinical and environmental isolates of *Aspergillus flavus* from a cluster of cutaneous infections in a neonatal intensive care unit. *J Clin Microbiol*. 2000;38(10):3612-3618.

117. Mahieu LM, De Dooy JJ, Van Laer FA, et al. A prospective study on factors influencing *Aspergillus* spore load in the air during renovation works in a neonatal intensive care unit. *J Hosp Infect*. 2000;45(3):191-197.

118. Groll AH, Jaeger G, Allendorf A, et al. Invasive pulmonary aspergillosis in a critically ill neonate: Case report and review of invasive aspergillosis during the first 3 months of life. *Clin Infect Dis*. 1998;27(3):437-452.

119. Mennink-Kersten MA, Klont RR, Warris A, et al. *Bifidobacterium* lipoteichoic acid and false ELISA reactivity in *Aspergillus* antigen detection. *Lancet*. 2004;363(9405):325-327.

120. Siemann M, Koch-Dorfler M, Gaude M. False-positive results in premature infants with the Platelia *Aspergillus* sandwich enzyme-linked immunosorbent assay. *Mycoses*. 1998;41(9–10):373-377.

121. Perzigian RW, Faix RG. Primary cutaneous aspergillosis in a preterm infant. *Am J Perinatol*. 1993;10(4):269-271.

122. Walsh TJ, Seibel NL, Arndt C, et al. Amphotericin B lipid complex in pediatric patients with invasive fungal infections. *Pediatr Infect Dis J*. 1999;18(8):702-708.

123. Herbrecht R, Denning DW, Patterson TF, et al. Voriconazole versus amphotericin B for primary therapy of invasive aspergillosis. *N Engl J Med*. 2002;347(6):408-415.

124. Shouldice E, Fernandez C, McCully B, et al. Voriconazole treatment of presumptive disseminated *Aspergillus* infection in a child with acute leukemia. *J Pediatr Hematol Oncol*. 2003;25(9):732-734.

125. Dennis JE, Rhodes KH, Cooney DR, et al. Nosocomial *Rhizopus* infection (zygomycosis) in children. *J Pediatr*. 1980;96(5):824-828.

126. Mitchell SJ, Gray J, Morgan ME, et al. Nosocomial infection with *Rhizopus microsporus* in preterm infants: Association with wooden tongue depressors. *Lancet*. 1996;348(9025):441-443.

127. Todd NJ, Millar MR, Dealler SR, et al. Inadvertent intravenous infusion of Mucor during parenteral feeding of a neonate. *J Hosp Infect*. 1990;15(3):295-297.

128. Lewis LL, Hawkins HK, Edwards MS. Disseminated mucormycosis in an infant with methylmalonic aciduria. *Pediatr Infect Dis J*. 1990;9(11):851-854.

129. Ng PC, Dear PR. Phycomycotic abscesses in a preterm infant. *Arch Dis Child*. 1989;64(6):862-864.

130. Alexander P, Alladi A, Correa M, et al. Neonatal colonic mucormycosis—a tropical perspective. *J Trop Pediatr*. 2005;51(1):54-59.

131. Butugan O, Sanchez TG, Goncalez F, et al. Rhinocerebral mucormycosis: Predisposing factors, diagnosis, therapy, complications and survival. *Rev Laryngol Otol Rhinol (Bord)*. 1996;117(1):53-55.

132. Roden MM, Zaoutis TE, Buchanan WL, et al. Epidemiology and outcome of zygomycosis: A review of 929 reported cases. *Clin Infect Dis*. 2005;41(5):634-653.

133. Linder N, Keller N, Huri C, et al. Primary cutaneous mucormycosis in a premature infant: Case report and review of the literature. *Am J Perinatol*. 1998;15(1):35-38.

17

134. Herbrecht RV, Letscher-Bru V, Bowden RA, et al. Treatment of 21 cases of invasive mucormycosis with amphotericin B colloidal dispersion. *Eur J Clin Microbiol Infect Dis*. 2001;20(7):460-466.

135. Kontoyiannis DP, Lionakis MS, Lewis RE, et al. Zygomycosis in a tertiary-care cancer center in the era of *Aspergillus*-active antifungal therapy: A case-control observational study of 27 recent cases. *J Infect Dis*. 2005;191(8):1350-1360.

136. Ely EW, Peacock JE, Haponik EF, et al. Cryptococcal pneumonia complicating pregnancy. *Medicine (Baltimore)*. 1998;77(3):153-167.

137. Whitt SP, Koch GA, Fender B, et al. Histoplasmosis in pregnancy: Case series and report of transplacental transmission. *Arch Intern Med*. 2004;164(4):454-458.

138. Watts EA, Gard PD, Tuthill SW. First reported case of intrauterine transmission of blastomycosis. *Pediatr Infect Dis*. 1983;2(4):308-310.

139. Shetty SS, Harrison LH, Hajjeh RA, et al. Determining risk factors for candidemia among newborn infants from population-based surveillance: Baltimore, Maryland, 1998–2000. *Pediatr Infect Dis J*. 2005;24(7):601-604.

140. Rangel-Frausto MS, Wiblin T, Blumberg HM, et al. National epidemiology of mycoses survey (NEMIS): Variations in rates of bloodstream infections due to *Candida* species in seven surgical intensive care units and six neonatal intensive care units. *Clin Infect Dis*. 1999;29(2):253-258.

141. Stamos JK, Rowley AH. Candidemia in a pediatric population. *Clin Infect Dis*. 1995;20(3):571-575.

142. Feja KN, Wu F, Roberts K, et al. Risk factors for candidemia in critically ill infants: A matched case-control study. *J Pediatr*. 2005;147(2):156-161.

143. Huttova M, Hartmanova I, Kralinsky K, et al. *Candida* fungemia in neonates treated with fluconazole: Report of forty cases, including eight with meningitis. *Pediatr Infect Dis J*. 1998;17(11):1012-1015.

144. Ostrosky-Zeichner L, Kontoyiannis D, Raffalli J, et al. International, open-label, noncomparative, clinical trial of micafungin alone and in combination for treatment of newly diagnosed and refractory candidemia. *Eur J Clin Microbiol Infect Dis*. 2005;24(10):654-661.

145. Levine J, Bernard DB, Idelson BA, et al. Fungal peritonitis complicating continuous ambulatory peritoneal dialysis: Successful treatment with fluconazole, a new orally active antifungal agent. *Am J Med*. 1989;86(6 Pt 2):825-827.

146. Salvaggio MR, Pappas PG. Current concepts in the management of fungal peritonitis. *Curr Infect Dis Rep*. 2003;5(2):120-124.

147. Arfania D, Everett ED, Nolph KD, et al. Uncommon causes of peritonitis in patients undergoing peritoneal dialysis. *Arch Intern Med*. 1981;141(1):61-64.

148. Corbella X, Sirvent JM, Carratala J. Fluconazole treatment without catheter removal in *Candida albicans* peritonitis complicating peritoneal dialysis. *Am J Med*. 1991;90(2):277.

149. Bren A. Fungal peritonitis in patients on continuous ambulatory peritoneal dialysis. *Eur J Clin Microbiol Infect Dis*. 1998;17(12):839-843.

150. Stern WH, Tamura E, Jacobs RA, et al. Epidemic postsurgical *Candida parapsilosis* endophthalmitis. Clinical findings and management of 15 consecutive cases. *Ophthalmology*. 1985;92(12):1701-1709.

151. Perraut LE, Perraut LE, Bleiman B, et al. Successful treatment of *Candida albicans* endophthalmitis with intravitreal amphotericin B. *Arch Ophthalmol*. 1981;99(9):1565-1567.

152. Breit SM, Hariprasad SM, Mieler WF, et al. Management of endogenous fungal endophthalmitis with voriconazole and caspofungin. *Am J Ophthalmol*. 2005;139(1):135-140.

153. Fitzgerald E, Lloyd-Still J, Gordon SL. *Candida* arthritis. A case report and review of the literature. *Clin Orthop*. 1975;106:143-147.

154. Petrikkos G, Skiada A, Sabatakou H, et al. Case report. Successful treatment of two cases of postsurgical sternal osteomyelitis, due to *Candida krusei* and *Candida albicans*, respectively, with high doses of triazoles (fluconazole, itraconazole). *Mycoses*. 2001;44(9–10):422-425.

155. Smego RA, Perfect JR, Durack DT. Combined therapy with amphotericin B and 5-fluorocytosine for *Candida* meningitis. *Rev Infect Dis*. 1984;6(6):791-801.

156. Liu KH, Wu CJ, Chou CH, et al. Refractory candidal meningitis in an immunocompromised patient cured by caspofungin. *J Clin Microbiol*. 2004;42(12):5950-5953.

157. Fan-Havard P, O'Donovan C, Smith SM, et al. Oral fluconazole versus amphotericin B bladder irrigation for treatment of candidal funguria. *Clin Infect Dis*. 1995;21(4):960-965.

CHAPTER 18

The Use of Biomarkers for Detection of Early- and Late-Onset Neonatal Sepsis

Nader Bishara, MD

Sepsis is a frequent and serious problem in neonatal intensive care units, particularly in very low birth weight (VLBW) infants. The current gold standard for detection, a blood culture, is difficult and time-consuming and lacks sensitivity. More than 20% of all VLBW infants experience one or more episodes of late-onset sepsis (LOS, defined as any sepsis occurring after 5 days of age), and the median age for the first episode of LOS is 17 days of age.[1] Delaying treatment until symptoms arise can be life threatening. On the other hand, recurrent treatment with antimicrobial agents in infants who are not infected presents potential risks to these infants by furthering the development of resistant organisms.[2]

Despite the frequency with which life-threatening infections are encountered in neonatal intensive care units, a rapid, sensitive, and specific diagnostic test remains elusive. Fastidious organisms, maternal antibiotic treatment, small specimen volumes, and a 24- to 72-hour delay for definitive results make blood culture a less than ideal method of diagnosis. In previous studies, physiologic parameters such as temperature alterations and heart rate have been used to predict infection. Clinical scores, for example, the nosocomical sepsis (NOSEP) score, have been implemented to predict nosocomial infection.[3,4]

The search for an early biomarker of sepsis has led many researchers to evaluate a variety of biomarkers, singly or in small combinations. Newer technologies can now evaluate multiple biomarkers using small blood volumes.

Characteristics of the Ideal Biomarker

An ideal biomarker or group of biomarkers should possess certain laboratory and clinical characteristics. A biomarker should have an adequate window of opportunity for sampling, should be biochemically stable, and should require minimal transport and storage requirements. The analysis should be fully automated and able to be performed in a nonspecialized laboratory. From the clinical aspect, an ideal biomarker should have a well-defined cutoff value for differentiating noninfected from infected infants. It should have high sensitivity and high negative predictive value (>99%) and good specificity and positive predictive value (>85%). It should be able to reflect the progress of the disease and guide the use of antibiotics.[5] Table 18-1 demonstrates the accuracy of various biomarkers that have been evaluated for early-onset sepsis (EOS) and LOS.

Types of Biomarkers

Cytokines

Cytokines are cell signaling proteins that are secreted by numerous cells of the immune system and by glial cells of the nervous system. Cytokines have been classed

Table 18-1   ACCURACY OF VARIOUS BIOMARKERS FOR EARLY- AND LATE-ONSET SEPSIS

Biomarker	Sensitivity	Specificity	PPV	NPV
Cytokines IL-6[7,8]	67-89	89-96	84-95	72-91
Umbilical cord IL-6[9]	87-90	93	93	93-100
GCSF >200 pg/mL[17]	95	73	40	99
TNF[15]	83.3	80.6		
Chemokines CCL4 >140 pg/mL[18]	92	40		98
IL-8[5]	80-91	76-100	70-74	91-95
Free IL-8[21]	97			99
Urine IL-8 >75 pg/mg Cr[22]	92			
IP-10 >1250 pg/mL[23]	93	89		
Cell Surface Markers CD64	64-97	72-96	64-88	84-98
CD11b[24]				
Neutrophils	100	56		
Monocytes	86	94		
Acute Phase Proteins CRP[7]	60-82	93-96	95-100	75-87
SAA[25]	96	95	85	99
Procalcitonin[26]	82-100	87-100	86-98	93-100
IαIp[27]	89.5	99	95	98
Combination Biomarkers IL-6/IL-10/CCL5[13]	100	97	85	100
IL-6 and/or CRP[5]	93	88-96	86-95	95
IL-8 and/or CRP[5]	80	87	68	93

CCL4, C-C motif ligand-4; *CCL5*, C-C motif ligand-5; *Cr*, creatinine; *CRP*, C-reactive protein; *GCSF*, granulocyte colony-stimulating factor; *IαIp*, inter-alpha inhibitor protein; *IL*, interleukin; *IP-10*, interferon-γ–induced protein-10; *NPV*, negative predictive value; *PPV*, positive predictive value; *SAA*, serum amyloid A.

as lymphokines, interleukins, and chemokines on the basis of their presumed function, cell of secretion, or target of action. Because cytokines are characterized by considerable redundancy and pleiotropism, such distinctions, with few exceptions, are obsolete.[6] Table 18-2 summarizes the sources, actions, gene locations, and receptors of various cytokines and chemokines that have been evaluated in neonatal EOS and LOS.

Interleukin-6

Interleukin (IL)-6 is produced mainly by mononuclear phagocytic cells. It is also produced by T and B lymphocytes, fibroblasts, and hepatocytes. IL-6 enhances B cell differentiation into mature plasma cells and secretion of immunoglobulins and shares several activities with Interleukin-1 (IL-1), including production of acute phase proteins (APPs) and induction of pyrexia. IL-6 is the most important inducer of hepatocyte synthesis of APPs. In contrast to these pro-inflammatory effects, IL-6 mediates several anti-inflammatory effects. Whereas IL-1 and tumor necrosis factor (TNF) induce synthesis of each other, as well as of IL-6, IL-6 terminates this

Table 18-2   SUMMARY OF SOURCE, ACTION, AND RECEPTOR INTERACTION OF VARIOUS CYTOKINES AND CHEMOKINES THAT HAVE BEEN EVALUATED IN NEONATAL SEPSIS

Biomarker	Source	Action	Gene Location	Receptor
IL-1	Macrophages	Stimulation of T cells and antigen presenting cells B cell growth/antibody production	1	IL-1R
IL-2	Activated T cells	Proliferation of activated T cells	4	IL-2R
IL-6	Activated T cells	Initiates inflammatory response Stimulates production of acute phase proteins	5	IL-6R
IL-8	Macrophages	Neutrophil chemoattractant Stimulates angiogenesis	4	IL-8RA IL-8RB
IL-10	Activated T cells B cells Monocytes	Inhibits inflammatory and immune responses	1	IL-10RA
IL-12	Macrophages B cells	Stimulates IFN-γ and TNF production Antiangiogenic activity	4	IL-12R
IL-18	Macrophages	Induces IFN-γ production	9	IL-18R
CCL4	Macrophages	Chemoattractant for NK cells and monocytes	17	CCR5
CCL5	Activated T cells	Proliferation and activation of NK cells Chemotactic for T cells, eosinophils, and basophils	17	CCR5
GCSF	Macrophages	Granulopoiesis	11	GCSFR
TNF	Macrophages	Acute phase proteins Neutrophil chemoattractant	6	TNF-R1 TNF-R2
IFN-γ	NK cells	Antigen presentation of macrophages Leukocyte adhesion	10	IFNGR1 IFNGR2
IP-10	Monocytes	Monocyte/macrophage chemoattractant Promotes T cell adhesion Inhibits angiogenesis	4	CXCR3

CCL4, C-C motif ligand-4; *CCL5,* C-C motif ligand-5; *IFN-γ,* interferon-gamma; *IL,* interleukin; *IP-10,* interferon-γ–induced protein-10; *R,* receptor; *TNF,* tumor necrosis factor.

upregulatory inflammatory cascade and inhibits IL-1 and TNF synthesis. Furthermore, IL-6 stimulates synthesis of IL-1-receptor antagonist (IL-1ra). IL-6 levels are significantly elevated during sepsis, and this precedes the appearance of other cytokines. IL-6 has a short half-life, and its sensitivity decreases after 12 to 24 hours. IL-6 as a marker in the early phases of infection has been evaluated and has been found to have a sensitivity of 89% and a negative predictive value of 91% (compared with 60% and 75% for C-reactive protein [CRP], respectively).[7,8] Cord blood IL-6 levels were measured and were found to have high sensitivities and negative predictive values (87% to 100% and 93% to 100%, respectively).[9,10] In another study by Oguz and colleagues, IL-6 and CRP levels were evaluated in late-onset fungal and bacterial infections. IL-6 levels were markedly elevated in bacterial sepsis (38 vs. 392 ng/dL), and CRP levels were elevated in fungal sepsis (11 vs. 28 mg/L).[11]

Interleukin-10 Family

The interleukin-10 family includes IL-10, IL-19, IL-20, IL-22, IL-24, IL-26, IL-28, and IL-29. The principal routine function of IL-10 is to limit and ultimately terminate inflammatory responses.

IL-10 is capable of inhibiting the synthesis of pro-inflammatory cytokines such as interferon (IFN)-γ, IL-2, TNF, and granulocyte colony-stimulating factor (G-CSF) (Figure 18-1). IL-10 also displays potent abilities to suppress the antigen

18

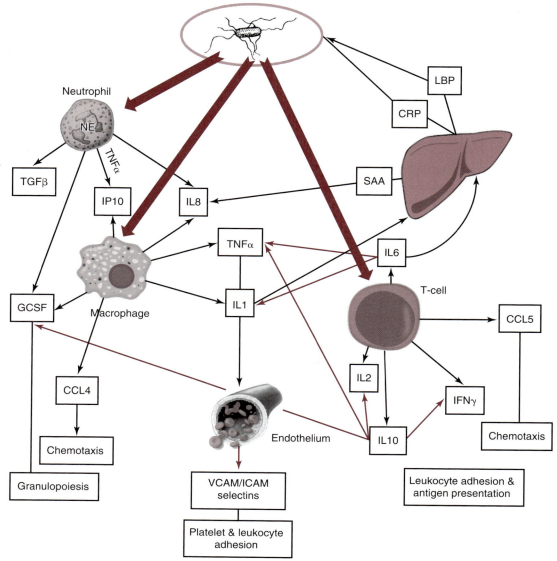

Figure 18-1   This figure illustrates the interactions of various biomarkers in response to an inflammatory stimulus. Black arrows are stimulatory and red arrows are inhibitory. *CCL4,* C-C motif ligand-4; *CCL5,* C-C motif ligand-5; *CRP,* C-reactive protein; *GCSF,* granulocyte colony-stimulating factor; *IαIp,* inter-alpha inhibitor protein; *ICAM,* intracellular adhesion molecule; *IFN-γ,* interferon-gamma; *IP-10,* interferon-γ–induced protein-10; *LBP,* lipopolysaccharide-binding protein; *NE,* neutrophil elastase; *SAA,* serum amyloid A; *TGF,* tumor growth factor; *TNF,* tumor necrosis factor; and *VCAM,* vascular adhesion molecule. Upon exposure to microorganisms, macrophages respond by producing interleukin (IL)-8, TNF, CCL4, and GCSF; this ultimately leads to granulopoiesis, chemotaxis, and stimulation of selectins, VCAM, and ICAM, resulting in leukocyte adhesion. T cells after activation release IL-6 (which inhibits both TNF and IL-1), IL-10, IFN-γ, and CCL5. CCL5 helps with chemotaxis, and IFN-γ facilitates leukocyte adhesion and antigen presentation to macrophages. IL-6 induces the production of acute phase proteins. The production of IL-10 from T cells mainly results in negative feedback to decrease the immune response and leads to inhibition of GCSF, IL-2, TNF, and IFN-γ. Neutrophils respond by production of neutrophil elastase, which, upon secretion, upregulates IL-8 and IP-10 production (under the effect of TNF) and induces the production of GCSF. Acute phase proteins are released mainly by hepatocytes. SAA induces production of IL-8. CRP binds to phosphocholine in bacterial cells, and LBP binds to the lipopolysaccharide (LPS) of microorganisms.

presentation capacity of antigen presenting cells. However, it is also stimulatory toward certain T cells and mast cells and stimulates B cell maturation and antibody production. Several studies have evaluated IL-10, mostly with IL-6 and other cytokines, as a biomarker for neonatal sepsis. Higher levels of IL-10, IL-6, and CRP were observed in neonates with sepsis, pneumonia, and necrotizing enterocolitis (NEC). Elevated IL-6 levels were observed at the onset of sepsis, and IL-10 was predominant 12 hours later. Markedly elevated IL-10 and CRP levels were associated with increased mortality.[12] Ng and associates measured IL-10, IL-6, and C-C ligand-5 (CCL5) levels at the time of clinical presentation and 24 hours afterward in VLBW infants with suspected infection requiring full sepsis screening. The model had a sensitivity of 100% and a specificity of 97% when cutoffs for IL-10 (>208 ng/dL), IL-6 (>168 ng/dL), and CCL5 (<3110 ng/dL) were used.[13] Test characteristics of IL-12 and IL-10 were evaluated by Sherwin and colleagues. At the time sepsis was first suspected, IL-12 had a sensitivity of 28% and a specificity of 99%, and IL-10 had a sensitivity of 17% and a specificity of 99%.[14]

Interleukin-1 Family

The IL-1 family includes IL-1α, IL-1β, and IL-1ra. IL-1α induces the release of TNF by endothelial cells and stimulates the secretion of APPs by hepatocytes. IL-1β is produced by activated macrophages and is an important mediator of inflammation. IL-1ra inhibits the activities of IL-1α and IL-1β. IL-1β has been evaluated in neonatal sepsis with controversial results,[15] in contrast to IL-1ra, which has been shown to be consistently increased in infected (concentrations of 6 to 30 ng/mL) compared with noninfected neonates (concentrations of 2 to 3 ng/mL). A 15-fold increase in IL-1ra levels was observed 2 days before sepsis was diagnosed.[16]

Tumor Necrosis Factor

TNF is one of the primary agents responsible for vascular, metabolic, and cellular responses to sepsis. It stimulates IL-6 production and has a broad spectrum of biologic actions on several types of target cells. Its usefulness as a diagnostic biomarker for neonatal sepsis is controversial. In one study, the sensitivity and specificity of TNF were 83.3% and 80.6%, respectively, on day 0. TNF levels correlated positively with CRP levels on day 0.[15]

Granulocyte Colony-Stimulating Factor

Granulocyte colony-stimulating factor (G-CSF) is a cytokine and a hematopoietic growth factor. It is produced by macrophages, endothelium, and several other immune cells. The G-CSF receptor is present on precursor cells in the bone marrow; in response to stimulation by G-CSF, it stimulates proliferation and differentiation of stem cells into mature granulocytes. It also stimulates their release into the bloodstream. G-CSF has been proposed to be a reliable biomarker for EOS in neonates. A concentration greater than 200 pg/mL has high sensitivity (95%) and a high negative predictive value (99%) for predicting early-onset sepsis.[17]

Chemokines

The major role of chemokines is to act as chemoattractants to guide the migration of cells. Cells that are attracted by chemokines follow a signal of increasing chemokine concentration toward the source of the chemokine. Members of the chemokine family are divided into four groups, depending on the spacing of their first two cysteine residues. Chemokines that have been evaluated in sepsis include C-C ligand motif (CC) chemokines and C-X-C ligand motif (CXC) chemokines.

CC Chemokines

The CC chemokines have two adjacent cysteines near their amino terminus. CC chemokines induce the migration of monocytes and other cell types such as natural killer (NK) cells and dendritic cells. CC chemokines that have been evaluated in neonatal sepsis include C-C motif ligand-4 (CCL4) and C-C motif ligand-5 (CCL5).

C-C Motif Ligand-4

CCL4, also known as macrophage inflammatory protein-1β, is a chemoattractant for NK cells, monocytes, and a variety of other immune cells. CCL4 induces the synthesis and release of other pro-inflammatory cytokines such as IL-1, IL-6, and TNF from fibroblasts and macrophages. CCL4 levels were evaluated in pediatric patients as an outcome biomarker for mortality in pediatric septic shock. Levels greater than 140 pg/mL yielded a sensitivity of 92% and a specificity of 40% for mortality. Serum levels less than 140 pg/mL had a negative predictive value for mortality of 98%.[18]

C-C Motif Ligand-5

CCL5, also known as RANTES (Regulated upon Activation, Normal T cell Expressed, and Secreted), is chemotactic for T cells, eosinophils, and basophils. It plays an important role in recruiting leukocytes into inflammatory sites. With the help of particular cytokines (IL-2 and IFN-γ) that are released by T cells, CCL5 induces the proliferation and activation of certain NK cells to form CC chemokine–activated killer cells. Królak-Olejnik and coworkers evaluated levels of CCL5 and melanoma growth stimulatory activity/growth-related oncogene-α (MGSA/GRO-α) concentrations in umbilical cord blood samples and compared values in preterm and term infants. Preterm neonates had lower CCL5 concentrations than term neonates, and CCL5 concentrations did not increase during infection. MGSA/GRO-α concentrations were constitutively higher in preterm than in term neonates, and sepsis events further increased concentrations in preterm neonates.[19] In a recent study, Shouman and associates measured levels of CCL5 and TNF in septic (early- and late-onset) neonates and demonstrated that CCL5 levels were markedly decreased, whereas levels of TNF were elevated.[20] The same findings were confirmed by Ng.[13]

CXC Chemokines

The two N-terminal cysteines of CXC chemokines are separated by one amino acid represented in this name with an "X."

Interleukin-8

Interleukin-8 (IL-8) is one of the major mediators of the inflammatory response. It is secreted by several cell types and functions as a chemoattractant and as a potent angiogenic factor. It is similar to IL-6 but has a longer half-life. Many studies have evaluated the use of IL-8 as an early-phase biomarker. Recent studies measured sensitivity and specificity ranges from 80% to 91% and from 76% to 100%, respectively.[5] IL-8 levels were markedly elevated in infants diagnosed with perinatal infection compared with controls on day 1 but not on day 4.[28] In a multicenter, randomized, controlled trial, applying serum cutoff values for IL-8 in combination with CRP reduced antibiotic use in neonates with suspected early-onset sepsis from 50% to 36%. However, in the IL-8 group, 14.5% of infected infants were not detected at the initial evaluation, compared with 17.3% in the non-infected group.[29] IL-8 is bound to leukocyte receptors, thus plasma IL-8 levels are not indicative of the total IL-8 secreted in response to infection. Orlikowsky and colleagues compared total IL-8 levels by processing whole blood with detergent to release cell-associated IL-8 and combine it with free IL-8. Sensitivity and negative predictive values increased from 71% to 97% and from 89% to 99%, respectively, at 6 hours after clinical suspicion of infection, and from 33% to 70% and from 66% to 80% at 24 hours.[21] Bentlin and coworkers measured elevated urine IL-8 levels in premature infants with culture-proven and suspected LOS in comparison with noninfected infants. Sensitivity was higher than that of serum IL-8 measurements, and testing was less invasive.[22]

Interferon γ–Induced Protein-10

Interferon γ–induced protein-10 (IP-10, also known as CXCL10) is expressed from a variety of cells, including monocytes, endothelial cells, keratinocytes, and fibroblasts. Neutrophils produce IP-10 in response to the combined stimulus of IFN-γ with TNF or bacterial lipopolysaccharide (LPS). This response is blocked by IL-10 and IL-4. IP-10 also promotes T cell adhesion to endothelial cells and inhibits angiogenesis and colony formation by the bone marrow. Ng and colleagues reported IP-10 levels that were significantly higher in infected neonates than in the noninfected group at 0 hours; IP-10 levels markedly decreased by 24 hours. IP-10 concentrations of 1250 pg/mL or greater could identify all infants with sepsis or NEC with sensitivity and specificity of 93% and 89%, respectively.[23]

Surface Markers

Measurement of cell-bound receptor molecules involved in inflammation has several advantages. The volume of blood needed to quantitate the cell surface markers with the use of whole-blood flow cytometry, is minimal compared with that needed to identify soluble markers (cytokines and chemokines). The sample size may be critical in VLBW infants. Assessing the cellular response to cytokines may be a better way of identifying early immunologic response to bacterial antigens. Moreover, circulating concentrations of cytokines and chemokines may not necessarily reflect their biologic activities at the cellular level. Attention has recently been directed to neutrophils cluster of differentiation 64 (CD64) and cluster of differentiation 11b (CD11b) as diagnostic biomarkers of sepsis.

CD64

Neutrophil surface CD64, under the influence of IFN-γ and other inflammatory cytokines, is quantitatively upregulated during infection and sepsis. The increase in surface density is directly proportional to the intensity of the cytokine stimulus. A recent study assessed the usefulness of neutrophil CD64 as a diagnostic marker for sepsis. Infants with sepsis episodes (culture proven and suspected) had higher CD64 indices (5.6 vs. 2.6). When CD64 indices were combined with absolute neutrophil count, sensitivity was 95% for diagnosing sepsis, and the negative predictive value was 93% for ruling out sepsis. For culture proven sepsis, CD64 had the highest sensitivity (80%) and specificity (79%).[30] In another study, two neutrophil markers (CD11b and CD64) and two lymphocyte surface markers (CD25 and CD45RO) were evaluated. CD64 had the highest sensitivity (97%), specificity (90%), and negative predictive value (99%) as a diagnostic marker for early-onset neonatal sepsis at the onset of infection and 24 hours later. When combined with IL-6 and CRP, sensitivity and negative predictive value increased to 100%.[31]

CD11b

Neutrophils express CD11b at very low concentrations in the nonactivated state. Within a few minutes of exposure to microbial products, CD11b expression is markedly increased. Earlier trials were unable to demonstrate its diagnostic value for prediction of late-onset infection in preterm infants. Turunen and coworkers suggested that daily measurement of neutrophil or monocyte CD11b/CD18 could identify cases before clinical suspicion.[24] In the infected group, CD11b expression gradually increased during the 3 days preceding sampling for blood culture. At the day of sampling, median expression of CD11b in neutrophils and monocytes was higher in the infected group than in the control group. For neutrophils, sensitivity and specificity were 100% and 56%, respectively, and for monocytes, 86% and 94%, respectively. In preterm infants with respiratory distress syndrome, neutrophil CD11b expression during the first day was higher than in cord blood or in preterm infants without mechanical ventilation.[24] CD11b expression decreased by 10 days of life. These findings may limit the usefulness of CD11b as an early marker for early-onset sepsis.

HLA-DR

Major histocompatibility complex (MHC) II cell surface receptor (HLA-DR) is one of the key cell surface molecules expressed on antigen presenting cells (monocytes, macrophages, and dendritic cells) and is responsible for antigen presentation to T cells and initiation of the inflammatory cascade during infection. Hallwirth and associates investigated the expression of HLA-DR as a marker for antigen presenting capability in VLBW, late preterm, and term infants. HLA-DR expression was significantly diminished in VLBW infants; this may lead to a reduced antigen presenting capacity and may contribute to the higher incidence of infection in this population.[32] In a recent study, monocyte HLA-DR expression was evaluated in neonates with LOS. The percentage of HLA-DR expressing monocytes was significantly lower in the nonsurvivor sepsis group (17%) than in the survivor sepsis group (45%). Patients with monocyte HLA-DR expression of 30% or less had lower survival rates and a 30-fold higher risk of mortality.[33] Use of HLA-DR in another study did not support the use of monocyte HLA-DR alone or in combination with other infection markers in the diagnosis of EOS and pneumonia in term neonates.[34]

Other Cell Surface Markers

Other surface markers that have been evaluated include CD69 on NK cells and CD25 and CD69 on T cells. Upregulation of CD69 on NK cells was the most sensitive marker for neonatal sepsis (sensitivity 81%). CD69 and CD25 expression was significantly upregulated on T cells in 11 of 17 and 10 of 17 patients, respectively. A combination of CD45RA/CD45RO and CD45RO identified 11 of 16 infected patients. Measurement of CD69 expression on NK cells with CD45RA, CD45RO, CD25, and CD69 expression on T cells resulted in a significant increase in at least two inflammatory markers from infected patients.[35] In premature infants, an increase in lymphocyte antigens (CD3, CD19, CD25, CD26, CD71, and CD69) and neutrophil antigens (CD11b, CD11c, CD13, CD15, CD33, and CD66b) is seen in response to infection. CD33, CD66b, and CD19 levels were significantly elevated in both culture proven and suspected sepsis groups.[36] The diagnostic usefulness of these markers requires further evaluation because detection requires monoclonal antibodies that are not readily available.

Acute Phase Proteins

Acute phase proteins (APPs) is the generic name given to a group of approximately 30 different biochemically and functionally unrelated proteins. These proteins are secreted mainly by hepatocytes, and their levels in serum may be increased (positive APP) or reduced (e.g., albumin is a negative APP) approximately 90 minutes after the onset of a systemic inflammatory reaction. During the inflammatory process, cytokines, mainly IL-6, TNF, and INF-γ, are produced by macrophages, monocytes, and other cells. These cytokines influence APP production in hepatocytes, and IL-6 is the major inducer of APP. In neonatal sepsis, CRP, serum amyloid A (SAA), and procalcitonin (PCT) are most extensively studied.

C-Reactive Protein

C-reactive protein (CRP) is a nonspecific APP that binds to phosphocholine on microorganisms. It is postulated that CRP assists in enhancing phagocytosis by macrophages and in complement binding of damaged cells. It also plays an important role in innate immunity. CRP is widely used in neonatal intensive care units (NICUs) for monitoring treatment in LOS. CRP concentrations usually are not elevated at the time of clinical presentation, but delayed elevation occurs 8 to 10 hours after the onset of symptoms. CRP has a half-life of 19 hours, which may increase exponentially during an acute phase response. Several studies have shown its high specificity in neonatal sepsis. The range of sensitivity for EOS is 43% to 90%, and ranges of specificity for EOS and LOS are 70% to 78% and 93% to 100%, respectively.[37] Serial measurements of CRP concentrations are useful in ruling out sepsis and can help clinicians in deciding to discontinue antibiotic treatment in equivocal cases when levels are normal for 48 hours.[38] CRP levels usually are elevated after surgery, following recent immunizations, and in gastroschisis, which may limit its use in those conditions.[5,39] Other markers including serum amyloid-A and procalcitonin are more accurate in predicting neonatal sepsis especially in LOS, however, CRP continues to be used in NICUs. There is no established standard of practice for the use of CRP in neonates. Some authors use it as a screening tool to rule out the presence of sepsis while others support using serial CRP levels as an early diagnostic tool for confirming the presence of sepsis, some authors use CRP to monitor response to therapy and to guide duration of antibiotic use and others do not use it at all. CRP may be beneficial as a biomarker in clinically stable neonates.

Serum Amyloid A

Serum amyloid A (SAA) is another APP that has been investigated recently. It plays an important role in the inflammatory process and can stimulate the secretion of IL-8 from neutrophils. Arnon and colleagues evaluated the use of SAA in the detection of EOS. SAA levels in the sepsis group were significantly higher than in the nonseptic group at 0, 24, and 48 hours. In comparison with CRP, SAA levels increased earlier, reached higher levels, and returned more rapidly to normal values in infants with EOS. At the onset of sepsis, SAA had greater sensitivity (96% vs. 30%), specificity (95% vs. 98%), positive predictive value (85% vs. 78%), and negative predictive value (99% vs. 83%) when compared with CRP.[25] The same team of investigators studied SAA, CRP, and IL-6, along with clinical variables, in neonates with LOS and found similar results as for EOS. SAA at 10 µg/mL had the highest sensitivity at 0, 8, and 24 hours (95%, 100%, and 97%, respectively) after sepsis, as well as the greatest negative predictive value (97%, 100%, and 98%, respectively). Mortality in septic neonates was inversely correlated with SAA at 8 and 24 hours.[40] These studies suggest that SAA may be a better marker than CRP, especially during the early phase of infection.

Procalcitonin

Procalcitonin (PCT) is a peptide precursor of the hormone calcitonin. The level of PCT increases in response to a pro-inflammatory stimulus, especially of bacterial origin. The high PCT levels produced during infection are not followed by a parallel increase in calcitonin or serum calcium levels. A physiologic increase in PCT levels is noted during the first 2 days of life; this could be due to bacterial colonization of the gastrointestinal tract and translocation of endotoxin through the bowel wall. This physiologic increase is minor in comparison with that seen in bacterial infection. Further, noninfective perinatal events such as perinatal asphyxia, maternal pre-eclampsia, and intracranial hemorrhage may increase PCT concentrations.[41] A recent meta-analysis of 22 studies evaluated PCT for the diagnosis of EOS and LOS at different time points (birth, 0 to 12 hours, 12 to 24 hours, and 24 to 48 hours); all showed moderate accuracy ($Q^* = 0.79$, 0.86, 0.81, 0.82, and 0.77, respectively). PCT was more accurate than CRP for the diagnosis of LOS.[42]

Lipopolysaccharide-Binding Protein

Lipopolysaccharide-binding protein (LBP) is an APP similar to CRP and SAA; it is produced mainly by the liver. It binds to the lipopolysaccharide of bacteria to form a complex that interacts with the macrophage receptor and initiates the pro-inflammatory host response. After exposure to endotoxin, proinflammatory cytokines such as IL-6 peak 2-3 hours after exposure and decrease to normal values after 4-6 hours. CRP levels begin to rise 12-24 hours after exposure. Behrendt and colleagues argued that LBP may be able to fill a "diagnostic gap" between these biomarkers. LBP concentrations were markedly increased in preterm infants with EOS (median, 20 µg/mL) versus those without (median, 4.2 µg/mL). Further, LBP concentrations of preterm infants were comparable with those of term infants, and no significant effect of labor on LBP concentrations was observed.[43] In another study, serum LBP, LPS and soluble CD14, CRP, and PCT were measured on 2 consecutive days in critically ill neonates and children with and without sepsis. LBP concentration on the first day of suspected sepsis was a better marker than LPS, soluble CD14 (sCD14), PCT, and CRP in neonates younger than 48 hours and in children.[44]

Inter-Alpha Inhibitor Protein

Inter-alpha inhibitor proteins (IαIps) are a structurally related family of serine protease inhibitors found in human plasma. They are involved in many biologic activities, including inflammation, wound healing, and extracellular matrix stabilization. They also play important anti-inflammatory and regulatory roles in infection. Blood

IαIp levels in neonates, regardless of gestational age, were similar to those in adults.[45] Levels of IαIp were significantly lower in neonates with culture proven and suspected sepsis (121 μg/mL) than in nonseptic neonates (322 μg/mL). Sensitivity was 89.5%, specificity 99%, positive predictive value 95%, and negative predictive value 98%.[27]

Other Biomarkers

Thrombopoietin

Thrombocytopenia frequently occurs in septic neonates. Postulated mechanisms include increased platelet consumption, decreased platelet production, or a combination of the two. Platelet production is regulated by hematopoietic cytokines, including thrombopoietin (Tpo), IL-3, and IL-6, which act on the megakaryocyte, stimulating its proliferation and differentiation. In a recent study by Brown and colleagues, Tpo, circulating megakaryocyte progenitor concentrations (CMPs), and reticulated platelets were evaluated in septic neonates and neonates with NEC. Septic neonates had significantly elevated Tpo and CMP concentrations. The highest levels were associated with Gram-negative and presumed sepsis.[46]

Selectins

During inflammation, local release of IL-1 and TNF from damaged cells induces overexpression of selectins from endothelial cells (E- and P-selectins) and platelets (P-selectin) of nearby blood vessels. E- and P-selectins are components of an adhesion cascade that leads to leukocyte and platelet accumulation at sites of inflammation and injury. Elevations in serum and platelet P-selectin levels have been demonstrated in adult sepsis and septic shock, and in platelets in group B *Streptococcus* sepsis.[47] However, only elevated levels of E-selectin have been documented in neonatal sepsis.[48]

Neutrophil Elastase

In part as a result of E-selectin elevation, recruitment of neutrophils is another early component of the host response to infection. Neutrophil elastase (NE) is a major serine proteinase secreted by activated or damaged neutrophils. The intracellular function of this enzyme is the degradation of foreign microorganisms that are phagocytosed by the neutrophil. NE is emptied into the extracellular space, where it can also inactivate bacteria. Secretion of NE upregulates the expression of IL-6, IL-8, G-CSF, and transforming growth factor (TGF)-β, while promoting the degradation of IL-1 and IL-2. Several studies have documented NE as a potentially useful biomarker for neonatal sepsis.[49]

Adhesion Molecules

Intracellular adhesion molecule-1 (ICAM-1) and vascular adhesion molecule-1 (VCAM-1) are present in low concentrations in leukocyte and endothelial cell membranes. Upon cytokine stimulation (mainly IL-1 and TNF), the concentrations of ICAM-1 and VCAM-1 increase markedly. ICAM-1 is a ligand for integrin, a receptor found on leukocytes. When activated, leukocytes bind to endothelial cells via ICAM-1/integrin and VCAM-1/intergrin and then transmigrate into tissues. Concentrations of ICAM-1 and VCAM-1 were markedly elevated in septic neonates, regardless of their gestational age, but CRP levels were still normal. ICAM-1 levels increased in neonates with positive blood cultures and suspected sepsis; levels greater than 274 mg/mL correlated with positive blood cultures. VCAM-1 levels increased only slightly in culture proven sepsis.[50]

Microarray Assays

Individual biomarkers may lack adequate positive or negative predictive value. A combination of several biomarkers can enhance diagnostic accuracy in neonatal sepsis. Microarray assays and bead flow cytometry are newer technologies that allow identification of more than 100 analytes in a small sample volume. Kingsmore and colleagues used microarray assays to identify 142 serum proteins in clinically infected and noninfected neonates. P- and E-selectins, IL-2 soluble receptor alpha, IL-18, neutrophil elastase, urokinase plasminogen activator, and CRP were significantly altered in infected subjects.[51] Our investigative group used bead flow cytometry to measure 90 different biomarkers in infected (late-onset sepsis) and noninfected neonates at less than 32 weeks' gestation. Clinical and biomarker data were analyzed, and an algorithm was generated using data mining and machine-based learning software. The results identified markers that have been evaluated for infection in neonates, including CCL4, IL-1ra, IL-18, and Tpo. Other markers that have not been evaluated previously for neonatal sepsis, such as IL-15, plasminogen-activator inhibitor-1, and alpha-fetoprotein, appeared to be promising as potential markers.

Proteomics

Proteomics is the study of expressed proteins. It is more complicated than DNA-RNA–based technologies, largely owing to the fact that the proteome differs from cell to cell and is time dependent, but an organism's genome is constant. Proteomics is much more clinically relevant and easier to translate into diagnostic and therapeutic strategies. Recent advances in proteomic profiling such as surface-enhanced laser desorption/ionization have been used to identify host response proteins as markers for diagnosing a wide array of pathologic conditions such as intra-amniotic inflammation and neonatal sepsis.[52] A recent case-control study by Ng and colleagues used a proteomic approach to identify biomarkers for diagnosis of LOS and NEC in preterm infants. Plasma samples were collected at clinical presentation and were assessed for biomarker discovery and then were independently validated. Pro-apolipoprotein CII (Pro-apoC2) and a des-arginine variant of SAA were identified as potentially useful markers.[53] Biomarkers of all types have been used by generations of scientists, physicians, and researchers to study human disease. Several points should be considered before using biomarkers in clinical studies. Advantages of biomarkers include precision of measurement, objective assessment, and reliability as validity can be established. Disadvangates include timing, cost of analyses, storage, laboratory errors. Also, sometimes normal ranges are difficult to establish.

To date, no single biomarker or set of biomarkers has sufficient sensitivity and specificity to enable neonatologists to confidently withhold antimicrobial treatment of a sick neonate with suspected sepsis. The use of reliable biomarkers such as IL-6, IL-8, CD11b, and CD64, singly or in combination with an acute phase protein, would help clinicians in deciding whether to stop antimicrobial treatment early in noninfected neonates. It is unlikely that a single biomarker would possess all the aforementioned characteristics of the "ideal biomarker". The use of clinical signs in addition to panels of biomarkers customized for neonates will improve sensitivity and specificity and may ultimately provide a specific biosignature for infectious agents unique to the neonatal population.

References

1. Stoll B, Hansen N, Fanaroff A, et al. Late-onset sepsis in very low birth weight neonates: The experience of the NICHD Neonatal Research Network. *Pediatrics.* 2002;110:285-291.
2. Clark R, Bloom B, Spitzer A, et al. Empiric use of ampicillin and cefotaxime, compared with ampicillin and gentamicin, for neonates at risk for sepsis is associated with an increased risk of neonatal death. *Pediatrics.* 2006;117:67-74.
3. Dalgic N, Ergenekon E, Koc E, et al. NOSEP and clinical scores for nosocomial sepsis in a neonatal intensive care unit. *J Trop Pediatr.* 2006;52:226-227.
4. Griffin MP, Lake DE, Bissonette EA, et al. Heart rate characteristics: Novel physiomarkers to predict neonatal infection and death. *Pediatrics.* 2005;116:1070-1074.
5. Ng PC. Diagnostic markers of infection in neonates. *Arch Dis Child Fetal Neonatal Ed.* 2004;89: F229-F235.
6. Commins SP, Borish L, Steinke JW. Immunologic messenger molecules: Cytokines, interferons, and chemokines. *J Allergy Clin Immunol.* 2010;125:S53-S72.
7. Ng PC, Cheng SH, Chui KM, et al. Diagnosis of late onset neonatal sepsis with cytokines, adhesion molecule, and C-reactive protein in preterm very low birthweight infants. *Arch Dis Child Fetal Neonatal Ed.* 1997;77:F221-F227.

18

18

8. Mehr S, Doyle LW. Cytokines as markers of bacterial sepsis in newborn infants: A review. *Pediatr Infect Dis J.* 2000;19:879-887.

9. D'Alquen D, Kramer BW, Seidenspinner S, et al. Activation of umbilical cord endothelial cells and fetal inflammatory response in preterm infants with chorioamnionitis and funisitis. *Pediatr Res.* 2005;57:263-269.

10. Ng PC, Lam HS. Diagnostic markers for neonatal sepsis. *Curr Opin Pediatr.* 2006;18:125-131.

11. Oguz SS, Sipahi E, Dilmen U. C-reactive protein and interleukin-6 responses for differentiating fungal and bacterial aetiology in late-onset neonatal sepsis. *Mycoses.* 2011;54:212-216.

12. Romagnoli C, Frezza S, Cingolani A, et al. Plasma levels of interleukin-6 and interleukin-10 in preterm neonates evaluated for sepsis. *Eur J Pediatr.* 2001;160:345-350.

13. Ng PC, Li K, Leung TF, et al. Early prediction of sepsis-induced disseminated intravascular coagulation with interleukin-10, interleukin-6, and RANTES in preterm infants. *Clin Chem.* 2006;52:1181-1189.

14. Sherwin C, Broadbent R, Young S, et al. Utility of interleukin-12 and interleukin-10 in comparison with other cytokines and acute-phase reactants in the diagnosis of neonatal sepsis. *Am J Perinatol.* 2008;25:629-636.

15. Ucar B, Yildiz B, Aksit MA, et al. Serum amyloid A, procalcitonin, tumor necrosis factor-alpha, and interleukin-1beta levels in neonatal late-onset sepsis. *Mediators Inflamm.* 2008;2008:737141.

16. Kuster H, Weiss M, Willeitner AE, et al. Interleukin-1 receptor antagonist and interleukin-6 for early diagnosis of neonatal sepsis 2 days before clinical manifestation. *Lancet.* 1998;352:1271-1277.

17. Kennon C, Overturf G, Bessman S, et al. Granulocyte colony-stimulating factor as a marker for bacterial infection in neonates. *J Pediatr.* 1996;128:765-769.

18. Nowak JE, Wheeler DS, Harmon KK, et al. Admission chemokine (C-C motif) ligand 4 levels predict survival in pediatric septic shock. *Pediatr Crit Care Med.* 2010;11:213-216.

19. Krolak-Olejnik B, Beck B, Olejnik I. Umbilical serum concentrations of chemokines (RANTES and MGSA/GRO-alpha) in preterm and term neonates. *Pediatr Int.* 2006;48:586-590.

20. Shouman B, Badr R. Regulated on activation, normal T cell expressed and secreted and tumor necrosis factor-alpha in septic neonates. *J Perinatol.* 2009;30:192-196.

21. Orlikowsky TW, Neunhoeffer F, Goelz R, et al. Evaluation of IL-8-concentrations in plasma and lysed EDTA-blood in healthy neonates and those with suspected early onset bacterial infection. *Pediatr Res.* 2004;56:804-809.

22. Bentlin MR, de Souza Rugolo LM, Junior AR, et al. Is urine interleukin-8 level a reliable laboratory test for diagnosing late onset sepsis in premature infants? *J Trop Pediatr.* 2007;53:403-408.

23. Ng PC, Li K, Chui KM, et al. IP-10 is an early diagnostic marker for identification of late-onset bacterial infection in preterm infants. *Pediatr Res.* 2007;61:93-98.

24. Turunen R, Andersson S, Nupponen I, et al. Increased CD11b-density on circulating phagocytes as an early sign of late-onset sepsis in extremely low-birth-weight infants. *Pediatr Res.* 2005;57:270-275.

25. Arnon S, Litmanovitz I, Regev RH, et al. Serum amyloid A: An early and accurate marker of neonatal early-onset sepsis. *J Perinatol.* 2007;27:297-302.

26. Chiesa C, Panero A, Rossi N, et al. Reliability of procalcitonin concentrations for the diagnosis of sepsis in critically ill neonates. *Clin Infect Dis.* 1998;26:664-672.

27. Chaaban H, Singh K, Huang J, et al. The role of inter-alpha inhibitor proteins in the diagnosis of neonatal sepsis. *J Pediatr.* 2009;154:620-622.

28. Fotopoulos S, Mouchtouri A, Xanthou G, et al. Inflammatory chemokine expression in the peripheral blood of neonates with perinatal asphyxia and perinatal or nosocomial infections. *Acta Paediatr.* 2005;94:800-806.

29. Franz AR, Bauer K, Schalk A, et al. Measurement of interleukin 8 in combination with C-reactive protein reduced unnecessary antibiotic therapy in newborn infants: A multicenter, randomized, controlled trial. *Pediatrics.* 2004;114:1-8.

30. Bhandari V, Wang C, Rinder C, et al. Hematologic profile of sepsis in neonates: Neutrophil CD64 as a diagnostic marker. *Pediatrics.* 2008;121:129-134.

31. Ng PC, Li G, Chui KM, et al. Neutrophil CD64 is a sensitive diagnostic marker for early-onset neonatal infection. *Pediatr Res.* 2004;56:796-803.

32. Hallwirth U, Pomberger G, Pollak A, et al. Monocyte switch in neonates: high phagocytic capacity and low HLA-DR expression in VLBWI are inverted during gestational aging. *Pediatr Allergy Immunol.* 2004;15:513-516.

33. Genel F, Atlihan F, Ozsu E, et al. Monocyte HLA-DR expression as predictor of poor outcome in neonates with late onset neonatal sepsis. *J Infect.* 2010;60:224-228.

34. Ng PC, Li G, Chui KM, et al. Quantitative measurement of monocyte HLA-DR expression in the identification of early-onset neonatal infection. *Biol Neonate.* 2006;89:75-81.

35. Hodge G, Hodge S, Han P, et al. Multiple leucocyte activation markers to detect neonatal infection. *Clin Exp Immunol.* 2004;135:125-129.

36. Weinschenk NP, Farina A, Bianchi DW. Premature infants respond to early-onset and late-onset sepsis with leukocyte activation. *J Pediatr.* 2000;137:345-350.

37. Mishra UK, Jacobs SE, Doyle LW, et al. Newer approaches to the diagnosis of early onset neonatal sepsis. *Arch Dis Child Fetal Neonatal Ed.* 2006;91:F208-F212.

38. Polin RA. The "ins and outs" of neonatal sepsis. *J Pediatr.* 2003;143:3-4.

39. Ramadan G, Rex D, Okoye B, et al. Early high C-reactive protein in infants with open abdominal wall defects does not predict sepsis or adverse outcome. *Acta Paediatr.* 2010;99:126-130.

40. Arnon S, Litmanovitz I, Regev R, et al. The prognostic virtue of inflammatory markers during late-onset sepsis in preterm infants. *J Perinat Med*. 2004;32:176-180.
41. Turner D, Hammerman C, Rudensky B, et al. Procalcitonin in preterm infants during the first few days of life: Introducing an age related nomogram. *Arch Dis Child Fetal Neonatal Ed*. 2006;91: F283-F286.
42. Yu Z, Liu J, Sun Q, et al. The accuracy of the procalcitonin test for the diagnosis of neonatal sepsis: A meta-analysis. *Scand J Infect Dis*. 2010;42:723-733.
43. Behrendt D, Dembinski J, Heep A, et al. Lipopolysaccharide binding protein in preterm infants. *Arch Dis Child Fetal Neonatal Ed*. 2004;89:F551-F554.
44. Pavcnik-Arnol M, Hojker S, Derganc M. Lipopolysaccharide-binding protein, lipopolysaccharide, and soluble CD14 in sepsis of critically ill neonates and children. *Intensive Care Med*. 2007;33: 1025-1032.
45. Baek YW, Brokat S, Padbury JF, et al. Inter-alpha inhibitor proteins in infants and decreased levels in neonatal sepsis. *J Pediatr*. 2003;143:11-15.
46. Brown RE, Rimsza LM, Pastos K, et al. Effects of sepsis on neonatal thrombopoiesis. *Pediatr Res*. 2008;64:399-404.
47. Siauw C, Kobsar A, Dornieden C, et al. Group B streptococcus isolates from septic patients and healthy carriers differentially activate platelet signaling cascades. *Thromb Haemost*. 2006;95: 836-849.
48. Edgar JD, Gabriel V, Gallimore JR, et al. A prospective study of the sensitivity, specificity and diagnostic performance of soluble intercellular adhesion molecule 1, highly sensitive C-reactive protein, soluble E-selectin and serum amyloid A in the diagnosis of neonatal infection. *BMC Pediatr*. 2010;10:22.
49. Laskowska-Klita T, Czerwiska B, Maj-Pucek M. [Neutrophil elastase level in cord blood and diagnosis of infection in mature and premature neonates]. *Med Wieku Rozwoj*. 2002;6:13-21.
50. Figueras-Aloy J, Gomez-Lopez L, Rodriguez-Miguelez JM, et al. Serum soluble ICAM-1, VCAM-1, L-selectin, and P-selectin levels as markers of infection and their relation to clinical severity in neonatal sepsis. *Am J Perinatol*. 2007;24:331-338.
51. Kingsmore SF, Kennedy N, Halliday HL, et al. Identification of diagnostic biomarkers for infection in premature neonates. *Mol Cell Proteomics*. 2008;7:1863-1875.
52. Buhimschi CS, Bhandari V, Han YW, et al. Using proteomics in perinatal and neonatal sepsis: Hopes and challenges for the future. *Curr Opin Infect Dis*. 2009;22:235-243.
53. Ng PC, Ang IL, Chiu RW, et al. Host-response biomarkers for diagnosis of late-onset septicemia and necrotizing enterocolitis in preterm infants. *J Clin Invest*. 2010;120:2989-3000.

18

CHAPTER 19

Chorioamnionitis and Its Effects on the Fetus/Neonate: Emerging Issues and Controversies

Irina A. Buhimschi, MD, MMS, and Catalin S. Buhimschi, MD

- Introduction
- Controversies in Definition of Chorioamnionitis
- Emerging Evidence Linking Chorioamnionitis With Antenatal Fetal Injury
- Controversies in Determination of Neonatal Encephalopathy: Early-Onset Neonatal Sepsis vs. Antenatal and Intrapartum Hypoxia
- Intra-amniotic Infection/Inflammation and Systems Biology

The term *chorioamnionitis* was originally coined to depict "fever during labor." This concept centered on the premise that vaginal organisms ascend into the uterine cavity and trigger an inflammatory response. Hence, the concept of *clinical chorioamnionitis* included a wide variety of clinical manifestations such as maternal fever, uterine tenderness, and fetal tachycardia. As our understanding of infectious and inflammatory processes continued to improve, inherited limitations in the concept of chorioamnionitis began to emerge. Today, we know that a clear distinction should be made between clinical and histologic chorioamnionitis. That said, only a minor fraction of women exhibiting inflammatory changes in the fetal membranes or placenta exhibit symptoms of overt infection, including fever. In addition, a difference should be made between the notion of intra-amniotic infection and inflammation because not all intrauterine inflammatory processes are caused by microorganisms, and vice versa. Despite the silent course of most cases, intra-amniotic infection and/or inflammation is a pathologic process linked closely to preterm birth, which also raises considerably the risk for early-onset neonatal sepsis (EONS). Whether delivery occurs at term or before term, poor neurodevelopmental outcome is often encountered as a sequela of a pregnancy complicated by chorioamnionitis. By acting synergistically with prematurity, exposure of the fetus to intra-amniotic inflammation increases the risk for adverse neonatal outcomes, including intraventricular hemorrhage and cerebral palsy. Conversely, evidence suggests that chorioamnionitis may have a positive effect on lung maturation and on acceleration of surfactant production. However, the molecular mechanisms underlying the divergent effects of antenatal exposure to infection and/or inflammation on various fetal organ systems remain incompletely understood.

Similar to preterm birth, fetal injury should be viewed as a syndrome of many causes. Owing to common postnatal manifestations and overlapping pathogenic pathways, it is often difficult to identify the initiating trigger. For many reasons, it is critical to discriminate between insult inflicted by antenatal exposure of the fetus to infection/inflammation or to hypoxia. Therefore discovery of clinically and biologically relevant diagnostic markers able to identify pregnancies at risk for antenatal fetal damage remains a priority. These biomarkers should provide a clear image of the precise pathogenic process and molecular targets involved in each case of fetal injury. Elucidation of these events should permit prevention of human long-term disability and prioritization of health care resources at the societal level.

19

Introduction

Over the past three decades, interest has increased in fetal inflammation as an adaptive response triggered by infection. Accumulating evidence made us conclude that fetal inflammation plays a central role in maintenance of cellular homeostasis, although both an exaggerated response and lack of response to a microbial attack may lead to severe tissue damage. Implicitly, considerable progress has been made in our understanding of the process of chorioamnionitis as a determinant of neonatal outcome. However, controversies continue as to why and how the fetus becomes infected in the first place. The burden of discerning between fetal consequences secondary to an infection acquired in the antenatal versus intrapartum or postnatal period persists today as much as in 1961, when William Blanc published in the pages of *The Journal of Pediatrics* his manuscript entitled, "Pathways of Fetal and Early Neonatal Infection: Viral Placentitis, Bacterial and Fungal Chorioamnionitis."[1] At that time, a significant body of observational research had already accumulated to suggest that infection of the amniotic fluid, placenta, and fetal membranes can potentially extend to the fetus, causing sepsis in the absence of a maternal inflammatory response.[2-5] This work was published in journals geared primarily toward pediatricians and neonatologists. From this perspective, it is interesting to note that the 12th edition of *Williams Obstetrics,* which also appeared in 1961, does not include chorioamnionitis among its indexed subjects. It was not until the 18th edition of *Williams Obstetrics,* published in 1989, that the notion of chorioamnionitis was given proper consideration in relationship to intrauterine infection and preterm birth.[6]

Advances in immunology accelerated research progress in the field. As a consequence, the links among exposure of the fetus to infection, particularities of the inflammatory host response and downstream processes involved in preterm labor, preterm premature rupture of membranes (PPROM), and damage to fetal vital organs began to be increasingly clear. Given that the topic of chorioamnionitis has been extensively reviewed,[7-9] the aim of this chapter is not to recapitulate well-established facts. Herein, we will focus on a number of issues that have emerged recently with respect to the mechanisms through which chorioamnionitis damages the fetus, as well as issues that remain controversial and for which specific emphasis is needed at this time.

The term *chorioamnionitis* denotes infection and/or inflammation of the amniotic fluid, placenta, fetal membranes, and decidua. Particularities of this inflammatory process with respect to causative agents (often fastidious) and differential immune responses in the fetal versus the maternal compartment have created a level of challenge difficult to surpass using conventional approaches. Thus arose the need for and an opportunity to apply novel approaches such as high-throughput "-omics" discovery and systems biology to this topic. New strategies for diagnosis/treatment of affected pregnancies may improve neonatal outcomes.

Controversies in Definition of Chorioamnionitis

Bacterial Colonization Versus Infection

The first distinction that needs to be made is between colonization and infection. Because amniotic fluid is thought to be normally sterile, identification of microorganisms is implicitly considered evidence of infection (i.e., the pathogen invades the host tissues and causes signs and symptoms of illness). Colonization (i.e., a pathogen grows in the host without causing signs or symptoms of illness) may, on the other hand, occur normally in both placenta and fetal membranes. One study comparing the microbial and inflammatory status of the amniotic fluid with that of the placenta found high levels of colonization and bacterial contamination of fetal membranes and villous tissues.[10] From a clinical perspective, these observations bring a high level of complexity and uneasiness for correct interpretation of microbial test results gathered from the placenta after birth. Moreover, a high frequency of acute histologic inflammation was noted in patients with negative amniotic fluid cultures and absent intra-amniotic inflammation.[10] Although colonization would indicate the presence of bacteria without pathologic consequences, tissue contamination could be the result of factors related to amniocentesis, delivery, or the procedure applied for tissue collection. In the group of women with negative amniotic fluid microbial cultures, cesarean section seemed to be protective against a positive placental culture result. Overall, these observations lend support to the concept that a low level of bacterial colonization of the membranes or placenta exists, but that changes in the maternal, fetal, or intra-amniotic milieu facilitate conversion of colonization to pathologic infection.[10]

Although biologic compartments that are considered physiologically sterile may be intermittently colonized by bacteria, infection usually is precluded through a competent innate immune response. For example, bacterial DNA can be detected occasionally in the blood of healthy individuals with no clinical signs of infection.[11] The existence of this phenomenon was not necessarily proven for the amniotic fluid cavity, given the difficulties and ethical aspects involved in obtaining samples in a serial fashion. However, evidence suggests that in the second trimester, *Mycoplasma* spp. may reside silently in the gestational sac in the absence of clinical signs or symptoms of chorioamnionitis or of adverse perinatal outcomes.[12] Increasingly, colonization of the gestational sac by bacteria appears to be a likely possibility, although natural antimicrobials present in the fetal membranes and amniotic fluid seem to prevent development of an inflammatory reaction and even eradicate the infection.[13-15]

Intra-amniotic Infection, Intra-amniotic Inflammation, and Chorioamnionitis As Nonoverlapping Entities

As mentioned previously, a clear distinction should be established between intra-amniotic infection, inflammation, and the generalized term *chorioamnionitis*. Many publications use these terms interchangeably, which is arguably incorrect. Not all instances of intra-amniotic inflammation are caused by infection, and not all cases in which bacteria or bacterial footprints are detected in the amniotic cavity manifest clinical chorioamnionitis and/or significant neutrophil infiltration in reproductive tissues (histologic chorioamnionitis). Figure 19-1 presents a schematic view of the nonoverlapping nature of these entities.

Decidual bleeding (abruption) is an important cause of intra-amniotic inflammation in the absence of an infectious trigger.[16,17] Free hemoglobin, thrombin, globin-centered radicals, free iron, and bilirubin oxidation products can initiate/amplify inflammatory cytokine responses.[18,19] Cytokines such as interleukin (IL)-1β and IL-6 enhance the expression of leukocyte interactive proteins such as P-selectin, E-selectin, vascular adhesion molecule-1 (VCAM-1), and intracellular adhesion molecule-1 (ICAM-1) on the decidual vascular surface, causing vascular injury and neutrophil infiltration. This process facilitates access of diverse coagulation factors to the perivascular adventitial tissue factor, known as one of the most potent initiators of aberrant coagulation.[17,20] Specifically, the coagulation pathway is activated when circulating factor VII (FVII) gains access to decidual tissue factor and generates thrombin.[21] Release of free hemoglobin at the decidual level inactivates nitric oxide, leading to vasoconstriction and vasospasm.[19] In turn, these processes induce tissue hypoxia and reperfusion, further worsening the injury.[17] Collectively, all of this provides powerful evidence that inflammation shifts the decidual hemostatic mechanisms in favor of thrombosis.[22]

When zooming in on the process of infection-induced inflammation, it is important to recognize that the emergence of culture-independent methods of microbial identification adds a new layer of complexity to the distinction between colonization and infection. The cornerstone of culture-independent detection has been the use of the 16S rRNA gene sequence to identify and differentiate microbial species, and to determine the phylogenetic relationships between microorganisms.[23] The 16S rRNA genes, which usually are approximately 1500 bp in length, are highly conserved among bacterial and archaeal species, yet they are sufficiently diverse to allow differentiation among bacteria. Application of this technique led to the striking realization that cultivated organisms represented only a tiny fraction of species (<1%) in the environment.[24] In particular, several studies demonstrated that commonly

19

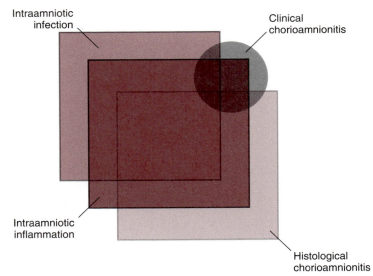

Figure 19-1 Venn diagram illustrating the nonoverlapping nature of several notions often collectively labeled as *chorioamnionitis*. Intra-amniotic infection is diagnosed by the presence of microorganisms in the amniotic cavity. Lack of a confining black border illustrates that the limits of this entity are technique dependent and are currently unknown. *Intra-amniotic inflammation* is defined as the presence of polymorphonucleated neutrophils (PMNs) in amniotic fluid above a relative cutoff, which itself is a subject of discussion. *Histologic chorioamnionitis* is defined as the presence of PMNs in the chorionic plate and/or fetal membranes. The numeric cutoff and tissue localization are also subjects of discussion. *Clinical chorioamnionitis*, which is the smallest entity, is defined as the presence of maternal fever, maternal or fetal tachycardia, uterine tenderness, and/or malodorous vaginal discharge.

used culturing methods are unable to detect the "true" prevalence of intra-amniotic infection. This may explain the commonly encountered discrepancies between the results of amniotic fluid culture and the presence of intra-amniotic inflammation.[25-30] A collaborative study from our group determined that as many as 60% of the organisms associated with intra-amniotic infection are uncultivated or difficult-to-cultivate bacteria.[30] Phylogenetic classification of the amniotic fluid species associated with intra-amniotic inflammation found that the most prevalent taxa were *Fusobacterium nucleatum* followed by *Shigella* spp. and *Leptotrichia* spp. *Fusobacterium nucleatum*, a Gram-negative anaerobe, is an opportunistic oral pathogen.[31] Intrauterine *F. nucleatum* has been suspected to originate from the oral cavity, where the species is ubiquitous.[32] It was previously proposed that after transient bacteremia, oral *F. nucleatum* translocates to the pregnant uterus and possibly to the fetus via the hematogenous route.[31] Animal studies in which hematogenous injection of orally related *F. nucleatum* resulted in its preferential localization to placental blood vessels, from which it crossed the endothelium to finally spread to the amniotic cavity, provide support for this hypothesis.

Although noninfectious triggers and uncultivated bacteria potentially explain why intra-amniotic inflammation is often identified in the absence of a positive Gram stain or microbial culture result, the reverse situation is also encountered. In such instances, bacterial invasion of the amniotic fluid is diagnosed at the time of the amniocentesis in the presence of only minimal or absent inflammation. In such clinical circumstances, histologic examination of the placenta or the umbilical cord for funisitis fails to reveal the expected inflammatory reaction. Although one may argue in favor of artifactual contamination of the amniotic fluid specimen, biologic explanations are possible. First, it is possible that sampling of the amniotic fluid occurred at a very incipient phase during the inflammatory response, and given the decision to induce delivery, no time remained for neutrophil recruitment. Second, intra-amniotic infection and inflammation are chronic processes that do not vary linearly from each other. Third, most of the neutrophils in the amniotic cavity are of fetal origin.[33] Thus intra-amniotic inflammation mostly reflects the fetal innate immune response, which varies remarkably from that of the adult, especially in premature fetuses. Inability of the premature fetus to mount a robust inflammatory response could serve as a reasonable explanation of why bacteria are present in the amniotic fluid in the absence of inflammation.

Unlike newborn sepsis, where in the immediate postnatal period progression to septic shock occurs rapidly with cardiovascular, respiratory, hepatic, and renal organ dysfunction, the clinical equivalents of fetal septic syndrome have been only minimally studied.[34-36] Still, it is agreed that a fetal systemic inflammatory response to infection could be characterized by bradycardia and neutropenia at birth.[37,38] If bradycardia would manifest antenatally as a nonreassuring fetal heart rate pattern, the equivalent of neutropenia resulting from bone marrow exhaustion would translate into a low amniotic fluid white blood cell count in the context of an infected amniocentesis specimen. It is known that the ability of neonatal granulocytes to degrade intracellularly phagocytosed bacteria and foreign particles is deficient compared with that of adult cells. If these qualitative deficiencies are extrapolated to the antenatal life, they may explain the excessive destruction of fetal neutrophils by bacteria, which is often encountered in infected amniotic fluid.[25] Last, dissemination of bacteria from the mother to the fetus via the hematogenous route may bypass the amniotic cavity and elicit a disproportionately low level of intra-amniotic inflammatory response compared with that of the fetus.[34] All of these scenarios underscore the complex nature of the interaction between microorganisms, amniotic cavity, and fetus, and the importance of keeping a clear distinction between infection and inflammation.

Clinical vs. Histologic Chorioamnionitis

Clinical chorioamnionitis is diagnosed in the presence of maternal fever, leukocytosis, tachycardia, uterine tenderness, and foul odor of the amniotic fluid. These clinical manifestations were described when the medical diagnosis relied solely on maternal signs and symptoms of the disease. Clinical chorioamnionitis occurs in 0.5% to 1% of all pregnancies.[39] With inclusion of amniocentesis as part of the clinical management of preterm labor, it became apparent that intra-amniotic infection is more frequently encountered. In 1974, Bobitt and Ledger performed quantitative cultures of amniotic fluid and were able to isolate bacteria in more than half of their subjects.[40] This was powerful evidence that unrecognized intrauterine infection might contribute to prematurity and neonatal sepsis. In a subsequent study, the same group concluded that fever occurs late in the natural progression of the intra-amniotic infectious process and is frequently absent in patients delivering preterm infants despite a positive bacterial culture.[41] The authors concluded by raising several important questions: "Should abdominal amniocentesis be performed in selected cases of idiopathic preterm labor? If bacterial contamination is recognized, what is the appropriate management—prompt delivery with antibiotic coverage or the use of antibiotics and uterine relaxants? What is the frequency of the problem, and how it is affected by socioeconomic factors?" Unfortunately, the answers to all of these questions remain unknown.

Examination of the placenta has virtually been the first modality to classify pathologically the large range of clinical entities linked to preterm birth and poor neurodevelopmental outcomes (e.g., infection, abruption, hypoxia). Significant focus has been placed on antenatal inflammatory processes.[42-44] The proximity of the placenta to the fetus, its common embryologic origin, and tissue availability for research have all facilitated a significant number of studies that have linked placental inflammatory lesions to short- and long-term neonatal outcomes such as cerebral palsy.[45] The major clinical disadvantage is that pathologic examination of the placenta is available only after birth. As a result, histologic biomarkers are irrelevant for the antenatal period of the affected fetus, because they do not allow initiation of therapies meant to prevent preterm birth or adverse neonatal outcomes. For

19

this reason, their overall usefulness involves postnatal counseling and research purposes.

Pathologic examination of the placenta has limitations inherent to the relatively large subjectivity in interpretation of histologic findings. First, inflammatory lesions responsible for similar outcomes are characterized by a high degree of heterogeneity and poor to moderate intraoperator and interoperator variability.[46] Second, the intricacy and redundancy of biologic processes responsible for cellular and tissue injury might lead to identical pathologic footprints in the context of distinctive triggers. Third, a mild degree of histologic chorioamnionitis may occur after normal labor at term without pathologic consequences for the newborn.[47,48] Thus a rigorous quantitative assessment of the severity of the inflammatory infiltrate is required.

Given previous studies that associated short- and long-term follow-up characteristics with distinct placental lesions,[46,49-52] our laboratory used the results of histologic examination of the placenta (as performed by a perinatal pathologist) as an intermediate outcome variable when evaluating the performance of new diagnostic tests. In keeping with the findings of other investigators, we have confirmed the nonoverlapping nature of histologic and clinical chorioamnionitis.[53-55] A significant proportion of women with histologic chorioamnionitis and/or "severe" intra-amniotic inflammation by a variety of amniotic fluid proteomics biomarkers lacked clinical signs of inflammation. Specifically, the prevalence of histologic chorioamnionitis (stages 1 to 3) in our study population was 64%.[53] Overall, a poor correlation was noted between clinical chorioamnionitis and the presence or severity of histologic chorioamnionitis. Almost 90% of women with histologic chorioamnionitis lacked signs or symptoms of clinical chorioamnionitis. Once again, our findings highlight the limited value of maternal clinical symptoms in predicting histologic inflammation in the placenta.

It is important to note that one of the converging points between intra-amniotic infection and abruption is histologic chorioamnionitis. In a recent study, acute lesions of chorioamnionitis and funisitis were frequently associated with histologic evidence of abruption (e.g., hematoma, fibrin deposition, compressed villi, hemosiderin-laden histiocytes).[56] This is especially important in the context where histologic (but not clinical) chorioamnionitis is a significant predictor of neonatal brain injury.[51]

Emerging Evidence Linking Chorioamnionitis With Antenatal Fetal Injury

Pathophysiologic Significance of Inflammation for the Fetus and the Newborn

Inflammation is a highly orchestrated process designed to guard and ensure the survivability of vertebrate organisms.[57,58] Host defense mechanisms are traditionally grouped into innate and adaptive immune processes. Innate immunity includes the inflammatory reactions of neutrophils and monocytes; adaptive immunity refers to lymphocyte responses that recognize specific microbial antigens. Both innate immunity and adaptive immunity have evolved phylogenetically to clear pathogens and prevent tissue injury by counteracting their damaging effects.[57] When properly controlled, the inflammatory response is beneficial, but when dysregulated, its effect can be detrimental.[59] Infection, bleeding, and trauma are well-recognized instigators of inflammation. For instance, studies derived from humans and from animal models of septic and hemorrhagic shock have shown that infection and bleeding are characterized by the acute release of a variety of inflammatory mediators, which often produce collateral damaging effects.[60,61]

Detection of microorganisms relies on pattern recognition receptors (PRRs), which are involved in microbe internalization by phagocytes (soluble and endocytic PRRs) and/or cell activation (signaling PRRs).[62] The most studied PRRs are Toll-like receptors (TLRs), which mitigate host defenses through engagement of ubiquitous constituents of the bacterial wall, known as pathogen-associated molecular patterns (PAMPs).[63,64] Unfortunately, the discriminatory ability of the innate immune system is imperfect. With respect to pregnancy, inappropriate control of the inflammatory course can lead to preterm birth, tissue damage, and even maternal and fetal death.[64-67] Evidence from humans[68] and from animal models of sepsis[69] suggests that intrauterine inflammation in response to infection may evolve silently. The fetus therefore is adversely affected by host defense mechanisms before the onset of signs and symptoms of preterm birth.[70] In such cases, prematurity is inappropriately cited as the only cause of perinatal mortality or morbidity.[71] This paradigm is supported by evidence that intra-amniotic inflammation superimposed on prematurity can lead to more devastating consequences for the neonate than prematurity alone.[69,72-74]

Strong correlations exist among the level of intrauterine and/or fetal inflammation (as reflected by elevated cytokine levels), histologic chorioamnionitis, and the incidence of perinatal complications, independent of gestational age at delivery.[67,75-78] Inflammatory cells are found in the lungs of neonates born to women with chorioamnionitis.[79] The end result is pneumonitis, which is considered an important contributor to bronchopulmonary dysplasia (BPD).[79] Other studies have established synergistic relationships between intrauterine inflammation and other important adverse neonatal outcomes, including intraventricular hemorrhage, necrotizing enterocolitis, retinopathy of prematurity, periventricular leukomalacia, and neurodevelopmental delays and cerebral palsy.[78,80-82]

A growing body of evidence supports the notion that cerebral palsy is preceded by a robust intra-amniotic inflammatory response.[67,80,83,84] Transfer of neurotoxic cytokines in the fetal systemic circulation is facilitated by inflammation-induced vascular injury, with funisitis being the histologic hallmark of fetal inflammation. Extension of the inflammatory process to the fetal central nervous system is frequently linked to brain injury.[85] The previous assertion is supported by evidence that bacterial endotoxins cause white matter injury in utero.[86] In humans, extremely low birth weight infants with sepsis are more likely to have adverse neurodevelopmental outcomes, and a link among sepsis, brain injury, and adverse outcomes has long been proposed.[87] Our group also demonstrated a link between neonatal sepsis and poor short- and long-term neurodevelopmental outcomes.[67] It is interesting to note that in our studies, neurologic damage was encountered even in the context of minimal intra-amniotic inflammation.[67]

Although the mechanisms by which inflammation injures the fetal central nervous system are not as well understood, several premises should be considered. The mechanisms mediating periventricular leukomalacia (PVL) in preterm infants with sepsis are postulated to include injury to pre-oligodendrocytes induced by free radicals (FRs), reactive oxygen species (ROS), and inflammatory cytokines.[87] Injury to endothelial cells induced by similar mechanisms adds to the damage, leading to multisystemic organ dysfunction.[88] In an animal model of inflammation-induced fetal damage, Burd and colleagues observed elevated brain cytokine levels and altered morphology of fetal cortex neurons with decreased microtubule-associated protein 2 (MAP2) staining, as well as decreased numbers of dendrites. If translated to humans, this finding has clinical relevance because dendrite morphology and plasticity likely represent the cellular response to learning and memory.[89] Our results indicate that this neuronal injury does not result from the process of parturition on an immature brain but rather is caused by activation of inflammatory pathways. Taken together, these observations suggest that whereas an adequate innate and adaptive immune response is critical for the survival of mother and child, excessive inflammation and FR/ROS production may lead to poor outcomes in newborns.[90]

Significance of Redox Homeostasis and Implications of Oxidative Stress in Fetal Injury

In all respiring organisms, the univalent reduction of dioxygen to water involves the addition of four electrons that can result in the formation of FR, such as superoxide anion ($O_2^{\bullet-}$) or the hydroxyl ($HO^{\bullet}$) radical, and partially reduced intermediates (nonradical ROS), such as hydrogen peroxide (H_2O_2) or hypochlorous acid (HOCl). Most living organisms have evolved well-integrated antioxidant defense mechanisms that scavenge FR/ROS, including superoxide dismutase (SOD), catalase, glutathione

(GSH) peroxidases, reduced GSH, β-carotene, uric acid, and vitamins C and E. The ratio between FR/ROS (oxidants) and antioxidants is defined as the redox balance.[91] The redox balance is continuously challenged by the external and internal environments and plays an important role in maintaining redox homeostasis. GSH, a tripeptide (γ-glutamyl-cysteinylglycine), is the most abundant intracellular thiol and a potent antioxidant.

FR/ROS is particularly dangerous for the preterm fetus and newborn because of its low antioxidant resources.[69] Deficiencies in SOD, catalase, and GSH peroxidase are reported in the lung tissues of premature infants who die of respiratory distress.[92] Lung levels of these three key antioxidant enzymes are directly proportional to gestational age at birth.[92] Compared with postnatal levels, fetal erythrocytes have lower concentrations of SOD.[93] Furthermore, GSH metabolism is altered in preterm infants who have an absolute GSH deficiency secondary to low levels of cysteine (the precursor amino acid for GSH).[94] These observations have led several authors to suggest that cysteine is an essential amino acid for premature infants.[95] What should be concluded from this is that the fetus, not just the newborn, is at increased risk for redox imbalance.[96-98]

The fetal brain with its high concentration of unsaturated fatty acids, high rate of oxygen consumption, and low concentration of antioxidants is particularly vulnerable to oxidative stress.[99] The pathophysiologic consequences of redox imbalance, irrespective of the initial source of FR/ROS, has particular relevance in perinatal biology because it may explain the common spectrum of neonatal complications in neonates exposed to hypoxia, hyperoxia, or excessive inflammation in utero.[100]

DAMPs and RAGE: "Missing Links" Between Oxidative Stress, Inflammation, and Fetal Cellular Injury

As opposed to PAMPs, which are microbial constituents, damage-associated molecular pattern molecules (DAMPs) are a pleiotropic group of endogenous proteins, which include among others the high-mobility group box-1 (HMGB1), S100 proteins, heat shock proteins, uric acid, and amyloids and altered matrix proteins (fibronectin fragments).[101-103] When released in excess in the extracellular compartment as a result of oxidative stress and cell injury or dysfunction, DAMPs become "danger signals" that activate pattern recognition receptors such as TLRs and the receptor for advanced glycation end-products (RAGE).[104] Most DAMPs have intracellular and extracellular functions. As intracellular molecules, DAMPs have roles in cell homeostasis that serve as chaperones, calcium-binding proteins, or chromatin-stabilizing molecules. Once actively released in the extracellular compartment as a result of loss of cell membrane integrity, they become danger signals.[105] Owing to their similarity to cytokines, these endogenous pro-inflammatory molecules have also been termed *alarmins*.[105] Acting through specialized receptors, including TLR-2, TLR-4, and RAGE, DAMPs recruit inflammatory cells, which in turn modulate the innate immune response and enhance the level of RAGE and TLR activation. An important feature of the RAGE receptor is that its expression is low in normal tissues but increases transcriptionally in environments where RAGE ligands such as DAMPs accumulate, escalating tissue damage in a spiral positive-feedback fashion.[106]

RAGE is a transmembrane receptor, a member of the immunoglobulin superfamily, present on numerous cells such as macrophages, endothelial cells, neurons, and smooth muscle cells.[107,108] RAGE was initially identified by its ability to engage advanced glycation end-products (AGEs). In time it became clear that a wide range of ligands can bind to RAGE, and that RAGE activation is a generalized feature of many chronic inflammatory conditions, including diabetes, rheumatoid arthritis, and arteriosclerosis.[107,109,110,111] The key role of an oxidant environment in fueling RAGE activation has been demonstrated.[112] A number of studies have shown that RAGE signaling is abrogated by an endogenous soluble truncated form of RAGE (soluble RAGE: sRAGE), which acts as a "decoy" by binding RAGE ligands. sRAGE derives from proteolytic cleavage of the membrane-bound RAGE.[113] The stimulus for RAGE shedding seems to involve HMGB1 binding to RAGE and the sheddase ADAM10.[113] Successful binding of a ligand to the extracellular domain of RAGE activates key cell signaling pathways such as nuclear factor (NF)-κB, mitogen-activated protein (MAP) kinases, and generation of FR/ROS.[111,114] NF-κB transactivation plays a pivotal role in parturition via induction of pro-inflammatory cytokines, prostaglandins, and matrix metalloproteases.[115] RAGE-mediated NF-κB activation initiated by DAMPs is unique because of its self-perpetuating and sustained nature, which overwhelms the autoregulatory inhibitory feedback loops.[116]

Our group discovered that two amniotic fluid S100 proteins (S100A12 and unbound S100A8) are biomarkers characteristic of intra-amniotic inflammation and impending preterm birth.[25,117] Given that S100A12 is a RAGE ligand, we reasoned that besides being biomarkers, these proteins participate in modulating the intra-amniotic inflammation process through activation of this system. Spearheaded by the proteomics findings, we were the first group to study the presence and regulation of the RAGE axis in human amniotic fluid.[118] We found that S100A12 is present in the amniotic fluid of women with intra-amniotic infection in direct relationship to the degree of inflammation and the severity of histologic chorioamnionitis and funisitis. Furthermore, we showed that S100A12 localized primarily on infiltrating inflammatory cells, and that advanced histologic chorioamnionitis was associated with elevated S100A12 mRNA levels in fetal membranes, but not in the placenta. Because fetal membranes express high levels of RAGE in amnion epithelial, decidual, and extravillous trophoblast cells in fetal membranes, we postulated that these are potential sites of RAGE signaling. We further found that compared with other biologic fluids, amniotic fluid is very rich in soluble-RAGE (sRAGE, natural inhibitor of RAGE activation). The sRAGE concentration in the amniotic cavity was gestational age–regulated, increasing about 100-fold from 15 weeks' up to 30 weeks' gestation. This observation led us to speculate that the low levels of endogenous sRAGE earlier in gestation (<30 weeks) may predispose to enhanced RAGE activation in the event of a DAMP challenge. Conversely, an excess of sRAGE later in gestation (>30 weeks) may act as a "natural blocker" of NF-κB activation via RAGE (Fig. 19-2). The gestational age dependence of the inhibitor molecule sRAGE may be one potential explanation for the higher incidence of infection-related preterm births and fetal damage at earlier gestational ages.[119]

In women with PPROM, antibiotic therapy has been shown to prolong pregnancy.[120,121] Yet the childhood outcome results of the ORACLE II clinical trial showed that prescription of antibiotics to women in preterm birth increased the risk of cerebral palsy.[122,123] This suggests that in certain fetuses, the short-term benefit may be falsely reassuring. Our model (Fig. 19-3) may provide a pathophysiologic mechanism for these findings: Antibiotics induce suppression of bacteria but do not eradicate PAMPs and DAMPs. In turn, PAMPs and DAMPs may continue to maintain actively the processes leading to fetal cellular damage. This concurs with data derived from animal models of sepsis, which demonstrated that that antibiotic-treated rats display higher plasma endotoxin levels than untreated animals.[124] Moreover, different antibiotics may induce the release of different forms of endotoxin, which may be lethal for sensitized animals. This may also explain why attempts to prevent preterm birth with antibiotic treatment in patients with bacterial vaginosis or trichomoniasis increased the rate of preterm birth or the risk of cerebral palsy.[125] In this context, suppression of labor may be detrimental by prolonging exposure of the fetus to the damaging environment.[126]

The Paradoxical Effect of Chorioamnionitis on Fetal Lung Maturation and Injury

A previous study showed a lower incidence of respiratory distress syndrome (RDS) among premature newborns delivered in the setting of chorioamnionitis.[127] In the long run, however, intra-amniotic inflammation and infection promote chronic lung disease by increasing the risk for BPD.[128] The mechanism is not well understood, and limitations to progress in these aspects include lack of consensus concerning the best definitions of chorioamnionitis, RDS, and BPD, as well as inability to accurately and objectively point to infection as an inflammatory trigger in fetuses that have been exposed antenatally. In this context, animal experiments have proved

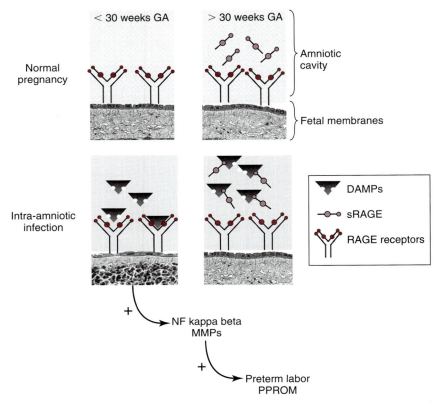

Figure 19-2 Schematic representation of the proposed interplay between S100A12 (also a damage-associated molecular pattern [DAMP] molecule) and the soluble receptor for advanced glycation end-products (sRAGE) circulating in amniotic fluid and RAGE receptors in fetal membranes in normal pregnancy versus pregnancy complicated by intra-amniotic infection. We propose that later in the course of pregnancy, excess sRAGE may function as a "natural blocker" of RAGE engagement by DAMPs, thus preventing the activation of nuclear factor (NF)-κB and of matrix metalloproteases implicated in preterm labor or preterm premature rupture of membranes (PPROM).

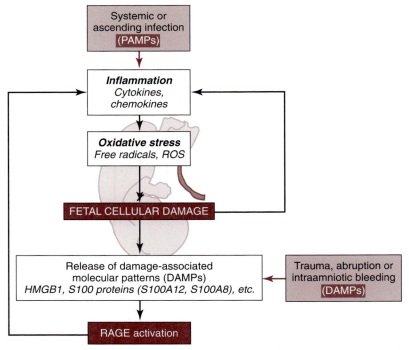

Figure 19-3 Working model illustrating the central role of damage-associated molecular pattern molecules (DAMPs) (alarmins) and the receptor for advanced glycation end-products (RAGE) in promoting cellular damage to the fetus exposed to inflammation and oxidative stress initiated by infection or by noninfectious triggers.

useful and for the most part have confirmed these observations in humans. In sheep, intra-amniotic injection of endotoxin and IL-1 induced fetal lung maturation with elevated mRNA levels for surfactant proteins (SPs) A through D—an effect that occurred independent of fetal cortisol levels.[129]

Recent studies have focused on the role of chorioamnionitis in aberrant fetal pulmonary angiogenesis leading to BPD. It was proposed that angiopoietin balance plays a pivotal role in the process. Angiopoeitin-2 (Ang-2) has been shown to destabilize vessels and is an important inducer of epithelial cell death in the neonatal lung.[130] Tracheal Ang-2 was noted to increase in neonates that develop BPD.[131] Angiopoietin-1 (Ang-1) and soluble tunica internal endothelial cell kinase 2 (sTie-2) are endogenous Ang-2 antagonists that stabilize newly formed vessels and reduce vascular leakage. Our group has shown that human amniotic fluid contains relatively high levels of Ang-1, Ang-2, and sTie-2.[34] As gestation progresses, the angiopoietin balance favors Ang-1 and sTie2 as opposed to Ang-2. In intra-amniotic inflammation, a relative increase in the amniotic fluid levels of Ang-1, Ang-2, and sTie2 occurs compared with expected levels for gestational age. This phenomenon appears to occur independent of changes in mRNA expression of these factors in the amniochorion or the placenta.[34] Bhandari and colleagues noted that infants who developed BPD or who died had increased Ang-2 in the first week of life.[130] Dexamethasone attenuated this effect. In a separate study, Thomas and coworkers measured the tracheal fluid level of Ang-2, which decreased over time.[132] These observations suggest that in utero, the fetus is exposed to higher concentrations of Ang-2 than those generated in the postnatal lung. Amniotic fluid Ang-2 could also have accounted for increased tracheal Ang-2 in the immediate postnatal period. The observed decreased Ang2/Ang1 ratio in tracheal fluid on postnatal days 5 to 7 was consistent with an inability of the newborn to sustain and adequately control the pro-angiogenic signal needed for lung development.[132] Additional studies are needed to explore the dual effect of intra-amniotic infection on lung angiogenic signals and their relationship to BDP.

Controversies in Determination of Neonatal Encephalopathy: Early-Onset Neonatal Sepsis vs. Antenatal and Intrapartum Hypoxia

Many newborns receive antibiotherapy based on nonspecific symptoms of suspected EONS and/or maternal risk factors (e.g., prematurity, intrapartum fever, chorioamnionitis, prolonged rupture of membranes).[133] The inability of clinicians to diagnose EONS on the basis of neonatal blood cultures is well recognized, and several explanations are available. First, the frequency of bloodstream infections fluctuates widely from 8% to 73% in the diagnosis of "presumed" EONS.[134] These data underscore the elusive nature of this clinical entity. Second, similar to intra-amniotic infection, microbiology laboratories search for only a narrow spectrum of pathogens. For example, culturing for *Ureaplasma* and *Mycoplasma* spp. is not part of a routine sepsis work-up in neonates. A study that evaluated the frequency of umbilical cord blood infections with these species found that 23% of newborns born at less than 32 weeks tested positive for these pathogens.[49] Third, it is plausible that analogous to intra-amniotic inflammation, the fetal and newborn insult is induced by additional uncultivated and difficult-to-cultivate species. Data supporting this premise have shown that 16S rRNA polymerase chain reaction (PCR) technology improves the accuracy of culture-based methods for diagnosis of neonatal sepsis.[135] Therefore in current clinical practice, microbiological laboratories are often unable to pinpoint a specific microbial agent. In these cases, the cause of fetal injury may be wrongfully attributed to antepartum and intrapartum hypoxia. Because infection and hypoxia-reperfusion injury overlap in terms of their clinical manifestations (i.e., antenatal heart rate abnormalities, postnatal seizures), such errors are easy to make.[34,136]

Salafia and associates hypothesized that "sensitization" of umbilical cord blood vessels by inflammatory cytokines alters the vasomotor response to mechanical compression during uterine contractions or fetal movement.[77] Our group analyzed the fetal heart rate patterns in a cohort of 87 fetuses delivered

19

in the context of presence or absence of histologic funisitis. We determined that an advanced grade of arteritis and phlebitis was associated with a higher fetal heart rate baseline and nonreactive, nonreassuring pattern at the time of initial evaluation. Figure 19-4 presents the relationship between abnormal fetal heart rate tracings and amniotic fluid biomarkers of intra-amniotic inflammation. All episodes of fetal tachycardia occurred in the context of severe intra-amniotic inflammation, infection, and funisitis and in most cases in the absence of maternal clinical chorioamnionitis. Once again, this highlights the relevance of a thorough evaluation of the intrauterine environment even in the absence of maternal signs or symptoms of chorioamnionitis.

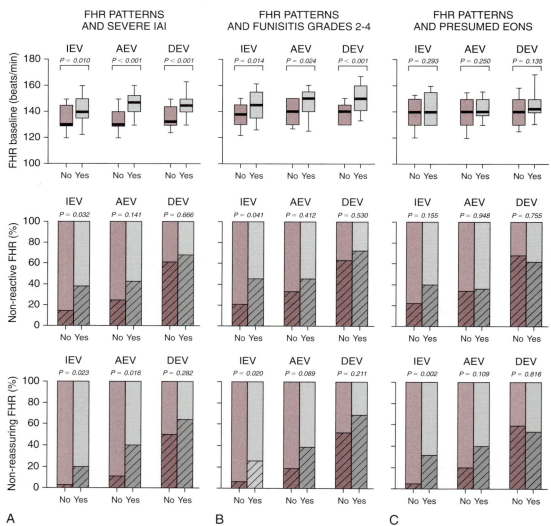

Figure 19-4 Fetal heart rate (FHR) monitoring patterns recorded from 87 singleton premature neonates delivered within 48 hours from amniocentesis (gestational age, 28.9 ± 3.3 weeks) were analyzed blindly using strict National Institute of Child Health and Human Development (NICHD) criteria. Strips were evaluated at three time points: at admission (initial evaluation [IEV]), at amniocentesis (AEV), and before delivery (DEV). Intra-amniotic inflammation (IAI) was established on the basis of a previously validated proteomic fingerprint (mass restricted (MR) score[25,117]). Diagnoses of histologic chorioamnionitis and early-onset neonatal sepsis (EONS) were based on well-recognized pathologic, clinical, and laboratory criteria. FHR baseline levels *(top)* and percentages of fetuses with nonreactive *(middle)* and/or nonreassuring *(bottom)* FHR are presented as a function of **(A)** severe intra-amniotic inflammation (MR score of 3 or 4; Yes, n = 51 vs. MR score of 0, 1, or 2; No, n = 36); **(B)** funisitis (grades 2 to 4; Yes, n = 33 vs. grades 0 to 1; No, n = 48); and **(C)** EONS (presumed and/or culture-confirmed; Yes, n = 26 vs. No, n = 60).

As discussed earlier, several of the pathogenic pathways leading to fetal injury initiated by infection and hypoxia overlap. Hypoxic-ischemic brain injury that occurs during the perinatal period is one of the most invoked causes of severe, long-term neurologic deficits in children.[85] However, the concept that cerebral palsy is due only to acquired insults such as perinatal asphyxia has been fundamentally challenged in the past decade. The current view is that a vast majority of injuries are the result of interplay between several risk factors such as genetic background, excitotoxicity, hypoxia, oxidative stress, and sepsis and an exacerbated inflammatory fetal and placental host response.[45,85] Discerning among these factors is important not only when formulating antenatal preventive or therapeutic strategies to avert cerebral palsy, but also within medico-legal contexts. With regard to the latter, clinical practice guidelines indicate the importance of evaluating umbilical cord blood gases and the acid-base status of the premature neonate at the time of birth for documentation or exclusion at fetal academia.[137,138] Furthermore, exclusion of other identifiable causes (e.g., trauma, coagulation disorder, infectious or genetic conditions) is vital before an anoxic intrapartum event is declared as the definitive cause of poor neurodevelopmental outcome. In most cases where hypoxia-ischemia is invoked as the cause of neonatal encephalopathy, no evidence of neonatal stroke is found, and no work-up of brain oxygenation or blood flow is completed. Because the correct choice of words is important, and until specific markers of intrapartum hypoxic injury are discovered and validated, a change in terminology that does not assume cause is necessary and has been advocated by experts.[139]

Intra-amniotic Infection/Inflammation and Systems Biology

Pregnancy by itself is a prototype biologic system. Its complexity results from the underlying presence of two genomes (maternal, fetal), the intrauterine environment as well as that external to the mother, growth and maturation of the fetus, and the dynamic and nonlinear interactions among system components.[140] One has to add the bacterial genome(s) to the equation, as well as the maternal and fetal host responses, to gain a glimpse of the challenge placed in front of us when we try to elucidate the topic here under review.

Reductionist approaches assume that conclusions about a system can be inferred by studying individual components alone (e.g., DNA or protein sequences) or as part of simpler systems (e.g., in vitro or animal models).[141] In contrast, systems biologists advocate that true features of each component can be grasped only in the context of their interactions with other components and only as part of the system under study.[142] Theoretical principles belonging to systems biology are far ahead compared with experimental tools available to scientists. Genomics, proteomics, transcriptomics, and interactomics are still in the phase of cataloguing system components. Focusing on a few pathways that appear randomly more significant than others seems to be the current trend. However, even with this approach, therapeutic targets unravel faster compared with hypothesis-driven methods, which often fail in clinical trials.[143] More important than the expensive and cutting-edge analytic instrumentation required for -omics discovery is the change in thinking that characterizes systems biology.

Heisenberg's Uncertainty Principle, one of the best known implications of quantum theory, dictates that any experiment aimed at understanding a living organism will interrupt its course, making it impossible to discriminate the truth from induced artifact.[144] In a more radical view, Heisenberg explained the Uncertainty Principle as a limitation of nature implying that the correct notions of quantum mechanics should be statistical probabilities rather than well-defined classical trajectories. Such a view rendered a turning point in physics, and life sciences and medicine are now starting to follow.[145] Regarding the fetus, the implications for advancing diagnostics and therapy through biomarker discovery and validation are huge. However, it is critical for our method of data analysis to also change and account for the lack of a "gold standard" for intra-amniotic infection, inflammation, chorioamnionitis, and neonatal sepsis. Instead of applying receiver-operating curve analysis to determine the sensitivity and specificity of a new biomarker to identify an elusive clinical entity (e.g., chorioamnionitis, presumed neonatal sepsis), novel statistical approaches able to compute diagnostic probabilities rather than certainties need to applied or developed.

References

1. Blanc WA. Pathways of fetal and early neonatal infection. Viral placentitis, bacterial and fungal chorioamnionitis. *J Pediatr.* 1961;59:473-496.
2. Hallendahl H, Beitr Z, Geburtsh U. Gynak. 1906; 10:320-324; as quoted by Slemons JM. Placental Bacteremia. *JAMA* 1915;65:1265.
3. Slemons JM. Placental bacteremia. *JAMA.* 1915;65:1265-1268.
4. Kobak AJ. Fetal bacteremia; a contribution to the mechanism of intrauterine infection and to the pathogenesis of placentitis. *Am J Obstet Gynecol.* 1930;19:299-316.
5. Wohlwill F, Bock HE. Uber Entzundungen der Placenta und fetale Sepsis. *Arch Gynakol.* 1929;135:271-319.
6. Cunningham FG, MacDonald PC, Gant NF. In: *Williams Obstetrics,* 18th ed. Norwalk, CT: Appleton and Lange; 1989:749-750.
7. Tita AT, Ramin SM. Intraamniotic infection (chorioamnionitis) (211). Topic last updated: May 31 2011. <http://www.uptodateonline.com> Accessed July 1, 2011.
8. Vrachnis N, Vitoratos N, Iliodromiti Z, et al. Intrauterine inflammation and preterm delivery. *Ann N Y Acad Sci.* 2010;1205:118-122.
9. Menon R, Taylor RN, Fortunato SJ. Chorioamnionitis—a complex pathophysiologic syndrome. *Placenta.* 2010;31:113-120.
10. Pettker CM, Buhimschi IA, Magloire LK, et al. Value of placental microbial evaluation in diagnosing intra-amniotic infection. *Obstet Gynecol.* 2007;109:739-749.
11. Moriyama K, Ando C, Tashiro K, et al. Polymerase chain reaction detection of bacterial 16S rRNA gene in human blood. *Microbiol Immunol.* 2008;52:375-382.
12. Markenson GR, Adams LA, Hoffman DE, et al. Prevalence of *Mycoplasma* bacteria in amniotic fluid at the time of genetic amniocentesis using the polymerase chain reaction. *J Reprod Med.* 2003;48:775-779.
13. King AE, Kelly RW, Sallenave JM, et al. Innate immune defenses in the human uterus during pregnancy. *Placenta.* 2007;28:1099-1106.
14. Pettker CM, Buhimschi CS, Dulay AT, et al. Antimicrobial properties of the amniotic fluid: A growth curve analysis of *E. coli. Am J Obstet Gynecol.* 2008;199:S148.
15. Dulay AT, Buhimschi CS, Zhao G, et al. Soluble TLR2 is present in human amniotic fluid and modulates the intraamniotic inflammatory response to infection. *J Immunol.* 2009;182:7244-7253.
16. Nath CA, Ananth CV, Smulian JC, et al. New Jersey-Placental Abruption Study Investigators. Histologic evidence of inflammation and risk of placental abruption. *Am J Obstet Gynecol.* 2007;197:319.e1-6.
17. Buhimschi CS, Schatz F, Krikun G, et al. Novel insights into molecular mechanisms of abruption-induced preterm birth. *Expert Rev Mol Med.* 2010;12:e35.
18. Cakmak H, Schatz F, Huang ST, et al. Progestin suppresses thrombin- and interleukin-1beta-induced interleukin-11 production in term decidual cells: Implications for preterm delivery. *J Clin Endocrinol Metab.* 2005;90:5279-5286.
19. Pyne-Geithman GJ, Morgan CJ, Wagner K, et al. Bilirubin production and oxidation in CSF of patients with cerebral vasospasm after subarachnoid hemorrhage. *J Cereb Blood Flow Metab.* 2005;25:1070-1077.
20. Levi M, van der Poll T. Inflammation and coagulation. *Crit Care Med.* 2010;38:S26-S34.
21. Lockwood CJ, Paidas M, Murk WK, et al. Involvement of human decidual cell–expressed tissue factor in uterine hemostasis and abruption. *Thromb Res.* 2009;124:516-520.
22. Esmon CT. Crosstalk between inflammation and thrombosis. *Maturitas.* 2008;61:122-131.
23. Weng L, Rubin EM, Bristow J. Application of sequence-based methods in human microbial ecology. *Genome Res.* 2006;16:316-322.
24. Riesenfeld CS, Schloss PD, Handelsman J. Metagenomics: Genomic analysis of microbial communities. *Annu Rev Genet.* 2004;38:525-552.
25. Buhimschi CS, Bhandari V, Hamar BD, et al. Proteomic profiling of the amniotic fluid to detect inflammation, infection, and neonatal sepsis. *PLoS Med.* 2007;4:e18.
26. Gardella C, Riley DE, Hitti J, et al. Identification and sequencing of bacterial rDNAs in culture-negative amniotic fluid from women in premature labor. *Am J Perinatol.* 2004;21:319-323.
27. Jalava J, Mäntymaa ML, Ekblad U, et al. Bacterial 16S rDNA polymerase chain reaction in the detection of intra-amniotic infection. *Br J Obstet Gynaecol.* 1996;103:664-669.
28. Hitti J, Riley DE, Krohn MA, et al. Broad-spectrum bacterial rDNA polymerase chain reaction assay for detecting amniotic fluid infection among women in premature labor. *Clin Infect Dis.* 1997;24:1228-1232.
29. Bearfield C, Davenport ES, Sivapathasundaram V, et al. Possible association between amniotic fluid micro-organism infection and microflora in the mouth. *BJOG.* 2002;109:527-533.
30. Han YW, Shen T, Chung P, et al. Uncultivated bacteria as etiologic agents of intra-amniotic inflammation leading to preterm birth. *J Clin Microbiol.* 2009;47:38-47.

19

31. Han YW, Redline RW, Li M, et al. *Fusobacterium nucleatum* induces premature and term stillbirths in pregnant mice: Implication of oral bacteria in preterm birth. *Infect Immun*. 2004;72: 2272-2279.
32. Madianos PN, Lieff S, Murtha AP, et al. Maternal periodontitis and prematurity. Part II. Maternal infection and fetal exposure. *Ann Periodontol*. 2001;6:175-182.
33. Sampson JE, Theve RP, Blatman RN, et al. Fetal origin of amniotic fluid polymorphonuclear leukocytes. *Am J Obstet Gynecol*. 1997; 176: 77-81.
34. Buhimschi CS, Abdel-Razeq S, Cackovic M, et al. Fetal heart rate monitoring patterns in women with amniotic fluid proteomic profiles indicative of inflammation. *Am J Perinatol*. 2008;25:359-372.
35. Letti Müller AL, Barrios Pde M, Kliemann LM, et al. Tei index to assess fetal cardiac performance in fetuses at risk for fetal inflammatory response syndrome. *Ultrasound Obstet Gynecol*. 2010;36: 26-31.
36. Azpurua H, Dulay AT, Buhimschi IA, et al. Fetal renal artery impedance as assessed by Doppler ultrasound in pregnancies complicated by intraamniotic inflammation and preterm birth. *Am J Obstet Gynecol*. 2009;200:203.e1-e11.
37. Baley JE, Stork EK, Warkentin PI, et al. Neonatal neutropenia. Clinical manifestations, cause, and outcome. *Am J Dis Child*. 1988;142:1161-1166.
38. Melvan JN, Bagby GJ, Welsh DA, et al. Neonatal sepsis and neutrophil insufficiencies. *Int Rev Immunol*. 2010;29:315-348.
39. Gibbs RS, Castillo MS, Rodgers PJ. Management of acute chorioamnionitis. *Am J Obstet Gynecol*. 1980;136:796-803.
40. Bobitt JR, Ledger WJ. Unrecognized amnionitis and prematurity: A preliminary report. *J Reprod Med*. 1977;19:8-12.
41. Bobitt JR, Ledger WJ. Amniotic fluid analysis. Its role in maternal neonatal infection. *Obstet Gynecol*. 1978;51:56-62.
42. Benirschke K. Examination of the placenta. *Obstet Gynecol*. 1961;18:309-333.
43. Naeye RL. Disorders of the placenta and decidua. In: *Disorder of the Placenta, Fetus and Neonate: Diagnosis and Clinical Significance*. St. Louis: Mosby; 1992:118-247.
44. Salafia CM, Weigl C, Silberman L. The prevalence and distribution of acute placental inflammation in uncomplicated term pregnancies. *Obstet Gynecol*. 1989;73:383-389.
45. Redline RW. Placental pathology and cerebral palsy. *Clin Perinatol*. 2006;33:503-516.
46. Redline RW, Faye-Petersen O, Heller D, et al. Amniotic infection syndrome: Nosology and reproducibility of placental reaction patterns. *Pediatr Dev Pathol*. 2003;6:435-448.
47. van Hoeven KH, Anyaegbunam A, Hochster H, et al. Clinical significance of increasing histologic severity of acute inflammation in the fetal membranes and umbilical cord. *Pediatr Pathol Lab Med*. 1996;16:731-744.
48. Salafia CM, Weigl C, Silberman L. The prevalence and distribution of acute placental inflammation in uncomplicated term pregnancies. *Obstet Gynecol*. 1989;73:383-389.
49. Goldenberg RL, Andrews WW, Goepfert AR, et al. Alabama Preterm Birth Study: Umbilical cord blood *Ureaplasma urealyticum* and *Mycoplasma hominis* cultures in very preterm newborn infants. *Am J Obstet Gynecol*. 2008;198:e1-e5.
50. Bejar R, Wozniak P, Allard M, et al. Antenatal origin of neurologic damage in newborn infants. I. Preterm infants. *Am J Obstet Gynecol*. 1988;159:357-363.
51. De Felice C, Toti P, Laurini RN, et al. Early neonatal brain injury in histologic chorioamnionitis. *J Pediatr*. 2001;138:101-104.
52. Grafe MR. The correlation of prenatal brain damage with placental pathology. *Neuropathol Exp Neurol*. 1994;53:407-415.
53. Buhimschi IA, Zambrano E, Pettker CM, et al. Using proteomic analysis of the human amniotic fluid to identify histologic chorioamnionitis. *Obstet Gynecol*. 2008;111:403-412.
54. Smulian JC, Shen-Schwarz S, Vintzileos AM, et al. Clinical chorio-amnionitis and histologic placental inflammation. *Obstet Gynecol*. 1999;94:1000-1005.
55. Heller DS, Rimpel LH, Skurnick JH. Does histologic chorioamnionitis correspond to clinical chorioamnionitis? *J Reprod Med*. 2008;53:25-28.
56. Elsasser DA, Ananth CV, Prasad V, et al. New Jersey-Placental Abruption Study Investigators. Diagnosis of placental abruption: Relationship between clinical and histopathological findings. *Eur J Obstet Gynecol Reprod Biol*. 2010;148:125-130.
57. Meeusen EN, Bischof RJ, Lee CS. Comparative T-cell responses during pregnancy in large animals and humans. *Am J Reprod Immunol*. 2001;46:169-179.
58. Martinon F, Mayor A, Tschopp J. The inflammasomes: Guardians of the body. *Annu Rev Immunol*. 2009;27:229-265.
59. Reddy RC, Chen GH, Tekchandani PK, et al. Sepsis-induced immunosuppression: From bad to worse. *Immunol Res*. 2001;24:273-287.
60. Cinel I, Opal SM. Molecular biology of inflammation and sepsis: A primer. *Crit Care Med*. 2009; 37:291-304.
61. Benhamou Y, Favre J, Musette P, et al. Toll-like receptors 4 contribute to endothelial injury and inflammation in hemorrhagic shock in mice. *Crit Care Med*. 2009;37:1724-1728.
62. Jeannin P, Jaillon S, Delneste Y. Pattern recognition receptors in the immune response against dying cells. *Curr Opin Immunol*. 2008;20:530-537.
63. Takeda K, Kaisho T, Akira S. Toll-like receptors. *Annu Rev Immun*. 2003;21:335-376.
64. Zähringer U, Lindner B, Inamura S, et al. TLR2 -promiscuous or specific? A critical re-evaluation of a receptor expressing apparent broad specificity. *Immunobiology*. 2008;213:205-224.

19

19

65. Brun-Buisson C, Doyon F, Carlet J, et al. Incidence, risk factors, and outcome of severe sepsis and septic shock in adults. A multicenter prospective study in intensive care units. French ICU Group for Severe Sepsis. *JAMA*. 1995;274:968-974.
66. Benirschke K, Robb JA. Infectious causes of fetal death. *Clin Obstet Gynecol*. 1987;30:284-294.
67. Buhimschi CS, Dulay AT, Abdel-Razeq S, et al. Fetal inflammatory response in women with proteomic biomarkers characteristic of intra-amniotic inflammation and preterm birth. *BJOG*. 2009;116:257-267.
68. Malaeb S, Dammann O. Fetal inflammatory response and brain injury in the preterm newborn. *J Child Neurol*. 2009;24:1119-1126.
69. Buhimschi IA, Buhimschi CS, Weiner CP. Protective effect of N-acetylcysteine against fetal death and preterm labor induced by maternal inflammation. *Am J Obstet Gynecol*. 2003;188:203-208.
70. Weiner CP, Lee KY, Buhimschi CS, et al. Proteomic biomarkers that predict the clinical success of rescue cerclage. *Am J Obstet Gynecol*. 2005;192:710-718.
71. Maalouf EF, Duggan PJ, Rutherford MA, et al. Magnetic resonance imaging of the brain in a cohort of extremely preterm infants. *J Pediatr*. 1999;35:351-357.
72. Lau J, Magee F, Qiu Z, et al. Chorioamnionitis with a fetal inflammatory response is associated with higher neonatal mortality, morbidity, and resource use than chorioamnionitis displaying a maternal inflammatory response only. *Am J Obstet Gynecol*. 2005;193:708-713.
73. Buhimschi IA, Buhimschi CS, Pupkin M, et al. Beneficial impact of term labor: Non-enzymatic antioxidant reserve in the human fetus. *Am J Obstet Gynecol*. 2003;189:181-188.
74. Jacobsson B. Infectious and inflammatory mechanisms in preterm birth and cerebral palsy. *Eur J Obstet Gynecol Reprod Biol*. 2004;115:159-160.
75. Dammann O, Leviton A. Inflammation, brain damage and visual dysfunction in preterm infants. *Semin Fetal Neonatal Med*. 2006;11:363-368.
76. Grigg J, Arnon S, Chase A, et al. Inflammatory cells in the lungs of premature infants on the first day of life. Perinatal risk factors and origin of cells. *Arch Dis Child*. 1993;69:40-43.
77. Salafia CM, Ghidini A, Sherer DM, et al. Abnormalities of the fetal heart rate in preterm deliveries are associated with acute intra-amniotic infection. *J Soc Gynecol Investig*. 1998;5:188-191.
78. Kaukola T, Herva R, Perhomaa M, et al. Population cohort associating chorioamnionitis, cord inflammatory cytokines and neurologic outcome in very preterm, extremely low birth weight infants. *Pediatr Res*. 2006;59:478-483.
79. Watterberg KL, Demers LM, Scott SM, et al. Chorioamnionitis and early lung inflammation in infants in whom bronchopulmonary dysplasia develops. *Pediatrics*. 1996;97:210-215.
80. Stoll BJ, Hansen NI, Adams-Chapman I, et al. National Institute of Child Health and Human Development Neonatal Research Network. Neurodevelopmental and growth impairment among extremely low-birth-weight infants with neonatal infection. *JAMA*. 2004;292:2357-2365.
81. Hitti J, Tarczy-Hornoch P, Murphy J, et al. Amniotic fluid infection, cytokines, and adverse outcome among infants at 34 weeks' gestation or less. *Obstet Gynecol*. 2001;98:1080-1088.
82. Murphy DJ, Sellers S, MacKenzie IZ, et al. Case control study of antenatal and intrapartum risk factors for cerebral palsy in very preterm singleton babies. *Lancet*. 1995;346:1449-1454.
83. Rouse DJ, Landon M, Leveno KJ, et al. NICHD Maternal-Fetal Medicine Units Network. The MFMU cesarean registry: Chorioamnionitis at term and its duration-relationship to outcomes. *Am J Obstet Gynecol*. 2004;91:211-216.
84. Martius JA, Roos T, Gora B, et al. Risk factors associated with early-onset sepsis in premature infants. *Eur J Obstet Gynecol Reprod Biol*. 1999;85:151-158.
85. Ferriero DM. Neonatal brain injury. *N Engl J Med*. 2004;351:1985-1995.
86. Duncan JR, Cock ML, Scheerlinck JP, et al. White matter injury after repeated endotoxin exposure in the preterm ovine fetus. *Pediatr Res*. 2002;52:941-949.
87. Leviton A, Dammann O, Durum SK. The adaptive immune response in neonatal cerebral white matter damage. *Ann Neurol*. 2005;58:821-828.
88. Hack CE, Zeerleder S. The endothelium in sepsis: Source of and a target for inflammation. *Crit Care Med*. 2000;29:S21-S27.
89. Burd I, Bentz AI, Chai J, et al. Inflammation-induced preterm birth alters neuronal morphology in the mouse fetal brain. *J Neurosci Res*. 2010;88:1872-1881.
90. Watterberg K. Anti-inflammatory therapy in the neonatal intensive care unit: Present and future. *Semin Fetal Neonatal Med*. 2006;21:1-7.
91. Fridovich I. Oxygen: Boon and bane. *Am Sci*. 1975;63:54-59.
92. Bazowska G, Jendryczo A. Antioxidant enzyme activities in fetal and neonatal lung: Lowered activities of these enzymes in children with RDS. *Ginekol Pol*. 1996;67:70-74.
93. Aliakbar S, Brown P, Bidwell D, et al. Human erythrocyte superoxide dismutase in adults, neonates and normal, hypoxemic and chromosonally abnormal fetuses. *Clin Biochem*. 1993;26:109-115.
94. Jain A, Mehta T, Auld PA, et al. Glutathione metabolism in newborns: Evidence for glutathione deficiency in plasma, bronchoalveolar lavage fluid, and lymphocytes in prematures. *Pediatr Pulmonol*. 1995;20:60-66.
95. Zlotkin SH, Bryan MH, Anderson GH. Cysteine supplementation to cysteine-free intravenous feeding regimens in newborn infants. *Am J Clin Nutr*. 1981;34:914-923.
96. Varsila E, Pitkanen O, Hallman M, et al. Immaturity-dependent free radical activity in premature infants. *Pediatr Res*. 1994;36:55-59.
97. Kelly FJ. Free radical disorders of preterm infants. *Br Med Bull*. 1993;49:668-678.
98. Perrone S, Negro S, Tataranno ML. Oxidative stress and antioxidant strategies in newborns. *J Matern Fetal Neonatal Med*. 2010;23:63-65.

99. Halliwell B. Reactive oxygen species and the CNS. *J Neurochem*. 1992;59:1609-1623.
100. Buhimschi IA, Weiner CP. Oxygen free radicals and disorders of pregnancy. *Fetal Matern Med Rev*. 2001;12:273-298.
101. Medzhitov R. Origin and physiological roles of inflammation. *Nature*. 2008;454:428-435.
102. Foell D, Wittkowski H, Roth J. Mechanisms of disease: A 'DAMP' view of inflammatory arthritis. *Nat Clin Pract Rheumatol*. 2007;3:382-390.
103. Su SL, Tsai CD, Lee CH, et al. Expression and regulation of Toll-like receptor 2 by IL-1beta and fibronectin fragments in human articular chondrocytes. *Osteoarthritis Cartilage*. 2005;13:879-886.
104. Lotze MT, Zeh HJ, Rubartelli A, et al. The grateful dead: Damage-associated molecular pattern molecules and reduction/oxidation regulate immunity. *Immunol Rev*. 2007;220:60-81.
105. Oppenheim JJ, Tewary P, de la Rosa G, et al. Alarmins initiate host defense. *Adv Exp Med Biol*. 2007;601:185-194.
106. Yan SF, Ramasamy R, Naka Y, et al. Glycation, inflammation, and RAGE: A scaffold for the macro-vascular complications of diabetes and beyond. *Circ Res*. 2003;93:1159-1169.
107. Hofmann MA, Drury S, Fu C, et al. RAGE mediates a novel proinflammatory axis: A central cell surface receptor for S100/calgranulin polypeptides. *Cell*. 1999;97:889-901.
108. Stern D, Yan SD, Yan SF, et al. Receptor for advanced glycation endproducts: A multiligand receptor magnifying cell stress in diverse pathologic settings. *Adv Drug Deliv Rev*. 2002;54:1615-1625.
109. Mohamed AK, Bierhaus A, Schiekofer S, et al. The role of oxidative stress and NF-kappaB activation in late diabetic complications. *Biofactors*. 1999;10:157-167.
110. Yan SD, Chen X, Fu J, et al. RAGE and amyloid-beta peptide neurotoxicity in Alzheimer's disease. *Nature*. 1996;382:685-691.
111. Chavakis T, Bierhaus A, Nawroth PP. RAGE (receptor for advanced glycation end products): A central player in the inflammatory response. *Microbes Infect*. 2004;6:1219-1225.
112. Miyata T, Hori O, Zhang J, et al. The receptor for advanced glycation end products (RAGE) is a central mediator of the interaction of AGE-beta2microglobulin with human mononuclear phago-cytes via an oxidant-sensitive pathway. Implications for the pathogenesis of dialysis-related amyloi-dosis. *J Clin Invest*. 1996;98:1088-1094.
113. Raucci A, Cugusi S, Antonelli A, et al. A soluble form of the receptor for advanced glycation end-products (RAGE) is produced by proteolytic cleavage of the membrane-bound form by the sheddase a disintegrin and metalloprotease 10 (ADAM10). *FASEB J*. 2008;22:3716-3727.
114. Baeuerle PA, Baltimore D. I kappa B: A specific inhibitor of the NF-kappa B transcription factor. *Science*. 1988;242:540-546.
115. Lindstrom TM, Bennett PR. The role of nuclear factor kappa B in human labour. *Reproduction*. 2005;130: 569-581.
116. Bierhaus A, Schiekofer S, Schwaninger M, et al. Diabetes-associated sustained activation of the transcription factor NF-B. *Diabetes*. 2001;50:2792-2809.
117. Buhimschi IA, Christner R, Buhimschi CS. Proteomic biomarker analysis of amniotic fluid for identification of intra-amniotic inflammation. *BJOG*. 2005;112:173-181.
118. Buhimschi IA, Zhao G, Pettker CM, et al. The receptor for advanced glycation end products (RAGE) system in women with intraamniotic infection and inflammation. *Am J Obstet Gynecol*. 2007;196:181.e1-e13.
119. Watts D, Krohn M, Hillier S, et al. The association of occult amniotic fluid infection with gestational age and neonatal outcome among women in preterm labor. *Obstet Gynecol*. 1992;79:351-357.
120. Johnston MM, Sanchez-Ramos L, Vaughn AJ, et al. Antibiotic therapy in preterm premature rupture of membranes: A randomized, prospective, double-blind trial. *Am J Obstet Gynecol*. 1990;163:743-747.
121. ACOG Committee on Practice Bulletins-Obstetrics. Bulletin No. 80: PPROM. Clinical management guidelines for obstetrician-gynecologists. *Obstet Gynecol*. 2007;109:1007-1019.
122. Kenyon SL, Pike K, Jones DR, et al. Childhood outcomes after prescription of antibiotics to pregnant women with preterm rupture of the membranes: 7-year follow-up of the ORACLE I trial. *Lancet*. 2001;357:979-988.
123. Kenyon SL, Pike K, Jones DR, et al. Childhood outcomes after prescription of antibiotics to pregnant women with spontaneous preterm labour: 7-year follow-up of the ORACLE II trial. *Lancet*. 2008;372:1319-1327
124. Holzheimer RG. Antibiotic induced endotoxin release and clinical sepsis: A review. *J Chemother*. 2001;1:159-172.
125. Klebanoff MA, Carey JC, Hauth JC, et al. Failure of metronidazole to prevent preterm delivery among pregnant women with asymptomatic *Trichomonas vaginalis* infection. *N Engl J Med*. 2001;345:487-493.
126. Buhimschi IA, Buhimschi CS, Weiner CP. Acute versus chronic inflammation: What makes the intra-uterine environment "unfriendly" to the fetus? From free radicals to proteomics. *Am J Reprod Immunol*. 2003;49:328.
127. Kramer BW, Kallapur S, Newnham J, et al. Prenatal inflammation and lung development. *Semin Fetal Neonatal Med*. 2009;14:2-7.
128. Bhandari A, Panitch HB. Pulmonary outcomes in bronchopulmonary dysplasia. *Semin Perinatol*. 2006;30:219-226.
129. Willet KE, Kramer BW, Kallapur SG, et al. Intra-amniotic injection of IL-1 induces inflammation and maturation in fetal sheep lung. *Am J Physiol Lung Cell Mol Physiol*. 2002;282:L411-L420.

19

19

130. Bhandari V, Choo-Wing R, Lee CG, et al. Hyperoxia causes angiopoietin 2-mediated acute lung injury and necrotic cell death. *Nat Med.* 2006;12:1286-1293.
131. Aghai ZH, Faqiri S, Saslow JG, et al. Angiopoietin 2 concentrations in infants developing broncho-pulmonary dysplasia: Attenuation by dexamethasone. *J Perinatol.* 2008;28:149-155.
132. Thomas W, Seidenspinner S, Kramer BW, et al. Airway angiopoietin-2 in ventilated very preterm infants: Association with prenatal factors and neonatal outcome. *Pediatr Pulmonol.* 2011;46:777-784.
133. Yancey MK, Duff P, Kubilis P, et al. Risk factors for neonatal sepsis. *Obstet Gynecol.* 1996;87:188-194.
134. Buttery JP. Blood cultures in newborns and children: Optimising an everyday test. *Arch Dis Child Fetal Neonatal Ed.* 2002;87:F25-F28.
135. Jordan JA, Durso MB, Butchko AR, et al. Evaluating the near-term infant for early onset sepsis: Progress and challenges to consider with 16S rDNA polymerase chain reaction testing. *J Mol Diagn.* 2006;8:357-363.
136. Ohlin A, Björkqvist M, Montgomery SM, et al. Clinical signs and CRP values associated with blood culture results in neonates evaluated for suspected sepsis. *Acta Paediatr.* 2010;99:1635-1640.
137. ACOG Committee on Obstetric Practice. ACOG Committee Opinion No. 348, November 2006: Umbilical cord blood gas and acid-base analysis. *Obstet Gynecol.* 2006;108:1319-1322.
138. Leviton A, Allred E, Kuban KC, et al. ELGAN Study Investigators. Early blood gas abnormalities and the preterm brain. *Am J Epidemiol.* 2010;172:907-916.
139. Dammann O, Ferriero D, Gressens P. Neonatal encephalopathy or hypoxic-ischemic encephalopathy? Appropriate terminology matters. *Pediatr Res.* 2011;70:1-2.
140. Tinoco Jr I, Gonzalez Jr RL. Biological mechanisms, one molecule at a time. *Genes Dev.* 2011;25:1205-1231.
141. Szathmáry E, Jordán F, Pál C. Molecular biology and evolution. Can genes explain biological complexity? *Science.* 2001;292:1315-1316.
142. Strange K. The end of "naive reductionism": Rise of systems biology or renaissance of physiology? *Am J Physiol Cell Physiol.* 2005;288:C968-C974.
143. Hackam DG, Redelmeier DA. Translation of research evidence from animals to humans. *JAMA.* 2006;296:1731-1732.
144. Heisenberg W. *Physikalische Prinzipien der Quantentheorie, Leipzig: Hirzel English translation The Physical Principles of Quantum Theory.* Chicago: University of Chicago Press; 1930.
145. Strippoli P, Canaider S, Noferini F, et al. Uncertainty principle of genetic information in a living cell. *Theor Biol Med Model.* 2005;2:40.e1-e6.

Index

Page numbers followed by "f" indicate figures, and "t" indicate tables